International
REVIEW OF
Neurobiology
Volume 83

International
REVIEW OF
Neurobiology
Volume 83

SERIES EDITORS

RONALD J. BRADLEY
Department of Psychiatry, College of Medicine
The University of Tennessee Health Science Center
Memphis, Tennessee, USA

R. ADRON HARRIS
Waggoner Center for Alcohol and Drug Addiction Research
The University of Texas at Austin
Austin, Texas, USA

PETER JENNER
Division of Pharmacology and Therapeutics
GKT School of Biomedical Sciences
King's College, London, UK

EDITORIAL BOARD

Epilepsy in Women: The Scientific Basis for Clinical Management

EDITED BY

BARRY E. GIDAL
School of Pharmacy & Department of Neurology
University of Wisconsin
Madison, Wisconsin, USA

CYNTHIA L. HARDEN
Department of Neurology
Leonard M. Miller School of Medicine
University of Miami
Miami, Florida, USA

ELSEVIER

AMSTERDAM • BOSTON • HEIDELBERG • LONDON
NEW YORK • OXFORD • PARIS • SAN DIEGO
SAN FRANCISCO • SINGAPORE • SYDNEY • TOKYO
Academic Press is an imprint of Elsevier

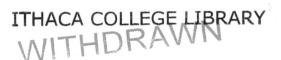

Academic Press is an imprint of Elsevier
360 Park Avenue South, New York, NY 10010-1700
525 B Street, Suite 1900, San Diego, California 92101-4495, USA
32 Jamestown Road, London NW1 7BY, UK

This book is printed on acid-free paper.

For information on all Academic Press publications
visit our Web site at www.elsevierdirect.com

ISBN-13: 978-0-12-374276-6

PRINTED AND BOUND IN THE UNITED STATES OF AMERICA
08 09 10 11 12   9 8 7 6 5 4 3 2 1

CONTENTS

CONTRIBUTORS xiii
PREFACE xvii

Gender Differences in Pharmacological Response
GAIL D. ANDERSON

  I. Introduction 2
 II. Pharmacokinetics 2
III. Pharmacodynamics 7
 IV. Conclusions 8
     References 8

Epidemiology and Classification of Epilepsy: Gender Comparisons
JOHN C. MCHUGH AND NORMAN DELANTY

   I. Introduction 12
  II. Classification of Epilepsy and Seizures 12
 III. Methodology of Epidemiologic Studies in Epilepsy 14
  IV. Gender Differences in Epidemiology of Epilepsy 14
   V. Summary 23
      References 24

Hormonal Influences on Seizures: Basic Neurobiology
CHERYL A. FRYE

    I. Introduction 28
   II. Organizing Effects of Androgens-Sex Differences in Seizures 30
  III. Activational Effects of Androgens on Seizures 31
   IV. Hypothalamic–Pituitary–Gonadal Axis Factors and Seizures 33
    V. Reproductive Events and Seizures 36
   VI. Mechanisms of 3α, 5α-THP Through GABA Receptors 47
  VII. Acute Stress-Induced Steroid Biosynthesis and Seizures 50
 VIII. Developmental Differences in Stress-Induced Steroids 52
   IX. Other Factors that may Underlie Differences in Sensitivity to Steroids ... 54

    X. A Review of Progestins, Absence Seizures, and Mechanisms of Action   55
   XI. Interactions Between AEDs and Steroid Hormones   56
  XII. Summary   57
        References   59

Catamenial Epilepsy

Patricia E. Penovich and Sandra Helmers

    I. Introduction   80
   II. Normal Female Neuroendocrine Cycle   80
  III. Definition and Epidemiology   81
   IV. Proposed Mechanisms   83
    V. Treatment Strategies   85
   VI. Conclusion   87
        References   88

Epilepsy in Women: Special Considerations for Adolescents

Mary L. Zupanc and Sheryl Haut

    I. Introduction   92
   II. Epidemiology   93
  III. Hormones and Epilepsy   93
   IV. Epilepsy and Reproductive Health   94
    V. Bone Health   97
   VI. Psychosocial Considerations   98
  VII. Selected Comorbidities   101
 VIII. Patient Management   102
   IX. Conclusions   106
        References   106

Contraception in Women with Epilepsy: Pharmacokinetic Interactions, Contraceptive Options, and Management

Caryn Dutton and Nancy Foldvary-Schaefer

    I. Introduction   114
   II. Knowledge of Pregnancy Risk and Practice of Contraception in
        Women with Epilepsy   115
  III. Pharmacology of Combined Oral Contraceptives   116
   IV. Hormonal Contraceptive–AED Interactions   117
    V. Other Hormonal Contraceptives and Their Known or Potential
        Interactions with AEDs   122
   VI. Contraceptive Methods Without AED Interaction   125
  VII. Counseling and Management of Contraception in Women
        Requiring AED Prescription   128

VIII. Summary 130
       References 130

Reproductive Dysfunction in Women with Epilepsy: Menstrual Cycle Abnormalities, Fertility, and Polycystic Ovary Syndrome

JÜRGEN BAUER AND DÉIRDRE COOPER-MAHKORN

  I. Introduction 136
 II. Puberty and Menopause in Women with Epilepsy 138
III. Fertility of Women with Epilepsy... 139
 IV. Evaluation of Women with Epilepsy for Reproductive
      Endocrine Disorders 141
  V. Polycystic Ovary Syndrome 144
 VI. Final Remarks and Conclusions 148
      References 151

Sexual Dysfunction in Women with Epilepsy: Role of Antiepileptic Drugs and Psychotropic Medications

MARY A. GUTIERREZ, ROMILA MUSHTAQ, AND GLEN STIMMEL

  I. Effect of Psychotropic and Antiepileptic Drugs on Sexual Function 157
 II. Treatment Strategies for Female Sexual Dysfunction 163
      References 165

Pregnancy in Epilepsy: Issues of Concern

JOHN DETOLEDO

  I. Approach to Assessment... 170
 II. Conclusion 178
      References 178

Teratogenicity and Antiepileptic Drugs: Potential Mechanisms

MARK S. YERBY

  I. Introduction 182
 II. Historical Aspects 182
III. Is Increased Fetal Risk Related to Maternal Epilepsy
      or to AED Exposure?.. 183
 IV. The Role of Maternal Epilepsy as a Confounder for Teratogenic Risk ... 184
  V. Type and Pattern of AED-Related Malformations 185
 VI. Potential Mechanisms of AED-Related Teratogenicity 186

VII. Folate Deficiency as a Potential Mechanism of AED-Induced
      Teratogenicity.. 190
VIII. NTDs and VPA Exposure 192
  IX. Carbamazepine and NTDs.. 195
   X. Phenobarbital Teratogenicity..................................... 196
  XI. Conclusions 196
       References... 197

Antiepileptic Drug Teratogenesis: What are the Risks for Congenital Malformations and Adverse Cognitive Outcomes?

CYNTHIA L. HARDEN

   I. Introduction.. 206
  II. Criteria for High-Quality Studies that Assess AED-Related
       Teratogenesis 206
 III. The Risk of MCMs with AEDs Overall Among WWE........................ 207
  IV. Are Some AEDs Associated with More Risk of MCMs than Others? 208
   V. Polytherapy Versus Monotherapy MCM Risk 209
  VI. Relationship of Dose to Malformations............................. 209
 VII. AED-Specific MCMs.. 209
VIII. AED-Related Cognitive Teratogenesis.................................. 210
  IX. Minor Malformations... 211
   X. Conclusions 211
       References.. 212

Teratogenicity of Antiepileptic Drugs: Role of Pharmacogenomics

RAMAN SANKAR AND JASON T. LERNER

   I. Introduction.. 215
  II. Drug Metabolism 218
 III. Genetics.. 221
  IV. Conclusion 223
       References.. 223

Antiepileptic Drug Therapy in Pregnancy I: Gestation-Induced Effects on AED Pharmacokinetics

PAGE B. PENNELL AND COLLIN A. HOVINGA

   I. Introduction.. 228
  II. Seizure Frequency and AED Concentrations 228
 III. AEDs During Pregnancy 229
  IV. Summary... 237
       References.. 237

Antiepileptic Drug Therapy in Pregnancy II: Fetal and Neonatal Exposure

COLLIN A. HOVINGA AND PAGE B. PENNELL

I.	Introduction	242
II.	Factors Influencing Anticonvulsant Distribution to the Neonate	242
III.	Quantifying AED Exposures	245
IV.	Review of AEDs and Transplacental and Lactation Exposures	247
V.	Summary	254
	References	255

Seizures in Pregnancy: Diagnosis and Management

ROBERT L. BEACH AND PETER W. KAPLAN

I.	Introduction	260
II.	AED Pharmacokinetics in Pregnancy	262
III.	Seizures in Nonepileptic Patients During Pregnancy	262
IV.	Eclampsia	265
	References	268

Management of Epilepsy and Pregnancy: An Obstetrical Perspective

JULIAN N. ROBINSON AND JANE CLEARY-GOLDMAN

I.	Introduction	274
II.	Preconception	274
III.	Assessment of Seizure Control	275
IV.	Considerations for Antiseizure Medicine Management During Pregnancy	275
V.	Prenatal Vitamins and Seizure Disorder	276
VI.	Prenatal Care	277
VII.	Screening for Fetal Abnormalities	277
VIII.	Obstetrical Risks and Management During Labor	278
IX.	Conclusion	281
	References	282

Pregnancy Registries: Strengths, Weaknesses, and Bias Interpretation of Pregnancy Registry Data

MARIANNE CUNNINGTON AND JOHN MESSENHEIMER

I.	Introduction	284
II.	Background	285
III.	Design of a Pregnancy Registry	286
IV.	A Brief History of AED Pregnancy Registries	290
V.	Impact of Registry Design on Data Interpretation	293

VI.   Interpretation of Signals 299
VII.   The Future 302
       References.. 303

Bone Health in Women With Epilepsy: Clinical Features and Potential Mechanisms

ALISON M. PACK AND THADDEUS S. WALCZAK

I.   Introduction.. 306
II.   Bone Physiology 306
III.   Assessment of Bone Health.. 308
IV.   Fracture Risk in Persons with Epilepsy.. 311
V.   AED Effects on Bone 313
VI.   Potential Mechanisms to Explain Changes in Bone Health in
       Persons with Epilepsy... 316
VII.   Treatment 321
VIII. Conclusion and Recommendations 322
       References.. 323

Metabolic Effects of AEDs: Impact on Body Weight, Lipids and Glucose Metabolism

RAJ D. SHETH AND GEORGIA MONTOURIS

I.   Introduction.. 329
II.   Body Weight and AEDs 330
III.   Lipid Metabolism and AEDs.. 335
IV.   Metabolic Acidosis 340
V.   Renal Stones 342
       References.. 343

Psychiatric Comorbidities in Epilepsy

W. CURT LAFRANCE, Jr., ANDRES M. KANNER, AND BRUCE HERMANN

I.   Comorbid Disorders in Epilepsy... 348
II.   Depression in Epilepsy 350
III.   Treatment of Depression in Epilepsy 353
IV.   Anxiety Disorders in Epilepsy 355
V.   Psychosis of Epilepsy.. 357
VI.   Attention Deficit Disorders and Behavior Disturbances........................ 362
VII.   Psychosocial Consequences for Women with Epilepsy 365
VIII. Nonepileptic Seizures... 366
IX.   Treatment of NES.. 369
X.   Conclusions 373
       References.. 374

Issues for Mature Women with Epilepsy
Cynthia L. Harden

I.	Introduction	386
II.	Premature Ovarian Failure: Early Onset Perimenopause and Menopause	386
III.	Changes in Seizures Related to Perimenopause and Menopause	387
IV.	Hormone Replacement Therapy in Women with Epilepsy	389
V.	Menopause and HRT in Animal Seizure Models	391
VI.	AED Treatment in the Elderly	392
VII.	Conclusion	393
	References	394

Pharmacodynamic and Pharmacokinetic Interactions of Psychotropic Drugs with Antiepileptic Drugs
Andres M. Kanner and Barry E. Gidal

I.	Introduction	398
II.	The Use of Antidepressant Drugs in Epilepsy	399
III.	Anxiolytic Drugs	405
IV.	Lithium	406
V.	CNS Stimulants	407
VI.	Other Treatment for ADHD: Atomoxetine	408
VII.	Antipsychotic Drugs	410
VIII.	Concluding Remarks	413
	References	413

Health Disparities in Epilepsy: How Patient-Oriented Outcomes in Women Differ from Men
Frank Gilliam

References	419

Index	421
Contents of Recent Volumes	433

CONTRIBUTORS

Numbers in parentheses indicate the pages on which the authors' contributions begin.

Gail D. Anderson (1), Health Science Complex H-361A, University of Washington, Box 357630, Seattle, Washington 98195, USA

Jürgen Bauer (135), Department of Epileptology, Bonn University Hospital, D-53105 Bonn, Germany

Robert L. Beach (259), Department of Neurology, Upstate Medical University, Syracuse, New York 13210, USA

Jane Cleary-Goldman (273), Englewood Hospital, Maternal Fetal Medicine, Englewood, NJ 07631, USA

Déirdre Cooper-Mahkorn (135), Department of Epileptology, Bonn University Hospital, D-53105 Bonn, Germany

Marianne Cunnington (283), GlaxoSmithKline Research and Development, Harlow, United Kingdom

Norman Delanty (11), Department of Neurology, Beaumont Hospital, Dublin 9, Ireland

John DeToledo (169), Waked Forest University, School of Medicine, Medical Center Boulevard, Winston Salem, NC, 27157

Caryn Dutton (113), University of Wisconsin School of Medicine and Public Health, Madison, Wisconsin 53704, USA

Nancy Foldvary-Schaefer (113), Cleveland Clinic Lerner College of Medicine of Case Western Reserve University, Cleveland, Ohio 44195, USA

Cheryl A. Frye (27), Departments of Psychology, Biology, and Centers for Neuroscience and Life Sciences Research, The University at Albany-State University of New York, Albany, New York 12222, USA

Barry E. Gidal (397), School of Pharmacy and Department of Neurology, University of Wisconsin, Madison, Wisconsin, USA

Frank Gilliam (417), Department of Neurology, Columbia University Medical Center, Comprehensive Epilepsy Center, New York 10032, USA

Mary A. Gutierrez (157), Department of Pharmacology and Outcomes Sciences, Loma Linda University School of Pharmacy, Loma Linda, California 92350, USA

Cynthia L. Harden (205, 385), Department of Neurology, Leonard M. Miller School of Medicine, University of Miami, Miami, Florida, USA

Sheryl Haut (91), Comprehensive Epilepsy Management Center, Montefiore Medical Center, Albert Einstein College of Medicine, New York 10467, USA

Sandra Helmers (79), Emory University School of Medicine, Georgia 30322, USA

Bruce Hermann (347), University of Wisconsin, Madison, Wisconsin 53972, USA

Collin A. Hovinga (227, 241), Departments of Clinical Pharmacy and Pediatrics, University of Tennessee Health Science Center, LeBonheur Children's Medical Center, Memphis, Tennessee 38105, USA

Andres M. Kanner (347, 397), Rush Epilepsy Center, Chicago, Illinois 60612, USA; Rush University Medical Center, Chicago, Illinois, USA

Peter W. Kaplan (259), Department of Neurology, Johns Hopkins University School of Medicine, Johns Hopkins Bayview Medical Center, Baltimore, Maryland 21224, USA

W. Curt LaFrance, Jr., (347), Brown Medical School, Rhode Island Hospital, Departments of Psychiatry and Neurology, Providence, Rhode Island 02903, USA

Jason T. Lerner (215), David Geffen School of Medicine at UCLA, Mattel Children's Hospital at UCLA, Los Angeles, California 90095-1752, USA

John C. McHugh (11), Department of Neurology, Beaumont Hospital, Dublin 9, Ireland

John Messenheimer (283), GlaxoSmithKline Research and Development, North Carolina, USA

Georgia Montouris (329), Department of Neurology, Boston University Medical Center, Boston, Massachusetts 02118, USA

Romila Mushtaq (157), Medical College of Wisconin, Milwaukee, Wisconin 53226, USA

Alison M. Pack (305), Columbia University, New York, NY 10032, USA

Page B. Pennell (227, 241), Emory Epilepsy Program, Emory University School of Medicine, Atlanta, Georgia 30322, USA

Patricia E. Penovich (79), Minnesota Epilepsy Group PA, Department of Neurology, University of Minnesota, Minnesota 55102, USA

Julian N. Robinson (273), Brigham and Women's Hospital, Maternal-Fetal Medicine, Bostan, Massachusetts 02115, USA

Raman Sankar (215), David Geffen School of Medicine at UCLA, Mattel Children's Hospital at UCLA, Los Angeles, California 90095-1752, USA

Raj D. Sheth (329), Department of Neurology, University of Wisconsin, Madison, Wisconsin 53792, USA

Glen Stimmel (157), University of Southern California Schools of Pharmacy and Medicine, Los Angeles, California 90089, USA

Thaddeus S. Walczak (305), MINCEP Epilepsy Care, Minnea Polis, MN 55416, USA

Mark S. Yerby (181), North Pacific Epilepsy Research, Portland, Oregon 97210, USA

Mary L. Zupanc (91), Department of Neurology and Pediatrics, Division of Pediatric Neurology, Pediatric Comprehensive Epilepsy Program, Children's Hospital of Wisconsin, Medical College of Wisconsin, Milwaukee, Wisconsin 53226, USA

PREFACE

This book, "*Epilepsy in Women: The Scientific Basis for Clinical Management*," was inspired by the growing body of scientific information that has direct impact on the care of women with epilepsy. For this book, we sought to answer a seemingly simple question, that being "what is special about gender and antiepileptic drug use?" To address this question, we have been fortunate enough to assemble a panel of experts from both the basic neurobiological and pharmaceutical sciences, as well as adult neurology, pediatric neurology, and obstetrics communities. Our charge to these authors was to summarize the current state of scientific opinion, but yet provide the reader with pragmatic advice on the care of women with epilepsy.

We recognized that there are a number of both basic physiological and clinical issues that are quite specific to women. For example, gender may influence both the neurobiology of seizures and the pharmacologic response to medication. These same neurobiological considerations are clearly important when making clinical decisions regarding antiepileptic drug (AED) treatment, particularly with respect to issues surrounding sexuality, contraception, and reproductive function. Importantly, clinical issues may change over the course of a woman's lifetime, and therefore we will also address issues such as catamenial epilepsy, psychiatric comorbidities as well as unique considerations in both the adolescent and mature woman. Recognizing that AED treatment may carry the potential for metabolic adverse effects, this book will also address current perspectives surrounding bone health, weight changes, and glucose and lipid metabolism.

A topic of critical interest to the medical community at large has been that of teratogenicity and optimization of AED pharmacotherapy during pregnancy. As discussed herein, management of epilepsy during pregnancy is multifaceted, with scientific insight and data that is continually evolving. Three chapters discuss aspects of teratogenesis of AEDs, including mechanisms, the role of pharmacogenomics, and evidence from recent prospective, population-based studies regarding the absolute and relative risks of AED teratogenesis. The influence of physiological changes seen in pregnancy upon AED disposition is discussed not only from a pharmacokinetic perspective but also from a clinical standpoint, with particular attention paid to potential neonatal and fetal exposure to these medications.

As with all provocative clinical summaries, more questions may be raised than answered at times; such is the dynamic nature of science.

The editors are awed by the generous expertise, perspicacity, and scientific passion evident in the contributions to this book. We are also grateful for the balanced yet personal perspective of each author, which lends true clinical nuance as well as scientific evidence to the guidance provided. We hope that you find this book both practical and provocative.

BARRY E. GIDAL
CYNTHIA L. HARDEN

GENDER DIFFERENCES IN PHARMACOLOGICAL RESPONSE

Gail D. Anderson

Health Science Complex H-361A, University of Washington, Box 357630,
Seattle, Washington 98195, USA

I. Introduction
II. Pharmacokinetics
   A. Size Matters
   B. Absorption
   C. Distribution
   D. Metabolism
   E. Transporters
   F. Renal Elimination
III. Pharmacodynamics
   A. Long QT Syndrome
   B. Idiosyncratic Reactions
IV. Conclusions
   References

Female sex has been shown to be a risk factor for clinically relevant adverse drug reactions. Is the increased risk due to sex differences in pharmacokinetics, in pharmacodynamics, or did females receive more medications and higher mg/kg doses than males? Recent studies suggest that all of the above may play a role.

Generally, males weigh more than females, yet few drugs are dosed based on body weight. Drug concentrations are dependent on the volume of distribution (Vd) and clearance (Cl). Both parameters are dependent on body weight for most drugs independent of sex differences. Females have a higher percent body fat than males which can affect the Vd of certain drugs. Renal clearance of unchanged drug is decreased in females due to a lower glomerular filtration. Sex differences in activity of the cytochrome P450 (CYP) and uridine diphosphate glucuronosyltransferase (UGT) enzymes and renal excretion will result in differences in Cl. There is evidence for females having lower activity of CYP1A2, CYP2E1, and UGT; higher activity of CYP3A4, CYP2A6, and CYP2B6; and no differences in CPY2C9 and CYP2D6 activity. Pharmacodynamic changes can affect both the desired therapeutic effect of a drug as well as its adverse effect profile. The most widely reported sex difference is the higher risk in females for drug-induced long QT syndrome, with two-thirds of all cases of drug-induced torsades occurring in

1

females. Females also have a higher incidence of drug-induced liver toxicity, gastrointestinal adverse events due to NSAIDs, and allergic skin rashes.

In conclusion, at the minimum, it is important to take into account size and age as well as co-morbidities in determining the appropriate drug regiment for females, as well as males. There are still large gaps in our knowledge of sex differences in clinical pharmacology and significantly more research is needed.

I. Introduction

Gender-based research has increased significantly in the last decade, identifying significant differences in disease prevalence as well as pharmacokinetic and pharmacodynamic differences in drug treatments. Female sex has been shown to be a risk factor for clinically relevant adverse drug reactions with a 1.5- to 1.7-fold greater risk of developing an adverse drug reaction compared to male patients (Fattinger *et al.*, 2000; Tran *et al.*, 1998). Is this due to sex differences in pharmacokinetics (relationship between dose and concentration), differences in pharmacodynamics (relationship between concentration and effect), or do females just receive more medications and higher mg/kg doses than males? Recent studies suggest that all of the above may play a role.

II. Pharmacokinetics

A. Size Matters

Initial drug concentrations after a bolus dose or loading dose (C_0), and maximum peak concentrations (C_{max}) are dependent on the volume of distribution (Vd) as shown in Eqs. (1) and (2), respectively. Average steady-state concentrations (C^{ss}) are dependent on clearance (Cl) as shown in Eq. (3). For the majority of drugs, Vd and Cl are dependent on body weight; yet few drugs are dosed based on body weight. Generally, males weigh more than females. Therefore, based on differences in body weight alone, females often receive higher mg/kg doses which results in higher concentration and drug exposure than males irrespective of other pharmacokinetic differences described below.

$$C_0 = \frac{\text{Dose}}{\text{Vd}} \qquad (1)$$

$$C_{\max} = \frac{\text{Dose}}{\text{Vd}(1 - e^{-(\text{Cl/Vd})\tau})} \tag{2}$$

$$C^{ss} = \frac{F \times (D/t)}{\text{Cl}} \tag{3}$$

The Food and Drug Administration (FDA) reviewed 300 new drug applications between 1995 and 2000 (http://www.fda.gov/fdac/features/2005/405_sex.html). Of the 163 that included a sex analysis, 20% of drugs had a significant sex difference in pharmacokinetics with 11 drugs having greater than a 40% difference between males and females. Yet, no dosing recommendations were made based on sex for any of the products. Based on a prospective drug surveillance study of hospitalized patients, Domecq *et al.* (1980) estimated that 93% of the adverse reactions in females and 83% in males may be dose dependent suggesting that the higher mg/kg doses females receive are clinically significant.

B. Absorption

There is limited evidence of sex difference in absorption and/or bioavailability. In a small study evaluating the effects of food on the absorption of enteric coated aspirin, females had a significantly longer gastric residence time and a significantly delayed absorption with a meal (Mojaverian *et al.*, 1987). Females have lower gastric alcohol dehydrogenase which results in an increased bioavailability (percent absorbed) and significantly higher ethanol concentrations in females compared to males receiving the same weight corrected amount (Frezza *et al.*, 1990).

Prior to 1993, women were rarely included in bioequivalence trials based on the assumption that including women would result in significantly higher intersubject variability resulting in a need for a larger sample size. This resulted in the sex-related analysis by the FDA of 26 bioequivalence studies including 94 data sets (Chen *et al.*, 2000). In over a third of the data sets, there was greater than a 20% sex-related difference in area under the concentration time curve (AUC) or maximum concentration ($C_{\max}$). Weight correction alone reduced the difference to 15% of the studies. For the drugs with sex-related differences, not adjusting for weight resulted in 20–88% higher AUC in females compared to males. For drugs with narrow therapeutic ranges and/or steep dose–concentration curves, this may result in significantly increased adverse events in females compared to males. Even within a group of females, not taking into account body weight can alter efficacy. Holt *et al.* (2005) found that if a woman was greater than 70.5 kg, she had a 1.6 greater risk of oral contraceptive (OC) failure. With a low dose OC and weight greater than 86 kg, the relative risk increased to greater than 2-fold.

C. DISTRIBUTION

Females have a higher percent body fat than males, which can affect the Vd of certain drugs. For example, females have larger weight corrected Vd for diazepam, midazolam, and vancomycin, and a smaller Vd for alprazolm and ethanol (Anderson, 2005). Vd is important for determining loading doses [Eq. (1)] and can affect the C_{max}, the elimination half-life ($T_{1/2}$), and duration of effect. For example, a larger Vd will result in a decreased C_{max}, an increased $T_{1/2}$, and an increased duration of effect when the same dose is given to a female compared to a male.

$$T_{1/2} = \frac{0.693 \times \text{Vd}}{\text{Cl}} \tag{4}$$

D. METABOLISM

Sex differences in the activity of hepatic enzymes, drug transporters, and renal excretion will result in differences in clearance (elimination). The most common families of enzymes involved in drug metabolism are the cytochrome P450 (CYP), uridine diphosphate glucuronosyltransferase (UGT), and N-acetyl-transferase (NAT) enzymes. The primary function of the hepatic enzymes is twofold; the metabolism of endogenous compounds, like steroids and the detoxification of exogenous compounds like drugs. CYP are a multigene superfamily of enzymes primarily found in the liver, but also found in the gastrointestinal tract, lungs, and kidneys to a lesser extent. The individual isozymes are composed of three major families, CYP1, CYP2, and CYP3, with specific isozymes involved in the hepatic metabolism of most drugs: CYP1A2, CYP2A6, CYP2B6, CYP2C8, CYP2C9, CYP2C19, CYP2D6, CYP2E1, and CYP3A4 (Wrighton and Stevens, 1992). The AEDs metabolized predominately by one or more CYPs include carbamazepine (CYP3A4, CYP1A2, CYP2C8), diazepam (CYP2C19, CYP3A4), ethosuximide (CYP3A4), and phenytoin (CYP2C9, CYP2C19). UGTs are a group of isozymes located in the hepatic endoplasmic reticulum and consist of two major subfamilies, UGT1 and UGT2 (Burchell et al., 1995). The UGT1 subfamily catalyzes the conjugation of a variety of xenobiotic phenols and bilirubin, but generally do not catalyze steroid conjugation. UGT2 isozymes primarily catalyze steroid and bile acid glucuronidation, but also drugs. The UGT isozymes involved in the glucuronidation of lamotrigine and lorazepam are

UGT1A4 and UGT2B7, respectively. The UGT isozymes responsible for conjugation of the MHD, the active metabolite of oxcarbazepine, have not been identified.

The activity of hepatic enzymes is dependent on genetic, physiological, and environmental effects. Genetic polymorphisms in the expression of several CYP enzymes are responsible for clinically significant effects on the efficacy and toxicity of drugs predominately metabolized by the enzymes involved. The polymorphisms are genetically inherited as an autosomal recessive trait. As the genes involved in the CYP proteins are not X-linked, the incidence of polymorphism in the populations would not be expected to be sex dependent. However, genetics also controls the amount (or activity) of the enzymes. There are sex-dependent differences in the activity of the CYP and UGT enzymes. There is evidence for females having lower activity of CYP1A2, CYP2E1, and the UGTs; higher activity of CYP3A4, CYP2A6, and CYP2B6; and no significant differences in CPY2C9, CYP2D6, and NAT2 activity (Anderson, 2005). There is also evidence of an interaction between ethnicity and sex in the activity of CYP2C19 and CYP2B6. The CYP2C19 activity in females has been reported to be higher or lower than males dependent on the ethnicity of the population studied; however, concurrent oral contraceptive use was not reported. Concurrent oral contraceptive use has been shown to decrease the activity of CYP1A2, CYP2B6, and CYP2C19 and increase the activity of CYP2A6 and UGT and therefore may be a confounder in the large population studies evaluating sex-dependent differences. CYP2B6 activity was higher in females than males and was three- to fivefold higher in Hispanic females than Caucasian or African American females (Table I). Because of wide intersubject variability in the activity of the metabolic enzymes, the clinical significance of the sex- and ethnic-dependent difference in hepatic metabolism is not fully understood.

E. Transporters

P-glycoprotein (Pgp) is a drug transporter protein belonging to the ATP-binding cassette (ABC) membrane protein family. Functioning as a transmembrane pump, Pgp is a significant transporter in normal tissues, including the placenta, brain, intestine, testes, the liver, and kidneys. Pgp decreases absorption and increases the renal clearance of specific xenobiotics. Many substrates of CYP3A4 are also substrates of Pgp and the contradictory sex differences found with CYP3A4 have been hypothesized due to sex-dependent differences in Pgp (Cummins et al., 2002). Pgp activity was significantly lower in livers obtained from females compared to males in one study (Schuetz et al., 1995) but not others (Wolbold et al., 2003).

TABLE I

Sex Differences in Hepatic Enzymes, P-Glycoprotein, and Renal Elimination

	Sex effect	Effect of oral contraceptive	Effect of hormone replacement therapy
P-glycoprotein	F < M		
CYP3A4	F > M		
CYP2C9	F = M		
CYP2C19[a]	–	Inhibits	
CYP2D6	F = M		
CYP1A2	F < M	Inhibits	Induces
CYP2A6	F > M	Induces	
CYP2B6	F > M	Inhibits	Inhibits
UGTs	F < M	Induces	
NAT2	F = M		
Renal elimination	F < M		

[a]Sex differences have been reported dependent on ethnicity of populations studied; however, studies may be confounded by unreported oral contraceptive use.

F. Renal Elimination

Renal clearance of unchanged drug is also decreased in females due to a lower glomerular filtration rate. Glomerular filtration rate is 10% lower in females than males after correction for body size and age (Gross *et al.*, 1992). The oral clearance of digoxin, a drug predominately eliminated by renal elimination, is 12–14% lower in females than males. Digoxin is also a substrate for Pgp. As described above, males may have higher amounts of Pgp than females, which would theoretically also result in an increased bioavailability and decreased renal clearance in females. A recent study demonstrated that females treated with digoxin for heart failure had a higher rate of death compared to placebo; however, males did not (Rathore *et al.*, 2002). There was a small, but statistical difference in digoxin concentration in a subset of the study population where concentrations were available. A *post hoc* analysis of the trial demonstrated that these higher serum digoxin concentrations were associated with increased mortality (Rathore *et al.*, 2003).

Females also have decreased renal clearance of several types of antibiotics that are predominately eliminated unchanged in the urine, including vancomycin, ceftazidime, and cefepime (Anderson, 2005). Therefore, renal clearance of drugs will be lower in females than males and lowest in older females (Schwartz, 2007). Evaluating creatinine clearance and adjusting dose especially in older women receiving AEDs eliminated predominantly by renal excretion (gabapentin, pregabalin, vigabatrin) is important to prevent adverse events.

III. Pharmacodynamics

Pharmacodynamic changes can affect both the desired therapeutic effect of a drug as well as its adverse effect profile. For example, females have a higher incidence of drug-induced liver toxicity, gastrointestinal adverse events due to NSAIDs, allergic skin rashes, and drug-induced torsades.

A. LONG QT SYNDROME

The higher risk in females for drug-induced long QT syndrome is the most widely reported sex difference. Two-thirds of all cases of drug-induced torsades occur in females (Drici and Clement, 2001; Makkar et al., 1993). Female sex is associated with a longer corrected QT (QT_c) interval at baseline and a more significant effect of QT_c prolonging drugs. For example, quinidine causes a 44% higher change in the slope of the QT_c interval in females compared to males (Rodriguez et al., 2001). Studies in rabbits have suggested that the presence of male sex hormones may be responsible for the shorter QT interval in males (Liu et al., 2003). The presence of drugs that prolong the QT interval and/or induce torsade de pointes with substantial evidence for a sex difference include amiodarone, bepridil, disopyramide, ibutilide, quinidine, sotalol, erythromycin, pentamidine, terfenadine, chlorpromazine, and pimozide (Drici and Clement, 2001).

B. IDIOSYNCRATIC REACTIONS

Skin reactions are the most frequently reported adverse drug reactions in both males and females, with antibiotics responsible for the majority of reports (Fattinger et al., 2000; Tran et al., 1998). Of the adverse drug reactions reported, females report a higher incidence of rash than males. There is a higher use of antibiotics in females. However, studies controlling for use still found a higher incidence. In general, drug-induced rashes are considered idiosyncratic, that is, not related to the pharmacology of the drugs and no obvious relationship to dose. There are significant sex differences in immunoreactivity. Seventy-five percent of those affected by autoimmune diseases are women. Osteoarthritis, rheumatoid arthritis, fibromyalgia effect women disproportionately (Buckwalter and Lappin, 2000). Some disorders, like systemic lupus erythematosus (SLE), have a 9:1 female to male ratio (Rider and Abdou, 2001). Women have stronger immune responses, produce more antibodies and auto-antibodies (Whitacre et al., 1999). There is also evidence that sex hormones influence the course of autoimmune diseases. For example, SLE starts after puberty, fluctuates with menstrual cycle, and flares during pregnancy (Rider and Abdou, 2001).

The risk of drug-induced rash for nevirapine and efavirenz is six- to eightfold higher in females than males (Umeh and Currier, 2005). In a study evaluating patients with a history of penicillin allergy, of sixty-four patients with a positive penicillin skin test, 83% were females (Park *et al.*, 2007). Female patients receiving lamotrigine had a 1.8-fold higher risk of developing a rash than males (Wong *et al.*, 1999). The incidence of carbamazepine rash was not found to be higher in females in small clinical studies (Konishi *et al.*, 1993; Kramlinger *et al.*, 1994). In a large-scale study evaluating the predictors of AED-induced rash that occurred in 262 of 1649 patients receiving AEDs, female sex was a predictor of rash in the univariate analysis (twofold higher risk); however, in the multivariant analysis, only the history of another AED rash was statistically significant (Arif *et al.*, 2007). The rate of rash was five times greater in patients with a history of another AED rash.

Drug-induced liver disease is the most frequent adverse drug reaction leading to withdrawal of a drug from the market. Seventy-four percent of drug-induced acute liver failure occurs in females (Miller, 2001; Zimmerman, 2000). None of the AEDs are direct hepatotoxins. Generally, hepatoxicity with carbamazepine, phenytoin, and lamotrigine occurs as part of a hypersensitivity syndrome also consisting of fever, rash, lymphadenopathy, and eosinophilia (Dreifuss and Langer, 1987; Overstreet *et al.*, 2002). Valproate therapy is associated with a transient elevation in liver function test in 15–30% of patients and a rare, fatal hepatotoxicity not associated with hypersensitivity (Dreifuss *et al.*, 1987). In contrast to non-AED-induced toxicity, liver toxicity due to AEDs does not appear to occur preferentially in females.

IV. Conclusions

Despite mandates by the National Institutes of Health (NIH) and FDA requiring the inclusion of women and minorities in clinical studies, the analysis of outcome is not carried out consistently with only a small percentage of studies analyzed by sex (Vidaver *et al.*, 2000). There are still large gaps in our knowledge of sex differences in clinical pharmacology. At a minimum, it is important to take into account size (body weight) and age as well as co-morbidities in determining the appropriate drug regiment for both males and females.

References

Anderson, G. D. (2005). Sex and racial differences in pharmacological response: Where is the evidence? Pharmacogenetics, pharmacokinetics, and pharmacodynamics. *J. Womens Health (Larchmt)* **14,** 19–29.

Arif, H., Buchsbaum, R., Weintraub, D., Koyfman, S., Salas-Humara, C., Bazil, C. W., Resor, S. R., Jr., and Hirsch, L. J. (2007). Comparison and predictors of rash associated with 15 antiepileptic drugs. *Neurology* **68,** 1701–1709.

Buckwalter, J. A., and Lappin, D. R. (2000). The disproportionate impact of chronic arthralgia and arthritis among women. *Clin. Orthop. Relat. Res.* **372,** 159–168.

Burchell, B., Brierley, C. H., and Rance, D. (1995). Specificity of human UDP-glucuronosyltransferases and xenobiotic glucuronidation. *Life Sci.* **57,** 1819–1831.

Chen, M. L., Lee, S. C., Ng, M. J., Schuirmann, D. J., Lesko, L. J., and Williams, R. L. (2000). Pharmacokinetic analysis of bioequivalence trials: Implications for sex-related issues in clinical pharmacology and biopharmaceutics. *Clin. Pharmacol. Ther.* **68,** 510–521.

Cummins, C. L., Wu, C. Y., and Benet, L. Z. (2002). Sex-related differences in the clearance of cytochrome P450 3A4 substrates may be caused by P-glycoprotein. *Clin. Pharmacol. Ther.* **72,** 474–489.

Domecq, C., Naranjo, C. A., Ruiz, I., and Busto, U. (1980). Sex-related variations in the frequency and characteristics of adverse drug reactions. *Int. J. Clin. Pharmacol. Ther. Toxicol.* **18,** 362–366.

Dreifuss, F. E., and Langer, D. H. (1987). Hepatic considerations in the use of antiepileptic drugs. *Epilepsia* **28**(Suppl. 2), S23–S29.

Dreifuss, F. E., Santilli, N., Langer, D. H., Sweeney, K. P., Moline, K. A., and Menander, K. B. (1987). Valproic acid hepatic fatalities: A retrospective review. *Neurology* **37,** 379–385.

Drici, M. D., and Clement, N. (2001). Is gender a risk factor for adverse drug reactions? The example of drug-induced long QT syndrome. *Drug Saf.* **24,** 575–585.

Fattinger, K., Roos, M., Vergeres, P., Holenstein, C., Kind, B., Masche, U., Stocker, D. N., Braunschweig, S., Kullak-Ublick, G. A., Galeazzi, R. L., Follath, F., *et al.* (2000). Epidemiology of drug exposure and adverse drug reactions in two Swiss departments of internal medicine. *Br. J. Clin. Pharmacol.* **49,** 158–167.

Frezza, M., di Padova, C., Pozzato, G., Terpin, M., Baraona, E., and Lieber, C. S. (1990). High blood alcohol levels in women. The role of decreased gastric alcohol dehydrogenase activity and first-pass metabolism. *N. Engl. J. Med.* **322,** 95–99.

Gross, J. L., Friedman, R., Azevedo, M. J., Silveiro, S. P., and Pecis, M. (1992). Effect of age and sex on glomerular filtration rate measured by ^{51}Cr-EDTA. *Braz. J. Med. Biol. Res.* **25,** 129–134.

Holt, V. L., Scholes, D., Wicklund, K. G., Cushing-Haugen, K. L., and Daling, J. R. (2005). Body mass index, weight, and oral contraceptive failure risk. *Obstet. Gynecol.* **105,** 46–52.

Konishi, T., Naganuma, Y., Hongo, K., Murakami, M., Yamatani, M., and Okada, T. (1993). Carbamazepine-induced skin rash in children with epilepsy. *Eur. J. Pediatr.* **152,** 605–608.

Kramlinger, K. G., Phillips, K. A., and Post, R. M. (1994). Rash complicating carbamazepine treatment. *J. Clin. Psychopharmacol.* **14,** 408–413.

Liu, X. K., Katchman, A., Whitfield, B. H., Wan, G., Janowski, E. M., Woosley, R. L., and Ebert, S. N. (2003). *In vivo* androgen treatment shortens the QT interval and increases the densities of inward and delayed rectifier potassium currents in orchiectomized male rabbits. *Cardiovasc. Res.* **57,** 28–36.

Makkar, R. R., Fromm, B. S., Steinman, R. T., Meissner, M. D., and Lehmann, M. H. (1993). Female gender as a risk factor for torsades de pointes associated with cardiovascular drugs. *JAMA* **270,** 2590–2597.

Miller, M. A. (2001). Gender-based differences in the toxicity of pharmaceuticals—The Food and Drug Administration's perspective. *Int. J. Toxicol.* **20,** 149–152.

Mojaverian, P., Rocci, M. L., Jr., Conner, D. P., Abrams, W. B., and Vlasses, P. H. (1987). Effect of food on the absorption of enteric-coated aspirin: Correlation with gastric residence time. *Clin. Pharmacol. Ther.* **41,** 11–17.

Overstreet, K., Costanza, C., Behling, C., Hassanin, T., and Masliah, E. (2002). Fatal progressive hepatic necrosis associated with lamotrigine treatment: A case report and literature review. *Dig. Dis. Sci.* **47,** 1921–1925.

Park, M. A., Matesic, D., Markus, P. J., and Li, J. T. (2007). Female sex as a risk factor for penicillin allergy. *Ann. Allergy Asthma Immunol.* **99,** 54–58.

Rathore, S. S., Curtis, J. P., Wang, Y., Bristow, M. R., and Krumholz, H. M. (2003). Association of serum digoxin concentration and outcomes in patients with heart failure. *JAMA* **289,** 871–878.

Rathore, S. S., Wang, Y., and Krumholz, H. M. (2002). Sex-based differences in the effect of digoxin for the treatment of heart failure. *N. Engl. J. Med.* **347,** 1403–1411.

Rider, V., and Abdou, N. I. (2001). Gender differences in autoimmunity: Molecular basis for estrogen effects in systemic lupus erythematosus. *Int. Immunopharmacol.* **1,** 1009–1024.

Rodriguez, I., Kilborn, M. J., Liu, X. K., Pezzullo, J. C., and Woosley, R. L. (2001). Drug-induced QT prolongation in women during the menstrual cycle. *JAMA* **285,** 1322–1326.

Schuetz, E. G., Furuya, K. N., and Schuetz, J. D. (1995). Interindividual variation in expression of P-glycoprotein in normal human liver and secondary hepatic neoplasms. *J. Pharmacol. Exp. Ther.* **275,** 1011–1018.

Schwartz, J. B. (2007). The current state of knowledge on age, sex, and their interactions on clinical pharmacology. *Clin. Pharmacol. Ther.* **82,** 87–96.

Tran, C., Knowles, S. R., Liu, B. A., and Shear, N. H. (1998). Gender differences in adverse drug reactions. *J. Clin. Pharmacol.* **38,** 1003–1009.

Umeh, O. C., and Currier, J. S. (2005). Sex differences in HIV: Natural history, pharmacokinetics, and drug toxicity. *Curr. Infect. Dis. Rep.* **7,** 73–78.

Vidaver, R. M., Lafleur, B., Tong, C., Bradshaw, R., and Marts, S. A. (2000). Women subjects in NIH-funded clinical research literature: Lack of progress in both representation and analysis by sex. *J. Womens Health Gend. Based Med.* **9,** 495–504.

Whitacre, C. C., Reingold, S. C., and O'Looney, P. A. (1999). A gender gap in autoimmunity. *Science* **283,** 1277–1278.

Wolbold, R., Klein, K., Burk, O., Nussler, A. K., Neuhaus, P., Eichelbaum, M., Schwab, M., and Zanger, U. M. (2003). Sex is a major determinant of CYP3A4 expression in human liver. *Hepatology* **38,** 978–988.

Wong, I. C. K., Mawer, G. E., and Sander, J. W. A. S. (1999). Factors influencing the incidence of lamotrigine-related skin rash. *Ann. Pharmacother.* **33,** 1037–1042.

Wrighton, S. A., and Stevens, J. C. (1992). The human hepatic cytochrome P450 involved in drug metabolism. *Crit. Rev. Toxicol.* **22,** 1–21.

Zimmerman, H. J. (2000). Drug-induced liver disease. *Clin. Liver Dis.* **4,** 73–96, vi.

EPIDEMIOLOGY AND CLASSIFICATION OF EPILEPSY: GENDER COMPARISONS

John C. McHugh and Norman Delanty

Department of Neurology, Beaumont Hospital, Dublin 9, Ireland

I. Introduction
II. Classification of Epilepsy and Seizures
III. Methodology of Epidemiologic Studies in Epilepsy
IV. Gender Differences in Epidemiology of Epilepsy
    A. Incidence of Epilepsy
    B. Prevalence of Epilepsy
    C. Gender Differences in Specific Epilepsy Syndromes
    D. Prognosis in Epilepsy
    E. Mortality in Epilepsy
    F. Status Epilepticus
V. Summary
    Glossary
    References

Epilepsy is a common disease. The cumulative lifetime risks for epilepsy and for any unprovoked seizure are 3.1% and 4.1%, respectively, in industrialized countries. Estimates of annual incidence of epilepsy are as high as 43 cases per 100,000 of the population in so-called developed countries, and are almost double this figure in the developing world. Within this there is a growing appreciation of gender differences in the epidemiology of epilepsy and of specific epilepsy syndromes.

In 1993, the International League Against Epilepsy (ILAE) proposed simplified classification guidelines to facilitate epidemiologic work in epilepsy, and to allow meaningful comparison between studies undertaken at different times and in different parts of the world. Since then, a number of national studies have been completed, adding to the existing data of already well-established databases such as the Rochester Epidemiology Project.

There is broad agreement between studies that females have a marginally lower incidence of epilepsy and unprovoked seizures than males. This difference is usually attributed to males' greater exposure to risk factors for lesional epilepsy and acute symptomatic seizures. On the other hand, idiopathic generalized epilepsies (IGEs), which may represent some 15–20% of all epilepsies, are more common among females. Also, the behavior of some common epilepsy syndromes

INTERNATIONAL REVIEW OF
NEUROBIOLOGY, VOL. 83
DOI: 10.1016/S0074-7742(08)00002-0

11

such as mesial temporal sclerosis may differ between genders with isolated auras more common among females and secondary seizure spread more likely in males. Trends toward gender differences are also seen in other important aspects of epilepsy. These include the incidence of status epilepticus (more common in men), incidence of sudden unexpected death in epilepsy (SUDEP), prognosis, and mortality.

I. Introduction

Over the last number of decades, a pattern has emerged in relation to gender difference in the epidemiology of epilepsy worldwide. It appears overall that epilepsy is slightly more common in males than in females. Beyond this, however, it seems that certain epilepsy syndromes have a greater association with females, and that sometimes the same epilepsy syndrome may behave differently in women than in men. This has implications both for prognosis and for our understanding of seizure pathophysiology. Before going into details of these interesting differences, it is important to briefly review the classification of epilepsy, and to explain some methodological principles that are important in interpreting epidemiologic studies of epilepsy.

II. Classification of Epilepsy and Seizures

Classification of seizures and epilepsy syndromes is an important part of clinical work. Appropriate classification relies on detailed history and a collateral account, neurologic examination, and the interpretation of specialized tests— notably electroencephalography (EEG) and neuroimaging. Accurate classification allows for optimal medical therapy of a seizure disorder and provides important prognostic information for the patient. From an etiological viewpoint, classification and "phenotyping" of epilepsies is an essential step in the process of understanding the pathophysiology of different epilepsy syndromes, particularly in relation to genetic research. The classification used most commonly in clinical practice is the International League Against Epilepsy (ILAE) classification of epileptic seizures (1981) and of epilepsy syndromes (1989), which are based on both clinical and EEG information. From an epidemiologic perspective, there are a number of limitations associated with the 1981 and 1989 classifications, notably the requirement for EEG. This has restricted their use and has led to their misapplication in a number of epidemiologic reports, prompting the ILAE to propose new simplified guidelines, which do not require EEG (Commission on Epidemiology and Prognosis, ILAE, 1993).

In 1993, the ILAE proposed guidelines for the classification of epilepsy for the purposes of epidemiologic studies. In this document, they provided clear consensus definitions of a number of important basic terms including seizure, epilepsy, and status epilepticus. They further defined the concepts of "active" epilepsy as well as "epilepsy in remission (with and without medication)." They outlined a simple schema for the classification of seizures, and the presentation of risk factors in epidemiological work (see Fig. 1).

In the epidemiologic classification, seizures are classified as either partial or generalized. Seizures are said to be "unclassified" if insufficient information exists to determine if the onset was focal or generalized. Epilepsies are grouped according to etiology, which may be known or unknown, and may be associated with a

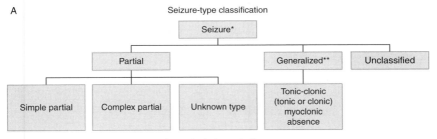

*Based on history, seizure semiology, and neurological examination.
**When seizures are secondarily generalized, they should be referred to as partial seizures.

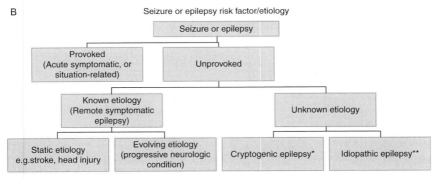

*Cryptogenic epilepsy includes both partial and generalized epilepsies, where no cause has been found and the syndrome does not satisfy criteria for an idiopathic epilepsy **Idiopathic epilepsy – this refers to a group of epilepsy syndromes that are defined by strict clinical and electrographic criteria as defined by the ILAE (1989)

FIG. 1. ILAE classification of (A) seizures and (B) etiologic risk factors in the 1993 Guidelines for Epidemiologic Studies in Epilepsy.

static or an evolving neurological condition. The ILAE report appends lists of risk factors for each of these etiological groups. For unknown etiologies, a distinction is made between idiopathic epilepsies (a strictly defined group of epilepsies with a presumed genetic basis) and cryptogenic epilepsies (see Fig. 1). A number of epidemiologic studies have now been completed using this scheme and will be discussed below.

III. Methodology of Epidemiologic Studies in Epilepsy

A number of problems have been described in relation to published epidemiologic studies of epilepsy (Sander and Shorvon, 1987). Broadly, these center around problems of case ascertainment and nonuniformity of case definition. This relates to: the definition of epilepsy itself (often not stated in studies); the inclusion or exclusion of febrile, neonatal, or acute symptomatic seizures; classification of same-day seizures as single or multiple events; and definition and inclusion of "active epilepsy" versus "epilepsy in remission." Another problem is inaccurate classification of seizure syndromes (see above), which is often evidenced in published studies by the suspiciously low number of "unclassified" seizures in the results (Sander and Shorvon, 1987). Many studies are unclear as to the level of investigation undertaken to establish etiology for seizures, which clearly affects the accuracy of classification. Problems relating to the misuse of basic epidemiologic measures have also been criticized (Commission on Epidemiology and Prognosis, ILAE, 1993).

A systematic review and quantitative meta-analysis of all incidence studies published between 1966 and 2002 in relation to epilepsy and unprovoked seizures found that variation in methodology (and in subsequently published incidence rates) was high among the studies, and that overall methodological quality was low (Kotsopoulos *et al.*, 2002). It is for these reasons that one must be vigilant when viewing and comparing studies of epilepsy epidemiology. The discussion below on gender differences is made in the light of these comments, and a glossary of terminology is included at the end.

IV. Gender Differences in Epidemiology of Epilepsy

A. INCIDENCE OF EPILEPSY

Incidence studies are especially useful in epilepsy epidemiology because they give information on etiology and prognosis of epilepsy and seizures. They are methodologically demanding however, and are ideally planned prospectively or are derived from rigorously maintained population-based records such as the database of the Rochester epidemiologic project in Minnesota.

The estimated median incidence of epilepsy is 43.4/100,000 among industrialized countries and 68.7/100,000 in the developing world according to a recent meta-analysis (Kotsopoulos *et al.*, 2002). The Rochester data show a cumulative incidence of 3.1% for epilepsy up to 74 years of age, and of 4.1% for an unprovoked seizure of any kind. Age-specific incidence figures demonstrate bimodal distribution in industrialized countries with an initial peak in childhood and a later peak after the age of 55. In industrialized countries, the highest incidences are now seen in people over 75 years of age, reflecting improvements in care of the elderly (Hauser *et al.*, 1993) (Fig. 2). This "U-shaped curve" is not a feature in developing countries, where higher rates of epilepsy are found in children and young adults with relatively lower incidences in the elderly (Mac *et al.*, 2007; Medina *et al.*, 2005).

It appears worldwide that females have a marginally smaller annual incidence of epilepsy than males: 46.2 and 50.7/100,000, respectively, in the review by Kotsopoulos *et al.* (2002). This gender difference may be multifactorial but it is usually attributed to the greater exposure of males to risk factors for remote symptomatic epilepsy and acute symptomatic seizures, particularly head injury, stroke, and CNS infection. Alcohol-related seizures and remote alcohol-related epilepsies are also significantly more common in men, and account for much of this gender difference as observed in two studies from Jallon and colleagues in Geneva and in the Island of Martinique (Jallon *et al.*, 1997, 1999).

The EPIMART and EPIGEN studies were both year-long prospective incidence studies based on the 1993 ILAE epidemiologic classification. They have similar methodologies and are therefore appropriate to compare. EPIGEN was a

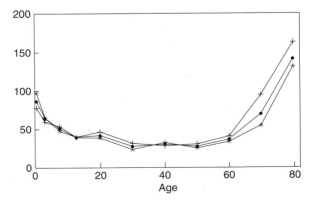

FIG. 2. Age- and gender-specific incidence/100,000 of epilepsy in Rochester, Minnesota, 1935–1984. Total (solid circles), male (plus signs), female (stars). From Hauser *et al.* (1993).

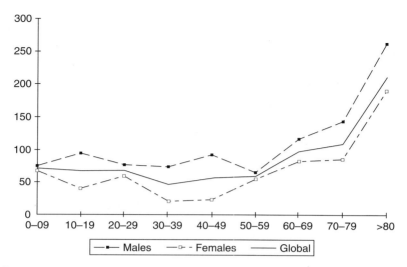

FIG. 3. Age-adjusted incidence/100,000 of first epileptic seizures in the canton of Geneva, Switzerland. Age is represented on the x-axis. Males, broken line squares; females, broken line and open squares; global, solid line. From Jallon *et al.* (1997).

Swiss project centered around Geneva, and EPIMART was conducted on the French Caribbean Island, Martinique (Jallon *et al.*, 1997, 1999). Both studies revealed a greater incidence of acute symptomatic seizures and epilepsy in male patients. Age-adjusted incidence of first seizure, which included both provoked and unprovoked seizures, was 56.8/100,000 population for women, and 88.4/100,000 for men in EPIGEN (Fig. 3), with a twofold increased incidence of male epilepsy in EPIMART. Alcohol was associated with 18% of the total number of seizures in EPIMART and 13% in EPIGEN. In EPIMART, alcohol withdrawal accounted for 30.1% of provoked seizures (69.8% of them in males), and chronic alcoholism was identified as a contributing cause of 48.6% of unprovoked seizures of remote-symptomatic etiology.

Table I summarizes the findings of the EPIMART, EPIGEN, and EPISOUSSE (a pediatric incidence study from Tunisia) reports and compares them to the incidence of unprovoked seizures in Rochester, Minnesota.

It is interesting that the studies from Rochester found a male predominance both for generalized and partial epilepsies, although epilepsies characterized by absence seizures were more common in females (Figs. 4 and 5). Most recent reports would challenge this early finding, and will be discussed below.

How does age-specific incidence vary between genders? In the Rochester study, the pattern of age-adjusted incidences was similar for males and females, with a slight female excess observed within the first five years of life, and a male excess thereafter with the widest gender gap observed in the oldest age groups

TABLE I
GENDER DIFFERENCES IN FOUR STUDIES OF FIRST SEIZURE ONSET

	Incidence of first seizure per 100,000		
	Male	Female	All
Hauser et al. (1993)[a]	49	41	44
Jallon et al. (1997) Switzerland	88.4	56.8	69.4
Jallon et al. (1999) Martinique	107.6	55.4	80.5
Dogui et al. (2003) Tunisia	103.8	100.4	102.1

[a]The study of Hauser et al. excludes acute symptomatic seizures.

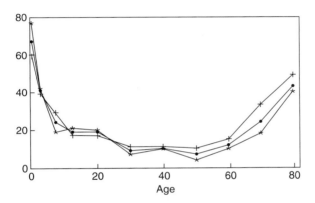

FIG. 4. Age- and gender-specific incidence/100,000 of generalized onset epilepsy in Rochester, Minnesota, 1935–1984. Total (solid circles), male (plus signs), female (stars). From Hauser et al. (1993).

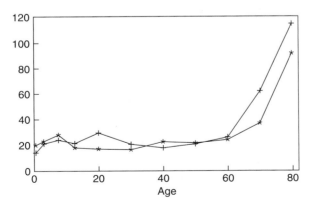

FIG. 5. Age- and gender-specific incidence/100,000 of partial epilepsy in Rochester, Minnesota, 1935–1984. Male (plus signs), female (stars). From Hauser et al. (1993).

consistent with the greater risks for lesional epilepsy in elderly males. Within this, generalized epilepsies are more common in females in the first year of life, after which incidences for both genders converge and remain similar until 45 years, when a slight male excess becomes apparent (Fig. 4). Generalized epilepsy syndromes characterized by absence seizures were diagnosed typically in childhood and early adulthood, as was the greatest incidence of generalized myoclonic epilepsies. Generalized epilepsies with first presentation in the adult and elder populations were mostly characterized by generalized tonic–clonic seizures alone. Partial epilepsies are similarly sex distributed during childhood and early adulthood but incidence again becomes higher in males after the age of 65 (Fig. 5).

B. Prevalence of Epilepsy

Prevalence studies provide information on disease burden within a population and are useful for planning health care and resource planning. There are more published epilepsy prevalence studies than incidence studies in the literature. Generally, case ascertainment is easier for prevalence than for incidence studies, but their methodologies are often flawed (Sander and Shorvon, 1997).

Estimates of epilepsy prevalence in the developed world vary between 4 and 10 per thousand of population (Jallon, 1997). In the developing world, they range from 17 to 57/1000 in South America, 5.2 to 43/1000 in African countries, and from 1.5 to 14/1000 in Asia (Mac et al., 2007). In the majority of studies, a slight male preponderance is once again seen. Table II summarizes a selection of gender-specific prevalence studies from Europe and Asia.

C. Gender Differences in Specific Epilepsy Syndromes

While the small overall preponderance of epilepsy in males seems well established, it has recently been realized that the group of idiopathic generalized epilepsies (IGEs) is more common in females (Christensen et al., 2005). IGEs (formerly considered as primary generalized epilepsies) are an overlapping group of epilepsy syndromes that are defined by strict clinical and electrographic criteria. They are generally believed to have an underlying genetic causation (Jallon and Latour, 2005). IGEs probably represent 15–20% of all epilepsy syndromes although it is recognized that they are often misclassified in population-based epidemiologic studies due to lack of EEG data. A summary of IGE syndromes is presented in Table III.

Although it is difficult to establish consistent incidence and prevalence figures for IGEs, a female predominance has been shown in several studies. Childhood absence epilepsy (CAE) is generally reported to be 2–5 times more common in

TABLE II

PREVALENCE (PER 1000) OF EPILEPSY BY GENDER IN EUROPE AND ASIA

Country	Males	Females	Age
Italy	5.5	4.9	All ages
Iceland	5.2	4.3	All ages
China	3.6	2.5	All ages
Turkey	8.7	6.3	All ages
India	4.4	3.4	All ages
Pakistan	9.2	10.9	All ages
Nepal	6.8	7.9	All ages
India	5.9	5.5	All ages
Finland	7.4	5.2	Adults
Sweden	5.8	5.3	Adults
Estonia	6.9	4.0	Adults
Estonia	3.8	3.2	Children
Sweden	4.0	4.5	Children
Norway	6.0	4.2	Children
Finland	4.1	3.8	Children
Lithuania	4.7	3.8	Children
Singapore	3.5	3.5	Children

After Forsgren *et al.* (2005a) and Mac *et al.* (2007). Note that methodologies differ widely among studies and that the chosen European prevalences are for cases of "active" epilepsy.

TABLE III

IDIOPATHIC GENERALIZED EPILEPSY (IGE) SYNDROMES

Idiopathic generalized epilepsy syndromes
• Childhood absence epilepsy (CAE)
• Juvenile absence epilepsy (JAE)
• Juvenile myoclonic epilepsy (JME)
• Epilepsy with generalized tonic–clonic seizures on awakening (EGTCA)
• Idiopathic generalized epilepsy with tonic–clonic seizures only (IGTC)

females: 2.5% of epilepsy syndromes in boys compared to 11.4% in girls, in the Norwegian prevalence study by Waaler *et al.* (2000). Both juvenile absence epilepsy (JAE) and juvenile myoclonic epilepsy (JME) are more common among females than males, and a report from Denmark by Christensen and colleagues showed significant gender differences for IGE using two separate population-based databases. He showed that JAE was three times more common in females, whereas JME was 1.5 times more common in females than males. These workers also noted that the female predominance for IGE was maximal between the ages of 15 and 50 years suggesting that sex hormones may be responsible for the difference, which therefore decline following menopause. One retrospective study reported a significant association between female gender and epilepsy with generalized seizures upon awakening (Mullins *et al.*, 2007).

For focal epilepsies, Briellman *et al.* (1999)reported an equal gender distribution of hippocampal sclerosis between males and females. However, Janszky *et al.* (2004) reported that the expression of focal epilepsy due to mesial temporal sclerosis is different in females than in males; with females more likely to experience isolated auras than males, and males more likely to have secondary generalization of seizures. They also found that electrographic lateralization of seizures was more likely to be ipsilateral to the side of hippocampal sclerosis in female patients. Although there is no clear mechanistic explanation for this, it suggests a gender-specific difference in seizure threshold which correlates with the observation that generalized tonic–clonic seizures (although not IGEs) are more common in men (Hauser *et al.*, 1993).

D. PROGNOSIS IN EPILEPSY

Prognosis in epilepsy relates both to the likelihood of premature death and to the likelihood of remission from seizures. The National General Practice Study of Epilepsy (NGPSE) was a large prospective population-based study in the UK, which began in 1984 and ascertained all cases of first seizure from primary care attendances and case records (Cockerell *et al.*, 1997). After six months, patients were classified as having definite epilepsy (based on a history of recurrent seizures preceding the index seizure and review of medical records), or probable epilepsy. There was excellent retention of the overall study population over 9 years of follow-up with only 33 of 792 patients completely lost to follow-up in this time. For those patients with definite epilepsy, 86% had achieved a 3-year remission from seizures, and 68% a 5-year remission, with over half of all patients showing evidence of a so-called "terminal remission" from seizures at 9 years (i.e., they remained in remission of 5 years or more at the 9-year follow-up mark). It is presumed that a majority of these patients were in remission with antiepileptic drug (AED) treatment. Epilepsy characterized by generalized seizure types and epilepsy without known cause (including both cryptogenic and idiopathic epilepsies) had a greater proportion of remission. Gender was not reported as a significant outcome variable in this study.

One retrospective review identified a poorer prognosis for female patients following surgery for temporal lobe epilepsy (Burneo *et al.*, 2006). This finding should be viewed cautiously, however, as it was identified retrospectively as a consequence of multiple comparisons within the same data set and has not been replicated in any other study.

E. Mortality in Epilepsy

Studies of mortality in epilepsy show that there is an increase in mortality in patients with epilepsy relative to a normal control population. This increased risk varies but is generally between two- and threefold in community-based population studies. Higher risk is identified for subgroups of patients with severe epilepsy and for those with remote symptomatic epilepsy, and the highest mortality risk is seen among children with epilepsy and neurological disability from birth [standardized mortality ratio (SMR) up to 50 in different studies] (Forsgren et al., 2005b).

The age-specific distribution for mortality risk in epilepsy resembles the "U-shaped" curve for incidence with bimodal peaks reflecting high mortality in the elderly, and in very young children, mainly due to underlying disease. Excess mortality risk in epilepsy is accounted for by different factors and includes both seizure-related and non-seizure-related causes and is greater for males than females (Table IV). Cerebrovascular disease, heart disease, accidents, neoplasms (including non-primary brain tumors), and pneumonia are all important causes of death associated with epilepsy. The risk of suicide is increased among patients with epilepsy and may be particularly so among the newly diagnosed. One population-based study in Iceland identified an almost sixfold increased risk for suicide in men but not women (Rafnsson et al., 2001).

Sudden unexpected death in epilepsy (SUDEP) is the most common seizure-related cause of death in adolescence and young adulthood and accounts for 7–17% of deaths among all patients with epilepsy in this age group. The incidence of SUDEP appears to be 1–2/1000 in most hospital-ascertained cohorts of chronic epilepsy, with higher rates observed in presurgical and refractory groups. A lesser incidence is observed in population-based incidence cohorts of epilepsy, which generally include milder cases. Despite early reports suggesting a male preponderance of SUDEP, most recent studies do not show a gender difference for the

TABLE IV
Mortality in Populations with Epilepsy by Gender

Country, year (reference)	Males SMR (95% CI[a])	Females SMR (95% CI[a])
Warsaw, Poland, 1974 (4)	20 (NR)	1.4 (NR)
Rochester, Minnesota, USA, 1980 (5)	2.1 (1.5–2.8)	1.6 (1.1–2.2)
United Kingdom, 1994 (6)	2.7 (NR)	3.4 (NR)
Iceland, 1997 (7)	1.4 (0.9–2.2)[b]	1.0 (0.4–2.2)[b]
Sweden, 2000 (9)	2.7 (1.8–3.9)	2.3 (1.4–3.7)

[a]95% confidence interval.
[b]Idiopathic cases.
From Forsgren et al. Epidepsia 2005, 46: 18–27.
NR, not reported; SMR, standardized mortality ratio.

incidence of SUDEP. A greater number of male SUDEP cases ware identified in the study of Nilsson and colleagues but specific incidence of SUDEP was equal for men and women (1.4/1000/year) when the case number was compared to the total patient population (in which there also existed a greater number of males). The greater number of male cases in this study possibly relates to ascertainment bias in that cases were ascertained from patients admitted to hospital, and the authors speculate that other disorders leading to admission (such as alcoholism, which is more common in males) may account for the gender difference.

Important risk factors for SUDEP include seizure burden and age at onset of epilepsy. A tenfold increased risk of SUDEP is seen among patients, who have more than 50 seizures per year, when compared to those with less than two seizures a year. Early onset of epilepsy is associated with an eightfold increased risk of SUDEP than late-onset disease. Frequency of AED dose changes, and the extent of AED polytherapy is an independent risk factor for SUDEP. The former association appears to be stronger for females than for males, whereas age of onset and seizure frequency are weaker risk associations in females than in males (Nilsson et al., 1999). One risk factor that was exclusive to females in Nilsson's study was co-prescription of neuroleptic drugs, which conferred a tenfold risk increase in women but not in men.

F. STATUS EPILEPTICUS

The incidence of status epilepticus is lower in females than in males. This has been shown in a number of studies, notably in a retrospective population-based incidence study from Rochester, and a prospective population-based study from Switzerland (Hesdorffer et al., 1998). In the study of Coyetaux et al. (2000) from Switzerland, the age-adjusted rate for status epilepticus was 7.8/100,000 for females and 12.1/100,000 for males. This is lower than the incidence in Rochester (18.3/100,000), where again the rate was almost two times higher in males than females (Fig. 6).

The predominant etiology for status epilepticus in both studies was acute symptomatic seizures, and the major seizure syndrome was focal. Hesdorffer and colleagues proposed that the greater incidence of status epilepticus in men could be partially explained by this fact, as men are at greater risk of acute symptomatic and remote symptomatic insults (cerebrovascular disease, head trauma, alcoholism, CNS infections) than women. The authors also speculated upon a gender difference in seizure threshold possibly mediated by the GABA-sensitive substantia nigra, which is under the influence of sex hormones, and which may be involved in the expression of seizures.

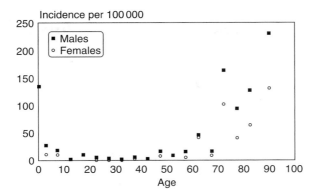

FIG. 6. Age-specific incidence of status epilepticus by gender in Rochester, Minnesota, 1965–1984. From Hesdorffer *et al.* (1998).

V. Summary

In summary, epilepsy is overall slightly more common in males than in females, largely relating to males' greater risk exposure to causes of lesional epilepsy. Mortality is also increased for males than females, although SUDEP appears to have an equal gender incidence. IGEs are more common in females.

Glossary

Given the stated importance of accurate and consistent terminology within epidemiological studies a glossary of terms is included here, which comprises selected clinical and epidemiological concepts referred to within this chapter. The definitions are reproduced from the 1997 report of the ILAE commission on epidemiology and prognosis in epilepsy. Terms that have been clearly defined in the main text are omitted.

Status epilepticus: A single epileptic seizure >30 min in duration or a series of epileptic seizures during which function is not regained between ictal events in more than 30-min period.

Active epilepsy: A prevalent case of active epilepsy is defined as a person with epilepsy who has had at least one epileptic seizure in the previous 5 years, regardless of AED treatment. A case under treatment is someone with the diagnosis of epilepsy receiving AEDs on prevalence day.

Epilepsy in remission with treatment: A prevalent case of epilepsy with no seizures for 25 years with AED treatment at the time of ascertainment.

Epilepsy in remission without treatment: A prevalent case of epilepsy with no seizures for 25 years and without AED treatment at the time of ascertainment.

Single or isolated seizure: One or more epileptic seizures occurring in a 24-h period.

Generalized seizures: A seizure is considered generalized when clinical symptomatology provides no indication of an anatomic localization and no clinical evidence of focal onset. The three main subtypes are generalized convulsive seizures, generalized nonconvulsive seizures, and myoclonic seizures.

Partial seizures: A seizure should be classified as partial when there is evidence of a clinical partial onset, regardless of whether the seizure is secondarily generalized.

Unclassified seizures: The term unclassified seizures should be used when it is impossible to classify seizures owing to lack of adequate information.

Idiopathic epilepsies: The term idiopathic is used herein as defined by the ILAE and must be reserved for certain partial or generalized epileptic syndromes with particular clinical characteristics and with specific EEG findings and should not be used to refer to epilepsy or seizures without obvious cause.

Cryptogenic epilepsies: The term cryptogenic is used to include partial or generalized unprovoked seizures or epilepsies in which no factor associated with increased risk of seizures has been identified. This group includes patients who do not conform to the criteria for the symptomatic or idiopathic categories.

Incidence: The number of new cases of epilepsy occurring during a given time interval, usually 1 year, in a specified population.

Cumulative incidence: The individual's risk of developing epilepsy by a certain time, for example, the time a specified age is reached.

Point prevalence: The proportion of patients with epilepsy in a given population at a specified time (usually a specific day: the prevalence day). Inclusion criteria should be specified (i.e., active epilepsy, epilepsy in remission with treatment, epilepsy in remission without treatment).

Period prevalence: The proportion of patients with epilepsy in a given population during a defined time interval (e.g., 1 year).

Standardized mortality ratio: The ratio of observed number of deaths in a population with epilepsy to that expected based on the age- and sex-specific mortality rates in a reference population.

References

Briellmann, R. S., Jackson, G. D., Mitchell, L. A., Fitt, G. J., Kim, S. E., and Berkovic, S. F. (1999). Occurrence of hippocampal sclerosis: Is one hemisphere or gender more vulnerable? *Epilepsia* **40,** 1816–1820.

Burneo, J. G., Black, L., Martin, R., Devinsky, O., Pacia, S., Faught, E., Vasquez, B., Knowlton, R. C., Luciano, D., Doyle, W., Najjar, S., and Kuzniecky, R. I. (2006). Race/ethnicity, sex, and socioeconomic status as predictors of outcome after surgery for temporal lobe epilepsy. *Arch. Neurol.* **63,** 1106–1110.

Christensen, J., Kjeldsen, M. J., Andersen, H., Friis, M. L., and Sidenius, P. (2005). Gender differences in epilepsy. *Epilepsia* **46,** 956–960.

Cockerell, O. C., Johnson, A. L., Sander, W. A. S., and Shorvon, S. D. (1997). Prognosis of epilepsy: A review and further analysis of the first nine years of the British National general practice study of epilepsy, a prospective population-based study. *Epilepsia* **38,** 31–46.

Coeytaux, A., Jallon, P., Galobardes, B., and Morabia, A. (2000). Incidence of status epilepticus in French-speaking Switzerland: (EPISTAR). *Neurology* **55,** 693–697.

Commission on Classification and Terminology of the International League Against Epilepsy (1981). Proposal for revised clinical and electroencephalographic classification of epileptic seizures. *Epilepsia* **22,** 489–501.

Commission on Classification and Terminology of the International League Against Epilepsy (1989). Proposal for revised classification of epilepsies and epileptic syndromes. *Epilepsia* **30,** 389–399.

Commission on Epidemiology and Prognosis, International League Against Epilepsy (1993). Guidelines for epidemiologic studies on epilepsy. *Epilepsia* **34**(4), 592–596.

Dogui, M., Jallon, P., Tamallah, J. B., Sakly, G., Trabelsi, M. A., Khalifa, K., Yacoub, M., and Abroug, S. (2003). Episousse: Incidence of newly presenting seizures in children in the Region of Sousse, Tunisia. *Epilepsia* **44,** 1441-1444.

Forsgren, L., Beghi, E., Oun, A., and Sillanpaa, M. (2005a). The epidemiology of epilepsy in Europe— A systematic review. *Eur. J. Neurol.* **12,** 245–253.

Forsgren, L., Hauser, W. A., Olafsson, E., Sander, J. W. A. S., Sillanpaa, M., and Tomson, T. (2005b). Mortality of epilepsy in developed countries: A review. *Epilepsia* **46**(Suppl. 11), 18–27.

Hauser, W. A., Annegers, J. F., and Kurland, L. T. (1993). Incidence of epilepsy and unprovoked seizures in Rochester, Minnesota: 1935–1984. *Epilepsia* **34**(3), 453–468.

Hesdorffer, D. C., Logroscino, G., Cascino, G., Annegers, J. F., and Hauser, W. A. (1998). Incidence of status epilepticus in Rochester Minnesota, 1965–1984. *Neurology* **50,** 735–741.

ILAE Commission Report (1997). The epidemiology of the epilepsies: Future directions. International league against epilepsy. *Epilepsia* **38,** 614–618.

Jallon, P. (1997). ILAE workshop report: Epilepsy in developing countries. *Epilepsia* **38**(10), 1143–1151.

Jallon, P., and Latour, P. (2005). Epidemiology of idiopathic generalized epilepsies. *Epilepsia* **46**(Suppl 9), 10–14.

Jallon, P., Goumaz, M., Haenggeli, C., and Morabia, A. (1997). Incidence of first epileptic seizures in the canton of Geneva, Switzerland. *Epilepsia* **38**(5), 541–552.

Jallon, P., Smadja, D., Cabre, P., Le Mab, G., Bazin, M., and EPIMART Group, M. (1999). EPIMART: Prospective incidence study of epileptic seizures in newly referred patients in a French Caribbean Island (Martinique). *Epilepsia* **40,** 1103–1109.

Janszky, J., Schulz, R., Janszky, I., and Ebner, A. (2004). Medial temporal lobe epilepsy: Gender differences. *J. Neurol. Neurosurg. Psychiatr.* **75,** 773–775.

Kotsopoulos, I. A. W., van Merode, T., Kessels, F. G. H., deKrom, M. C. T. F. M., and Knotterus, J. A. (2002). Systematic review and meta-analysis of incidence studies of epilepsy and unprovoked seizures. *Epilepsia* **43,** 1402–1409.

Mac, T. L., Tran, D. S., Quet, F., Odermatt, P., Preux, P. M., and Tan, C. T. (2007). Epidemiology, aetiology, and clinical management of epilepsy in Asia: A systematic review. *Lancet Neurol.* **6,** 533–543.

Medina, M. T., Reyna, M. D., Martinez, L., Osorio, J. R., Estrada, A. L., Zuniga, C., Cartagena, D., Collins, J. S., and Holden, K. R. (2005). Prevalence, incidence, and eriology of epilepsies in rural honduras. The Salama study. *Epilepsia* **46,** 124–131.

Mullins, G. M., O'Sullivan, S. S., Neligan, A., McCarthy, A., McNamara, B., Galvin, R. J., and Sweeney, B. J. (2007). A study of idiopathic generalised epilepsy in an Irish population. *Seizure* **16,** 204–210.

Nilsson, L., Farahmand, B. Y., Persson, P. G., Thiblin, I., and Tomson, T. (1999). Risk factors for sudden unexpected death in epilepsy: A case control study. *Lancet* **353,** 888–893.

Rafnsson, V., Olafsson, E., Hauser, W. A., and Gudmundsson, G. (2001). Cause-specific mortality in adults with unprovoked seizures. A population-based incidence cohort study. *Neuroepidemiology* **4,** 232–236.

Sander, J. W. A. S., and Shorvon, S. D. (1987). Incidence and prevalence studies in epilepsy and their methodological problems: A review. *J. Neurol. Neurosurg. Psychiatr.* **50,** 829–839.

Waaler, P. E., Blom, B. H., Skeidsvoll, H., and Mykletun, A. (2000). Prevalence, classification, and severity of epilepsy in children in Western Norway. *Epilepsia* **41,** 802–810.

HORMONAL INFLUENCES ON SEIZURES: BASIC NEUROBIOLOGY

Cheryl A. Frye

Departments of Psychology, Biology, and Centers for Neuroscience
and Life Sciences Research, The University at Albany-State
University of New York, Albany, New York 12222, USA

I. Introduction
II. Organizing Effects of Androgens-Sex Differences in Seizures
III. Activational Effects of Androgens on Seizures
IV. Hypothalamic–Pituitary–Gonadal Axis Factors and Seizures
V. Reproductive Events and Seizures
   A. Estrogen and Seizures
   B. Progesterone and Seizures
   C. Progesterone Metabolites and Seizures
   D. Biosynthesis/Metabolism of 3α, 5α-THP
   E. Variations in 3α, 5α-THP
   F. Effects of Postmenopausal Hormone Therapy
VI. Mechanisms of 3α, 5α-THP Through GABA Receptors
VII. Acute Stress-Induced Steroid Biosynthesis and Seizures
VIII. Developmental Differences in Stress-Induced Steroids
   A. Chronic Stress-Induced Changes in Seizures
IX. Other Factors that may Underlie Differences in Sensitivity to Steroids
X. A Review of Progestins, Absence Seizures, and Mechanisms of Action
XI. Interactions Between AEDs and Steroid Hormones
XII. Summary
   References

There are sex differences and effects of steroid hormones, such as androgens, estrogens, and progestogens, that influence seizures. Androgens exert early organizational and later activational effects that can amplify sex/gender differences in the expression of some seizure disorders. Female-typical sex steroids, such as estrogen (E_2) and progestins, can exert acute activational effects to reduce convulsive seizures and these effects are mediated in part by the actions of steroids in the hippocampus. Some of these anticonvulsive effects of sex steroids are related to their formation of ligands which have agonist-like actions at γ-aminobutyric acid ($GABA_A$) receptors or antagonist actions at glutamatergic receptors. Differences in stress, developmental phase, reproductive status, endocrine status, and treatments, such as anti-epileptic drugs (AEDs), may alter levels of these ligands and/ or the function of target sites, which may mitigate differences in sensitivity to,

INTERNATIONAL REVIEW OF
NEUROBIOLOGY, VOL. 83
DOI: 10.1016/S0074-7742(08)00003-2

27

and/or tolerance of, steroids among some individuals. The evidence implicating sex steroids in differences associated with hormonal, reproductive, developmental, stress, seizure type, and/or therapeutics are discussed.

I. Introduction

Steroid hormones can influences seizures. In support, there are gender-dependent discrepancies in the incidence of some seizure disorders. Furthermore, the occurrence of some epileptiform activity in women is greatest during times of hormonal flux, as during the premenstrual and perimenopausal periods, suggesting that gender differences in brain structure or gonadal steroids may mitigate vulnerability to seizures.

It is important to understand the role of steroids in seizure disorders. Antiepileptic drugs (AEDs) are the most common treatment for epilepsy. Use of AEDs enable about 60% of people to remain seizure-free, another 20% achieve partial control of seizures, but the remaining 20% are not responsive to AEDs (Shorvon, 1996). New therapeutic approaches are needed as adjunctive therapies for those that are resistant to the existing AEDs and to help those with intractable epilepsy achieve control. As such, steroids may represent an important therapeutic target. Thus, this chapter reviews some of the basic neurobiological findings about the role of steroids in seizure processes.

Investigators hoping to understand the nature of these differences have attempted to develop animal models looking at the effect of sex/gender and gonadal hormone milieu on seizures. In studies using rats as a model, females typically exhibit less ictal-like behavior than do their male conspecifics. However, in studies where effects are determined in relation to day of estrus, reductions in seizures occur during the afternoon of proestrus, when the ovarian hormones, estrogen (E_2) and progesterone (P_4), are at their peak, rather than in diestrous when these same hormones are at their lowest. For example, proestrous females show reduced kainic acid and/or pentylenetetrazol (PTZ)-induced seizures than do diestrous females or males (Frye and Bayon, 1998a, 1999c; Rhodes and Frye, 2004a). These data, in addition to findings from human and animal studies that there are opposing effects of E_2 (proconvulsant) and P_4 (anticonvulsant) on seizures, suggest that attenuation of epileptiform activity during proestrus may be due in part to high endogenous levels of E_2 and P_4, each of which can modulate specific neurotransmitter systems known to mediate seizures. Levels of these hormones fluctuate throughout the menstrual cycle, and, in some women with epilepsy, these fluctuations may be related to the occurrence of seizures around the time of menses or an increase in seizures in relation to the menstrual cycle, also known as catamenial epilepsy. Thus, the nature of E_2 and P_4's effects on seizures will be discussed further in this chapter.

Given that organizational sex/gender differences and activation by gonadal steroids play an important role in mediating seizure status, the next question becomes where in the brain are these effects manifested. The most common type of epilepsy, temporal lobe epilepsy (McNamara, 1994), involves the amygdala and the hippocampus (Lothman *et al.*, 1991). Animal models of pilocarpine-induced seizures produce neuropathology very similar to that observed in people, including status epilepticus (SE) and damage to the hippocampus, amygdala, and entorhinal cortex (Bruton *et al.*, 1994; Covolan and Mello, 2000; Fujikawa, 1996; Margerison and Corsellis, 1966; Turski *et al.*, 1983). These brain regions are sensitive to hormones, trophic effects of hormones are observed in these regions, and these regions also have steroid receptors (Hagihara *et al.*, 1992; Leranth *et al.*, 2003; Meyer *et al.*, 1978; Simerly *et al.*, 1990; Shughrue *et al.*, 1997; Weiland *et al.*, 1997). Although steroid receptors have been localized to these regions, there may be steroid receptor-dependent and -independent effects that are relevant for steroid modulation of ictal processes.

What are some of the actions that steroids may exert in these and other brain regions to influence seizures? Steroid hormones have several different mechanisms in the central nervous system (CNS). First, there is the classical genomic mechanism in which the steroids bind to intracellular steroid receptors. Steroids can have traditional actions through their cognate intracellular receptors to mediate gene transcription, DNA, and posttranscriptional processes, such as protein synthesis (McEwen and Woolley, 1994). The classical hormone nuclear receptors for E_2 and P_4 are present in neurons and uniquely distributed in limbic and hypothalamic regions of the brain (Pfaff *et al.*, 1976). For E_2, both α and β isoforms of the E_2 receptor have been identified in the human brain (Osterlund *et al.*, 2000a,b). In animal studies, these receptor isoforms have been localized throughout the brain and specifically to regions involved in memory/learning and reproductive behaviors, such as the hippocampus and hypothalamus (Shughrue *et al.*, 1997). Second, more recent research has demonstrated that steroids can also produce rapid effects on excitability and synaptic function through direct membrane mechanisms, such as ligand-gated ion channels and neurotransmitter transporters (Boulware *et al.*, 2005; Wong *et al.*, 1996). One of the differences between actions involving the classical genomic mechanism and the membrane actions of steroids is that actions at cognate steroid receptors involve a response time on the order of several minutes, hours, or days, unlike membrane mechanism, which can occur within seconds to minutes.

This chapter discusses the influence of hormones in epilepsy with an emphasis on female-typical sex steroids. First, evidence that androgens may exert early organizational and activational effects that give rise to sex/gender differences in the expression of some seizure and/or developmental disorders is discussed.

Second, findings that E_2 and progestins may have acute activational effects on seizures are presented. Third, the potential substrates (brain areas and mechanisms within them) that mediate the effects of these female-typical sex steroids on seizures are described. Fourth, findings relevant for hormone-replacement therapies are summarized. Fifth, possible reasons for differences in sensitivity and/or tolerance to steroids among some individuals, and with reproductive status, are discussed. Sixth, effects of steroids in absence epilepsy versus convulsant seizures are considered. Finally, the relevance of these findings for treatments strategies, in particular AEDs, are mentioned. Although some results of relevant clinical studies are described as appropriate, the emphasis of this chapter is on the basic research regarding the neurobiological effects of female-typical sex steroids on seizures.

II. Organizing Effects of Androgens-Sex Differences in Seizures

Sex steroid hormones play fundamental roles in the development and function of the CNS and contribute to differences in the structure and function of the brains of male and female animals and people (Panzica and Melcangi, 2004). It is now widely accepted that gonadal steroids exert their effects on physiology and behavior by organizing the brain early in development (organizational effects) and by activating brain systems and behavior starting at puberty (activational effects) (reviewed in McCarthy and Konkle, 2005). Evidence of sex difference, which are primarily due to organizing effects of androgens, on seizures are discussed first.

Females are less vulnerable to some types of seizures than are males. Females, compared to males, are less likely to experience developmentally regulated seizures, such as febrile seizures and infantile spasms, and the incidence of syndromes, such as Landau–Kleffner syndrome and Lennox–Gastaut syndrome, are lower in females compared to males (International League Against Epilepsy; Hauser et al., 1993). The occurrence of these sex differences early in development proximate to times when sexual differentiation occurs suggest that the effects may be in part due to early organizing effects of androgens.

One model that has been used to investigate the neurobiological substrates associated with sex differences in seizure susceptibility is infusions of muscimol, a γ-aminobutyric acid ($GABA_A$) receptor agonist, to the substantia nigra pars reticulata (SNR). Using this approach, Velíšková and colleagues have found that the SNR is an important brain region that mediates some sex-differences in seizure susceptibility (Galanopoulou et al., 2003a; Iadarola and Gale, 1981; Moshé et al., 1992; Ravizza et al., 2003). Infusions of muscimol to the SNR at postnatal day 15 (PND15), produce seizures among male, but not female, rats (Velíšková and Moshé, 2001). By PND15 and in adulthood, female rats have more GABA and $GABA_A\alpha1$ subunit receptor mRNA in the SNR than do their male counterparts

(Ravizza *et al.*, 2003). These findings suggest that sex differences in seizure suscep- tibility occur early in development and may be somewhat independent of the activational effects of steroids that begin to be secreted at puberty.

Testosterone (T) has profound masculinizing effects during early development that can influence the male nervous system to be more seizure susceptible. If the natural surge in T that occurs on the day of birth is blocked in male rats by castration (i.e., removal of the primary endogenous source of T), then the female pattern of reduced seizure susceptibility develops. This effect is reversed if T is administered at the same time that rats are castrated on the day of birth (Giorgi *et al.*, 2006; Velíšek *et al.*, 2006; Velíšková and Moshé, 2001). Among female rats, the male-typical pattern of increased seizure vulnerability is observed if female rats are administered exogenous T on the day of birth (Breedlove *et al.*, 1982; Velíšková and Moshé, 2001). These findings suggest that androgens can have organizational effects on brain development to increase sensitivity to some proconvulsant stimuli.

Organizational effects of androgens on seizures may be mediated in part through their actions at intracellular androgen receptors (ARs). T and its metab- olite, dihydrotestosterone (DHT), act primarily on ARs (Grisham *et al.*, 2002). ARs have been localized to the SNR (Giorgi *et al.*, 2006; Velíšek *et al.*, 2006; Velíšková and Moshé, 2001). Blocking effects of the early T surge on its actions at ARs by early postnatal administration of flutamide, an AR antagonist, has a "demasculinization" effect on seizure susceptibility. Together these findings sug- gest that T has actions through ARs that differentiate the SNR and seizure susceptibility. In addition to the effects of androgens to organize sex differences in the brain that influence seizures, there is also evidence that androgens can have activational effects that modulate seizures.

III. Activational Effects of Androgens on Seizures

Androgens, male-typical sex steroid hormones, such as T and its metabolites, E_2 and DHT, were identified in the early part of the last century (Tausk, 1984), and exert reciprocal effects related to seizures. That is, androgens influence seizures and seizures influence androgen levels. Among some men with epilepsy, hypogo- nadism, sexual interest, reproductive function, and plasma T levels are low (Herzog, 1991, 1998; Isojarvi *et al.*, 1995; Murialdo *et al.*, 1994). Anti-epileptic drugs, such as carbamazepine and phenytoin, can decrease free plasma T levels (Duncan *et al.*, 1999; Isojarvi *et al.*, 1989; Panesar *et al.*, 1996; Rosenbrock *et al.*, 1999; Stoffel-Wagner *et al.*, 1998), but removal of the epileptogenic tissue can normalize plasma T levels even when AEDs are continued (Bauer *et al.*, 2000a). These findings suggest that seizures may influences androgen status independent of AEDs.

Among some men with epilepsy, androgen levels may contribute to reproductive dysfunction and seizure dysregulation. For example, there are significantly higher serum E_2 levels and lower free T to E_2 ratios in men with epilepsy that have reduced sexual function than in either men with epilepsy or nonepileptic control subjects that do not have problems in sexual function (Murialdo *et al.*, 1995). E_2 can lower male sexual interest and function (Herzog *et al.*, 1991) and may contribute to seizure dysregulation (Herzog *et al.*, 2004a, 2005). In support, the combination of T and the aromatase inhibitor, testolactone (which minimizes conversion of T to E_2) improves reproductive/sexual function and reduces seizure frequency significantly more than T treatment alone in AED-treated hyposexual men with complex partial seizures (Herzog *et al.*, 1998). These findings underscore the importance of considering endogenous levels of sex steroids, and their ratio with other sex steroids, and how they together may influence seizures and other steroid-dependent behaviors, such as reproduction.

T has anticonvulsant effects in animal models. T administration to castrated rats increases the threshold to seizures produced by electroshock, electrical kindling of the amygdala, or kainic acid (Edwards *et al.*, 1999a; Mejias-Aponte *et al.*, 2002; Woolley *et al.*, 1961). However, there is variability in the effects of T on seizures that may be related to relative levels of proconvulsant aromatized metabolites versus anticonvulsant 5α-reduced metabolites that are produced (Hardy, 1970; Nicoletti *et al.*, 1985). The role of T's 5α-reduced metabolites in mediating seizures is discussed below.

T's anticonvulsant actions may involve formation of its 5α-reduced metabolites. The first step in T's metabolism is its irreversible reduction by 5α-reductase isoenzymes, which leads to the formation of DHT, which can block N-methyl-d-aspartate (NMDA) transmission and may thereby have antiseizure effects (Pouliot *et al.*, 1996). DHT is then further reduced, an effect which is catalyzed by 3α-hydroxysteroid dehydrogenase (3α-HSD), resulting in the synthesis of 3α-androstan-17β-diol (3α-diol). 3α-Diol administration to rats attenuates kainic acid, PTZ, picrotoxin, β-carboline, and perforant pathway stimulation-induced seizures (Frye, 2006; Frye and Reed, 1998; Reddy, 2004; Rhodes and Frye, 2004a). 3α-Diol is a positive allosteric modulator of $GABA_A$ receptors (Frye *et al.*, 1996a; Gee, 1988; Jorge-Rivera *et al.*, 2000), which allows GABA to bind more effectively to its receptor. 3α-Diol may also reduce the binding of convulsants to $GABA_A$ receptors, by displacing *t*-butylcicyclophophorothioate, a compound that is used to assess the allosteric site of picrotoxin (Gee, 1988).

3α-Diol may be a biologically relevant, endogenous antiseizure agent for some people with epilepsy. 3α-Diol is normally excreted in urine and is present in serum and the brain (Callies *et al.*, 2000; Poór *et al.*, 2004; Rittmaster *et al.*, 1989; Slaunwhite and Sandberg, 1958). Among men with epilepsy, levels of this neuroactive steroid are particularly low (Herzog *et al.*, 2004a, 2005, 2006). 3α-Diol is also an androgenic neurosteroid, and like the pregnane neuroactive steroid that will be discussed later, it is produced in the brain and can have profound anticonvulsant effects. Lastly, although androgens are considered male-typical steroids, androgens, and 3α-diol, in particular, are biologically active and have clear anticonvulsant effects in females (Frye and Bayon, 1999b; Frye and Reed, 1998; Frye et al., 1996a–e).

We have investigated the effects of seizures on androgen-dependent hippo-campal and hypothalamic functions in an animal model. Male rats were administered on PND10, the chemoconvulsant, pilocarpine 60 mg/kg, IP, which induces SE, saline vehicle, or no manipulation. As adults, androgen-dependent behaviors that are indicative of hippocampal (anxiety behavior) and hypothalamic (social behavior) function was assessed before and after administration of pilocarpine (100 mg/kg IP). E_2, T, DHT, and 3α-diol levels in hippocampus and hypothalamus were then measured by radioimmunoassay. There were differences among the four groups in seizure severity scores. Rats that received pilocarpine on PND10 and in adulthood had higher seizure scores [according to Racine's (1972) 5-point scale] than did those administered saline on PND10 and pilocarpine as adults, rats with no perinatal manipulations and pilocarpine in adulthood, or rats with neither PND10 nor adult pilocarpine. Manipulation of pilocarpine or saline on PND10 decreased hypermotor effects of adult pilocarpine that were observed in the number of beam breaks made for 5 min when rats were placed in an activity monitor and in the number of total squares entered in the open field. Manipulation of pilocarpine or saline on PND10 decreased anti-anxiety behavior, which was amplified by pilocarpine administration in adulthood. Pilocarpine administration early, and later in life, decreased the duration of time spent in social contact and the number of sexual contacts and 3α-diol levels in the hypothalamus and hippcampus. These findings suggest that seizure-related disruption of 3α-diol in the hippocampus and/or hypothalamus may underlie dysregulation of anxiety, social, and/or reproductive behavior. See Table I.

IV. Hypothalamic–Pituitary–Gonadal Axis Factors and Seizures

As discussed above, there are gender/sex differences, and evidence for androgenic hormones, to influence seizure processes. One hallmark of the sexual dimorphism of the brain is whether the hypothalamic–pituitary–gonadal axis (HPG) responds to gonadotropins in a cyclic, female-typical pattern or a tonic male-typical pattern. Notably, the function of the HPG that gives rise to the menstrual cycle is linked to differences in patterns of seizures among some women with epilepsy (Bäckström, 1976; Herzog et al., 1997; Laidlaw, 1956). In order to discuss the role of the HPG in seizures, we first review the neuroendocrine control of the HPG axis.

TABLE I

Mean (+Standard Error of the Mean) Seizure Scores (Top), Motor Behavior (Middle Top), Anxiety Behavior (Middle), Social/Reproductive Behavior (Middle), and Endocrine Measures (Bottom), of Male Rats That Were Administered Saline on Postnatal Day 10 (PND10) and Pilocarpine (100 mg/kg IP) in Adulthood (Left Column), Pilocarpine on PND10 and in Adulthood (Middle Left Column), No Manipulation on PND10 and Pilocarpine in Adulthood (Middle Right), or No Manipulation on PND10 or in Adulthood (Right Column)

	PND10 saline, adult pilocarpine ($n = 10$)		PND10 pilocarpine, adult pilocarpine ($n = 10$)		PND10 no manipulation, adult pilocarpine ($n = 10$)		PND10 no manipulation, adult no manipulation ($n = 10$)	
	Pre-	Post-	Pre-	Post-	Pre-	Post-	Pre-	Post-
Seizure behavior								
Seizure score	na	2.0 + 0.1	na	2.8 + 0.2	na	1.8 + 0.1	na	na
Motor behavior								
Beam breaks in activity monitor	510 + 56	621 + 55	645 + 80	733 + 51	683 + 71	988 + 80	545 + 35	685 + 55
Total entries in the open field	175 + 15	44 + 6	192 + 11	63 + 9	167 + 12	128 + 19	157 + 12	80 + 12
Anxiety behavior								
Central entries	28 + 5	6 + 2	43 + 7	10 + 2	13 + 2	15 + 3	22 + 5	28 + 4
Open arm time	16 + 7	17 + 6	12 + 3	27 + 6	32 + 7	24 + 7	50 + 8	19 + 7
Social and reproductive behavior								
Social interaction time	60 + 6	56 + 4	60 + 8	50 + 3	83 + 5	72 + 5	71 + 5	73 + 5
# Sexual contacts	6 + 2	2 + 2	4 + 1	2 + 2	8 + 3	6 + 2	8 + 2	15 + 3
Endocrine measures								
	hippo	hyp	hippo	hyp	hippo	hyp	hippo	hyp
E2 (pg/mg)	2 + 1	1 + 1	1 + 1	1 + 1	1 + 1	1 + 1	1 + 1	1 + 1
T (ng/mg)	6 + 1	7 + 1	8 + 1	7 + 1	7 + 1	8 + 2	7 + 2	8 + 3
DHT (ng/mg)	5 + 1	5 + 1	5 + 1	5 + 1	5 + 3	5 + 2	5 + 2	5 + 3
3α-Diol (ng/mg)	2 + 1	1 + 1	1 + 1	1 + 1	3 + 1	3 + 2	4 + 1	4 + 1

"Pre-" refers to behavioral indices prior to adult manipulation and "Post-" indicates outcomes after manipulations in adulthood.

The HPG is controlled by neurons in the hypothalamus that synthesize gonadotropin-releasing hormone (GnRH), which can activate neurons in the diagonal band of Broca, organum vasculosum of the lamina terminalis, and preoptic area to coordinate secretion of GnRH into the hypophysial-portal vasculature (Silverman et al., 2002). The median eminence releases GnRH in a pulsatile fashion, which regulates the production and release of the gonadotropins, luteinizing hormone (LH), and follicle stimulating hormone (FSH) from the anterior pituitary, which in turn controls gonadal steroidogenesis (Everett, 1994; Levine and Ramirez, 1982). Thus, pulsatile release of GnRH is essential for normal HPG and reproductive function.

The HPG axis may be disrupted in some people with epilepsy. Among women with epilepsy, evidence of HPG dysregulation includes an increased incidence of reproductive endocrine disorders, such as anovulatory and/or inadequate luteal phase cycles (Bilo et al., 1988; Herzog et al., 1986). Reproductive endocrine dysfunctions, such as polycystic ovary syndrome (Herzog et al., 2003) and hypogonadotropic hypogonadism (Herzog et al., 1986), which are associated with altered pulsatile release LH, are more common among individuals with temporal lobe epilepsy. These reproductive endocrine dysfunctions may be due in part to acute or chronic effects of epilepsy (and/or the use of AEDs, which will be discussed at the end of this chapter). First, among people with epilepsy, after generalized tonic/clonic seizures, there are postictal increases in secretion of the hypothalamic peptide, prolactin, for up to 20 min (Pritchard et al., 1983; Trimble, 1978), and serum LH (in males and females) and FSH (in women) can remain elevated for up to 60 min (Dana-Haeri et al., 1983). Second, there are also chronic changes in LH pulse frequency among women and men with temporal lobe epilepsy (Bilo et al., 1991; Drislane et al., 1994; Herzog et al., 1990). Third, abnormal afferents to the hypothalamus and/or changes in neurotransmitters could also lead to alterations in GnRH release. Fourth, seizures are exacerbated during periods of anovulation and low P_4 (Backstrom, 1976; Herzog et al., 1997). Because of the inherent challenges of addressing these factors in people, findings from animal models are discussed below.

Animal models of epilepsy in which seizures spontaneously occur subsequent to kindling or chemoconvulsants have provided insight into the etiology of alterations in hormone secretion. The amygdala and hippocampus have efferent projections to the hypothalamus, a brain region that is essential for reproductive function (Price, 2003; Renaud and Hopkins, 1977). Stimulation and/or lesion of the hippocampus and/or amygdala influence neurons in the hypothalamus and modulate gonadotropin release (Brown-Grant and Raisman, 1972; Carrer et al., 1978; Kawakami and Terasawa, 1972; Velasco and Taleisnik, 1971). For example, amygdala kindling produces acyclicity, cystic ovarian follicules, pituitary hypertrophy, and supraphysiological levels of E_2 in serum (Edwards et al., 1999b). Infusions of kainic acid to the amygdala decrease GnRH fibers in a region of the hypothalamus (Friedman *et al.*, 2002). In temporal lobe epilepsy, gliosis and neuronal loss in the hilus, CA1, and CA3 regions of the hippocampus and the amygdala (Tauck and Nadler, 1985; Tuunanen *et al.*, 1996) are seen which may lead to increased excitatory circuits (Tauck and Nadler, 1985), loss of inhibitory GABAergic neurons (Tuunanen *et al.*, 1996), and reduced synaptic inhibition (Buckmaster and Dudek, 1997; Kobayashi and Buckmaster, 2003), which may increase ictal activity and directly or indirectly alter the GnRH system (Glass and Dragunow, 1995; Gore and Terasawa, 2001; Hong *et al.*, 1988; Negro-Vilar *et al.*, 1979; Ojeda *et al.*, 1982; Simon *et al.*, 1984; Tasker and Dudek, 1991). Thus, data from animal models supports the notion that seizure activity and/or the progression of epilepsy disrupts function of the hypothalamus, which may lead to chronic reproductive endocrine disorders.

Given that these anovulatory and/or inadequate luteal phase cycles associated with reproductive endocrine dysfunction may exacerbate seizures (Backstrom *et al.*, 1976; Mattson *et al.*, 1981), an important question is whether improving endocrine function can attenuate seizure activity. It has been demonstrated that achieving control of seizures, through surgery or anti-epileptic drugs, reduces reproductive endocrine dysfunction (Bauer *et al.*, 2000b; Bilo *et al.*, 1991; Herzog *et al.*, 1986; Meo *et al.*, 1993). As another example, clomiphene, a drug that can induce gonadotropin secretion and ovulatory cycles among anovulatory women (if they do not have primary pituitary or ovarian failure), improves seizure control among some women (Cantor, 1984). In a study of 12 women with partial seizures, 10 women had an improvement in their seizures with clomiphene therapy (Herzog, 1988). However, clomiphene also acts as an E_2 antagonist and may produce some effects on seizures due to these effects. Thus, discussed below is how seizures can change with reproductive cycles and the role of female-typical sex steroids, E_2 and P_4.

V. Reproductive Events and Seizures

It has long been acknowledged that seizures do not occur randomly, but that they can cluster. There are reports of seizure frequencies being higher every 3–6 weeks in about a third of men and women with epilepsy (Almqvist, 1955; Tauboll *et al.*, 1991). It was from observations of temporal rhythmicity in seizure patterns, which in some cases aligned with the menstrual cycle, that catamenial epilepsy was first considered. It is now generally accepted that, among women with epilepsy, reproductive events can influence seizure susceptibility. Periods of heightened hormonal variability, that is, menarche (Lennox and Lennox, 1960), premenstrual periods (Laidlaw, 1956; Newmark and Penry, 1980), pregnancy and postpartum (Knight and Rhind, 1975; Schmidt *et al.*, 1985), and peri-menopause

(Sallusto and Pozzi, 1964; Turner, 1907), increase vulnerability to seizures among some women with seizure disorder. Thus, reproductive cycles can influence seizures in part due to changes in gonadal hormones.

Natural changes in reproductive status associated with differences in gonadal hormones produce marked alterations in ictal behaviors. Findings from women with catamenial epilepsy suggest that seizure frequency is greater when E_2 levels are higher and decreased when plasma levels of P_4 are low (Backstrom, 1976; Herzog et al., 1997). In ovariectomized rats, a similar relationship is observed (Edwards et al., 1999a). Although there is ample evidence for E_2 to be proconvulsant, and P_4 to be anticonvulsant, emerging evidence suggests that each of these steroids may also exert the opposite effects, as well.

A. ESTROGEN AND SEIZURES

Over 150 years ago, the effects of estrogens on seizures were originally described (Gowers, 1881; Locock, 1857). Since then, emphasis has been placed on seizure occurrence increasing when there are natural, cyclic elevations in the E_2:P_4 ratio, such as occurs around menarche (Klein et al., 2003; Rosciszewska, 1975), the perimenstrum (Herzog et al., 1997; Laidlaw, 1956; Logothetis et al., 1959; Mattson and Cramer, 1985), or perimenopausal (Abbasi et al., 1999; Harden et al., 1999; Rosciszewska, 1978) periods. Intravenous administration of conjugated E_2 to 16 women produced seizures in 4 and epileptiform discharges in 11 of these women (Logothetis et al., 1958). The use of E_2-based contraceptives was reported to increase ictal activity (Bickerstaff, 1975; Herzog et al., 1991; Logothetis et al., 1959). Circulating E_2 levels are also unusually high among some individuals with seizure disorder (Herzog et al., 1991). Finally, treatment with an anti-estrogenic agent reduced focal paroxysmal epileptiform discharges (Sharf et al., 1969). Together, these clinical findings suggest that E_2 is proconvulsant.

Findings from animal models have supported the premise that E_2 has proconvulsant effects. The threshold to electroshock or kindling-induced ictal activity is lower during proestrus when there are high levels of circulating E_2 (Edwards et al., 1999b; Woolley and Timiras, 1962a). Systemic administration of E_2 lowers the threshold to electroshock, kindling, PTZ, kainic acid, and ethyl chloride–induced seizures (Hom and Buterbaugh, 1986; Logothetis and Harner, 1960; Nicoletti et al., 1985; Spiegel and Wycis, 1945; Woolley and Timiras, 1962a). Furthermore, central or intravenous E_2 administration to rabbits increases spontaneous electrical activity (Hardy, 1970; Logothetis and Harner, 1960; Marcus et al., 1966). Despite these findings, which indicate that E_2 has proconvulsant effects, there are other reports that suggest that E_2 can have antiseizure effects.

The regimen of E_2 seems to influence the nature of its effects on seizures. Chronic administration of E_2 that produce low physiological E_2 levels (2–10 μg to rats) increases the threshold to clonic seizures and reduces mortality from kainic acid (Hoffman *et al.*, 2003; Velíšková *et al.*, 2000). However, in another experiment, neither 2, 6, nor 20 μg E_2 decreased seizure threshold or severity, but 40 μg had proconvulsant effects (Nicoletti *et al.*, 1985; Reibel *et al.*, 2000; Stitt and Kinnard, 1968). We have shown that the nature of E_2's effects on seizures may be in part related to the capacity of physiological concentrations of E_2 to enhance the synthesis of progestins, which as will be discussed further below, are anticonvulsant (Frye and Rhodes, 2005). Thus, there is some indication that physiological E_2 levels may be anticonvulsant and supraphysiological E_2 levels may be proconvulsant.

Another factor that may influence E_2's effects on seizures is its actions on various CNS substrates. E_2 positively modulates $GABA_A$ receptor and potentiates non-NMDA glutamatergic transmission (English and Sweatt, 1997; Kim *et al.*, 2002; Silva *et al.*, 1992; Smith and McMahon, 2006). Interestingly, E_2 reduces seizures associated with $GABA_A$ or NMDA. In support, picrotoxin-, cyclosporin A-, NMDA-, or kainic acid–induced seizures are decreased by E_2 (Kalkbrenner and Standley, 2003; Schwartz-Giblin *et al.*, 1989; Tominaga *et al.*, 2001; Velíšková *et al.*, 2000). In contrast, seizure activity produced by chemoconvulsants that activate the cholinergic system, such as pilocarpine or flurothyl, are not altered by E_2 (Galanopoulou *et al.*, 2003b; Velíšek *et al.*, 1999). E_2 administration to female rats can downregulate serotonin receptor, 5HT1A, in the limbic system (Osterlund and Hurd, 1998) and upregulate 5HT2A receptors in the cortex (Moses-Kolko *et al.*, 2003; Summer and Fink, 1995), substrates that in the bed nucleus of the stria terminalis mediate opposing effects on seizures (Levita *et al.*, 2004). Thus, the diversity of actions and substrates for E_2 need to be further explored in order to fully understand E_2's role in mediating seizures.

B. PROGESTERONE AND SEIZURES

The antiseizure properties of P were described by Selye in 1941 over 60 years ago (Selye, 1941). Since then, it has been well documented that elevations in endogenous or exogenous P_4 can increase the threshold and decrease the magnitude of seizure activity in animal models (Hom and Buterbaugh, 1986; Nicoletti *et al.*, 1985; Spiegel and Wycis, 1945; Wilson, 1992). Indeed, concentrations of P_4 over reproductive cycles, such as the estrous cycle, pregnancy, and postpartum, are inversely related to seizure activity (Frye and Bayon, 1998b, 1999c). Removal of the primary endogenous source of P_4, the ovaries, increases seizures and reinstatement of P_4 (4.0 mg/kg SC) produces the opposite effects to reduce kainic acid, PTZ, and perforant pathway-induced seizures in ovx rats (Frye and Bayon, 1998a, 1999;

Frye *et al.*, 1998). Furthermore, direct administration of P_4 to the brain has anti-seizure effects. In cats, application of P_4 to the cortex inhibited electrical discharges from a penicillin focus (Landgren *et al.*, 1978). In rats, application of P_4 to the hippocampus reduces PTZ-induced seizures (Rhodes and Frye, 2004b). Thus, in animal models, P_4 has clear, well-demonstrated anticonvulsant effects.

Evidence that P_4 has antiseizure effects also comes in part from examination of the effects on catamenial exacerbation of seizures. Among women with cata-menial epilepsy, seizures are typically less frequent during the mid-luteal phase when P_4 levels are highest (Mattson and Cramer, 1985; Mattson *et al.*, 1981); however, there are three distinct patterns of catamenial epilepsy (Herzog *et al.*, 2004b, 1997). First, among women with normal ovulatory cycles, some experi-ence increases in seizure frequency during the perimenstrual phase which has been attributed to the withdrawal of P_4 (Laidlaw, 1956). Second, other women with normal ovulatory cycles have increases in seizure frequency during the preovulatory phase, which may be due to the surge of E_2 which is unopposed by P_4 until ovulation occurs (Backstrom, 1976). Third, among women with inadequate luteal phase cycles, seizure frequency can be increased during the midfollicular phase compared with the other phases, which may be due in part to less than normal P_4 secretion during the second half of the cycle, irrespective of ovulation (Herzog *et al.*, 1997). Thus, there is heterogeneity in the manner in which catamenial epilepsy is expressed.

Intravenous administration of P_4 benefits some women with catamenial epilepsy to reduce spontaneous epileptiform discharges. In support, of seven women with partial seizures that were infused intravenously with P_4, and had serum P_4 levels increased to that typically seen during the luteal phase, four experienced decreases in interictal spikes in their EEG (Backstrom *et al.*, 1984). Notably, the latency of intravenously administered P_4 to decrease epileptic dis-charge frequency was ~1–2 h. One explanation that was provided for this time-frame was that P_4's antiseizure effects may be mediated in part through actions of its metabolites, which have depressant effects in the CNS.

Oral administration of natural P_4 can enhance seizure control of some women with catamenial epilepsy. In a study of eight women with inadequate luteal phase cycles, six women experienced improved control over the catamenial exacerba-tion of intractable complex partial seizures with P_4 lozenges (Herzog, 1986, 1995). Similarly, micronized P_4 therapy reduced catamenial seizures among 19 of 25 women with complex partial or secondary generalized seizures (Herzog, 1995). Two explanations for the beneficial effects of P_4 therapy have been provided. First, steroid hormones and AEDs are both metabolized by hepatic enzymes. P_4 therapy may represent an increase in the substrate for these liver enzymes, which then reduces the degradation of AEDs, which thereby enhances their therapeutic efficacy. Second, as alluded to above, depressant actions in the CNS of P_4's metabolites may underlie the anticonvulsant effects of P_4. Indeed, oral synthetic progestins, which do not readily metabolize to antidepressant progestins, have not demonstrated antiseizure effects in clinical investigations, whereas those that can be metabolized do (Hall, 1977). Thus, metabolism of P_4 may be important for some of its anticonvulsant effects.

C. Progesterone Metabolites and Seizures

Although P_4 is a precursor to many neuroactive steroids, recent investigations of metabolites of P_4 have revealed that the anticonvulsant actions of P_4 are due, at least in part, to its metabolite 3α-hydroxy-5α-pregnan-20-one (3α,5α-THP). P_4 is metabolized by actions of the 5α-reductase isoenzymes to form 5α-dihydropro-gesterone (DHP) which is then metabolized by 3α-HSD into 3α,5α-THP. In 1941, Selye reported that 3α,5α-THP had anticonvulsant effects and this has been verified in many other laboratories since then (Belelli *et al.*, 1989; Concas *et al.*, 1996). Male rats treated with 3α,5α-THP (2.5 mg/kg) prior to perforant pathway stimulation show a reduction in tonic–clonic and partial seizure activity (Frye, 1995). Although P_4 and 3α,5α-THP (4.0 mg/kg SC) similarly reduce kainic acid or perforant pathway-induced seizures in ovx rats (Frye and Scalise, 2000), P_4's anticonvulsant effects have a longer latency and correspond with increases in 3α,5α-THP levels. Over the estrous cycle and pregnancy, the threshold for chemoconvulsant-induced seizures is more directly correlated with 3α,5α-THP than P_4 levels (Frye and Bayon, 1998a). Inhibition of P_4's metabolism to 3α,5α-THP by administration of 5α-reductase inhibitors, such as finasteride, or a genetic deficiency in the 5α-reductase type I enzyme, attenuates P_4's anticonvulsant effects (Frye *et al.*, 2002; Kokate *et al.*, 1999). Together these data suggest that the 5α-reduced metabolites of P_4 are at least partially responsible for P_4's anticon-vulsant effects.

In our laboratory, we have been investigating for some time the role of progestins in mediating ictal activity in various animal models. We have done so by determining effects on seizure threshold of administration of chemoconvul-sants (in this case PTZ; 70 mg/kg) and manipulating and/or measuring levels of P_4 and 3α,5α-THP. Rats that have low P_4 and 3α,5α-THP levels due to endoge-nous variations (diestrous phase of estrous cycle) or extirpation of the ovaries experience more seizures when administered PTZ than do rats with high P_4 and 3α,5α-THP levels due to endogenous variations (proestrous phase of estrous cycle; Table II) or systemic (Table III) or intrahippocampal (Table IV) P_4 or 3α,5α-THP administration to ovariectomized rats. Given the longer latencies and fewer number of seizures coincide with elevations in 3α,5α-THP, irrespective of P_4 levels, in the hippocampus, these findings suggest that P_4's antiseizure effects are related to the capacity to form 3α,5α-THP in the hippocampus. Notably, blocking P_4's conversion to 3α,5α-THP in the hippocampus by administering a

TABLE II

Latencies to (Top), and Number of (Top Middle), Tonic Seizures of ovx Control (Left Column; $N = 10$), Diestrous (Middle Column; $N = 10$), or Proestrous Rats (Right Column; $N = 10$)

	Ovx control	Diestrous	Proestrous
Seizure behavior after PTZ			
Latency to tonic seizures (s)	82 + 12	194 + 27	330 + 70
# of Tonic seizures	2 + 1	2 + 1	1 + 1
Endocrine measures			
Hippocampal P_4 levels (ng/g)	2 + 1	2 + 1	10 + 2
Hippocampal 3α,5α-THP levels (ng/g)	2 + 1	2 + 1	12 + 2

Hippocampal P_4 (bottom middle) and 3α,5α-THP (bottom) of ovx control (left column; $n = 5$), diestrous (middle column; $n = 4$), or proestrous rats (right column; $n = 7$).

TABLE III

Latencies to (Top), and Number of (Top Middle), Tonic Seizures of ovx Control Administered SC Vehicle (ovx Control, Left Column; $N = 10$), Progesterone (P4) (SC P, Middle Column; $N = 10$), or 3α,5α-THP (SC 3α,5α-THP, Right Column; $N = 10$)

	Ovx control	SC P_4	SC 3α,5α-THP
Seizure behavior after PTZ			
Latency to tonic seizures (s)	160 + 80	398 + 94	435 + 87
# of tonic seizures	2 + 1	1 + 1	1 + 1
Endocrine measures			
Hippocampal P_4 levels (ng/g)	2 + 1	9 + 2	2 + 2
Hippocampal 3α,5α-THP levels (ng/g)	2 + 1	8 + 2	8 + 2

Hippocampal P_4 (bottom middle) and 3α,5α-THP (bottom) of ovx control (left column; $n = 6$), P_4 (middle column; $n = 9$), or 3α,5α-THP-administered rats (right column; $n = 4$).

TABLE IV

Latencies to (Top), and Number of (Top Middle), Tonic Seizures of ovx Control Administered Intrahippocampal Cholesterol (ovx Control, Left Column; $N = 10$), Progesterone (Hippocampal P_4, Middle Column; $N = 10$), or 3α,5α-THP (Hippocampal 3α,5α-THP, Right Column; $N = 10$)

	Cholesterol control	Hippocampal P_4	Hippocampal 3α, 5α-THP
Seizure behavior after PTZ			
Latency to tonic seizures (s)	90 + 12	185 + 37	512 + 45
# of tonic seizures	3 + 1	1 + 1	0 + 0
Endocrine measures			
Hippocampal P_4 levels (ng/g)	2 + 1	8 + 2	2 + 2
Hippocampal 3α,5α-THP levels (ng/g)	2 + 1	5 + 2	9 + 2

Hippocampal P (bottom middle) and 3α,5α-THP (bottom) of cholesterol control (left column; $n = 5$), hippocampal P (middle column; $n = 6$), or hippocampal 3α,5α-THP-administered rats (right column; $n = 2$).

5α-reductase inhibitor finasteride obviates the antiseizure effects of P_4 (Table V), which indicates that formation of 3α,5α-THP is essential for P's anticonvulsive effects.

D. Biosynthesis/Metabolism of 3α, 5α-THP

The CNS acts both as a target and a source of sex steroids and of their metabolites. Sex steroids produced by the gonads have profound organizational and activational effects on the developing and adult nervous systems, respectively. Furthermore, some steroids, called neurosteroids in reference to their site of formation—the CNS, are synthesized within the brain and peripheral nerves and can produce some of their functional effects through paracrine actions at local targets (Baulieu, 1997). Neuroactive steroids are those steroids that produce their functional effects through actions in the CNS subsequent to production within or outside of the CNS (Paul and Purdy, 1992). Neuro(active) steroids can mediate many diverse neuroendocrine functions, including release of GnRH

TABLE V

Latencies to (Top), and Number of (Top Middle), Tonic Seizures of ovx Control Administered Intrahippocampal Cholesterol (ovx Control, Left Column; $N = 10$), SC Progesterone (SC P_4, Left Middle Column; $N = 10$), SC P_4 and Intrahippocampal Finasteride (SC P_4 and Intrahippocampal Finasteride, Middle Right Column; $N = 10$), or Intrahippocampal Finasteride ($N = 10$; Right Column)

Seizures after PTZ	Ovx control	SC P_4	SC P_4 and intrahippocampal finasteride	Intrahippocampal finasteride
Seizure behavior after PTZ				
Latency to tonic seizures (s)	105 + 22	403 + 62	98 + 15	125 + 17
# Tonic seizures	3 + 1	1 + 1	3 + 3	2 + 2
Endocrine measures				
Hippocampal P_4 levels (ng/g)	2 + 1	11 + 2	12 + 3	2+ 2
Hippocampal 3α,5α-THP levels (ng/g)	2 + 2	10 + 2	3 + 2	2 + 2

Hippocampal P_4 (bottom middle) and 3α,5α-THP (bottom) of intrahippocampal cholesterol (ovx control, left column; $n = 2$), SC P_4 (SC P, left middle column; $n = 2$), SC P_4 and intrahippocampal finasteride (SC P_4 and Intrahippocampal finasteride, middle right column; $n = 2$), or intrahippocampal finasteride ($n = 2$; right column).

(el-Etr *et al.*, 1995; Vincens *et al.*, 1994), LH, and FSH (Brann *et al.*, 1990), and ovulation inhibition (Genazzani *et al.*, 1995). Neuro(active) steroids also influence female sexual behavior (Frye *et al.*, 1996b; McCarthy *et al.*, 1995; reviewed in Frye, 2001; reviewed in Frye *et al.*, 2006a; Frye and Rhodes, 2006a) and mitigate stress responses (Purdy *et al.*, 1991). Our lab has been focused on characterizing the functional effects of neuro(active) steroids and, in particular, their role in mediating seizure processes and associated functions. Described below are the route of biosynthesis of neuro(active) steroids.

Neurosteroids are produced by *de novo* steroidogenesis from cholesterol in the brain (Baulieu, 1997; Baulieu and Robel, 1990; the pathway for neurosteroidogenesis is shown in Fig. 1). In support, neurosteroids accumulate in the brains of animals that are castrated and/or adrenalectomized and therefore lack peripheral glands as a source of steroid secretion (Corpechot *et al.*, 1981; Robel *et al.*, 1987). Neurosteroidogenesis involves cholesterol's conversion to pregnenolone by the cytochrome P450 side-chain cleavage enzyme (*P450scc:CYP11A1*), which is the first and rate-limiting enzyme in steroid biosynthesis (Hu *et al.*, 2004). The gene for *CYP11A1* is expressed in the CNS of rats during neonatal development (Ukena *et al.*, 1998). The 3β-HSD steroidogenic enzyme catalyzes the dehydrogenation and isomerization of pregnenolone into P$_4$ (Payne and Hales, 2004). *3βHSD* messenger RNA and enzymatic activity expression have been reported in the CNS of several vertebrates (Sanne and Krueger, 1995; Ukena *et al.*, 1999a). The expression of *3βHSD* increases during the neonatal period in rats, indicating an increase of P$_4$ formation during neonatal life (Ukena *et al.*, 1999b). In addition to production of P$_4$ in the brain by these enzymes, there are other enzymes in the brain that convert P$_4$ (irrespective of its source being *de novo* or peripheral) to 3α,5α-THP.

P$_4$ is converted to DHP by actions of the steroid 5α-reductase enzymes, which is the rate-limiting enzyme of its conversion to 3α,5α-THP. The 5α-reductase enzyme is expressed as two isozymes, 5α-reductase 1 and 5α-reductase 2, which are both present in different brain regions, including cerebral cortex (Sanchez *et al.*, 2005, 2006; Torres and Ortega, 2003a, 2006). The type 1 isoform, which is constitutively expressed in the rodent CNS at all stages of brain development (Melcangi *et al.*, 1998), may play a role in protecting neurons from excessive glucocorticoids that may induce apoptosis (Mahendroo *et al.*, 1997; Poletti *et al.*, 1998). DHP is then converted by the 3α-hydrosteroid dehydrogenase enzymes to form 3α,5α-THP. Notably, the conversion of DHP to 3α,5α-THP is dynamic and labile, such that 3α,5α-THP can oxidize to form DHP, which can subsequently be reduced back to 3α,5α-THP. 3α,5α-THP is synthesized in brain, ovaries, testes, and adrenals from P$_4$ by steroidogenic enzymes 5α-reductase and 3α-HSD, with the former being the rate-limiting enzyme of the reaction (Bernardi *et al.*, 1998; Corpéchot *et al.*, 1993; Genazzani *et al.*, 2000, 2002; Marx *et al.*, 2003). Given the

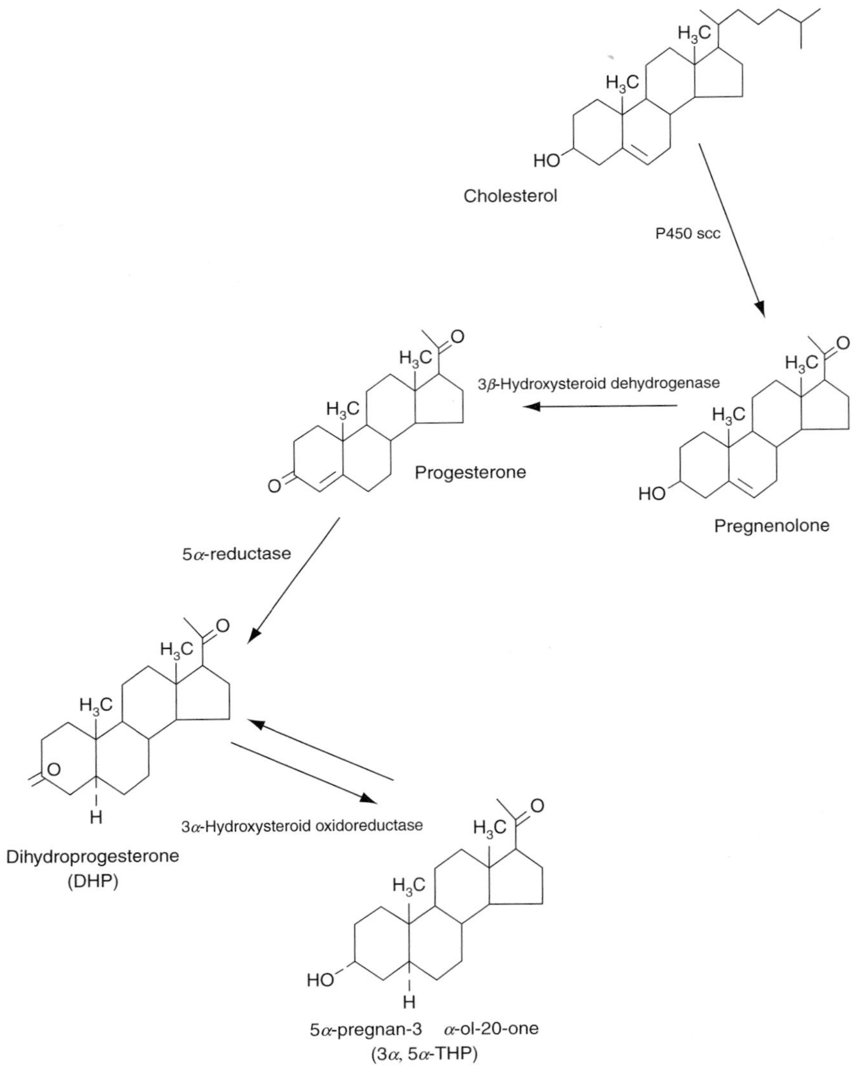

FIG. 1. Illustration of the pathway through which progestogen biosynthesis and metabolism occurs. Cholesterol produced *de novo* can be converted by P450 Side Chain Cleavage (P450$_{SCC}$) enzymes to form pregnenolone, which is subsequently metabolized by 3β-hydroxysteroid dehydrogenase to progesterone. Progesterone produced *de novo* in the brain, or from peripheral sources, can then metabolized to dihydroprogesterone (DHP) and 5α-pregnan-3α-ol-20-one (3α,5α-THP), by actions of 5α-reductase and 3α-hydroxysteroid oxidoreductase, respectively.

profound impact of 3α,5α-THP on ictal processes, normative variations in levels of 3α,5α-THP over reproductive cycles are discussed below.

E. Variations in 3α, 5α-THP

Although 3α,5α-THP is synthesized *de novo* in the CNS from cholesterol, plasma 3α,5α-THP in women predominantly originates from the corpus luteum (Ottander *et al.*, 2005). Over the menstrual cycle, circulating levels of 3α,5α-THP covary with P_4. During the luteal phase, 3α,5α-THP is higher (4 nmol/L; Wang *et al.*, 2001) than in the follicular phase (<1 nmol/L; Bicikova *et al.*, 1995; Genazzani *et al.*, 1998; Mellon, 1994; Purdy *et al.*, 1990; Wang *et al.*, 2001). During pregnancy, P_4 and 3α,5α-THP rise throughout gestation and peak in the third trimester, with plasma levels of 3α,5α-THP between 50 and 100 nmol/L (Hill *et al.*, 2001; Luisi *et al.*, 2000). Within 1 h of delivery, maternal serum 3α,5α-THP decreases significantly (Hill *et al.*, 2001). Concentrations of P_4 and 3α,5α-THP also vary in the brain (Bixo *et al.*, 1995; Purdy *et al.*, 1991). A postmortem study showed that women in the luteal phase had significantly higher brain concentrations of 3α,5α-THP than did postmenopausal controls (Bixo *et al.*, 1997). There were regional differences with 3α,5α-THP levels being highest 14–21 ng/g, in the substantia nigra and basal hypothalamus (Bixo *et al.*, 1997). Indeed, an important question is whether some of these natural fluctuations in 3α,5α-THP may underlie cyclic differences in seizure processes.

There has begun to be some investigations that suggest changes in 3α,5α-THP with menopause may contribute to seizure (dys)control. After ovulation, the corpus luteum produces P_4. The number of anovulatory cycles increases with aging. In the six years before menopause, about 10% of cycles are characterized by ovulation whereas, in younger women, about 60% of cycles are characterized by ovulation (Rannevik *et al.*, 1995). Although postmenopausal women have significantly lower serum concentrations of P_4 (typically less than 2 nmol/L) than do their younger counterparts, 3α,5α-THP levels are not different between postmenopausal women and younger women during the follicular phase (Genazzani *et al.*, 1998). The ratio of 3α,5α-THP to P_4 is reduced among postmenopausal women than in their younger counterparts (de Wit *et al.*, 2001). During menopause, dysregulation in the levels of 3α,5α-THP and other neurosteroids (Pearlstein, 1995) has been associated with depression and other mood disorders (Girdler *et al.*, 2001). These findings, together with the notion that adrenal activity increases with aging, suggest that adrenal, rather than ovarian P_4, may be the major source of circulating 3α,5α-THP among postmenopausal women.

Although fluctuations in plasma and brain concentrations of neuroactive steroids induced by physiological, pharmacological, or pathological conditions may result in alterations in seizure threshold (Biggio *et al.*, 2001; Concas *et al.*, 1999), it is a challenge to parcel out the relative contributions of these endocrine glands in people. Thus, findings from animal models and basic research has been particularly informative in delineating the role of neuron(active) steroids in seizure processes.

F. Effects of Postmenopausal Hormone Therapy

In addition to normal endogenous differences in steroids associated with reproductive status having an influence on seizure susceptibility, hormone therapies associated with reproductive senescence may also influence seizure susceptibility in part due to effects of $3\alpha,5\alpha$-THP. E_2 and conjugated equine estrogen (CEE) are used by some postmenopausal women to manage physical (vasomotor symptoms, atrophic vaginitis) (Campbell and Whitehead, 1977; MacLennan et al., 2001; Wiklund et al., 1993) and mental (Ditkoff et al., 1991; Sherwin, 1988; Sherwin and Gelfand, 1989) climacteric symptoms. The nature of the E_2 regimen can influence the production of $3\alpha,5\alpha$-THP. For example, levels of $3\alpha,5\alpha$-THP in plasma increase more with transdermal versus oral E_2 therapy (Bernardi et al., 2003). This is likely due to the very high levels of the 5α-reductase enzyme that are present in skin (reviewed in Andersson, 2001; Hoppe et al., 2006) and the enhancing effects of E_2 on the activity of this enzyme (Cheng and Karavolas, 1973; Malendowicz, 1976; Resko et al., 1986; Vongher and Frye, 1999). Although E_2 can influence $3\alpha,5\alpha$-THP production, and thereby alter seizures status, E_2 therapy is typically combined with progestins for women with an intact uterus to limit the risk of endometrial hyperplasia and/or carcinoma (Voigt et al., 1991; Whitehead, 1978).

When progestin therapy is combined with E_2, there are even more dramatic effects on $3\alpha,5\alpha$-THP levels. As expected, when natural P_4 was administered transvaginally after E_2, $3\alpha,5\alpha$-THP concentrations are further increased (Andréen et al., 2005; Wihlbäck et al., 2005). Sequential replacement of E_2 and progestins, to mimic the normal menstrual cycle, can result in increases in progestins followed by withdrawal (Andréen et al., 2003; Björn et al., 2000). However, the nature of the beneficial effects of reinstatement and adverse effects of withdrawal are influenced by the progestin regimen utilized. In general, replacement with natural P_4 seems to have the most favorable effect on seizures. Use of P_4 suppositories and lozenges decreases seizure frequency by 68% and 55%, respectively (Herzog, 1986, 1995). In contrast, replacement with medroxyprogesterone acetate (MPA, aka Provera) had either no effect or reduces seizure frequency by 30% (Herzog, 1999; Mattson et al., 1984). Notably, MPA has only modest effect to increase $3\alpha,5\alpha$-THP and may decrease conversion of P_4 to $3\alpha,5\alpha$-THP (Belelli and Herd, 2003).

We have directly compared the antiseizure effects of P_4, DHP, $3\alpha,5\alpha$-THP and MPA and analyzed whether formation of $3\alpha,5\alpha$-THP is involved in these effects. Ovx adult rats were administered P_4, $3\alpha,5\alpha$-THP, MPA, or vehicle prior to a subthreshold regimen of kainic acid (7 mg/kg b.w.), which did not produce seizures but did result in excitotoxic cell death in the hilus of the hippocampus. P_4, DHP, or $3\alpha,5\alpha$-THP prevented kainic acid–induced neuronal loss and increased the levels of DHP and $3\alpha,5\alpha$-THP in plasma and hippocampus. In contrast, MPA neither prevented kainic acid–induced neuronal loss nor increased DHP and $3\alpha,5\alpha$-THP levels. The administration of the 5α-reductase inhibitor finasteride prevented the increase in the levels of DHP and $3\alpha,5\alpha$-THP in plasma and hippocampus as a result of P_4 administration and abolished the neuroprotective effect of P_4. Administration of indomethacin, a 3α-HSD inhibitor, blocked the neuroprotective effect of both DHP and $3\alpha,5\alpha$-THP, suggesting that both metabolites are necessary for the neuroprotective effects of P_4. These findings suggest that P_4 is neuroprotective against kainic acid excitotoxicity but MPA is not, and that P_4's metabolism to DHP and/or $3\alpha,5\alpha$-THP is necessary for the neuroprotective effects of progestins.

VI. Mechanisms of 3α, 5α-THP Through GABA Receptors

The GABA transmitter system is the major inhibitory system in the mammalian CNS (Rang *et al.*, 1995). Central GABAergic transmission plays a key role in controlling neuronal excitability and in regulating reactivity to rapid changes in environmental conditions that may lead to neuronal excitation (Barbaccia *et al.*, 2001). $3\alpha,5\alpha$-THP is among the most potent known ligands of $GABA_A$/benzodiazepine receptor complex (GBRs) in the CNS. $3\alpha,5\alpha$-THP enhances muscimol and flunitrazepam binding and inhibits *t*-butyl bicyclophosphorothionate binding in rat brain membranes, and also enhances muscimol-stimulated chloride flux in intact neurons (Turner *et al.*, 1989). Furthermore, in electrophysiological studies, $3\alpha,5\alpha$-THP potentiates GBR chloride currents (Hawkinson *et al.*, 1994; Park-Chung *et al.*, 1999; Peters *et al.*, 1988; Turner and Simmonds, 1989; Twyman and Macdonald, 1992).

GBRs are composed of five subunits and contain binding sites for GABA and clinically important drugs such as benzodiazepines, barbiturates, (neuro)steroids, most anesthetic agents, ethanol, and anticonvulsants. $3\alpha,5\alpha$-THP's effects to potentiate GBR activity are believed to underlie its anticonvulsant action (Belelli *et al.*, 1989; Paul *et al.*, 1992). Benzodiazepines and their congeners, which act as positive allosteric modulators of GBRs, have antiseizure effects in people and may participate in the mitigation of neuronal excitability. $3\alpha,5\alpha$-THP regulates GBRs in a manner similar to barbiturates (Majewska, 1992; Paul and Purdy, 1992) and may, therefore, participate in the regulation of neuronal excitability. These drugs modulate the GABA-induced chloride ion flux by interacting with separate and distinct allosteric binding sites (Sieghart, 1995). Although the binding site(s) for 3α,5α-THP on GBRs differs from those of benzodiazepines, barbiturates, and picrotoxin (Gee *et al.*, 1995; Lan *et al.*, 1991), 3α,5α-THP has agonist-like effects at GBRs that are similar to that of sedative hypnotic drugs, such as benzodiazepines and barbiturates (Majewska, 1992; Paul and Purdy, 1992). 3α,5α-THP facilitates GABA-mediated responses by increasing both chloride channel opening time and frequency (Brussaard *et al.*, 1999; Kokate *et al.*, 1994; Martin and Dunn, 2002; Reddy and Rogawski, 2002).

Several studies have indicated that there are chronic effects of neuroactive steroids to modulate GBRs. Pregnancy or long-term treatment with P_4 can upregulate the density of GBRs and increases affinity for GABA and benzodiazepines in a region-specific manner (Canonaco *et al.*, 1989; Concas *et al.*, 1999; Gavish *et al.*, 1987). There are also reports of downregulation of GABA's ability to stimulate $^{36}Cl^-$ uptake and reductions in the efficacy of benzodiazepines and/or neurosteroids (Costa *et al.*, 1995; Yu and Ticku, 1995). These and other findings that suggest that sensitivity to neuroactive steroids may change with reproductive status (Sundström *et al.*, 1997, 1998).

Chronic exposure to neuroactive steroids may also have direct effects on GBR function, in part through changes in subunit composition. GBR function depends upon the combination of 18 subunits (α 1–6, β 1–4, δ, ε, γ 1–3, π, and ρ 1–2) (Hedblom and Kirkness, 1997; Hevers and Luddens, 1998; Mehta and Ticku, 1999). 3α,5α-THP selectively interacts with γ2 $GABA_A$ receptor subunit. Increasing amounts of circulating 3α,5α-THP, during pregnancy, induce a decrease of γ2L subunit mRNA in the cerebral cortex and in the hippocampus, which return to control values around delivery, when 3α,5α-THP levels decrease (Concas *et al.*, 1999). Additionally, chronic P_4 treatment downregulates the expression of γ2L and γ subunit mRNAs, in cultures of mammalian cerebellar granule cells (Follesa *et al.*, 2000). Conversely, persistent reduction in the brain concentrations of 3α,5α-THP in rats is associated with increased abundance of GBR γ2L and γ2S subunit mRNAs in cerebral cortex (Follesa *et al.*, 2002). Although these findings suggest that plasticity in GBRs with reproductive status and/or hormone exposure may contribute to changes in ictal activity, this relationship requires further investigation.

We have investigated whether anticonvulsive effects of 3α,5α-THP require actions at GBRs and/or NMDA receptors (see Fig. 2). This was done by administering P_4 to ovariectomized rats alone or in conjunction with systemic administration of, or intrahippocampal infusions of, bicuculline, a $GABA_A$ receptor antagonist, prior to PTZ administration. As Table VI, shows the antiseizure effects of progestins are attenuated by blocking their ability to act at $GABA_A$ receptors. Notably, actions at $GABA_A$ receptors are unlikely the only substrates as blocking NMDA receptors systemically or in the hippocampus with MK-801 also attenuate the anticonvulsive effects of progestins (Table VII).

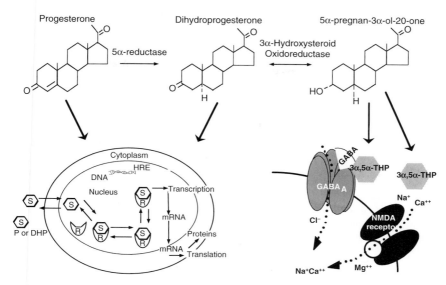

FIG. 2. Progesterone (P) and its 5-reduced metabolite, dihydroprogesterone (DHP), bind with high affinity to cognate, intracellular progestin receptors. However, the product of P and DHP, 5α-pregnan-3α-ol-20-one (3α,5α-THP), is devoid of activity at intracellular progestin receptors in physiological concentrations. 3α,5α-THP does effectively modulate function of GABAA and glutamate receptors (as well as other neurotransmitter receptors).

TABLE VI

Top Reflects Latencies to (Top), and Number of (Top Middle), Tonic Seizures of ovx Rats Administered SC Vehicle (Left Column; $N = 10$), SC P_4 and Saline (SC P_4, Left Middle Column; $N = 10$), SC P_4 + Bicuculline (Middle Right; $N = 10$), or SC Bicuculline (Right Column; $N = 10$)

Seizures after PTZ	Ovx control and vehicle	SC P_4 and vehicle	SC P_4 and bicuculline	Bicuculline
SC vehicle or biculline and seizure behavior after PTZ				
Latency to tonic seizures (s)	$185 + 25$	$455 + 37$	$173 + 25$	$178 + 20$
# Tonic seizures	$3 + 1$	$1 + 1$	$2 + 2$	$2 + 2$
Hippocampal vehicle or biculline and seizure behavior after PTZ				
Latency to tonic seizures (s)	$211 + 12$	$425 + 57$	$188 + 32$	$192 + 17$
# Tonic seizures	$3 + 1$	$1 + 1$	$3 + 3$	$3 + 3$

Bottom depicts latencies to (top), and number of (top middle), tonic seizures of ovx rats administered intrahippocampal vehicle (left column; $n = 10$), SC P_4 and intrahippocampal saline (left middle column; $n = 10$), SC P_4 + intrahippocampal bicuculline (middle right; $n = 10$), or intrahippocampal bicuculline (right column; $n = 10$).

TABLE VII

Top Reflects Latencies to (Top), and Number of (Top Middle), Tonic Seizures of ovx Rats Administered SC Vehicle (Left Column; $N = 10$), SC P_4 and Saline (SC P_4, Left Middle Column; $N = 10$), SC P_4 + MK-801 (Middle Right; $N = 10$), or SC MK-801 (Right Column; $N = 10$)

Seizures after PTZ	Ovx control and vehicle	SC P_4 and vehicle	SC P_4 and MK-801	MK-801
SC vehicle or MK-801 and seizure behavior after PTZ				
Latency to tonic seizures (s)	$198 + 32$	$488 + 59$	$140 + 44$	$194 + 42$
# Tonic seizures	$3 + 1$	$1 + 1$	$3 + 2$	$3 + 2$
Hippocampal vehicle or MK-801 and seizure behavior after PTZ				
Latency to tonic seizures (s)	$188 + 21$	$469 + 59$	$201 + 48$	$188 + 12$
# Tonic seizures	$3 + 1$	$1 + 1$	$3 + 3$	$3+ 3$

Bottom depicts latencies to (top), and number of (top middle), tonic seizures of ovx rats administered intrahippocampal vehicle (left column; $n = 10$), SC P_4 and intrahippocampal saline (left middle column; $n = 10$), SC P_4 + intrahippocampal MK-801 (middle right; $n = 10$), or intrahippocampal MK-801 (right column; $n = 10$).

VII. Acute Stress-Induced Steroid Biosynthesis and Seizures

Changes in progestins are not only associated with reproductive status but are also produced by stress. Exposure to stressors can induce a broad range of behavioral and physiological responses, including changes in hypothalamic–pituitary–adrenal (HPA) axis function (Mormède et al., 2002), the primary mediator of neuroendocrine stress responses (Selye, 1936). For example, stress leads to increases in P_4 secretion among adult intact and castrated male rats, which implies a role of the adrenal gland in the P_4 response to stress (Andersen et al., 2004, 2005; Persengiev et al., 1991; Schaeffer and Aron, 1987). In the adrenal cortex, progestin biosynthesis is increased by adrenocorticotropic hormone (ACTH) via cAMP-induced stimulation of steroidogenesis (Besman et al., 1989; Torres et al., 2001). Because diazepam binding inhibitor, an endogenous ligand to central and peripheral benzodiazepine receptors, has been implicated in the regulation of adrenal steroidogenesis and it is expressed in the brain, it was proposed that stress increases $3\alpha,5\alpha$-THP levels in both the adrenal gland and brain (Krueger and Papadopoulos, 1990; Mukhin et al., 1989; Purdy et al., 1991). The first report of acute stress altering neurosteroidogenesis involved forced swimming and showed that this produced time-dependent increases in P_4 and $3\alpha,5\alpha$-THP in brain and plasma of rats (Purdy et al., 1991). There has subsequently been many reports of changes in plasma and brain neurosteroids and levels of 5α-reductase isoenzymes in rodents under different acute and chronic stress situations (Barbaccia et al., 2001; Biggio et al., 1996, 2000).

These findings are relevant for people. For example, acute stressors, such as alcohol exposure, increase plasma levels of $3\alpha,5\alpha$-THP among adolescent boys and girls (Torres and Ortega, 2003b, 2004). These stress-induced increases in $3\alpha,5\alpha$-THP and other neurosteroids, such as 3α-diol, may serve to dampen stress-induced HPA function (Erskine and Kornberg, 1992; Patchev et al., 1996) and produce agonist-like actions at $GABA_A$ receptors (Frye et al., 1996a,b; Gee, 1988; reviewed in Frye et al., 2006a). Indeed, various acute stress situations (carbon dioxide exposure, forced swimming, exposure to a new environment) produce a rapid and reversible downregulation of $GABA_A$ receptor function (Andrews et al., 1992; Biggio, 1983; Biggio et al., 1980, 1981; Concas et al., 1987; Drugan et al., 1989; File et al., 1993; Medina et al., 1983; Serra et al., 1991). Thus, stress may alter seizure susceptibility, perhaps in part due to altering secretion of $3\alpha,5\alpha$-THP, and/or other neurosteroids.

We examined whether progestins' antiseizure effects requires HPA feedback. We have investigated effects of progestins to mediate seizures of sham or adrenalectomized (ADX) rats. Female Long-Evans rats were ovx, ADX, or sham-ADX and one-week later were administered P_4, RU5020, or $3\alpha,5\alpha$-THP (4 mg/kg, SC) 3 h prior to PTZ (70 mg/kg, IP)-induced seizures. P_4 and $3\alpha,5\alpha$-THP can bind to glucocorticoid and mineralicorticoid receptors (Ing, 2005); however, RU5020, does not bind well to glucocorticoid receptors (Zhang et al., 2005). P_4, RU5020, or $3\alpha,5\alpha$-THP significantly reduced the number of tonic seizures of sham, but not ADX rats, compared to vehicle administration. We also examined whether replacement of corticosterone, the stress hormone which is produced by the adrenals, could reinstate progestins' antiseizure effects in ADX rats. ADX rats had access to corticosterone (25 mg/ml) or vehicle in their drinking water for 4 days prior to administration of P_4, RU5020, $3\alpha,5\alpha$-THP, or vehicle, as above. The number of PTZ-induced seizures was modestly reduced by corticosterone-replacement among rats administered P_4 or RU5020, but not those administered $3\alpha,5\alpha$-THP or vehicle. Plasma corticosterone levels were higher in sham ADX rats administered vehicle; whereas progestin-administered rats showed basal levels of corticosterone, irrespective of ADX condition. Levels of $3\alpha,5\alpha$-THP in the hippocampus were increased in P_4- and $3\alpha,5\alpha$-THP-administered, rats, but not RU5020- or vehicle-administered, rats, irrespective of ADX condition. Together, these data suggest that progestins' modulation of seizure activity may involve effects on the HPA axis. However, given that $3\alpha,5\alpha$-THP is modified in the brain after stress (Purdy et al., 1991; Torres and Ortega, 2003a), and seizures represent a profound stressor, it is also likely that $3\alpha,5\alpha$-THP levels are modified by seizures. See Table VIII.

Findings from our laboratory suggest that seizures may alter steroid secretion. To date, we have primarily investigated this in male rats and focused on differences in androgens. For example, PTZ-induced seizures increase T levels, have no effect on DHT, and decrease 3α-diol levels, in the hippocampus of intact

TABLE VIII

Mean Number of Tonic Seizures Following Pentylenetetrazol (PTZ; 70 mg/kg IP) When Administered to Ovariectomized Rats Administered Vehicle, Progesterone (P_4; 4 mg/kg), 3α,5α-THP (4 mg/kg) or RU5020 ($N = 10$ grp) with Intact Adrenals (Top Panel), Adrenals Removed (Middle Panel) or Adrenals Removed and Corticosterone Replaced (Bottom Panel)

Seizures after PTZ	Vehicle	P_4	3α,5α-THP	RU5020
Ovx/sham ADX # Tonic seizures	2	1	1	1
Ovx/complete ADX # Tonic seizures	3	2	2	2
Ovx/ADX/corticosterone replacement # Tonic seizures	2	1	1	1

(but not GDX) middle-aged Long Evans rats compared to that of their counterparts that were administered vehicle (reviewed in Rhodes and Frye, 2004a). Administration of kainic acid reduces the expression in the hippocampus of 5α-reductase, the enzyme necessary for T's metabolism to DHT, which is then converted to 3α-diol. Together these findings suggest that seizures may reduce 3α-diol secretion in the hippocampus either due to cell loss in this region and/or by decreasing 5α-reductase enzyme activity. Either the former or latter scenario would also be expected to alter 3α,5α-THP in the hippocampus. Furthermore, the differences observed between intact and GDX rats imply that changes in steroids associated with seizures may be linked to the HPG function. For these reasons, it is important to consider the effects of endocrine and/or developmental status when investigating effects of seizures on steroid secretion.

VIII. Developmental Differences in Stress-Induced Steroids

There is evidence that adrenocortical secretion following stress differs as a function of gonadal and developmental status. Prepubertal male rats, compared to adult male rats, exposed to intermittent foot shock (Goldman et al., 1973), ether vapors (Vazquez and Akil, 1993), or restraint (Romeo et al., 2004a), have a corticosterone response that takes at least 45–60 min longer to return to baseline. Similarly, among female rats, there is differential adrenocortical secretion of P_4 in prepubertal and adult females. Ovx prepubertal females show higher and more prolonged stress-induced P_4 secretion compared to ovx adults (Romeo et al., 2004b). It is currently unknown whether P_4 modulates HPA axis reactivity; however, P_4 is rapidly converted to 3α,5α-THP, which can dampen stress-induced ACTH secretion (Patchev *et al.*, 1996). Moreover, steroids, such as T and E_2, can shift HPA responsiveness (Viau, 2002). These data suggest that differential exposure of the prepubertal and adult brain to steroids following stressors are likely to modulate the physiology and behavior of the organism differently before and after pubertal maturation. The physiological and behavioral significance of a greater and more prolonged stress-induced adrenocortical response in prepubertal compared adult males is presently unknown, but may influence seizure susceptibility and/or the course of epilepsy.

A. CHRONIC STRESS-INDUCED CHANGES IN SEIZURES

Results of studies, which have manipulated the HPA by altering early life stress exposure, reveal evidence for effects on seizures. Early life stress produces persistent effects on the hippocampus, the structure critically involved in limbic epilepsy, and can alter the course of some epilepsies (Fenoglio *et al.*, 2006; Mirescu *et al.*, 2004). Prenatal and early life stressors reduce the seizure threshold to adult exposure to chemoconvulsant (Frye and Bayon, 1999a; Frye *et al.*, 2006b) and electrical kindling epileptogenesis (Edwards *et al.*, 2002). Exposure to an early postnatal stress not only confers an enhanced vulnerability to limbic epileptogenesis in adulthood but also impairs hippocampal morphology and neurogenesis (Mirescu *et al.*, 2004; Schmitz *et al.*, 2002), produces HPA axis hyper-reactivity (reviewed in Weinstock, 2001), reduced response to gonadal hormones (Frye and Orecki, 2002a,b), and increases anxiety and depressive-like behavior (Frye and Wawrzycki, 2003; Sanchez *et al.*, 2001). Some of the former factors may also mediate effects of early life stress on seizures. In support, as infant rats, maternal separation stress has synergistic effects with PTZ on seizure duration, hippocampal neuronal degeneration and, as adults, hippocampal-dependent learning (Huang *et al.*, 2002). We have shown that maternal separation also reduces hippocampal-dependent learning independent of seizure status (Frisone *et al.*, 2002). As such, we subsequently examined effects of 1-h neonatal isolation on PNDs 2–9 followed by lithium-pilocarpine–induced SE at day 10. We found that this was associated with a lower seizure threshold to pilocarpine-induced seizures in adulthood and also lower levels of $3\alpha,5\alpha$-THP (Frye *et al.*, 2006b). Commensurate with this, others have demonstrated that rats that experience maternal separation and SE, compared to those who experienced SE only, have greater corticosterone release following SE and worse performance in hippocampally mediated memory in adulthood (Lai *et al.*, 2006). A glucocorticoid synthesis inhibitor given after SE corrected the lowered seizure threshold, suggesting the neonatal isolation effect was at least partly mediated by corticosterone and HPA function. Thus, effects of early life stress on vulnerability to limbic function and epileptogenesis, may be mediated in part by stress-induced steroid secretion.

The mechanisms underlying sequelae of early life stressors are complex and ill-understood. Seizures can produce changes in function of NMDA and GABA$_A$ receptors, gene transcription, dentate gyrus apoptosis and neurogenesis, mossy fiber sprouting and axonal reorganization, and result in hippocampal sclerosis (Sutula and Ockuly, 2005). There is a range of candidate mechanisms through which maternal separation could produce these effects (Mirescu *et al.*, 2004; Pryce *et al.*, 2005; Sanchez *et al.*, 2001), including the central CRH-circuit (Corticotrophin releasing hormone) (Sanchez *et al.*, 2001) and the HPA axis. CRH is involved in the pathogenesis of early life seizures (Baram and Hatalski, 1998). Corticosterone affects hippocampal electrophysiology and electrical kindling (Taher *et al.*, 2005). Further research is needed to determine whether increased seizure vulnerability persists into aging, the potential underlying mechanisms, and whether effects can be generalized to nonhuman primates and people, and relevance to the neuropsychiatric comorbidities of epilepsy.

IX. Other Factors that may Underlie Differences in Sensitivity to Steroids

In addition to reproductive, developmental, and/or stress status influencing neuroactive steroids, changes in the GABA$_A$ system may also mitigate some of these effects. GABA$_A$ receptor agonists such as benzodiazepines, barbiturates, alcohol, and 3α,5α-THP exert biphasic effects, such that at high and low concentrations produce divergent effects on the function of many GABA$_A$ receptors in several regions of the CNS (Beauchamp *et al.*, 2000; Carl *et al.*, 1990; Fish *et al.*, 2001; Masia *et al.*, 2000; Miczek *et al.*, 1997, 2003; Norberg *et al.*, 1987; Sundström *et al.*, 1998; Wenzel *et al.*, 2002). These differential effects may be due to inhibition of some inhibitory neurons that are less sensitive to GABA agonists and thus requiring higher concentrations of GABA$_A$ agonists for GABA-enhancing effect. Decreases in sensitivity may be due to stress, hormonal status, or prior experience with hormone therapy and/or GABA$_A$ agonists influencing responses in certain CNS regions as a result of changes in GABA$_A$ receptor subunits. For example, changes in the α4 subunit of GABA$_A$ receptors in the hippocampus of rats is seen with repeated cycles of P$_4$ withdrawal (Gulinello *et al.*, 2001) or long-term stress (Concas *et al.*, 1988). Together these findings suggest that increased sensitivity to steroids and/or GABA$_A$ agonists may be related to prior steroid exposure and changes in GABA$_A$ receptor subunits.

It is also possible that tolerance to neuroactive steroids can develop, which may influence seizure susceptibility. Following withdrawal from benzodiazepines or barbiturates, tolerance occurs. Prolonged exposure to, and withdrawal from, 3α,5α-THP may also produce tolerance. In some studies, rodents show tolerance after repeated 3α,5α-THP exposure (Czlonkowska *et al.*, 2001; Marshall *et al.*, 1997;

Palmer *et al.*, 2002; Zhu *et al.*, 2004), but in other studies tolerance did not occur (Damianisch *et al.*, 2001; Kokate *et al.*, 1996; Reddy and Rogawski, 2000). Exposure of GABA$_A$ receptors to endogenous 3α,5α-THP during the luteal phase of the menstrual cycle could underlie decreases in sensitivity to steroids of some women with catamenial epilepsy. Furthermore, increases in 3α,5α-THP from the adrenals during chronic stress could downregulate GABA$_A$ receptors and produce tolerance (Barbaccia *et al.*, 1998, 2001; Droogleever Fortuyn *et al.*, 2004; Purdy *et al.*, 1991). During the luteal phase, 3α,5α-THP from corpus luteum is added to the steroids from the adrenals (Ottander *et al.*, 2005). Considering these factors together, it has been proposed that some women with catamenial epilepsy have developed (cross) tolerance to neuroactive steroids (and/or other GABA$_A$ agonists) which produces increased seizure suspectibility at the end of the luteal phase when 3α,5α-THP declines and withdrawal occurs. Thus, the role of tolerance to neuroactive steroids in the etiology and/or therapeutic management of seizure disorders require further investigation.

X. A Review of Progestins, Absence Seizures, and Mechanisms of Action

The findings discussed above largely support a protective role of progestins on seizure susceptibility, but there is evidence that progestins may have different effects to aggravate absence epilepsy. In a case study, absence epilepsy was exacerbated by P$_4$ administration (Grunewald *et al.*, 1992). In an animal model, systemic acute administration of P$_4$, but not E$_2$, increased the number and total duration of spike-wave discharges (a hallmark of absence epilepsy; Budziszewska *et al.*, 1999). During the estrous cycle, spike-wave discharges increase during proestrus, when the levels of P$_4$ are naturally enhanced (Van Luijtelaar *et al.*, 2001). Increases of spike-wave discharges after acute administration of P$_4$ seem to be due to the GABA-agonist like actions of 3α,5α-THP (Budziszewska *et al.*, 1999). The effects of P$_4$ on spike-wave discharges were antagonized by finasteride, a 5α-reductase inhibitor, which did not produce effects alone (Van Luijtelaar *et al.*, 2003). Moreover, RU 38486, a progestin receptor antagonist, did not block effects of P$_4$ on spike-wave discharges (Budziszewska *et al.*, 1999), implying that P$_4$'s effects were likely due to actions at neurotransmitters, rather than steroid, receptor targets (Van Luijtelaar *et al.*, 2001). Thus, in contrast to the protective effects of progestins in convulsive epilepsy (Frye and Scalise, 2000; Kokate *et al.*, 1994), P$_4$ aggravates epileptoform activity of the spike-wave discharges type.

Although P$_4$ typically aggravates absence epilepsy, during pregnancy, which is characterized by high progestin levels, an attenuation of absence epilepsy is observed. It has been proposed that increased functioning of GABA in the cortex, concomitant with downregulation of GABA$_A$ receptors in the lateral thalamic nucleus might underlie these opposite effects on absence epilepsy during pregnancy. Increases in progestins during pregnancy alter expression, density, plasticity, and sensitivity of $GABA_A$ receptors in some cortical and limbic structures (Brussaard and Koksma, 2002; Brussaard et al., 1999; Concas et al., 1999; Weizman et al., 1997). These effects may be related to changes in expression of $GABA_A$ receptor subunit genes (Morrell, 1999) or the balance between endogenous phosphatase and protein kinase C activity. In support of the latter, during pregnancy, $GABA_A$ receptors in the supraoptic nucleus are sensitive to $3\alpha,5\alpha$-THP in part due to a constitutively high level of phosphatase activity. At parturition, release of oxytocin contributes to higher level of phosphorylation, which may lead to $3\alpha,5\alpha$-THP insensitivity of $GABA_A$ receptors (Brussaard and Koksma, 2002). Chronic exposure to P_4, as occurs during pregnancy, has effects to upregulate and downregulate $GABA_A$ receptors respectively in cortical and ventral lateral thalamic regions, which are central in thalamo-cortical oscillations of spike-wave discharges (Avanzini and Marescaux, 1991; Canonaco et al., 1989; Meeren et al., 2002). It is possible that positive modulation of GABA receptors in cortex may prevent hyperexcitability, which underlies spike-wave discharges (Gloor et al., 1979; Kostopoulos, 2000). Perhaps simultaneous effects to enhance in cortex, and downregulate in the lateral thalamic nucleus, $GABA_A$ receptors may produce opposite effects during pregnancy than are typically observed for P_4 to enhance spike-wave discharges. These effects and actions of $3\alpha,5\alpha$-THP at other glutamatergic (NMDA), cholinergic, and/or opioid (Melcangi and Panzica, 2001) substrates which are involved in absence epilepsy (Berdiev et al., 2000; Coenen et al., 1992; Lason et al., 1994) should also be considered.

XI. Interactions Between AEDs and Steroid Hormones

Not only do hormones influence seizure susceptibility, and seizures influence hormones, but AEDs can also alter steroid metabolism and/or reproductive function (Frye, 2005). Some anti-epileptic drugs induce cyctochrome P450 (e.g., phenytoin and carbamazapine), which stimulates sex hormone-binding globulin production and metabolism of adrenal and sex steroid hormones, thereby reducing hormone levels in the circulation (Macphee et al., 1988; Morrell et al., 2001; Stoffel-Wagner et al., 1998). Other drugs, such as valproate, inhibit steroid hormone metabolism, which increases the level of circulating androgens (Isojarvi et al., 2004; Morrell, 2003). It is a challenge to investigate the endocrine effects of AEDs in clinical populations because one does not want to undermind the beneficial therapeutic effects of AEDs, even if they have negative side-effects. Thus, we have begun to investigate the consequences of AED administration to male rats on androgen-dependent anxiety, cognitive, and social/reproductive behavior.

We have investigated the effects on intact male rats of administration of saline, phenytoin (50 mg/kg), or valproate (325 mg/kg) for 1.5, 15, or 30 days. After the designated time period, rats were trained in the object recognition task, then tested for anxiety behavior in the open field, and for social/sexual interactions. This was followed by testing in the object recognition task. Rats that were administered the enzyme-inducing AED phenytoin for 15 or 30, but not 1.5, days demonstrated less anti-anxiety behavior (central entries) in the open field. Phenytoin for 1.5, 15, or 30 days decreased object recognition learning and memory. Phenytoin for 15 or 30 days also increased the latency and decreased the number of social and sexual contacts. Notably, these regimen of phenytoin and valproate both increased the latency to, and decreased the incidence of, PTX-induced myoclonus, but valproate appears to do so with more untoward behavioral effects. See Table IX.

XII. Summary

There are sex differences and effects of steroid hormones, such as androgens, estrogen, and progestins, that influence seizures. Some of the capacity for anticonvulsive effects of these steroids may be related to their formation of ligands which have agonist-like actions at $GABA_A$ receptors or antagonist actions at glutamate receptors. These steroids can also have deleterious effects on seizures, due to withdrawal, changes they exert at $GABA_A$ and/or glutamate receptors or other targets, or sensitivity of the type of seizure (convulsive vs. absence). Many factors can influence steroid hormone secretion including developmental and stress status, and even therapeutics, such as AEDs. Thus, given the need for more effective anticonvulsant therapies, the interactions between hormonal/reproductive, developmental, and stress status, seizure experience, and therapeutics need to be investigated further.

Acknowledgments

Some of the research described from our lab was supported by The Epilepsy Foundation of America and was made possible by the efforts of trainees including Dr. Madeline Rhodes, Alicia Walf, Jason Paris, Janet Heuring, and others.

TABLE IX

Mean (+ Standard Error of the Mean) Anxiety (Top), Cognitive (Middle Top), Social/Reproductive (Middle Bottom), and Seizure (Bottom) Behavior of Male Rats that were Administered Saline, Phenytoin (50 mg/kg), or Valproate (325 mg/kg) for 1.5 (Left Panel), 15 (Middle Panel), or 30 Days (Right Panel)

	1.5 day exposure			15 day exposure			30 day exposure		
	Saline (n = 5)	Phenytoin (n = 5)	Valproate (n = 5)	Saline (n = 10)	Phenytoin (n = 10)	Valproate (n = 10)	Saline (n = 10)	Phenytoin (n = 5)	Valproate (n = 5)
Anxiety behavior									
Total entries in the open field	274 + 49	311 + 19	281 + 34	199 + 22	152 + 31	150 + 32	189 + 34	178 + 47	164 + 47
Central entries in open field	87 + 27	86 + 11	79 + 17	47 + 9	28 + 10	29 + 7	78 + 14	42 + 17	75 + 23
Cognitive behavior									
% of time spent with novel object	53 + 9	27 + 15	53 + 16	64 + 9	34 + 10	48 + 7	48 + 4	30 + 5	44 + 10
Social and reproductive behavior									
Latency to social interaction	478 + 122	445 + 86	484 + 75	64 + 55	112 + 22	36 + 4	40 + 8	185 + 51	43 + 11
# of bouts social interaction	3 + 1	3 + 1	3 + 1	6 + 1	3 + 1	7 + 1	6 + 1	3 + 1	7 + 1
# Sexual contacts	1 + 1	1 + 1	1 + 1	2 + 1	1 + 1	2 + 1	3 + 1	1 + 1	3 + 1
Seizure behavior									
Latency to myoclonus	89 + 25	152 + 112	201 + 135	94 + 5	116 + 15	121 + 14	110 + 16	144 + 22	153 + 48
Incidence of myoclonus	16 + 4	12 + 4	11 + 4	4 + 1	3 + 1	3 + 1	4 + 1	2 + 1	2 + 1

References

Abbasi, F., Krumholz, A., Kittner, S. J., and Langenberg, P. (1999). Effects of menopause on seizures in women with epilepsy. *Epilepsia* **40,** 205–210.
Almqvist, R. (1955). The rhythm of epileptic attacks and its relationship to the menstrual cycle. *Acta Psychiatr. Neurol. Scand. Suppl.* **105,** 1–116.
Andersen, M. L., Bignotto, M., Machado, R. B., and Tufik, S. (2004). Different stress modalities result in distinct steroid hormone responses by male rats. *Braz. J. Med. Biol. Res.* **37,** 791–797.
Andersen, M. L., Martins, P. J., D'Almedia, V., Bignotto, M., and Tufik, S. (2005). Endocrinological and catecholaminergic alterations during sleep deprivation and recovery in male rats. *J. Sleep Res.* **14,** 83–90.
Andersson, S. (2001). Steroidogenic enzymes in skin. *Eur. J. Dermatol.* **4,** 293–295.
Andréen, L., Bixo, M., Nyberg, S., Sundström-Poromaa, I., amd Bäckström, T. (2003). Progesterone effects during sequential hormone replacement therapy. *Eur. J. Endocrinol.* **148**(5), 571–577.
Andréen, L., Sundström-Poromaa, I., Bixo, M., Andersson, A., Nyberg, S., and Bäckström, T. (2005). Relationship between allopregnanolone and negative mood in postmenopausal women taking sequential hormone replacement therapy with vaginal progesterone. *Psychoneuroendocrinology* **30,** 212–224.
Andrews, N., Zharkowsky, A., and File, S. E. (1992). Acute stress down regulates benzodiazepine receptors: Reversal by diazepam. *Eur. J. Pharmacol.* **210,** 247–251.
Avanzini, G., and Marescaux, C. (1991). Genetic animal models for generalized non convulsive epilepsies and new antiepileptic drugs. *Epilepsy Res. Suppl.* **3,** 29–38.
Bäckström, T. (1976). Epilepsy in women. Oestrogen and progesterone plasma levels. *Experientia* **32,** 248–249.
Bäckström, T., Carstensen, H., and Sodergard, R. (1976). Concentration of estradiol, testosterone and progesterone in cerebrospinal fluid compared with plasma unbound and total concentrations. *J. Steroid Biochem.* **7,** 469–472.
Bäckström, T., Zetterlund, B., Blom, S., and Romano, M. (1984). Effects of intravenous progesterone infusions on the epileptic discharge frequency in women with partial epilepsy. *Acta Neurol. Scand.* **69,** 240–248.
Baram, T. Z., and Hatalski, C. G. (1998). Neuropeptide-mediated excitability: A key triggering mechanism for seizure generation in the developing brain. *Trends Neurosci.* **21,** 471–476.
Barbaccia, M. L., Concas, A., Serra, M., and Biggio, G. (1998). Stress and neurosteroids in adult and aged rats. *Exp. Gerontol.* **33,** 697–712.
Barbaccia, M. L., Serra, M., Purdy, R. H., and Biggio, G. (2001). Stress and neuroactive steroids. *Int. Rev. Neurobiol.* **46,** 243–272.
Bauer, J., Stoffel-Wagner, B., Flügel, D., Kluge, M., Schramm, J., Bidlingmaier, F., and Elger, C. E. (2000a). Serum androgens return to normal after temporal lobe epilepsy surgery in men. *Neurology* **55,** 820–824.
Bauer, J., Stoffel-Wagner, B., Flugel, D., Kluge, M., and Elger, C. E. (2000b). The impact of epilepsy surgery on sex hormones and the menstrual cycle in female patients. *Seizure* **9,** 389–393.
Baulieu, E. E. (1997). Neurosteroids: Of the nervous system, by the nervous system, for the nervous system. *Recent Prog. Horm. Res.* **52,** 1–32.
Baulieu, E. E., and Robel, P. (1990). Neurosteroids: A new brain function? *J. Steroid Biochem. Mol. Biol.* **493,** 395–403.
Beauchamp, M. H., Ormerod, B. K., Jhamandas, K., Boegman, R. J., and Beninger, R. J. (2000). Neurosteroids and reward: Allopregnano-lone produces a conditioned place aversion in rats. *Pharmacol. Biochem. Behav.* **67,** 29–35.
Belelli, D., and Herd, M. B. (2003). The contraceptive agent Provera enhances GABA(A) receptor-mediated inhibitory neurotransmission in the rat hippocampus: Evidence for endogenous neuro-steroids. *J. Neurosci.* **23,** 10013–10020.

Belelli, D., Bolger, M. B., and Gee, K. W. (1989). Anticonvulsant profile of the progesterone metabolite 5 alpha-pregnan-3 alpha-ol-20-one. *Eur. J. Pharmacol.* **166,** 325–329.

Berdiev, R. K., Chepurnov, S. A., Chepurnova, N. E., van Luijtelaar, E. L. J. M., and Coenen, A. M. L. (2000). "Effects of Neuropeptide Galanin on Spike-Wave Discharges in WAG/Rij Rats." pp. 71–78. Nijmegen University Press, Nijmegen.

Bernardi, F., Salvestroni, C., Casarosa, E., Nappi, R. E., Lanzone, A., Luisi, S., Purdy, R. H., Petraglia, F., and Genazzani, A. R. (1998). Aging is associated with changes in allopregnanolone concentrations in brain, endocrine glands and serum in male rats. *Eur. J. Endocrinol.* **138,** 316–321.

Bernardi, F., Pieri, M., Stomati, M., Luisi, S., Palumbo, M., Pluchino, N., Ceccarelli, C., and Genazzani, A. R. (2003). Effect of different hormonal replacement therapies on circulating allopregnano-lone and dehydroepiandrosterone levels in postmenopausal women. *Gynecol. Endocrinol.* **17,** 65–77.

Besman, M. J., Yanagibashi, K., Lee, T. D., Kawamura, M., Hall, P. F., and Shively, J. E. (1989). Identification of des-(Gly-Ile)-endozepine as an effector of corticotropin-dependent adrenal steroidogenesis: Stimulation of cholesterol delivery is mediated by the peripheral benzodiazepine receptor. *Proc. Natl. Acad. Sci. USA.* **86,** 4897–4901.

Bicikova, M., Lapcik, O., Hampl, R., Starka, L., Knuppen, R., Haupt, O., and Dibbelt, L. (1995). A novel radioimmunoassay of allopregnano-lone. *Steroids* **60,** 210–213.

Bickerstaff, E. (1975). "Neurological Complications of Oral Contraceptives." Clarendon Press, Oxford.

Biggio, G. (1983). The action of stress, U-carbolines, diazepam and Ro 15–1788 on GABA receptors in the rat brain. *In* "Benzodiazepine Recognition Site Ligands: Biochemistry and Pharmacology." pp. 105–117. Raven Press, New York, NY.

Biggio, G., Corda, M. G., Dermontis, G., Rossetti, Z., and Gessa, G. L. (1980). Sudden decrease in cerebellar GABA binding induced by stress. *Pharmacol. Res. Commun.* **12,** 489–493.

Biggio, G., Corda, M. G., Concas, A., Dermontis, G., Rossetti, Z., and Gessa, G. L. (1981). Rapid changes in GABA binding induced by stress in different areas of the rat brain. *Brain Res.* **229,** 363–369.

Biggio, G., Concas, A., Mostallino, M. C., Purdy, R. H., Trabucchi, M., and Barbaccia, M. L. (1996). Inhibition of GABAergic transmission enhances neurosteroid concentrations in the rat brain. *In* "The Brain: Source and Target for Sex Steroid Hormones." pp. 43–62. Informa Healthcare, New York, NY.

Biggio, G., Barbaccia, M. L., Follesa, P., Serra, M., Purdy, R. H., and Concas, A. (2000). Neurosteroids and GABAA receptor plasticity. *In* "GABA in the Nervous System." pp. 207–232. Lippincott Williams & Wilkins, Philadelphia, PA.

Biggio, G., Follesa, P., Sanna, E., Purdy, R. H., and Concas, A. (2001). GABAA-receptor plasticity during long-term exposure to and withdrawal from progesterone. *Int. Rev. Neurobiol.* **46,** 207–241. Review.

Bilo, L., Meo, R., Nappi, C., Annunziato, L., Striano, S., Colao, A. M., Merola, B., and Buscaino, G. A. (1988). Reproductive endocrine disorders in women with primary generalized epilepsy. *Epilepsia* **29,** 612–619.

Bilo, L., Meo, R., Valentino, R., Buscaino, G. A., Striano, S., and Nappi, C. (1991). Abnormal pattern of luteinizing hormone pulsatility in women with epilepsy. *Fertil. Steril.* **55,** 705–711.

Bixo, M., Bäckström, T., Winblad, B., and Andersson, A. (1995). Estradiol and testosterone in specific regions of the human female brain in different endocrine states. *J. Steroid Biochem. Mol. Biol.* **55,** 297–303.

Bixo, M., Andersson, A., Winblad, B., Purdy, R. H., and Bäckström, T. (1997). Progesterone, 5alphapregnane-3, 20-dione and 3alpha-hydroxy-5alpha-pregnane-20-one in specific regions of the human female brain in different endocrine states. *Brain Res.* **764,** 173–178.

Björn, I., Bixo, M., Nöjd, K. S., Nyberg, S., and Bäckström, T. (2000). Negative mood changes during hormone replacement therapy: A comparison between two progestogens. *Am. J. Obstet. Gynecol.* **183**(6), 1419–1426.

Boulware, M. I., Weick, J. P., Becklund, B. R., Kuo, S. P., Groth, R. D., and Mermelstein, P. G. (2005). Estradiol activates group I and II meta-botropic glutamate receptor signaling, leading to opposing influences on cAMP response element-binding protein. *J. Neurosci.* **25**, 5066–5078.

Brann, D. W., Putnam, C. D., and Mahesh, V. B. (1990). Gamma-aminobutyric acidA receptors mediate 3 alpha-hydroxy-5 alpha-pregnan-20-one-induced gonadotropin secretion. *Endocrinology* **126**, 1854–1859.

Breedlove, S. M., Jacobson, C. D., Gorski, R. A., and Arnold, A. P. (1982). Masculinization of the female rat spinal cord following a single injection of testosterone propionate but not estradiol benzoate. *Brain Res.* **237**(1), 173–181.

Brown-Grant, K., and Raisman, G. (1972). Reproductive function in the rat following selective destruction of afferent fibres to the hypothalamus from the limbic system. *Brain Res.* **46**, 23–42.

Brussaard, A. B., and Koksma, J. J. (2002). Short-term modulation of GABAA receptor function in the adult female rat. *Prog. Brain Res.* **139**, 31–42.

Brussaard, A. B., Devay, P., Leyting-Vermeulen, J. L., and Kits, K. S. (1999). Changes in properties and neurosteroid regulation of GABAergic synapses in the SO nucleus during the mammalian female reproductive cycle. *J. Physiol.* **516**, 513–524.

Bruton, C. J., Stevens, J. R., and Frith, C. D. (1994). Epilepsy, psychosis, and schizophrenia: Clinical and neuropathologic correlations. *Neurology* **44**, 34–42.

Buckmaster, P. S., and Dudek, F. E. (1997). Network properties of the dentate gyrus in epileptic rats with hilar neuron loss and granule cell axon reorganization. *J. Neurophysiol.* **77**, 2685–2696.

Budziszewska, B., Van Luijtelaar, G., Coenen, A., Leskiewicz, M., and Lason, W. (1999). Effects of neurosteroids on spike-wave discharges in the genetic epileptic WAG/Rij rat. *Epilepsy Res.* **33**, 23–29.

Callies, F., Arlt, W., Siekmann, L., Hubler, D., Bidlingmaier, F., and Allolio, B. (2000). Influence of oral dehydroepiandrosterone (DHEA) on urinary steroid metabolites in males and females. *Steroids* **65**, 98–102.

Campbell, S., and Whitehead, M. (1977). Oestrogen therapy and the menopausal syndrome. *Clin. Obstet. Gynaecol.* **4**, 31–47.

Canonaco, M., O'connor, L. H., Pfaff, D. W., and McEwen, B. S. (1989). Longer term progesterone treatment induces changes of GABAA receptor levels in forebrain sites in the female hamster: Quantative autoradiography study. *Exp. Brain Res.* **77**, 407–411.

Cantor, B. (1984). Induction of ovulation with clomiphene citrate. *In* "Gynecology and Obstetrics" (J. J. Sciarri, Ed.), Vol. 5, pp. 1–7. Harper and Rowe, Philadelphia, PA.

Carl, P., Högskilde, S., Nielsen, J. W., Sörensen, M. B., Lindholm, M., Karlen, B., and Bäckström, T. (1990). Pregnanolone emulsion. A preliminary pharmacokinetic and pharmacodynamic study of a new intravenous anaesthetic agent. *Anaesthesia* **45**, 189–197.

Carrer, H. F., Whitmoyer, D. I., and Sawyer, C. H. (1978). Effects of hippocampal and amygdaloid stimulation on the firing of preoptic neurons in the proestrous female rat. *Brain Res.* **142**, 363–367.

Cheng, Y. J., and Karavolas, H. J. (1973). Conversion of progesterone to 5α-pregnane-3,20-dione and 3α-hydroxy-5α-pregnan-20-one by rat medical basal hypothalami and the effects of estradiol and stage of estrous cycle on the conversion. *Endocrinology* **93**(5), 1157–1162.

Coenen, A. M. L., Drinkenburg, W. H. I. M., Inoue, M., and van Luijtelaar, E. L. J. M. (1992). Genetic models of absence epilepsy, with emphasis on the WAG/Rij strain of rats. *Epilepsy Res.* **12**, 75–86.

Concas, A., Mele, S., and Biggio, G. (1987). Foot shock stress decreases chloride efflux from rat brain neurosynaptosomes. *Eur. J. Pharmacol.* **135**, 423–427.

Concas, A., Serra, M., Atsoggiu, T., and Biggio, G. (1988). Foot-shock stress and anxiogenic beta-carbolines increase t-[35S]butylbicyclo-phosphorothionate binding in the rat cerebral cortex, an effect opposite to anxiolytics and gamma-aminobutyric acid mi-metics. *J. Neurochem.* **51,** 1868–1876.

Concas, A., Mostallino, M. C., Perra, C., Lener, R., Roscetti, G., Barbaccia, M. L., Purdy, R. H., and Biggio, G. (1996). Functional correlation between allopregnanolone and [35 S]TBPS binding in the brain of rats exposed to isoniazid, pentylenete-trazol or stress. *Br. J. Pharmacol.* **118,** 839–846.

Concas, A., Follesa, P., Barbaccia, M. L., Purdy, R. H., and Biggio, G. (1999). Physiological modulation of GABA receptor plasticity by progesterone metabolites. *Eur. J. Pharmacol.* **375,** 225–235.

Corpechot, C., Robel, P., Axelson, M., Sjövall, J., and Baulieu, E. E. (1981). Characterization and measurement of dehydroepiandrosterone sulfate in rat brain. *Proc. Natl. Acad. Sci. USA* **78,** 4704–4707.

Corpéchot, C., Young, J., Calvel, M., Wehrey, C., Veltz, J. N., Touyer, G., Mouren, M., Prasad, V. V., Banner, C., Sjövall, J., *et al.* (1993). Neurosteroids: 3 Alpha-hydroxy-5 alpha-pregnan-20-one and its precursors in the brain, plasma, and steroidogenic glands of male and female rats. *Endocrinology* **133,** 1003–1009.

Costa, A. M., Spence, K. T., Smith, S. S., and French-Mullen, J. M. (1995). Withdrawal from the endogenous steroid progesterone results in GABAA currents insensitive to benzodiazepine modulation in rats CA1 hippocampus. *J. Neurophysiol.* **74,** 464–469.

Covolan, L., and Mello, L. E. (2000). Temporal profile of neuronal injury following pilocarpine or kainic acid-induced status epilepticus. *Epilepsy Res.* **39,** 133–152.

Czlonkowska, A. I., Krzascik, P., Sienkiewicz-Jarosz, H., Siemiatkowski, M., Szyndler, J., Maciejak, P., Bidzinski, A., and Plaznik, A. (2001). Tolerance to the anticonvulsant activity of midazolam and allopregnanolone in a model of picrotoxin seizures. *Eur. J. Pharmacol.* **425,** 121–127.

Damianisch, K., Rupprecht, R., and Lancel, M. (2001). The influence of subchronic administration of the neurosteroid allopregnanolone on sleep in the rat. *Neuropsychopharmacology* **25,** 576–584.

Dana-Haeri, J., Trimble, M., and Oxley, J. (1983). Prolactin and gonadotrophin changes following generalised and partial seizures. *J. Neurol. Neurosurg. Psychiatry* **46,** 331–335.

de Wit, H., Schmitt, L., Purdy, R., and Hauger, R. (2001). Effects of acute progesterone administration in healthy postmenopausal women and normally-cycling women. *Psychoneuroendocrinology* **26,** 697–710.

Ditkoff, E. C., Crary, W. G., Cristo, M., and Lobo, R. A. (1991). Estrogen improves psychological function in asymptomatic postmenopausal women. *Obstet. Gynecol.* **18,** 991–995.

Drislane, F. W., Coleman, A. E., Schomer, D. L., Ives, J., Levesque, L. A., Seibel, M. M., and Herzog, A. G. (1994). Altered pulsatile secretion of luteinizing hormone in women with epilepsy. *Neurology* **44,** 306–310.

Droogleever Fortuyn, H. A., van Broekhoven, F., Span, P. N., Bäckström, T., Zitman, F. G., and Verkes, R. J. (2004). Effects of PhD examination stress on allopregnanolone and cortisol plasma levels and peripheral benzodiazepine receptor density. *Psychoneuroendocrinology* **93,** 1341–1344.

Drugan, R. C., Morrow, A. L., Weizman, R., Weizman, A., Deutsch, S. I., Crawley, J. N., and Paul, S. M. (1989). Stress-induced behavioural depression in the rat is associated with a decrease in GABA receptor-mediated chloride ion flux and brain benzodiazepine receptor occupancy. *Brain Res.* **487,** 45–51.

Duncan, S., Blacklaw, J., Beastall, G. H., and Brodie, M. J. (1999). Antiepileptic drug therapy and sexual function in men with epilepsy. *Epilepsia* **40,** 197–204.

Edwards, H. E., Burnham, W. M., Mendonca, A., Bowlby, D. A., and MacLusky, N. J. (1999a). Steroid hormones affect limbic afterdischarge thresholds and kindling rates in adult female rats. *Brain Res.* **838,** 136–150.

Edwards, H. E., Burnham, W. M., Ng, M. M., Asa, S., and MacLusky, N. J. (1999b). Limbic seizures alter reproductive function in the female rat. *Epilepsia* **40,** 1370–1377.

Edwards, H. E., Burnham, W. M., Mendonca, A., Bowlby, D. A., and MacLusky, N. J. (1999c). Steroid hormones affect limbic afterdischarge thresholds and kindling rates in adult female rats. *Brain Res.* **838,** 136–150.

Edwards, H. E., Dortok, D., Tam, J., Won, D., and Burnham, W. M. (2002). Prenatal stress alters seizure thresholds and the development of kindled seizures in infant and adult rats. *Horm. Behav.* **42,** 437–447.

el-Etr, M., Akwa, Y., Fiddes, R. J., Robel, P., and Baulieu, E. E. (1995). A progesterone metabolite stimulates the release of gonadotropin-releasing hormone from GT1–1 hypothalamic neurons via the gammaaminobutyric acid type A receptor. *Proc. Natl. Acad. Sci. USA* **92,** 3769–3773.

English, J. D., and Sweatt, J. D. (1997). A requirement for the mitogen-activated protein kinase cascade in hippocampal long term potentiation. *J. Biol. Chem.* **272,** 19103–19106.

Erskine, M. S., and Kornberg, E. (1992). Stress and ACTH increase circulating concentrations of 3 alpha-androstanediol in female rats. *Life Sci.* **51,** 2065–2071.

Everett, J. W. (1994). Pituitary and hypothalamus: Perspectives and overview. *In* "The Physiology of Reproduction." pp. 1509–1526. Academic Press, London, New York, and San Diego.

Fenoglio, K. A., Brunson, K. L., and Baram, T. Z. (2006). ippocampal neuroplasticity induced by early-life stress: Functional and molecular aspects. *Front. Neuroendocrinol.* **27,** 180–192.

File, S. E., Zangrossi, H., and Andrews, N. (1993). Novel environment and cat odor change GABA and 5HT release and uptake in the rat. *Pharmacol. Biochem. Behav.* **45,** 931–934.

Fish, E. W., Faccidomo, S., DeBold, J. F., and Miczek, K. A. (2001). Alcohol, allopregnanolone and aggression in mice. *Psychopharmacology (Berl)* **153,** 473–843.

Follesa, P., Serra, M., Cagetti, E., Pisu, M. G., Porta, S., Floris, S., Massa, F., Sanna, E., and Biggio, G. (2000). Allopregnanolone synthesis in cerebellar granule cells: Roles in regulation of GABAA receptor expression and function during progesterone treatment and withdrawal. *Mol. Pharmacol.* **57,** 1262–1270.

Follesa, P., Porcu, P., Sogliano, C., Cinus, M., Biggio, F., Mancuso, L., Mostallino, M. C., Paoletti, A. M., Purdy, R. H., Biggio, G., and Concas, A. (2002). Changes in GABAA receptor gamma 2 subunit gene expression induced by long-term administration of oral contraceptives in rats. *Neuropharmacology* **42,** 325–336.

Friedman, M. N., Geula, C., Holmes, G. L., and Herzog, A. G. (2002). GnRH-immunoreactive fiber changes with unilateral amygdala-kindled seizures. *Epilepsy Res.* **52,** 73–77.

Frisone, D. F., Frye, C. A., and Zimmerberg, B. (2002). Social isolation stress during the third week of life has age-dependent effects on spatial learning in rats. *Behav. Brain Res.* **128,** 153–160.

Frye, C. A. (2005). Ovarian hormones: Their effects on cortical excitation and influences on epileptogenesis. *In* "Epilepsy and Ovarian Hormones" (C. L. Harden, Ed.), Part 1 of the Epilepsy and Female Reproductive Milestones: Topics Spanning a Lifetime series, *Neurology* 64 (9): [CD E-sert]. CME: Emory University; Release Date: May 2005; End Date: May 31, 2008.

Frye, C. A. (2006). Role of androgens in epilepsy. *Expert Rev. Neurother.* **6,** 1061–1075.

Frye, C. A., and Bayon, L. E. (1998a). Seizure activity is increased in endocrine states characterized by decline in endogenous levels of the neurosteroid 3 alpha,5 alpha-THP. *Neuroendocrinology* **68,** 272–280 Erratum in: Neuroendocrinology 68, 436.

Frye, C. A., and Bayon, L. E. (1998b). Increased seizure activity following precipitous decline in endogenous 3α,5α-THP. *Neuroendocrinology* **68,** 272–280.

Frye, C. A., and Bayon, L. E. (1999a). Prenatal stress reduces the effectiveness of the neurosteroid 3 alpha,5 alpha-THP to block kainic-acid-induced seizures. *Dev. Psychobiol.* **34,** 227–234.

Frye, C. A., and Bayon, L. E. (1999b). Mating stimuli influence endogenous variations in the neurosteroids 3alpha,5alpha-THP and 3alpha-Diol. *J. Neuroendocrinol.* **11,** 839–847.

Frye, C. A., and Bayon, L. E. (1999c). Cyclic withdrawal from endogenous and exogenous progesterone increases kainic acid and perforant pathway induced seizures. *Pharmacol. Biochem. Behav.* **62**(2), 315–321.

Frye, C. A., and Orecki, Z. A. (2002a). Prenatal stress alters reproductive responses of rats in behavioral estrus and paced mating of hormone-primed rats. *Horm. Behav.* **42**, 472–483.

Frye, C. A., and Orecki, Z. A. (2002b). Prenatal stress produces deficits in socio-sexual behavior of cycling, but not hormone-primed, Long-Evans rats. *Pharmacol. Biochem. Behav.* **3**, 53–60.

Frye, C. A., and Reed, T. A. (1998). Androgenic neurosteroids: Anti-seizure effects in an animal model of epilepsy. *Psychoneuroendocrinology* **23**, 385–399.

Frye, C. A., and Rhodes, M. E. (2005). Estrogen-priming can enhance progesterone's anti-seizure effects in part by increasing hippocampal levels of allopregnanolone. *Pharmacol. Biochem. Behav.* **81**, 907–916.

Frye, C. A., and Rhodes, M. E. (2006). Infusions of 5alpha-pregnan-3alpha-ol-20-one (3alpha,5alpha-THP) to the ventral tegmental area, but not the substantia nigra, enhance exploratory, anti-anxiety, social and sexual behaviours and concomitantly increase 3alpha,5alpha-THP concentrations in the hippocampus, diencephalon and cortex of ovariectomised oestrogen-primed rats. *J. Neuroendocrinol.* **18**(12), 960–975.

Frye, C. A., Rhodes, M. E., Walf, A., and Harney, J. (2002). Progesterone reduces pentylenetetrazol-induced ictal activity of wild-type mice but not those deficient in type I 5alpha-reductase. *Epilepsia.* 43 Suppl **5**:14–17.

Frye, C. A., and Scalise, T. J. (2000). Anti-seizure effects of progesterone and 3 á,5 á-THP in kainic acid and perforant pathway models of epilepsy. *Psychoneuroendocrinology* **25**, 407–420.

Frye, C. A., and Wawrzycki, J. (2003). Effect of prenatal stress and gonadal hormone condition on depressive behaviors of female and male rats. *Horm. Behav.* **44**, 319–326.

Frye, C. A., Duncan, J. E., Basham, M., and Erskine, M. S. (1996a). Behavioral effects of 3 alpha-androstanediol. II: Hypothalamic and preoptic area actions via a GABAergic mechanism. *Behav. Brain Res.* **79**, 119–130.

Frye, C. A., McCormick, C. M., Coopersmith, C., and Erskine, M. S. (1996b). Effects of paced and non-paced mating stimulation on plasma progesterone, 3 alpha-diol and corticosterone. *Psychoneuroendocrinology* **21**, 431–439.

Frye, C. A., Van Keuren, K. R., and Erskine, M. S. (1996c). Behavioral effects of 3 alpha-androstanediol. I: Modulation of sexual receptivity and promotion of GABA-stimulated chloride flux. *Behav. Brain Res.* **79**, 109–118.

Frye, C. A., Van Keuren, K. R., Rao, P. N., and Erskine, M. S. (1996d). Analgesic effects of the neurosteroid 3 alpha-androstanediol. *Brain Res.* **709**, 1–9.

Frye, C. A., Van Keuren, K. R., Rao, P. N., and Erskine, M. S. (1996e). Progesterone and 3 alpha-androstanediol conjugated to bovine serum albumin affects estrous behavior when applied to the MBH and POA. *Behav. Neurosci.* **110**, 603–612.

Frye, C. A., Scalise, T., and Bayon, L. E. (1998). Finasteride blocks the reduction in ictal activity produced by exogenous estrous cyclicity. *J. Neuroendocrin.* **10**, 291–296.

Frye, C. A. (1995). The neurosteroid 3 alpha, 5 alpha-THP has antiseizure and possible neuroprotective effects in an animal model of epilepsy. *Brain Res.* **696**(1–2), 113–120.

Frye, C. A., Rhodes, M. E., Petralia, S. M., Walf, A. A., Sumida, K., and Edinger, K. L. (2006a). 3alpha-hydroxy-5alpha-pregnan-20-one in the midbrain ventral tegmental area mediates social, sexual, and affective behaviors. *Neuroscience* **138**, 1007–1014.

Frye, C. A., Rhodes, M. E., Raol, Y. H., and Brooks-Kayal, A. R. (2006b). Early postnatal stimulation alters pregnane neurosteroids in the hippocampus. *Psychopharmacology (Berl)* **186**, 343–350.

Fujikawa, D. G. (1996). The temporal evolution of neuronal damage from pilocarpine-induced status epilepticus. *Brain Res.* **725**, 11–22.

Galanopoulou, A. S., Kyrozis, A., Claudio, O. I., Stanton, P. K., and Moshé, S. L. (2003a). Sex-specific KCC2 expression and GABA(A) receptor function in rat substantia nigra. *Exp. Neurol.* **183,** 628–637.

Galanopoulou, A. S., Alm, E. M., and Velíšková, J. (2003b). Estradiol reduces seizure-induced hippocampal injury in ovariectomized female but not in male rats. *Neurosci. Lett.* **342,** 201–205.

Gavish, M., Weizman, A., Moussa, B. H., Okun, Y., and Okun, F. (1987). Regulation of central and peripheral benzodiazepinee receptors in progesterone-treated rats. *Brain Res.* **409,** 386–390.

Gee, K. W. (1988). Steroid modulation of the GABA/benzodiazepine receptor-linked chloride ionophore. *Mol. Neurobiol.* **2,** 291–317.

Gee, K. W., McCauley, L. D., and Lan, N. C. (1995). A putative receptor for neurosteroids on the GABA$_A$ receptor complex: The pharmacological properties and therapeutic potential of epalons. *Crit. Rev. Neurobiol.* **9,** 207–227.

Genazzani, A. R., Palumbo, M. A., de Micheroux, A. A., Artini, P. G., Criscuolo, M., Ficarra, G., Guo, A. L., Benelli, A., Bertolini, A., Petraglia, F., *et al.* (1995). Evidence for a role for the neurosteroid allopregnanolone in the modulation of reproductive function in female rats. *Eur. J. Endocrinol.* **133**(3), 375–380.

Genazzani, A. R., Petraglia, F., Bernardi, F., Casarosa, E., Salvestroni, C., Tonetti, A., Nappi, R. E., Luisi, S., Palumbo, M., Purdy, R. H., and Luisi, M. (1998). Circulating levels of allopregnanolone in humans: Gender, age, and endocrine influences. *J. Clin. Endocrinol. Metab.* **83**(6), 2099–2103.

Genazzani, A. R., Bernardi, F., Stomati, M., Monteleone, P., Luisi, S., Rubino, S., Farzati, A., Casarosa, E., Luisi, M., and Petraglia, F. (2000). Effects of estradiol and ealoxifene analog on brain, adrenal and serum allopregnanolone content in fertile and ovariectomized female rats. *Neuroendocrinology* **72,** 162–170.

Genazzani, A. D., Luisi, M., Malavasi, B., Strucchi, C., Luisi, S., Casarosa, E., Bernardi, F., Genazzani, A. R., and Petraglia, F. (2002). Pulsatile secretory characteristics of allopregnanolone, a neuroactive steroid, during the menstrual cycle and in amenorrheic subjects. *Eur. J. Endocrinol.* **146,** 347–356.

Giorgi, F. S., Velíšková, J., Chudomel, O., Kyrozis, A., and Moshé, S. L. (2006). The role of substantia nigra pars reticulata in modulating clonic seizures is determined by testosterone levels during the immediate postnatal period. *Neurobiol Dis.* **25,** 73–79.

Girdler, S., Straneva, P., Light, K., Pedersen, C., and Morrow, L. (2001). Allopregnanolone levels and reactivity to mental stress in premenstrual dysphoric disorder. *Biol. Psychiatry* **49,** 788–797.

Glass, M., and Dragunow, M. (1995). Neurochemical and morphological changes associated with human epilepsy. *Brain Res. Brain Res. Rev.* **21**(1), 29–41.

Gloor, P., Pellegrini, A., and Kostopoulos, G. K. (1979). Effects of changes in cortical excitability upon the epileptic bursts in generalized penicillin epilepsy of the cat. *Electroencephalogr. Clin. Neurophysiol.* **46,** 274–289.

Goldman, L., Winget, C., Hollingshead, G. W., and Levine, S. (1973). Postweaning development of negative feedback in the pituitary-adrenal system of the rat. *Neuroendocrinology* **12,** 199–211.

Gore, A. C., and Terasawa, E. (2001). Neural circuits regulating pulsatile luteinizing hormone release in the female guinea-pig: Opioid, adrenergic and serotonergic interactions. *J. Neuroendocrinol.* **13** (3), 239–248.

Gowers, W. R. (1881). "Epilepsy and other Chronic Convulsive Diseases." J. A. Churchill, London.

Grisham, W., Lee, J., McCormick, M. E., Yang-Stayner, K., and Arnold, A. P. (2002). Antiandrogen blocks estrogen-induced masculinization of the song system in female zebra finches. *J. Neurobiol.* **51,** 1–8.

Grunewald, R. A., Aliberti, V., and Panayiotopoulos, C. P. (1992). Exacerbation of typical absence seizures by progesterone. *Seizure* **1,** 137–138.

Gulinello, M., Gong, Q. H., Li, X., and Smith, S. S. (2001). Short-term exposure to a neuroactive-steroid increases alpha4 GABA(A) receptor subunit levels in association with increased anxiety in the female rat. *Brain Res.* **910**(1–2), 55–66.

Hagihara, K., Hirata, S., Osada, T., Hirai, M., and Kato, J. (1992). Distribution of cells containing progesterone receptor mRNA in the female rat di- and telencephalon: An *in situ* hybridization study. *Brain Res. Mol. Brain Res.* **14,** 239–249.

Hall, S. M. (1977). Treatment of menstrual epilepsy with a progesterone-only oral contraceptive. *Epilepsia* **18,** 235–236.

Harden, C. L., Pulver, M. C., Ravdin, L., and Jacobs, A. R. (1999). The effect of menopause and perimenopause on the course of epilepsy. *Epilepsia* **40,** 1402–1407.

Hauser, W. A., Annegers, J. F., and Kurland, L. T. (1993). Incidence of epilepsy and unprovoked seizures in Rochester, Minnesota: 1935–1984. *Epilepsia* **34,** 453–468.

Hawkinson, J. E., Kimbrough, C. L., Belelli, D., Lambert, J. J., Purdy, R. H., and Lan, N. C. (1994). Correlation of neuroactive steroid modulation of [35 S]t-butylbicyclophosphorothionate and [3 H]flunitrazepam binding and ã −aminobutyric acidA receptor function. *Mol. Pharmacol.* **46,** 977–985.

Hedblom, E., and Kirkness, E. F. (1997). A novel class of GABA receptor A subunit in tissues of the reproductive system. *J. Biol. Chem.* **272,** 15346–15350.

Herzog, A. G. (1986). Intermittent progesterone therapy and frequency of complex partial seizures in women with menstrual disorders. *Neurology* **36**(12), 1607–1610.

Herzog, A. G. (1988). Clomiphene therapy in epileptic women with menstrual disorders. *Neurology* **38,** 432–434.

Herzog, A. G. (1991). Reproductive endocrine considerations and hormonal therapy for men with epilepsy. *Epilepsia* **32**(6), 34–37.

Herzog, A. G. (1995). Progesterone therapy in women with complex partial and secondary generalized seizures. *Neurology* **45,** 1660–1662.

Herzog, A. G., Seibel, M. M., Schomer, D. L., Vaitukaitis, J. L., and Geschwind, N. (1986). Reproductive endocrine disorders in women with partial seizures of temporal lobe origin. *Arch. Neurol.* **43**(4), 341–346.

Herzog, A. G., Drislane, F. W., Schomer, D. L., Levesque, L. A., Ives, J., Blume, H. W., Dubuisson, D., and Cosgrove, G. R. (1990). Abnormal pulsatile secretion of luteinizing hormone in men with epilepsy: Relationship to laterality and nature of paroxysmal discharges. *Neurology* **40**(10), 1557–1561.

Heroz, A. G., Levesque, L. A., Drislane, F. W., Ronthal, M., and Schomer, D. L. (1991). Phenytoin-induced elevation of serum estradiol and reproductive dysfunction in men with epilepsy. *Epilepsia* **32**(4), 550–553.

Herzog, A. G., Klein, P., and Ransil, B. J. (1997). Three patterns of catamenial epilepsy. *Epilepsia* **38,** 1082–1088.

Herzog, A. G., Klein, P., and Jacobs, A. R. (1998). Testosterone versus testosterone and testolactone in treating reproductive and sexual dysfunction in men with epilepsy and hypogonadism. *Neurology* **50,** 782–784.

Herzog, A. G., Coleman, A. E., Jacobs, A. R., Klein, P., Friedman, M. N., Drislane, F. W., and Schomer, D. L. (2003). Relationship of sexual dysfunction to epilepsy laterality and reproductive hormone levels in women. *Epilepsy Behav.* **4**(4), 407–413.

Herzog, A. G., Drislane, F. W., Schomer, D. L., Pennell, P. B., Bromfield, E. B., Kelly, K. M., Farina, E. L., and Frye, C. A. (2004a). Differential effects of antiepileptic drugs on sexual function and reproductive hormones in men with epilepsy: Interim analysis of a comparison between lamotrigine and enzyme-inducing antiepileptic drugs. *Epilepsia* **45**(7), 764–768.

Herzog, A. G., Harden, C. L., Liporace, J., Pennell, P., Schomer, D. L., Sperling, M., Fowler, K., Nikolov, B., Shuman, S., and Newman, M. (2004b). Frequency of catamenial seizure exacerbation in women with localization-related epilepsy. *Ann. Neurol.* **56,** 431–434.

Herzog, A. G., Drislane, F. W., Schomer, D. L., Pennell, P. B., Bromfield, E. B., Dworetzky, B. A., Farina, E. L., and Frye, C. A. (2005). Differential effects of antiepileptic drugs on sexual function and hormones in men with epilepsy. *Neurology* **65**(7), 1016–1020.

Herzog, A. G., Drislane, F. W., Schomer, D. L., Pennell, P. B., Bromfield, E. B., Dworetzky, B. A., Farina, E. L., and Frye, C. A. (2006). Differential effects of antiepileptic drugs on neuroactive steroids in men with epilepsy. *Epilepsia* **47**(11), 1945–1948.

Hevers, W., and Luddens, H. (1998). The diversity of GABAA receptors: Pharmacological and electrophysiological properties of GABAA channel subtypes. *Mol. Neurobiol.* **18**, 35–86.

Hill, M., Bicikova, M., Parizek, A., Havlikova, H., Klak, J., Fajt, T., Meloun, M., Cibula, D., Cegan, A., Sulcova, J., Hampl, R., and Starka, L. (2001). Neuroactive-steroids, their precursors and polar conjugates during parturition and postpartum in maternal blood: 2. Time profiles of pregnanolone isomers. *J. Steroid Biochem. Mol. Biol.* **78**(1), 51–57.

Hoffman, G. E., Moore, N., Fiskum, G., and Murphy, A. Z. (2003). Ovarian steroid modulation of seizure severity and hippocampal cell death after kainic acid treatment. *Exp. Neurol.* **182**, 124–134.

Hom, A. C., and Buterbaugh, G. G. (1986). Estrogen alters the acquisition of seizures kindled by repeated amygdala stimulation or pentylenetetrazol administration in ovariectomized female rats. *Epilepsia* **27**, 103–108.

Hong, J. S., McGinty, J. F., Grimes, L., Kanamatsu, T., Obie, J., and Mitchell, C. L. (1988). Seizure-induced alterations in the metabolism of hippocampal opioid peptides suggest opioid modulation of seizure-related behaviors. *NIDA Res. Monogr.* **82**, 48–66.

Hoppe, U., Holterhus, P. M., Wunsch, L., Jocham, D., Drechsler, T., Thiele, S., Marschke, C., and Hiort, O. (2006). Tissue-specific transcription profiles of sex steroid biosynthesis enzymes and the androgen receptor. *J. Mol. Med.* **84**(8), 651–659.

Hu, M. C., Hsu, H. J., Guo, I. C., and Chung, B. C. (2004). Function of CYP11A1 in animal models. *Mol. Cell. Endocrinol.* **215**(1–2), 95–100.

Huang, L. T., Holmes, G. L., Lai, M. C., Hung, P. L., Wang, C. L., Wang, T. J., Yang, C. H., Liou, C. W., and Yang, S. N. (2002). Maternal deprivation stress exacerbates cognitive deficits in immature rats with recurrent seizures. *Epilepsia* **43**, 1141–1148.

Iadarola, M. J., and Gale, K. (1981). Cellular compartments of GABA in brain and their relationship to anticonvulsant activity. *Mol. Cell. Biochem.* **39**, 305–330.

Ing, N. H. (2005). Steroid hormones regulate gene expression posttranscriptionally by altering the stabilities of messenger RNAs. *Biol. Reprod.* **72**(6), 1290–1296.

Isojarvi, J. I., Pakarinen, A. J., and Myllyla, V. V. (1989). Effects of carbamazepine on the hypothalamic-pituitary-gonadal axis in male patients with epilepsy: A prospective study. *Epilepsia* **30**, 446–452.

Isojarvi, J. I., Repo, M., Pakarinen, A. J., Lukkarinen, O., and Myllyla, V. V. (1995). Carbamazepine, phenytoin, sex hormones, and sexual function in men with epilepsy. *Epilepsia* **36**, 366–370.

Isojärvi, J. I., Löfgren, E., Juntunen, K. S., Pakarinen, A. J., Päivänsalo, M., Rautakorpi, I., and Tuomivaara, L. (2004). Effect of epilepsy and antiepileptic drugs on male reproductive health. *Neurology* **62**(2), 247–253.

Jorge-Rivera, J. C., McIntyre, K. L., and Henderson, L. P. (2000). Anabolic steroids induce region- and subunit-specific rapid modulation of GABA(A) receptor-mediated currents in the rat forebrain. *J. Neurophysiol.* **83**, 3299–3309.

Kalkbrenner, K. A., and Standley, C. A. (2003). Estrogen modulation of NMDA-induced seizures in ovariectomized and non-ovariectomized rats. *Brain Res.* **964**, 244–249.

Kawakami, M., and Terasawa, E. (1972). Acute effect of neural deafferentation on timing of gonadotropin secretion before proestrus in the female rat. *Endocrinol. Jpn.* **19**(5), 449–459.

Kim, J. S., Kim, H. Y., Kim, J. H., Shin, H. K., Lee, S. H., Lee, Y. S., and Son, H. (2002). Enhancement of rat hippocampal long-term potentiation by 17 beta-estradiol i nvolves mitogen-activated protein kinase-dependent and -independent components. *Neurosci. Lett.* **332,** 65–69.

Klein, P., Van Passel-Clark, L. M., and Pezzullo, J. C. (2003). Onset of epilepsy at the time of menarche. *Neurology* **60,** 495–497.

Knight, A. H., and Rhind, E. G. (1975). Epilepsy and pregnancy: A study of 153 pregnancies in 59 patients. *Epilepsia* **16,** 99–110.

Kobayashi, M., and Buckmaster, P. S. (2003). Reduced inhibition of dentate granule cells in a model of temporal lobe epilepsy. *J. Neurosci.* **23**(6), 2440–2452.

Kokate, T. G., Svensson, B. E., and Rogawski, M. A. (1994). Anticonvulsant activity of neurosteroids: Correlation with ã-aminobutyric acid-evoked chloride current potentiation. *J. Pharmacol. Exp. Ther.* **270,** 1223–1229.

Kokate, T. G., Cohen, A. L., Karp, E., and Rogawski, M. A. (1996). Neuroactive steroids protect against pilocarpine- and kainic acid–induced limbic seizures and status epilepticus in mice. *Neuropharmacology* **35,** 1049–1056.

Kokate, T. G., Banks, M. K., Magee, T., Yamaguchi, S., and Rogawski, M. A. (1999). Finasteride, a 5alpha-reductase inhibitor, blocks the anticonvulsant activity of progesterone in mice. *J. Pharmacol. Exp. Ther.* **288**(2), 679–684.

Kostopoulos, G. (2000). Spike and wave discharges of absence seizures as a transformation of sleep spindles: The continuing development of a hypothesis. *Clin. Neurophysiol.* **111**(S2), 27–38.

Krueger, K. E., and Papadopoulos, V. (1990). Peripheral-type benzodiazepine receptors mediate translocation of cholesterol from outer to inner mitochondrial membranes in adrenocortical cells. *J. Biol. Chem.* **265,** 15015–15022.

Lai, M. C., Holmes, G. L., Lee, K. H., Yang, S. N., Wang, C. A., Wu, C. L., Tiao, M. M., Hsieh, C. S., Lee, C. H., and Huang, L. T. (2006). Effect of neonatal isolation on outcome following neonatal seizures in rats—the role of corticosterone. *Epilepsy Res.* **68**(2), 123–136.

Laidlaw, J. (1956). Catamenial epilepsy. *Lancet* **2,** 1235–1237.

Lan, N. C., Bolger, M. B., and Gee, K. W. (1991). Identification and characterization of a pregnane steroid recognition site that is functionally coupled to an expressed GABAA receptor. *Neurochem Res.* **16,** 347–356.

Landgren, S., Bäckström, T., and Kalistratov, G. (1978). The effect of progesterone on the spontaneous interictal spike evoked 'by the application of penicillin to the cat's cerebral cortex. *J. Neurol. Sci.* **36,** 119–133.

Lason, W., Przewlocka, B., Coenen, A., Przewlocki, R., and Van Luijtelaar, G. (1994). Effects of mu and delta opioid receptor agonists and antagonists on absence epilepsy in WAG/Rij rats. *Neuropharmacology* **33**(2), 161–166.

Lennox, W. G., and Lennox, M. A. (1960). Chapter 19: Sympathetic seizures. *In* "Epilepsy and Related Disorders."Vol. 2, pp. 638–658. Little Brown, Boston, MA.

Leranth, C., Petnehazy, O., and MacLusky, N. J. (2003). Gonadal hormones affect spine synaptic density in the CA1 hippocampal subfield of male rats. *J. Neurosci.* **23,** 1588–1592.

Levine, J. E., and Ramirez, V. D. (1982). Luteinizing hormone-releasing hormone release during the rat estrous cycle and after ovariectomy, as estimated with push-pull cannulae. *Endocrinology* **111,** 1439.

Levita, L., Hammack, S. E., Mania, I., Li, X. Y., Davis, M., and Rainnie, D. G. (2004). 5-hydroxytryptamine1A-like receptor activation in the bed nucleus of the stria terminalis: Electrophysiological and behavioral studies. *Neuroscience* **128,** 583–596.

Locock, C. (1857). Discussion of paper by EH Sieveking. Analysis of cases of epilepsy observed by the author. *Lancet 1* **52,** 527–528.

Logothetis, J., and Harner, R. (1960). Electrocortical activation by estrogens. *Arch. Neurol.* **3,** 290–297.

Logothetis, J., Harner, R., Morrell, F., *et al.* (1958). The role of estrogens in catamenial exacerbation of epilepsy. *Neurology (Minneap)* **9,** 352–360.

Logothetis, J., Harner, R., Morrel, F., and Torres, F. (1959). The role of estrogens in catamenial exacerbation of epilepsy. *Neurology* **9**(5), 352–360.

Lothman, E. W., Bertram, E. H., 3rd., and Stringer, J. L. (1991). Functional anatomy of hippocampal seizures. *Prog. Neurobiol.* **37**, 1–82.

Luisi, S., Petraglia, F., Benedetto, C., Nappi, R. E., Bernardi, F., Fadalti, M., Reis, F. M., Luisi, M., and Genazzani, A. R. (2000). Serum allopregnanolone levels in pregnant women: Changes during pregnancy, at delivery, and in hypertensive patients. *J. Clin. Endocrinol. Metab.* **85**(7), 2429–2433.

MacLennan, A., Lester, S., and Moore, V. (2001). Oral oestrogen re-placement therapy versus placebo for hot flushes. *Cochrane Database Syst. Rev.* **1**, CD002978.

Macphee, G. J., Larkin, J. G., Butler, E., Beastall, G. H., and Brodie, M. J. (1988). Circulating hormones and pituitary responsiveness in young epileptic men receiving long-term antiepileptic medication. *Epilepsia* **29**(4), 468–475.

Mahendroo, M. S., Cala, K. M., Landrum, D. P., and Russell, D. W. (1997). Fetal death in mice lacking 5alpha-Reductase type 1 caused by estrogen excess. *Mol. Endocrinol.* **11**, 917–927.

Majewska, M. D. (1992). Neurosteroids: Endogenous bimodal modulators of the GABAA receptor. Mechanism of action and physiological significance. *Prog. Neurobiol.* **38**, 379–395.

Malendowicz, L. K. (1976). Sex differences in adrenocortical structure and function. III. The effects of postpubertal gonadectomy and gonadal hormone replacement on adrenal cholesterol sidechain cleavage activity and on steroids biosynthesis by rat adrenal homogenates. *Endokrinologie* **67**, 26–35.

Marcus, E. M., Watson, C. W., and Goldman, P. L. (1966). Effects of steroids on cerebral electrical activity. *Arch. Neurol.* **15**, 521–532.

Margerison, J. H., and Corsellis, J. A. (1966). Epilepsy and the temporal lobes. A clinical, electroencephalographic and neuropathological study of the brain in epilepsy, with particular reference to the temporal lobes. *Brain* **89**, 499–530.

Marshall, F. H., Stratton, S. C., Mullings, J., Ford, E., Worton, S. P., Oakley, N. R., and Hagan, R. M. (1997). Development of tolerance in mice to the sedative effects of the neuroactive steroid minaxolone following chronic exposure. *Pharmacol. Biochem. Behav.* **58**, 1–8.

Martin, I. L., and Dunn, S. M. J. (2002). GABA receptors. Review written on request by Tocris, www.tocris.com.

Marx, C. E., VanDoren, M. J., Duncan, G. E., Lieberman, J. A., and Morrow, A. L. (2003). Olanzapine and clozapine increase the GABAergic neuroactive steroid allopregnanolone in rodents. *Neuropsychopharmacology* **28**, 1–13.

Masia, S. L., Perrine, K., Westbrook, L., Alper, K., and Devinsky, O. (2000). Emotional outbursts and posttraumatic stress disorder during intracarotid amobarbital procedure. *Neurology* **54**, 1691–1693.

Mattson, R. H., and Cramer, J. A. (1985). Epilepsy, sex hormones and antiepileptic drugs. *Epilepsia* **26**, S40–S51.

Mattson, R. H., Cramer, J. A., and Caldwell, B. V. (1981). Seizure frequency and the menstrual cycle: A clinical study. *Epilepsia* **22**, 242.

Mattson, R. H., Cramer, J. A., Caldwell, B. V., and Siconolfi, B. C. (1984). Treatment of seizures with medroxyprogesterone acetate: Preliminary report. *Neurology* **34**, 1255–1258.

McCarthy, M. M., and Konkle, A. T. (2005). When is a sex difference not a sex difference. *Front. Neuroendocrinol.* **26**, 85–102.

McCarthy, M. M., Felzenberg, E., Robbins, A., Pfaff, D. W., and Schwartz-Giblin, S. (1995). Infusions of diazepam and allopregnanolone into the midbrain central gray facilitate open-field behavior and sexual receptivity in female rats. *Horm. Behav.* **29**, 279–295.

McEwen, B. S., and Woolley, C. S. (1994). Estradiol and progesterone regulate neuronal structure and synaptic connectivity in adult as well as developing brain. *Exp. Gerontol.* **29**, 431–436.

McNamara, J. O. (1994). Cellular and molecular basis of epilepsy. *J. Neurosci.* **14**, 3413–3425.

Medina, J. H., Novas, M. L., Wolfman, C. N., Levi de Stein, M., and De Robertis, E. (1983). Benzodiazepine receptors in rat cerebral cortex and hippocampus undergo rapid and reversible changes alter acute stress. *Neuroscience* **9**, 331–335.

Meeren, H. K., Pijn, J. P., Van Luijtelaar, E. L., Coenen, A. M., and Lopes da Silva, F. H. (2002). Cortical focus drives widespread corticothalamic networks during spontaneous absence seizures in rats. *J. Neurosci.* **22**, 1480–1495.

Mehta, A. K., and Ticku, M. K. (1999). An update on GABA$_A$ receptors. *Brain Res. Rev.* **29**, 196–217.

Mejias-Aponte, C. A., Jimenez-Rivera, C. A., and Segarra, A. C. (2002). Sex differences in models of temporal lobe epilepsy: Role of testosterone. *Brain Res.* **944**, 210–218.

Melcangi, R. C., and Panzica, C. (2001). Steroids in the nervous system: Pandora's box? *Trends Neurosci.* **24**, 311–312.

Melcangi, R. C., Poletti, A., Cavarretta, I., Celotti, F., Colciago, A., Magnaghi, V., Motta, M., Negri-Cesi, P., and Martini, L. (1998). The 5α-reductase in the central nervous system: Expression and modes of control. *J. Steroid Biochem. Mol. Biol.* **65**, 295–299.

Mellon, S. H. (1994). Neurosteroids: Biochemistry, modes of action, and clinical relevance. *J. Clin. Endocrinol. Metab.* **78**, 1003–1008.

Meo, R., Bilo, L., Nappi, C., Tommaselli, A. P., Valentino, R., Nocerino, C., Striano, S, and Buscaino, G.A (1993). Derangement of the hypothalamic GnRH pulse generator in women with epilepsy. *Seizure* **2**, 241–252.

Meyer, G., Ferres-Torres, R., and Mas, M. (1978). The effects of puberty and castration on hippocampal dendritic spines of mice. A Golgi study. *Brain Res.* **155**, 108–112.

Miczek, K. A., DeBold, J. F., van Erp, A. M., and Tornatzky, W. (1997). Alcohol, GABA$_A$–benzodiazepine receptor complex, and aggression. *Recent Dev. Alcohol.* **13**, 139–171.

Miczek, K. A., Fish, E. W., and De Bold, J. F. (2003). Neurosteroids, GABA$_A$ receptors, and escalated aggressive behavior. *Horm. Behav.* **44**, 242–257.

Mirescu, C., Peters, J. D., and Gould, E. (2004). Early life experience alters response of adult neurogenesis to stress. *Nat. Neurosci.* **7**, 841–846.

Mormède, P., Courvoisier, H., Ramos, A., Marissal-Arvy, N., Ousova, O., Desautes, C., Duclos, M., Chaouloff, F., and Moisan, M. P. (2002). Molecular genetic approaches to investigate individual variations in behavioral and neuroendocrine stress responses. *Psychoneuroendocrinology* **27**, 563–583.

Morrell, M. J. (1999). Epilepsy and women: The science of why it is special. *Neurology* **53**, 42–47.

Morrell, M. J. (2003). Reproductive and metabolic disorders in women with epilepsy. *Epilepsia* **44**, 11–20.

Morrell, M. J., Flynn, K. L., Seale, C. G., Done, S., Paulson, A. J., Flaster, E. R., and Ferin, M. (2001). Reproductive dysfunction in women with epilepsy: Antiepileptic drug effects on sex-steroid hormones. *CNS Spectr.* **6**, 771–786.

Moses-Kolko, E. L., Berga, S. L., Greer, P. J., Smith, G., Cidis Meltzer, C., and Drevets, W. C. (2003). Widespread increases of cortical serotonin type 2A receptor availability after hormone therapy in euthymic postmenopausal women. *Fertil. Steril.* **80**, 554–911.

Moshé, S. L., Sperber, E. F., Brown, L. L., and Tempel, A. (1992). Age-dependent changes in substantia nigra GABA-mediated seizure suppression. *Epilepsy Res. Suppl.* **8**, 97–106.

Mukhin, A. G., Papadopoulos, V., Costa, E., and Krueger, K. E. (1989). Mitochondrial benzodiazepine receptors regulate steroid biosynthesis. *Proc. Natl. Acad. Sci. USA* **86**, 9813–9816.

Murialdo, G., Galimberti, C. A., Fonzi, S., Manni, R., Costelli, P., Parodi, C., Torre, F., Solinas, G. P., Polleri, A., and Tartara, A. (1994). Sex hormones, gonadotropins and prolactin in male epileptic subjects in remission: Role of the epileptic syndrome and of antiepileptic drugs. *Neuropsychobiology* **30**, 29–36.

Murialdo, G., Galimberti, C. A., Fonzi, S., Manni, R., Costelli, P., Parodi, C., Solinas, G. P., Amoretti, G., and Tartara, A., (1995). Sex hormones and pituitary function in male epileptic patients with altered or normal sexuality. *Epilepsia.* **36**(4), 360–5.

Negro-Vilar, A., Ojeda, S. A., and McCann, S. (1979). Catecholaminegric modulation of luteinizing hormone-releasing hormone release by median eminence terminals *in vitro*. *Endocrinology* **104**, 1749–1757.

Newmark, N. E., and Penry, J. K. (1980). Catamenial epilepsy: A review. *Epilepsia* **21**, 281–300.

Nicoletti, F., Speciale, C., Sortino, M. A., Summa, G., Caruso, G., Patti, F., and Canonico, P. L. (1985). Comparative effects of estradiol benzoate, the antiestrogen clomiphene citrate, and the progestin medroxyprogesterone acetate on kainic acid-induced seizures in male and female rats. *Epilepsia* **26**, 252–257.

Norberg, L., Wahlström, G., and Bäckström, T. (1987). The anaesthetic potency of 3 alpha-hydroxy-5 alphapregnan-20-one and 3 alpha-hydroxy-5 beta-pregnan-20-one determined with an intravenous EEG threshold method in male rats. *Pharmacol. Toxicol.* **61**, 42–47.

Ojeda, S., Nego-Vilar, A., and McCann, S. (1982). Evidence for involvement of a-adrenergic receptors in norepinephrine induced prostaglandin E2 and luteinizing hormone-releasing hormone release from the median eminence. *Endocrinology* **110**, 409–412.

Osterlund, M. K., and Hurd, Y. L. (1998). Acute 17 beta-estradiol treatment down-regulates serotonin 5HT1A receptor mRNA expression in the limbic system of female rats. *Brain Res. Mol. Brain Res.* **55**, 169–172.

Osterlund, M. K., Grandien, K., Keller, E., and Hurd, Y. L. (2000a). The human brain has distinct regional expression patterns of estrogen receptor alpha mRNA isoforms derived from alternative promoters. *J. Neurochem.* **75**(4), 1390–1397.

Osterlund, M. K., Gustafsson, J. A., Keller, E., and Hurd, Y. L. (2000b). Estrogen receptor beta (ERbeta) messenger ribonucleic acid (mRNA) expression within the human forebrain: Distinct distribution pattern to ERalpha mRNA. *J. Clin. Endocrinol. Metab.* **85**(10), 3840–3846.

Ottander, U., Sundström Poromaa, I., Bjurulf, E., Skytt, A., Bäckström, T., and Olofsson, J. I. (2005). Allopregnanolone and pregnanolone are produced by the human corpus luteum. *Mol. Cell. Endocrinol.* **239**, 37–44.

Pfaff, D. W., Gerlach, J. L., McEwen, B. S., Ferin, M., Carmel, P., and Zimmerman, E. A. (1976). Autoradiographic localization of hormone-concentrating cells in the brain of the female rhesus monkey. *J. Comp. Neurol.* **170**(3), 279–293.

Palmer, A. A., Moyer, M. R., Crabbe, J. C., and Phillips, T. J. (2002). Initial sensitivity, tolerance and cross-tolerance to allopregnanolone-and ethanol-induced hypothermia in selected mouse lines. *Psychopharmacology* **162**, 313–322.

Panesar, S. K., Bandiera, S. M., and Abbott, F. S. (1996). Comparative effects of carbamazepine and carbamazepine-10,11-epoxide on hepatic cytochromes P450 in the rat. *Drug Metab. Dispos.* **24**, 619–627.

Panzica, G. C., and Melcangi, R. C. (2004). "Steroids and the Nervous System." p. 1007. Annals of New York Academy of Science.

Park-Chung, M., Malayev, A., Purdy, R. H., Gibbs, T. T., and Farb, D. H. (1999). Sulfated and unsulfated steroids modulate ã-aminobutyric acid receptor A function through distinct sites. *Brain Res.* **830**, 72–87.

Patchev, V. K., Hassan, A. H., Holsboer, D. F., and Almeida, O. F. (1996). The neurosteroid tetrahydroprogesterone attenuates the endocrine response to stress and exerts glucocorticoid-like effects on vasopressin gene transcription in the rat hypothalamus. *Neuropsychopharmacology* **15**, 533–540.

Paul, S. M., and Purdy, R. H. (1992). Neuroactive steroids. *Faseb J.* **6**, 2311–2322.

Payne, A. H., and Hales, D. B. (2004). Overview of steroidogenic enzymes in the pathway from cholesterol to active steroid hormones. *Endocr. Rev.* **25**, 947–970.

Pearlstein, T. B. (1995). Hormones and depression: What are the facts about premenstrual syndrome, menopause, and hormone replacement therapy? *Am. J. Obstet. Gynecol.* **173**, 646–653.

Persengiev, S., Kanchev, L., and Vezenkova, G. (1991). Circadian patterns of melatonin, corticosterone, and progesterone in male rats subjected to chronic stress: Effect of constant illumination. *J. Pineal Res.* **11,** 57–62.

Peters, J. A., Kirkness, E. F., Callachan, H., Lambert, J. J., and Turner, A. J. (1988). Modulation of the GABA$_A$ receptor by depressant barbiturates and pregnane steroids. *Br. J. Pharmacol.* **94,** 1257–1269.

Poletti, A., Coscarella, A., Negri-Cesi, P., Colciago, A., Celotti, F., and Martini, L. (1998). 5 alpha-Reductase isozymes in the central nervous system. *Steroids* **63,** 246–251.

Poór, V., Juricskay, S., Gáti, A., Osváth, P., and Tényi, T. (2004). Urinary steroid metabolites and 11 â-hydroxysteroid dehydrogenase activity in patients with unipolar recurrent major depression. *J. Affect. Disord.* **81,** 55–59.

Pouliot, W. A., Handa, R. J., and Beck, S. G. (1996). Androgen modulates N-methyl-D-aspartate-mediated depolarization in CA1 hippocampal pyramidal cells. *Synapse* **23,** 10–19.

Price, J. L. (2003). Comparative aspects of amygdala connectivity. *Ann. N. Y. Acad. Sci.* **985,** 50–58.

Pritchard, P. B., III., Wannamaker, B. B., Sagel, J., Nair, R., and DeVillier, C. (1983). Endocrine function following complex partial seizures. *Ann. Neurol.* **14,** 27–32.

Pryce, C. R., Ruedi-Bettschen, D., Dettling, A. C., Weston, A., Russig, H., Ferger, B., and Feldon, J. (2005). Long-term effects of early-life environmental manipulations in rodents and primates: Potential animal models in depression research. *Neurosci. Biobehav. Rev.* **29,** 649–674.

Purdy, R. H., Moore, P. H., Jr., Rao, P. N., Hagino, N., Yamaguchi, T., Schmidt, P., Rubinow, D. R., Morrow, A. L., and Paul, S. M. (1990). Radioimmuno-assay of 3 alpha-hydroxy-5 alpha-pregnan-20-one in rat and human plasma. *Steroids* **55,** 290–296.

Purdy, R. H., Morrow, A. L., Moore, P. H., and Paul, S. M. (1991). Stress-induced elevations of gamma-aminobutyric acid type A receptor-active steroids in the rat brain. *Proc. Natl. Acad. Sci. USA* **88,** 4553–4557.

Racine, R. J. (1972). Modification of seizure activity by electrical stimulation. II. *Motor seizure. Electroencephalogr. Clin. Neurophysiol.* **32**(3), 281–294.

Rang, H., Dale, M., and Ritter, J. (1995). "Pharmacology." pp. 512–561. Churchill Livingstone, Edinburgh.

Rannevik, G., Jeppsson, S., Johnell, O., Bjerre, B., Laurell-Borulf, Y., and Svanberg, L. (1995). A longitudinal study of the perimenopausal transition: Altered profiles of steroid and pituitary hormones, SHBG and bone mineral density. *Maturitas* **21,** 103–113.

Ravizza, T., Friedman, L. K., Moshé, S. L., and Velíšková, J. (2003). Sex differences in GABA(A)ergic system in rat substantia nigra pars reticulata. *Int. J. Dev. Neurosci.* **21,** 245–254.

Reddy, D. S. (2004). Role of neurosteroids in catamenial epilepsy. *Epilepsy Res.* **62,** 99–118.

Reddy, D. S., and Rogawski, M. A. (2000). Chronic treatment with the neuroactive-steroid ganaxolone in the rat induces anticonvulsant tolerance to diazepam but not to itself. *J. Pharmacol. Exp. Ther.* **295,** 1241–1248.

Reddy, D. S., and Rogawski, M. A. (2002). Stress-induced deoxycorticosterone-derived neurosteroids modulate GABAA receptor function and seizure susceptibility. *J. Neurosci.* **22,** 3795–3805.

Reibel, S., Andre, V., Chassagnon, S., Andre, G., Marescaux, C., Nehlig, A., and Depaulis, A. (2000). Neuroprotective effects of chronic estradiol benzoate treatment on hippocampal cell loss induced by status epilepticus in the female rat. *Neurosci. Lett.* **281,** 79–82.

Renaud, L. P., and Hopkins, D. A. (1977). Amygdala afferents from the mediobasal hypothalamus: An electrophysiological and neuroanatomical study in the rat. *Brain Res.* **121**(2), 201–213.

Resko, J. A., Stadelman, H. L., and Handa, R. J. (1986). Control of 5α-reduction of testosterone in neuroendocrine tissues of female rats. *Biol. Reprod.* **34,** 870–877.

Rhodes, M. E., and Frye, C. A. (2004a). Androgens in the hippocampus can alter, and be altered by, ictal activity. *Pharmacol. Biochem. Behav.* **78,** 483–493.

Rhodes, M. E., and Frye, C. A. (2004b). Progestins in the hippocampus of female rats have antiseizure effects in a pentylenetetrazole seizure model. *Epilepsia* **45,** 1531–1538.

Rittmaster, R. S., Leopold, C. A., and Thompson, D. L. (1989). Androgen glucuronyl transferase activity in rat liver, evidence for the importance of hepatic tissue in 5 á-reduced androgen metabolism. *J. Steroid Biochem.* **33,** 1207–1212.

Robel, P., Bourreau, E., Corpechot, C., Dang, D. C., Halberg, F., Clarke, C., Haug, M., Schlegel, M. L., Synguelakis, M., and Vourch, C. (1987). Neurosteroids: 3 Beta-hydroxy-delta 5-derivatives in rat and 501 monkey brain. *J. Steroid Biochem.* **27,** 649–655.

Romeo, R. D., Lee, S. J., Chhua, N., McPherson, C. R., and McEwen, B. S. (2004a). Testosterone cannot activate an adult-like stress response in prepubertal male rats. *Neuroendocrinology* **79,** 125–132.

Romeo, R. D., Lee, S. J., and McEwen, B. S. (2004b). Differential stress reactivity in intact and ovariectomized prepubertal and adult female rats. *Neuroendocrinology* **80,** 387–393.

Rosciszewska, D. (1975). The course of epilepsy in girls at the age of puberty. *Neurol. Neurochir. Pol.* **9,** 597–602.

Rosciszewska, D. (1978). Menopause in women and its effects on epilepsy. *Neurol. Neurochir. Pol.* **12,** 315–319.

Rosenbrock, H., Hagemeyer, C. E., Singec, I., Knoth, R., and Volk, B. (1999). Testosterone metabolism in rat brain is differentially enhanced by phenytoin-inducible cytochrome P450 isoforms. *J. Neuroendocrinol.* **11,** 597–604.

Sallusto, L., and Pozzi, O. (1964). Relations between ovarian activity and the occurrence of epileptic seizures: Data on a clinical case. *Acta. Neurol.* **19,** 673–681.

Sanchez, M. M., Ladd, C. O., and Plotsky, P. M. (2001). Early adverse experience as a developmental risk factor for later psychopathology: Evidence from rodent and primate models. *Dev. Psychopathol.* **13,** 419–449.

Sanchez, P., Torres, J. M., and Ortega, E. (2005). Effects of dihydrotestosterone on brain mRNA levels of steroid 5alpha-Reductase isozymes in early postnatal life of rat. *Neurochem. Res.* **30,** 577–581.

Sanchez, P., Torres, J. M., Del Moral, R. G., and Ortega, E. (2006). Effects of testosterone on brain mRNA levels of steroid 5alpha-Reductase isozymes in early postnatal life of rat. *Neurochem. Int.* **49,** 626–630.

Sanne, J. L., and Krueger, K. E. (1995). Expression of cytochrome P450 side chain cleavage enzyme 514 and 3_-hydroxysteroid dehydrogenase in the rat central nervous system: A study by 515 polymerase chain reaction and *in situ* hybridization. *J. Neurochem.* **65,** 528–536.

Schaeffer, C., and Aron, C. (1987). Stress-related effects on the secretion of progesterone by the adrenals in castrated male rats presented to a stimulus male. Involvement of oestrogen. *Acta. Endocrinol.* **114,** 440–445.

Schmidt, D., Canger, R., and Avanzini, G. (1985). Change of seizure frequency in pregnant epileptic women. *J. Neurol. Neurosurg. Psychiatry* **46,** 751–755.

Schmitz, C., Rhodes, M. E., Bludau, M., Kaplan, S., Ong, P., Ueffing, I., Vehoff, J., Korr, H., and Frye, C. A. (2002). Depression: Reduced number of granule cells in the hippocampus of female, but not male, rats due to prenatal restraint stress. *Mol. Psychiatry* **7,** 810–813.

Schwartz-Giblin, S., Korotzer, A., and Pfaff, D. W. (1989). Steroid hormone effects on picrotoxin-induced seizures in female and male rats. *Brain Res.* **476,** 240–247.

Sherwin, B. B., and Gelfand, M. M. (1989). A prospective one-year study of estrogen and progestin in postmenopausal women: Effects on clinical symptoms and lipoprotein lipids. *Obstet. Gynecol.* **73,** 759–766.

Selye, H. (1936). A syndrome produced by diverse nocuous agents. *Nature* **138,** 32–33.

Selye, H. (1941). The antagonism between anesthetic steroid hormones and pentamethylenetetrazol (Metrazol). *J. Lab. Clin. Med.* **27,** 1051–1053.

Serra, M., Sanna, E., Concas, A., Foddi, C., and Biggio, G. (1991). Foot shock stress enhanced the increase of [35 S] TBPS binding in the rat cerebral cortex and the convulsions induced by isoniazid. *Neurochem. Res.* **16,** 17–22.

Sharf, M., Sharf, B., Bental, E., and Kuzminsky, T. (1969). The electroencephalogram in the investigation of anovulation and its treatment by clomiphene. *Lancet* **1,** 750–753.

Sherwin, B. B. (1988). Affective changes with estrogen and androgen replacement therapy in surgically menopausal women. *J. Affect. Disord.* **14,** 177–187.

Shorvon, S. D. (1996). The epidemiology and treatment of chronic and refractory epilepsy. *Epilepsia* **37**(Suppl. 2), S1–S3.

Shughrue, P. J., Lane, M. V., and Merchenthaler, I. (1997). Comparative distribution of estrogen receptor-alpha and -beta mRNA in the rat central nervous system. *J. Comp. Neurol.* **388,** 507–525.

Sieghart, W. (1995). Structure and pharmacology of gamma-aminobutyric acidA receptor subtypes. *Pharmacol. Rev.* **47,** 181–234.

Silva, A. J., Stevens, C. F., Tonegawa, S., and Wang, Y. (1992). Deficient hippocampal long-term potentiation in alpha-calcium-calmodulin kinase II mutant mice. *Science* **257,** 201–206.

Silverman, A. J., Asarian, L., Khalil, M., and Silver, R. (2002). GnRH, brain mast cells and behavior. *Prog. Brain Res.* **141,** 315–325.

Simerly, R. B., Chang, C., Muramatsu, M., and Swanson, L. W. (1990). Distribution of androgen and estrogen receptor mRNA-containing cells in the rat brain: An *in situ* hybridization study. *J. Comp. Neurol.* **294,** 76–95.

Simon, R. P., Aminoff, M. J., and Benowitz, N. L. (1984). Changes in plasma catecholamines after tonic-clonic seizures. *Neurology* **34,** 255–257.

Slaunwhite, W. R., Jr., and Sandberg, A. A. (1958). Metabolism of 4-C 14-testosterone in human subjects. III. Fate of androsterone and etiocholanolone. *J. Clin. Endocrinol. Metab.* **18,** 1056–1066.

Smith, C. C., and McMahon, L. L. (2006). Estradiol-induced increase in the magnitude of long-term potentiation is prevented by blocking NR2B-containing receptors. *J. Neurosci.* **26,** 8517–8522.

Spiegel, E., and Wycis, H. (1945). Anticonvulsant effects of steroids. *J. Lab. Clin. Med.* **30,** 947–953.

Stitt, S. L., and Kinnard, R. J. (1968). The effect of certain progestins and estrogen on the threshold of electrically-induced seizure patterns. *Neurology* **18,** 213–216.

Stoffel-Wagner, B., Bauer, J., Flugel, D., Brennemann, W., Klingmuller, D., and Elger, C. E. (1998). Serum sex hormones are altered in patients with chronic temporal lobe epilepsy receiving anticonvulsant medication. *Epilepsia* **39,** 1164–1173.

Summer, B. E., and Fink, G. (1995). Estrogen increases the density of 5-hydroxytryptamine(2A) receptors in cerebral cortex and nucleus accumbens in the female rat. *J. Steroid Biochem. Mol. Biol.* **54,** 15–20.

Sundström, I., Ashbrook, D., and Bäckström, T. (1997). Reduced benzo-diazepine sensitivity in patients with premenstrual syndrome: A pilot study. *Psychoneuroendocrinology* **22,** 25–38.

Sundström, I., Andersson, A., Nyberg, S., Ashbrook, D., Purdy, R. H., and Bäckström, T. (1998). Patients with premenstrual syndrome have a different sensitivity to a neuroactive-steroid during the menstrual cycle compared to control subjects. *Neuroendocrinology* **67,** 126–138.

Sutula, T., and Ockuly, J. (2005). Kindling, spontaneous seizures, and the consequences of epilepsy: More than a model. *In* "Models of Seizures and Epilepsy" (A. Pitkanen, P. Schwartzkroin, and S. Moshe, Eds.), pp. 395–406. Elsevier, Amsterdam.

Taher, T. R., Salzberg, M., Morris, M. J., Rees, S., and O'Brien, T. J. (2005). Chronic low-dose corticosterone supplementation enhances acquired epileptogenesis in the rat amygdale kindling model of TLE. *Neuropsychopharmacology* **30,** 1610–1616.

Tasker, J. G., and Dudek, F. E. (1991). Electrophysiology of GABA-mediated synaptic transmission and possible roles in epilepsy. *Neurochem. Res.* **16,** 251–262.

Tauboll, E., Lundervold, A., and Gjerstad, L. (1991). Temporal distribution of seizures in epilepsy. *Epilepsy Res.* **8,** 153–165.

Tauck, D. L., and Nadler, J. V. (1985). Evidence of functional mossy fiber sprouting in hippocampal formation of kainic acid-treated rats. *J. Neurosci.* **5,** 1016–1022.

Tausk, M. (1984). Androgens and anabolic steroids. *In* "Discoveries in Pharmacology; Haemodynamics, Hormones and Inflammation" (M. J. Parnham and J. Bruinvels, Eds.), Vol. 2, pp. 307–320. Elsevier, Amsterdam.

Tominaga, K., Yamauchi, A., Shuto, Y., Niizeki, M., Makino, K., Oishi, R., and Kataoka, Y. (2001). Ovariectomy aggravates convulsions and hippocampal gamma-aminobutyric acid inhibition induced by cyclosporin A in rats. *Eur. J. Pharmacol.* **430,** 243–249.

Torres, J. M., and Ortega, E. (2003a). Differential regulation of steroid 5alpha-Reductase isozymes expression by androgens in the adult rat brain. *Faseb J.* **17,** 1428–1433.

Torres, J. M., and Ortega, E. (2003b). Alcohol intoxication increases allopregnanolone levels in female adolescent humans. *Neuropsychopharmacology* **28,** 1207–1209.

Torres, J. M., and Ortega, E. (2004). Alcohol intoxication increases allopregnanolone levels in male adolescent humans. *Psychopharmacology* **172,** 352–355.

Torres, J. M., and Ortega, E. (2006). Steroid 5alpha-Reductase isozymes in the adult female rat brain: Central role of dihydrotestosterone. *J. Mol. Endocrinol.* **36,** 239–245.

Torres, J. M., Ruiz, E., and Ortega, E. (2001). Effects of CRH and ACTH administration on plasma and brain neurosteroid levels. *Neurochem. Res.* **26,** 555–558.

Trimble, M. R. (1978). Serum prolactin in epilepsy and hysteria. *Br. Med. J.* **2,** 1682.

Turner, D. M., Ransom, R. W., Yang, J. S., and Olsen, R. W. (1989). Steroid anesthetics and naturally occurring analogs modulate the ã-aminobutyric acid receptor complex at a site distinct from barbiturates. *J. Pharmacol. Exp. Ther.* **248,** 960–966.

Turner, J. P., and Simmonds, M. A. (1989). Modulation of the GABAA receptor complex by steroids in slices of rat cuneate nucleus. *Br. J. Pharmacol.* **96,** 409–417.

Turner, W. A. (1907). Epilepsy: Chapter 3. *In* "A Study of the Idiopathic Disease." pp. 41–64. MacMillan, London, UK.

Turski, W. A., Cavalheiro, E. A., Schwarz, M., Czuczwar, S. J., Kleinrok, Z., and Turski, L. (1983). Limbic seizures produced by pilocarpine in rats: Behavioural, electroencephalographic and neuropathological study. *Behav. Brain. Res.* **9,** 315–335.

Tuunanen, J., Halonen, T., and Pitkanen, A. (1996). Status epilepticus causes selective regional damage and loss of GABAergic neurons in the rat amygdaloid complex. *Eur. J. Neurosci.* **8,** 2711–2725.

Twyman, R. E., and Macdonald, R. L. (1992). Neurosteroid regulation of GABAA receptor single-channel kinetic properties of mouse spinal cord neurons in culture. *J. Physiol.* **456,** 215–245.

Ukena, K., Usui, M., Kohchi, C., and Tsutsui, K. (1998). Cytochrome P450 side-chain cleavage enzyme in the cerebellar Purkinje neuron and its neonatal change in rats. *Endocrinology* **139,** 137–147.

Ukena, K., Honda, Y., Inai, Y., Kohchi, C., Lea, R. W., and Tsutsui, K. (1999a). Expression and activity of 517 3_hydroxysteroid dehydrogenase/_5-4-isomerase in different regions of the avian brain. *Brain Res.* **140**(2), 536–542.

Ukena, K., Kohchi, C., and Tsutsui, K. (1999b). Expression and activity of 3_-hydroxysteroid dehydrogenase/520_5-_4-isomerase in the rat Purkinje neuron during neonatal life. *Endocrinology* **521140,** 805–813.

Van Luijtelaar, G., Budziszewska, B., Jaworska-Feil, L., Ellis, J., Coenen, A., and Lason, W. (2001). The ovarian hormones and absence epilepsy: A long term EEG study and pharmacological effects in a genetic absence epilepsy model. *Epilepsy Res.* **46,** 225–239.

Van Luijtelaar, G., Budziszewska, B., Tetich, M., and Lason, W. (2003). Finasteride inhibits the progesterone-induced spike-wave discharges in a genetic model of absence epilepsy. *Pharmacol. Biochem. Behav.* **75,** 889–894.

Vazquez, D. M., and Akil, H. (1993). Pituitary-adrenal response to ether vapor in the weanling animal: Characterization of the inhibitory effect of glucocorticoids on adrenocorticotropin secretion. *Pediatr. Res.* **34,** 646–653.

Velasco, M. E., and Taleisnik, S. (1971). Effects of the interruption of amygdaloid and hippocampal afferents to the medial hypothalamus on gonadotrophin release. *J. Endocrinol.* **51,** 41–55.

Velíšek, L., Velíková, J., Etgen, A. M., Stanton, P. K., and Moshé, S. L. (1999). Region-specific modulation of limbic seizure susceptibility by ovarian steroids. *Brain Res.* **842,** 132–138.

Velíšek, L., Velíšková, J., Giorgi, F. S., and Moshé, S. L. (2006). Sex-specific control of flurothyl-induced tonic-clonic seizures by the substantia nigra pars reticulate during development. *Exp. Neurol.* **201,** 203–211.

Velíšková, J., and Moshé, S. L. (2001). Sexual dimorphism and developmental regulation of substantia nigra function. *Ann. Neurol.* **50,** 596–601.

Velíšková, J., Velíšek, L., Galanopoulou, A. S., and Sperber, E. F. (2000). Neuroprotective effects of estrogens on hippocampal cells in adult female rats after status epilepticus. *Epilepsia* **41,** 30–35.

Viau, V. (2002). Functional cross-talk between the hypothalamic-pituitary-gonadal and –adrenal axes. *J. Neuroendocrinol.* **14,** 506–513.

Vincens, M., Li, S. Y., and Pelletier, G. (1994). Inhibitory effect of 5 beta-pregnan-3 alpha-ol-20-one on gonadotropin-releasing hormone gene expression in the male rat. *Eur. J. Pharmacol.* **260,** 157–162.

Voigt, L. F., Weiss, N. S., Chu, J., Daling, J. R., McKnight, B., and van Belle, G. (1991). Progestagen supplementation of exogenous oestrogens and risk of endometrial cancer. *Lancet* **338,** 274–277.

Vongher, J. M., and Frye, C. A. (1999). Progesterone in conjunction with estradiol has neuroprotective effects in an animal model of neurodegeneration. *Pharmacol. Biochem. Behav.* **64,** 777–785.

Wang, M., Bäckström, T., Sundström, I., Wahlström, G., Olsson, T., Zhu, D., Johansson, I. M., Björn, I., and Bixo, M. (2001). Neuroactive-steroids and central nervous system disorders. *Int. Rev. Neurobiol.* **46,** 421–459.

Weiland, N. G., Orikasa, C., Hayashi, S., and McEwen, B. S. (1997). Distribution and hormone regulation of estrogen receptor immunoreactive cells in the hippocampus of male and female rats. *J. Comp. Neurol.* **388,** 603–612.

Weinstock, M. (2001). Alterations induced by gestational stress in brain morphology and behaviour of the offspring. *Prog. Neurobiol.* **65,** 427–451.

Weizman, R., Dagan, E., Snyder, S. H., and Gavish, M. (1997). Impact of pregnancy and lactation on GABAA receptor and central-type and peripheral-type benzodiazepine receptors. *Brain Res.* **752,** 307–314.

Wenzel, R. R., Bartel, T., Eggebrecht, H., Philipp, T., and Erbel, R. (2002). Central-nervous side effects of midazolam during transesophageal echocardiography. *J. Am. Soc. Echocardiogr.* **15,** 1297–1300.

Whitehead, M. I. (1978). The effects of oestrogens and progestogens on the postmenopausal endometrium. *Maturitas* **1,** 87–98.

Wihlbäck, A. C., Nyberg, S., Bäckström, T., Bixo, M., and Sundström-Poromaa, I. (2005). Estradiol and the addition of progesterone increase the sensitivity to a neurosteroid in postmenopausal women. *Psychoneuroendocrinology* **30,** 38–50.

Wiklund, I., Karlberg, J., and Mattsson, L.Å. (1993). Quality of life of postmenopausal women on a regimen of transdermal estradiol therapy: A double-blind placebo-controlled study. *Am. J. Obstet. Gynecol.* **168,** 824–830.

Wilson, M.A. (1992). Influences of gender, gonadectomy, and estrous cycle on GABA/BZ receptors and benzodiazepine response in rats. *Brain Res. Bull.* **29**(2), 165–172.

Wong, M., Thompson, T. L., and Moss, R. L. (1996). Nongenomic actions of estrogen in the brain: Physiological significance and cellular mechanisms. *Crit. Rev. Neurobiol.* **10,** 189–203.

Woolley, D. E., and Timiras, P. S. (1962a). The gonad-brain relationship Effects of female sex hormones on electroshock convulsions in the rat. *Endocrinology* **70,** 196–209.

Woolley, D. E., and Timiras, P. S. (1962b). Estrous and circadian periodicity and electroshock convulsions in rats. *Am. J. Physiol.* **202,** 379–382.

Woolley, D. E., Tamiras, P. S., Rosenweig, M. R., Krech, D., and Bennett, E. L. (1961). Sex and strain in electroshock convulsion of the rat. *Nature* **190,** 15–516.

Yu, R., and Ticku, M. J. (1995). Chronic neurosteroid treatment produces functional heterologous uncoupling at the _-aminibutyric acid type A benzodiazepine receptor complex in mammalian cortical neurons. *Mol. Pharmacol.* **47,** 603–610.

Zhang, Z., Olland, A. M., Zhu, Y., Cohen, J., Berrodin, T., Chippari, S., Appavu, C., Li, S., Wilhem, J., Chopra, R., Fensome, A., Zhang, P., *et al.* (2005). Molecular and pharmacological properties of a potent and selective novel nonsteroidal progesterone receptor agonist tanaproget. *J. Biol. Chem.* **280,** 28468–28475.

Zhu, D., Birzniece, V., Bäckström, T., and Wahlström, G. (2004). Dynamic aspects of acute tolerance to allopregnanolone evaluated using anaesthesia threshold in male rats. *Br. J. Anaesth.* **93,** 560–567.

CATAMENIAL EPILEPSY

Patricia E. Penovich* and Sandra Helmers†

*Minnesota Epilepsy Group PA, Department of Neurology, University of Minnesota,
Minnesota 55102, USA
†Emory University School of Medicine, Georgia 30322, USA

I. Introduction
II. Normal Female Neuroendocrine Cycle
III. Definition and Epidemiology
IV. Proposed Mechanisms
   A. Brain Water Concentration
   B. AED Concentration Changes Due to Hepatic Induction
   C. Hormonal Effects
V. Treatment Strategies
   A. Acetazolamide Therapy
   B. Benzodiazepines
   C. Variable AED Dosing
   D. Clomiphene Therapy
   E. Progesterone Therapy
   F. Neuroactive Steroid Treatment
VI. Conclusion
   References

Catamenial epilepsy is defined by the cyclical seizure exacerbation seen in almost 40% of women with epilepsy. The pattern appears to be related to predominance of estrogen over progesterone during the pre-ovulatory and/or perimenstrual days of the ovulatory menstrual cycle or during the broad period between day 14 and menstruation in anovulatory cycles with inadequate luteal progesterone levels. Progesterone affects central nervous excitability in an "inhibitory" manner, slowing kindling and decreasing seizure susceptibility in animal models. Estrogen enhances kindling and decreases after discharge threshold. These neurosteroidal hormones alter the GABA-A receptor in cell cultures and in animal models. Treatment of this clinical syndrome has been empirical and reported in a small series of women. Progesterone therapy and possible new approaches with synthesized neurosteroids may offer a promising approach to improve seizure control in women with catamenial epilepsy.

INTERNATIONAL REVIEW OF
NEUROBIOLOGY, VOL. 83
DOI: 10.1016/S0074-7742(08)00004-4

79

I. Introduction

The cyclical nature of epilepsy with temporal relationship to the menstrual cycle is known as "catamenial" epilepsy. The earliest recorded observations were made by the ancient Greek physicians who described the monthly patterns ("kalamenios") as being related to the cycle of the moon (Temkin, 1971). Both Sir Charles Locock (1857) and Sir William Gowers (1881) described the relationship between the seizures and the menstrual cycle. This relationship continues to be observed and to present the patient and the physician with a challenging clinical problem.

II. Normal Female Neuroendocrine Cycle

The normal human menstrual cycle is the result of a highly integrated feedback loop involving the hypothalamus, the pituitary, and the ovaries (Fig. 1). The mediobasal hypothalamus secretes gonadotropin-releasing hormone (GnRH) in a pulsatile pattern into the portal system to the anterior pituitary. This results in pulsatile releases of follicle stimulating hormone (FSH) and luteinizing hormone (LH) that vary over the menstrual cycle. These pulses result in follicle development and subsequent luteal phase. FSH stimulates estradiol production in the ovary and the release from the ovarian granulosa cells of inhibin, a neuropeptide that feeds back to inhibit FSH secretion. LH stimulates the ovarian thecal cells to produce androgens that are metabolized to estradiol by the granulosa cells. The estradiol feeds back to inhibit the FSH and LH until an increase in midcycle estradiol concentration occurs. This results in an elevation of LH that produces oocyte maturation, the formation of the corpus luteum, and imminent ovulation. The corpus luteum produces progesterone. If there is no fertilization, the corpus luteum involutes and progesterone and estradiol production decline. The decline in these hormones results in menstruation. If the follicle does not develop and the corpus luteum is inadequate, there is no ovulation and the progesterone production fails to increase. This is termed an inadequate luteal cycle, which is recognized by a serum progesterone of <5 ng/ml. Estrogen concentration is then relatively unopposed. These cycle with inadequate luteal phases are typically shorter (<23 days) or longer (>35 days) cycles.

Herzog et al. (1997) evaluated these cyclical patterns (Fig. 2) in women with partial and/or secondarily generalized seizures. This work has been used to define the concept of a catamenial epilepsy pattern.

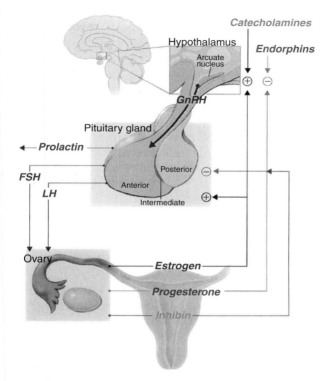

FIG. 1. The hypothalamic–pituitary–ovarian axis. Reprinted by permission: Foldvary-Schaefer N, Falcone T. "Catamenial Epilepsy, Pathophysiology, Diagnosis, and Management." Neurology 2003;61 (Suppl)2;S2–S15. Published by Lippincott Williams & Wilkins.

III. Definition and Epidemiology

Herzog *et al.* (1997) reported three patterns of catamenial seizure exacerbation after evaluating 184 women with refractory temporal lobe epilepsy. These observations were derived from analysis of seizure frequency data, menstrual diaries, and the results of mid-luteal progesterone levels (Fig. 2). He defined day 14 as beginning the luteal phase, the ovulatory phase as day 10 to day 13; the onset of menses is day 0. The C1 pattern is defined by increased seizures perimenstrually from day −3 to day +3. The C2 pattern is peri-ovulatory and occurs with seizure exacerbation occurring from day 10 to day 13. The C3 pattern is seen in women with inadequate luteal phases defined as progesterone levels <5 ng/ml resulting in anovulatory cycles. Seizures in the C3 pattern are increased throughout the period spanning day 10 to day 3. He calculated that the increase was about two times the baseline seizure frequency rate. This finding has defined the catamenial pattern to be an increase in seizure frequency of at least twice the baseline seizure frequency.

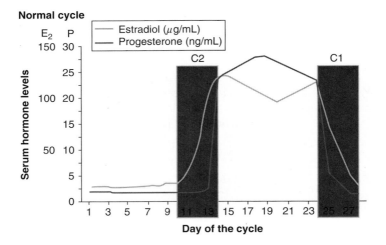

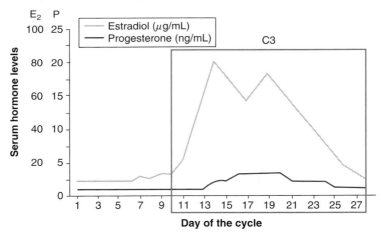

FIG. 2. Patterns of catamenial epilepsy. Perimenstrual (C1) and periovulatory (C2) exacerbations during normal cycles and entire second half of the cycle (C3) exacerbation during inadequate luteal phase cycles. Reprinted by permission: Herzog AG, Klein P, Ransil BJ. "Three Patterns of Catamenial Epilepsy." *Epilepsia*. Vol. 38, No. 10;1082–1088 (1997). Published by Wiley-Blackwell Publishing, Ltd.

The incidence of catamenial epilepsy reported in the literature spans a range of values depending on the population being studied, the number of menstrual cycles observed, and the timing of the cycle at the point of observation. A review by Foldvary-Schaefer and Falcone (2003) summarized these methodological and reporting differences, demonstrating a frequency of catamenial epilepsy between 9 and 78%.

Herzog *et al.* (2004) in a prospective multicenter study, evaluated 87 women over 3 cycles and confirmed the 3 catamenial patterns: women with C1 patterns (22.2%), C2 (10.6%), women with both C1 and C2 seizure exacerbation (10.6%), thus 43.4% had C1 and/or C2 patterns. In women with documented anovulatory cycles, the C3 pattern was seen in 39%. Morrell *et al.* (1998) reported that a catamenial pattern occurs more frequently in partial epilepsy than in generalized epilepsy.

IV. Proposed Mechanisms

A. Brain Water Concentration

Why seizures exacerbate at these times within the menstrual cycle is not fully understood. One mechanism suggested that body and brain water retention is responsible for the pattern, but this was not substantiated in a study that found no difference from controls for body weight, sodium metabolism, and total body water (Ansell and Clarke, 1956).

B. AED Concentration Changes Due to Hepatic Induction

Another theory proposes that the hepatic 450-system is induced by elevated gonadal steroid concentration in the days prior to menstruation (Krugers *et al.*, 1995; Woodbury, 1952). The elevated steroids induce the anti-epileptic drug (AED) metabolism and this produces a reduction in AED concentration for those drugs with inducible hepatic metabolism (Karkuzhali and Schomer, 1998; Kumar *et al.*, 1988; Shavit *et al.*, 1984). Herzog *et al.* (1997), however, saw no differences in enzyme-inducing or enzyme-inhibiting AED regimens. There are no studies to evaluate changes in AEDs that have no hepatic metabolism.

C. Hormonal Effects

The most plausible mechanisms involve the effect of the gonadal steroids directly on the central nervous system cells and neurotransmission. Reproductive steroids may act by receptor-mediated long latency genomic effects; receptor-mediated posttranscriptional intermediate latency effects; and direct membrane-mediated short latency effects (McEwen, 1991; Smith, 1989).

Estrogen and progesterone are highly lipophilic. When released into the circulation, they bind to Sex harmone binding globulin (SHBG) and are later bound to receptors at the target membrane. They diffuse into the cell and then bind to an intracellular receptor forming a hormone–receptor complex. This process occurs in the cytosol and subsequently the complexes are translocated into the nucleus. The hormone–receptor complex in the nucleus then binds to a target gene, which regulates the gene expression and protein products. This is a long latency effect.

Enzymatic conversion of progesterone to allopregnanolone does occur within the brain (Bixo et al., 1997). In the female rat, progesterone levels are high in the forebrain neocortex and decrease in puberty. Progesterone retards kindling in the rat and blocks behavioral seizures in fully kindled female rats (Edwards et al., 1999). An identifiable progesterone binding site is found on the GABA-A receptor. Progesterone increases seizure threshold (Backstrom, 1984; Majewska et al., 1986; Paul and Purdy, 1992).

Estradiol receptors are located throughout the central nervous system, stria terminalis, medial preoptic area, anterior hypothalamus, ventromedial nucleus of hypothalamus, median eminence, amygdala, midbrain, pituitary, hippocampal interneurons, and cortex (Loy, 1988; Pfaff and Kerner, 1973). In the mature rat, estrogen receptors are greatest in the limbic cortex. The hypothalamus receives direct connections from the amygdala, and the pituitary is directly influenced by the hypothalamus. Female rats kindled from the amygdala had high estradiol and prolactin levels (Edwards, 2000).

Estrogen is a potent pro-convulsant. The number of dendritic spines increases in the presence of estrogen. This increased cell-to-cell contact promotes hyper-synchronization and subsequently lowers seizure threshold. Estrogen potentiates excitatory post synaptic potentials (EPSPs) in the hippocampus. It blocks GABA-mediated transmission and produces increased neuronal firing and spontaneous discharges, alters glutamic acid decarboxylase, and decreases the synthesis rate of GABA-A subunits. It accelerates kindling and lowers the afterdischarge threshold in the amygdala at pre-ovulation and premenstruation times (Herzog, 1999b,c; Murialdo et al., 1997). In addition, generalized seizures disrupt normal ovarian cycling and repeated electroshock seizures delay the onset of puberty in juvenile rats. Intravenous administration of conjugated estrogens activates epileptiform discharges resulting in seizures.

In a rat model of catamenial epilepsy (Reddy et al., 2001), a pseudopregnant state was induced in immature rats by injecting them with gonadotropin. Allopregnanolone, the active metabolite of progesterone, is then decreased acutely by inhibition of the conversion of progesterone to allopregnanolone. This is accomplished by blocking 5α-reductase with finasteride. These rats subsequently exhibit increased sensitivity to subcutaneous pentylenetetrazol (PTZ) with decreased latency to seizure generation and a 35% decrease in seizure threshold to PTZ compared to the animal's baseline response and to control rate responses. Animals with chronically low allopregnanolone levels did not show this seizure susceptibility profile. This would confirm that the acute withdrawal from the elevated level of progestational compound is mechanistically important. The degree of progesterone elevation and the length of time the serum progesterone is elevated closely matches the human menstrual cycle. The authors postulate that there is an alteration in the GABA-A receptor or its properties. A human experience substantiates the validity of this model. A woman being treated with progesterone for control of catamenial seizures, experienced loss of seizure control when she was treated with finasteride which blocked the progesterone conversion to allopregnenolone (Herzog and Frye, 2003).

Maguire *et al.* (2005) demonstrates in mice that the δ GABA-A receptor is altered differently in the different estrous phases. This produces changes in the tonic inhibition and seizure susceptibility to intraperitoneal kainic acid injection. The animals were protected in late diestrus, a time of high progesterone and low estrogen concentrations. δ GABA receptors were upregulated, latency to seizure onset was longer, time in seizure was significantly less, and electrographic events were shorter.

A human teratocarcinoma cell line, NT2-N, shows morphology and function of a neuron after retinoic acid treatment (Pierson *et al.*, 2005). The cultures possess functional GABA receptors. Treatment with progesterone results in significant differences in GABA receptor subunits compared to the profile after estradiol exposure. This result is due to different mRNA expression after interaction with a nuclear progesterone receptor.

V. Treatment Strategies

A number of small series report treatments for catamenial epilepsy. To date there is not a large controlled, blinded trial of any treatment. There is one multicentered prospective study ongoing in the United States (Herzog *et al.*, 2004).

A. ACETAZOLAMIDE THERAPY

Acetazolamide continues to be used by many practitioners. Whether its mechanism of therapeutic effect is as a potent carbonic anhydrase inhibitor producing a metabolic acidosis, as a diuretic, or as a primary AED is uncertain. Lombroso and Forxythe (1960) reported no correlation of improvement in seizure frequency with bicarbonate levels. In a retrospective report, Lim (2001) noted a seizure reduction of 40% and seizure severity reduced by 30% with a low daily dose of acetazolamide. Recommended doses are 8–30 mg/kg/day up to a maximum of 1 g in 1–4 divided doses (Foldvary-Schaefer and Falcone, 2003). Side effects include paresthesia, dysgeusia, metabolic acidosis, fatigue, renal stones, and diuresis. Since tolerance to continuous administration is common, cyclic dosing may prevent development of tolerance.

B. Benzodiazepines

Benzodiazepines are used as AED therapy for catamenial seizure control. Tolerance to the AED effect is seen with this class of drugs. Therefore, intermittent use at the time of the seizure exacerbation is used by some. Clobazam is a 1,5-benzodiazepine with reportedly fewer adverse effects and less risk of tolerance than the classic 1,4 compounds. It is not available in the United States at this time. Feely *et al.* (1982) evaluated clobazam at 20 mg/day in a double-blind, placebo-controlled, and crossover trial. Women with refractory perimenstrual seizures were treated during one menstrual cycle for 10 days beginning 2–4 days prior to the anticipated menstrual onset. Seizure freedom or >50% reduction was the efficacy definition. Seventy-eight percent attained this response, although three patients responded only to a higher dose of 30 mg/day. This efficacy was maintained over 6–13 months without tolerance in patients evaluated for more than 1 year (Feely and Gibson, 1984). Dose recommendation is between 20 and 30 mg per day. Side effects are sedation and depression.

C. Variable AED Dosing

There are a few reports of improved catamenial seizure frequency when AED doses are adjusted in the perimenstrual period (Karkuzhali and Schomer, 1998). This manipulation is based on observations made by Logothetis *et al.* (1959) and Shavit *et al.* (1984) of variable phenytoin serum levels during the menstrual cycle. This variable dosing regimen requires a cooperative, compliant patient, since the doses may be adjusted several times during a menstrual cycle.

D. Clomiphene Therapy

Manipulation of the estrogen/progesterone ratio seems to offer a promising therapeutic approach. Historical use of clomiphene, an estrogen antagonist, was reported to reduce seizures by 87% in 10 of 12 women (Herzog, 1988).

E. Progesterone Therapy

Depot medroxyprogesterone in doses producing amenorrhea, 120–150 mg every 6–12 weeks, has had therapeutic success in small numbers of women (Fredrickson, 1996; Mattson, 1984) Side effects include hot flashes, irregular breakthrough bleeding and a delay in recovery of normal ovulatory cycles. Herzog (1995) reported a decrease in seizure frequency of 55% for complex partial seizures and secondarily generalized seizures with the use of natural

TABLE I
NATURAL PROGESTERONE[a] TREATMENT REGIMEN

	Dosing: three times daily		
	Day 1	If excessive sedation	If tolerated
Days 14–25	1/2	1/2	1
Days 26–27		1/4	1/2
Day 28		1/4	1/4
Day 29		Stop	Stop

[a]Extract of soy and yams compounded into lozenge form. Used by permission, personal communication from A. Herzog (2007).
If an early period occurs, start the three-day taper as per days 26–29.

progesterone lozenges taken on days 14–25 of the menstrual cycle (Table I) that was maintained in the responders over a three-year period (Herzog, 1999a). A prospective, multicentered, placebo-controlled trial of progesterone therapy in women with localization-related epilepsy is in progress (Herzog et al., 2004). The daily dose of natural progesterone should achieve a physiological luteal phase serum level of progesterone, between 5 and 25 ng/ml. Doses of 50–200 mg are given in three divided doses due to the short half-life. Side effects include sedation, depression, tiredness, breast tenderness, weight gain, and irregular vaginal bleeding. The progesterone therapy could induce concomitant AED hepatic metabolism. Synthetic progestins are not converted to allopregnanalone; this may explain the lack of success with this modality (Mattson, 1984).

F. NEUROACTIVE STEROID TREATMENT

Ganaxalone, 3α-hydroxy-3β-methyl-5α-pregnan-20-one, is a synthetic neuroactive steroid that modulates the GABA-A receptor at a site distinct from the benzodiazepine and barbiturate sites. It is an analogue of allopregnanalone. It is being developed as an AED and is presently in phase 3 pharmaceutical trials. Studies suggest this compound may have particular efficacy in patients with catamenial epilepsy patterns (McAuley et al., 2001; Reddy, 2004).

VI. Conclusion

Catamenial epilepsy is a common pattern of seizure occurrence in over one-third of women with both partial and generalized epilepsies. Seizure frequency increases in the pre-ovulatory and perimenstrual periods of the menstrual cycle. These patterns may contribute to the refractory course of some women. Although the exact mechanism is not completely understood, recent development of *in vitro* and *in vivo* models may elucidate the etiology. The modulation of the GABA-A receptor in response to progesterone and estrogen effects seems likely. There is no clear preferred mode of therapy for women with catamenial epilepsy. Therapeutic manipulation of the estrogen/progesterone ratio to decrease the estrogen effect or increase the progesterone effect in the central nervous system (CNS) appears most promising. The results of ongoing and future prospective controlled trials as well as designed therapies to modulate the GABA-A receptor, may improve therapeutic options and successful treatment of seizures that exacerbate at these times.

References

Ansell, B., and Clarke, E. (1956). Epilepsy and menstruation: The role of water retention. *Lancet* **2,** 1232–1235.

Backstrom, T., Zetterlund, B., Blom, S., and Romano, M. (2004). Effects of intravenous progesterone infusions on the epileptic discharge frequency in women with partial epilepsy. *Acta Neurologica Scand* **69,** 240–248.

Bixo, M., Andersson, A., Winblad, B., Purdy, R., and Backstrom, T. (1997). Progesterone, 5α-pregnane-3, 2-dione and 3α-hydroxy-5α-pregnane-2-one in specific regions of the human female brain in different endocrine states. *Brain Res.* **764,** 173–178.

Edwards, H. E., Burnham, W. M., Ng, M. M., Asa, S., and MacLusky, N. J. (1999). Limbic seizure alters reproduction function in the female rat. *Epilepsia* **40,** 1370–1377.

Edwards, H. E., MacLusky, N. J., and Burnham, W. M. (2000). The effect of seizures and kindling on reproductive hormones in the rat. *Neurosci. Biobehav. Rev.* **24**(7), 753–762.

Feely, M., and Gibson, J. (1984). Intermittent clobazam for catamenial epilepsy: Tolerance avoided. *J. Neurol. Neurosurg. Psychiatr.* **47,** 1279–1282.

Feely, M., Calvert, R., and Gibson, J. (1982). Clobazam in catamenial epilepsy: A model for evaluating anticonvulsants. *Lancet* **2,** 71–73.

Fredericksen, M. C. (1996). Depo medroxyprogesterone acetate contraception in women with medical problems. *J. Reprod. Med.* **41,** 414–418.

Foldvary-Schaefer, N., and Falcone, T. (2003). Catamenial epilepsy: Pathophysiology, diagnosis, and management. *Neurology* **61**(Suppl. 2), S2–S15.

Gowers, W. R. (1881). "Epilepsy and Other Chronic Convulsive Diseases. Their Causes, Symptoms, and Treatment." J & A, Churchill, London.

Herzog, A. G. (1988). Clomphene therapy in epileptic women with menstrual disorders. *Neurology* **38,** 432–434.

Herzog, A. G. (1995). Progesterone therapy in women with complex partial and secondarily generalized seizures. *Neurology* **45,** 1660–1662.

Herzog, A. G. (1999a). Progesterone therapy in women with epilepsy: A 3-year follow-up. *Neurology* **52,** 1917–1918.

Herzog, A. G. (1999b). Psychoneuroendocrine aspects of temporolimbic epilepsy, Part I: Brain, reproductive steroids and emotions. *Psychosomatics* **40,** 95–101.

Herzog, A. G. (1999c). Psychoneuroendocrine aspects of temporolimbic epilepsy, Part II: Epilepsy and reproductive steroid. *Psychosomatics* **40,** 102–108.

Herzog, A. G., and Frye, C. A. (2003). Seizure exacerbation associated with inhibition of progesterone metabolism. *Ann. Neurol.* **53,** 390–391.

Herzog, A. G., Klein, P., and Ransil, B. J. (1997). Three patterns of catamenial epilepsy. *Epilepsia* **38,** 1082–1088.

Herzog, A. G., Harden, C. L., Liporace, J., Pennel, P., *et al.* (2004). Frequency of catamenial seizure exacerbation in women with localization-related epilepsy. *Ann Neurol.* **56,** 431–434.

Karkuzhali, B., and Schomer, D. L. (1998). Weekly fluctuation and adjustment of antiepileptic drugs to treat catamenial seizures.. *Epilepsia* **39,** 179.

Krugers, H. J., Knollema, S., Kemper, R. H., TerHorst, G. J., and Kor, F. J. (1995). Down regulation of the hypothalamic–pituitary–adrenal axis reduces brain damage and number of seizures following hypoxia/ischaemia in rats. *Brain Res.* **690,** 41–47.

Kumar, N., Behari, M., Ahuja, G. K., and Jailkhani, B. L. (1988). Phenytoin levels in catamenial epilepsy. *Epilepsia* **29,** 155–158.

Lim, L. L., Foldvary, N., Mascha, E., and Lee, J. (2001). Acetazolamide in women with catamenial epilepsy. *Epilepsia* **42,** 746–749.

Locock, C. (1857). Analysis of fifty-two cases of epilepsy observed by the author. *In Med. Times Gaz.* **14,** 524–526.

Logothetis, J., Harner, R., Morrell, F., and Torres, F. (1959). The role of estrogens in catamenial exacerbation of epilepsy. *Neurology* **9,** 352–360.

Lombroso, C. T., and Forxythe, I. (1960). A long-term follow-up of acetazolamide in the treatment of epilepsy. *Epilepsia* **1,** 493–500.

Loy, R., Gerlach, J. L., and McEwen, B. S. (1988). Autoradiographic localization of estradiol-binding neurons in the rat hippocampal formation and entorhinal cortex. *Brain Res.* **46,** 245–251.

Maguire, J. L., Stell, B. M., Rafizadeh, M., and Mody, I. (2005). Ovarian cycle-linked changes in receptors mediating tonic inhibition after seizure susceptibility and anxiety. *Nat. Neurosci.* **8,** 797–804.

Majewska, M. D., Harrison, N. L., and Schwartz, R. D. (1986). Steroid hormone metabolites are barbiturate-like modulators of the GABA-A receptor. *Science* **232,** 1004–1007.

Mattson, R. H., Cramer, J. A., Caldwell, B. V., and Siconolfi, B. C. (1984). Treatment of seizures with medroxyprogesterone acetate: Preliminary report. *Neurology* **34,** 1255–1258.

McAuley, J. W., Moore, J. L., Reeves, A. L., *et al.* (2001). A pilot study of the neurosteriod ganaxolone in catamenial epilepsy: Clinical experience in two patients. *Epilepsia* **42,** 85.

McEwen, B. S. (1991). Nongenomic and genomic effects of steroids on neural activity. *Trends Pharmacol. Sci.* **12,** 141–147.

Morrell, M. J., Hamdy, S. F., Seale, C. G., and Springer, E. A. (1998). Self-reported reproductive history in women with epilepsy: Puberty onset and effects of menarche and menstrual cycle on seizures. *Neurology* **50,** 448.

Murialdo, G., Galimberti, C. A., Magri, F., *et al.* (1997). Menstrual cycle and ovary alterations in women with epilepsy on antiepileptic therapy. *J. Endocrinol. Invest.* **20,** 519–526.

Paul, S. M., and Purdy, R. H. (1992). Neuroactive steroids. *FASEB J.* **6,** 2311–2322.

Pfaff, D., and Kerner, M. (1973). Atlas of estradiol-concentrating cells in the central nervous system of the female rat. *J. Comp. Neurol.* **151,** 121–158.

Pierson, R. C., Lyons, A. M., and Greenfield, L. F. (2005). Gonadal steroids regulate GABA-$_A$ receptor subunit mRNA expression in NT2-N neurons. *Brain Res. Mol. Brain Res.* **138,** 105–115.

Reddy, D. S. (2004). Pharmacology of catamenial epilepsy. *Exp. Clin. Pharmacol.* **26,** 547–561.

Reddy, D. S., Kim, H., and Rogowski, M. A. (2001). Neurosteroid withdrawal model of perimenstrual catamenial epilepsy. *Epilepsia* **42,** 328–336.

Shavit, G., Lerman, P., Korczyn, A., Kivity, S., Bechar, M., and Gitter, S. (1984). Phenytoin pharmacokinetics in catamenial epilepsy. *Neurology* **34,** 959–961.

Smith, S. S. (1989). Estrogen administration increases neuronal responses to excitatory amino acids as a long-term effect. *Brain Res.* **503,** 354–357.

Temkin, O. (1971). "The Falling Sickness: A History of Epilepsy from the Greeks to the Beginnings of
    Modern Neurology." 2nd revised ed. Johns Hopkins Press, Baltimore.
Woodbury, D. M. (1952). Effect of adrenocortical steroids and adrenocorticotropic hormone on
    electroshock seizure threshold. *J. Pharmacol. Exp. Ther.* **105,** 27–36.

EPILEPSY IN WOMEN: SPECIAL CONSIDERATIONS FOR ADOLESCENTS

Mary L. Zupanc* and Sheryl Haut†

*Department of Neurology and Pediatrics, Division of Pediatric Neurology,
Pediatric Comprehensive Epilepsy Program, Children's Hospital of Wisconsin,
Medical College of Wisconsin, Milwaukee, Wisconsin 53226, USA
†Comprehensive Epilepsy Management Center, Montefiore Medical Center,
Albert Einstein College of Medicine, New York 10467, USA

I. Introduction
II. Epidemiology
III. Hormones and Epilepsy
IV. Epilepsy and Reproductive Health
  A. Menstrual Irregularities
  B. Polycystic Ovarian Syndrome/Polycystic Ovaries
  C. Sexual Dysfunction
  D. Effects of AEDs on Contraception
  E. Pregnancy
V. Bone Health
VI. Psychosocial Considerations
  A. Quality of Life
  B. School Performance
  C. Driving
  D. The Effect of Stigma
VII. Selected Comorbidities
  A. Depression and Suicide
  B. Migraine
VIII. Patient Management
  A. Choice of Antiepileptic Medication
  B. Choice of Contraception
  C. Nutrition
  D. Sports and Safety
  E. Compliance
  F. Sleep Deprivation
  G. The Adolescent Clinic
IX. Conclusions
  References

Adolescence is a time of many changes. It is a time of growing independence, physical and emotional change, accompanied by social insecurity. Girls tend to enter puberty ahead of their male peers, growing and changing physically. Our culture tells adolescents that they are still immature, but their bodies are saying otherwise. The adolescents are also becoming aware of themselves as individuals, separate from their parents, and are presented with the challenges of independent thinking and action.

If, in the midst of all of these changes, an adolescent is given the diagnosis of a chronic disease such as epilepsy, there is an additional burden. Often the adolescent must go through a variety of emotions, including shame, denial, anger, and sadness. Our role as medical providers is to provide some perspective to the illness and help guide our adolescent patient through the tumultuous emotions of grieving and acceptance. We must provide a foundation of assistance and emotional support, as well as medical knowledge. With a firm but compassionate hand, we can help them cope with their disorder.

In this chapter, Drs. Haut and Zupanc explore some of the unique considerations in adolescent women with epilepsy. The first part of the chapter deals with the epidemiologic diagnosis of epilepsy in adolescence, the effect of epilepsy on reproductive health, hormonal influences on epilepsy (including catamenial seizures), and the effects of antiepileptic drugs (AEDs) on hormones, contraception, and bone health. In the second part of the chapter, we deal with the very real psychosocial issues and comorbidities of epilepsy, including quality of life, school performance, depression, migraine headaches, social stigma, and lifestyle changes. In the final section, the authors suggest strategies for clinical patient management.

I. Introduction

Adolescence is a challenging phase of life, particularly superimposed on a backdrop of chronic illness. It is a time where peer pressure is paramount, independence is developing, driving and employment become possible, and exploration of relationships and sexuality begins (Devinsky et al., 1999; Sheth and Gidal, 2006). For many young women with epilepsy, navigating the developmental and psychosocial issues that beset the teenage years while at the same time living with the reality of seizures, medication, stigma, and restriction is particularly difficult. The additional burden of comorbidities such as depression further impacts daily function and quality of life for these young women. For these adolescents, it is imperative to take the time to discuss the implications of epilepsy with them and provide them with the knowledge and tools to succeed in gaining confidence and control of their lives.

II. Epidemiology

Epilepsy is a very common neurologic disorder during adolescence (Appleton *et al.*, 1997), with an incidence reported to be in the range of 21–39/100,000 (Camfield *et al.*, 1996; Hauser *et al.*, 1993) and a prevalence of 1.5–2% (Sheth *et al.*, 2004; Hauser, *et al.*, 1993). A number of important International League Against Epilepsy (ILAE)-classified age-specific syndromes have frequent onset during the teenage years, particularly idiopathic generalized epilepsies (IGE) such as juvenile absence epilepsy (JAE), juvenile myoclonic epilepsy (JME), and epilepsy with generalized tonic clonic seizures upon awakening (EGTCSA) (Engel for ILAE, 2001). Mesial temporal lobe epilepsy often begins in adolescence (Wheless and Kim, 2002), although localization-related epilepsy due to other structural lesions (focal cortical dysplasias; encephalomalacia; perinatal stroke) presents earlier in childhood (Nordli, 2001). In addition, many patients with childhood onset of epilepsy continue to have seizures throughout their teenage years.

While the overall incidence of epilepsy is slightly higher in males (Kotsopoulos *et al.*, 2002), this is not the case in adolescence, due to female predominance of IGE. Both JAE and JME (Christensen *et al.*, 2005) and more recently EGTCSA (Mullins *et al.*, 2007) are reported to be more common in females. Thus, the topic of epilepsy in the female adolescent is timely and clinically relevant.

III. Hormones and Epilepsy

The influence of hormones on epilepsy has been well described. The onset of certain epilepsy syndromes begins at the time of puberty; other epilepsy syndromes go into remission. Contrary to popular belief, menarche does not appear to exacerbate preexisting epilepsy. However, hormonal changes during the menstrual cycle can have a profound effect on seizure activity. Estrogen is a potent proconvulsant, whereas progesterone has anticonvulsant effects (Pfaff and McEwen, 1983; McEwen, 1998; Woolley and Schwartzkroin, 1998). The ratio of these two hormones probably influences the tendency of breakthrough seizures. With some young adolescent women, the highest risk for breakthrough seizures is either at the time of ovulation or right before menses, when the estrogen:progesterone ratio is at its peak. For other adolescent women, in particular those with anovulatory cycles, the risk for breakthrough seizures may persist throughout the cycle, most likely due to the unopposed action of estrogen (Herzog *et al.*, 1997).

Estimates of women with catamenial seizures vary greatly in the literature, perhaps reflecting how poorly we obtain an accurate menstrual history from our patients. The incidence of catamenial seizures has been reported to be as high as 75% of all women with epilepsy, including young adolescent women.

There is a significant potential for interaction between hormones and concurrent treatment with antiepileptic drugs (AEDs), especially those AEDs that alter hepatic microsomal enzymes of the cytochrome P450 enzyme system. These AEDs can affect not only endogenous hormones but also exogenous hormones typically found in contraception. Unfortunately, in two separate surveys, most physicians are not aware of this important AED:hormonal interaction. One survey involved more than 3500 primary care providers, including pediatricians and family practice physicians. The other survey interviewed neurologist and obstetricians. Their lack of this basic information was more surprising and concerning (Krauss et al., 1996; Morrell et al., 2000).

IV. Epilepsy and Reproductive Health

Young women with epilepsy are at risk for reproductive and endocrine disturbances, including polycystic ovarian syndrome, anovulatory cycles, menstrual irregularities, reduced fertility, sexual dysfunction, and premature menopause.

A. MENSTRUAL IRREGULARITIES

Women with epilepsy being treated with valproate had the highest rate of anovulatory cycles, significantly increased over all other AEDs. Women with primary generalized epilepsy who were taking valproate had a 55% chance of having anovulatory cycles (Morrell et al., 2002).

Physiologically, the anovulatory cycles are associated with endocrine and end-organ disturbances. Women with epilepsy have hypothalamic–pituitary dysfunction, including alterations in luteinizing hormone: follicle stimulating hormone (LH:FSH) ratios (Drislane et al., 1994; Herzog et al., 1986; Meo et al., 1993). In addition, women with epilepsy who are taking CYP450 enzyme-inducing AEDs (e.g., carbamazepine, phenobarbital, phenytoin) have significant reductions in sex steroid hormones, including testosterone, estradiol, and dihydroepiandrostenedione (Isojarvi et al., 1995; Levesque et al., 1986; Morrell et al., 2001; Stoffel-Wagner et al., 1998). Valproate is an inhibitor of the CYP450 enzyme system. Thus, women with epilepsy who are taking valproate have higher gonadal and adrenal androgen levels (Morrell et al., 2003; Murialdo et al., 1998). Women who are taking lamotrigine and gabapentin (two AEDs who do not alter the P450 enzyme system) do not demonstrate any changes in sex steroid hormone levels (Morrell et al., 2001, 2004).

B. Polycystic Ovarian Syndrome/Polycystic Ovaries

Polycystic ovarian syndrome (PCOS) is defined by hyperandrogenism, producing hirsutism, male pattern baldness, anovulatory cycles, and infertility. Polycystic ovaries are not required for PCOS; however, it is frequently found in association with these other findings. The requirement for a diagnosis of PCOS is serologic or phenotypic evidence of excess androgen, as well as anovulatory cycles. Polycystic ovaries may be an asymptomatic condition found in normal women of reproductive age, occurring in 20–25% (Clayton et al., 1992; Farquhar et al., 1994; Polson et al., 1988). PCOS is important to recognize as it does cause elevated androgens, abnormal lipid profile, abnormal LH: FSH ratio, and glucose intolerance, predisposing women to insulin resistant diabetes, atherosclerosis, cardiovascular disease, and an increased risk of endometrial cancer (Morrell et al., 2003).

In the general population, the risk of PCOS is estimated to be between 7 and 15%. In women with epilepsy, the risk of PCOS is higher. In women with epilepsy who are taking valproate, one report indicates that the risk of polycystic ovaries and hyperandrogenism is as high as 40% (Isojarvi et al., 1993; Morrell et al., 2004). In a prospective study of 94 women with epilepsy who were in the reproductive age, polycystic ovaries were detected in 26% of women with localization-related epilepsy, 41% of women with primary generalized epilepsy, and only 16% in the control population (Morrell et al., 2002). In this same study, women with epilepsy who were taking valproate had an even higher risk of polycystic ovaries than women with epilepsy who were taking other AEDs (Morrell et al., 2002). The polycystic ovaries may be a reversible condition. In a study conducted by Isojarvi, women with epilepsy who were taking valproate and had documented polycystic ovaries were changed to lamotrigine monotherapy. The polycystic ovaries rescinded in most women (Isojarvi et al., 1998).

The relative effect of epilepsy and antiepileptic medication on the production of polycystic ovaries and PCOS is debated and remains controversial. However, in at least one study, women with bipolar disorder who are taking valproate did not demonstrate abnormal menstrual cycle length, anovulatory cycles, or an increased risk of polycystic ovaries. Two other studies of women with bipolar disorder being treated with valproate did demonstrate an increased risk of polycystic ovaries and abnormal menstrual cycles (Rasgon et al., 2000; O'Donovan et al., 2002). In a primate study, primates without epilepsy who were given valproate at levels similar to adults with epilepsy did not demonstrate any menstrual cycle irregularities or polycystic ovaries (Ferin et al., 2003). Therefore, it appears that there is at least some effect of epilepsy on the relative risk for polycystic ovaries and polycystic ovarian syndrome. The antiepileptic medication, valproate, is probably a contributory factor that adds to this risk.

C. Sexual Dysfunction

Women with epilepsy do exhibit sexual dysfunction and diminished sexual arousal. Approximately 33% of women with epilepsy report dyspareunia, lack of vaginal lubrication, and vaginismus (Blumer and Walker, 1967; Demerdash *et al.*, 1991; Jensen, 1992; Morrell and Guldner, 1996). The cause of sexual dysfunction is probably multifactorial, but undoubtedly encompasses the social stigma of epilepsy as well as the effect of epileptiform discharges on the limbic structures. Adolescence is a time of emerging sexuality, and our patients will have concerns about their sexuality. These concerns add to the burden of epilepsy and should be addressed openly with the patient.

D. Effects of AEDs on Contraception

Young women with epilepsy who are taking CYP450 enzyme-inducing AEDs are at increased risk for oral contraception failure due to their induction of sex steroid hormones. As a result, if these women choose to take oral contraceptives (OCP), it is strongly recommended that they take an OCP preparation that contains at least 50 μg of estradiol (AAN Practice Parameter, 1998; Zahn *et al.*, 1998). This diminishes the risk of contraceptive failure. Unfortunately, in two recent surveys of health care providers, including neurologists and obstetricians/gynecologists, very few understood this basic concept (Krauss *et al.*, 1996; Morrell *et al.*, 2000).

In young adolescent women who are taking valproate, which inhibits the CYP 450 enzyme system, there is no need to readjust the OCP preparation. These women can be placed on a low estrogen preparation. Until recently, it was felt that women who were taking lamotrigine, a nonenzyme-inducing AED, could take any oral contraceptive without concern about an increased failure rate. However, in a small study of 16 women with epilepsy who were taking lamotrigine, the ethinylestradiol levels did not change significantly, but the levonorgestrel levels decreased slightly. None of the women ovulated and there were no contraceptive failures (Lamictal package insert, 2004). However, GlaxoSmithKline, the company who makes lamotrigine, has now released a disclaimer, stating that OCP may not be fully protective against pregnancy. Until further information is collected, the company has advocated using a backup form of contraception.

In adolescents, compliance for either AEDs or OCP is variable. Many adolescents cannot be relied upon to take their medication on a regular basis. The compliance rate for OCP is estimated to be low.

For adolescents, condoms are not uniformly accepted and do have higher contraceptive failure rates. Many OB-Gyn subspecialists recommend either depo-provera or the new copper T intrauterine device that has recently been approved for nulliparous women. Depo-provera is an excellent short-term solution, but it does carry an increased risk of osteoporosis if used chronically (Crawford *et al.*, 2002). In addition, just as with oral contraception, young adolescent women with epilepsy who are taking CYP450 enzyme-inducing AEDs need to receive their depo-provera injections more frequently than every three months, due to the induction of the sex steroid metabolism (Crawford, 2002; Zupanc, 2006).

Oral contraceptives can also have an effect on AEDs. Specifically, in women with epilepsy who are taking lamotrigine, there can be an induction of lamotrigine metabolism during the steroid-taking weeks. This can result in a significant reduction in the lamotrigine blood level—sometimes a decrease of 50%—placing patients at risk for breakthrough seizures (Sabers *et al.*, 2001, 2003). Furthermore, during the nonsteroid week of oral contraception, the lamotrigine blood levels may substantially increase, resulting in toxic side effects (Sabers *et al.*, 2001, 2003).

E. Pregnancy

Despite the difficulties of pregnancies in adolescents with epilepsy, the teenage pregnancy rate is notable and must be taken into account when counseling these patients. Although the topic of pregnancy in women with epilepsy is dealt with in another chapter of this book, there are a few unique considerations for adolescent women with epilepsy. Many of our adolescents have suboptimal nutrition, with poor calcium and vegetable intake. They are at risk for osteoporosis, folate deficiency, and microcytic anemia due to iron deficiency. Adolescent women with epilepsy should be counseled on the teratogenic risks of AEDs, the role of folate deficiency in producing minor and major fetal anomalies, and the changes that occur in AED levels with pregnancy. They should also be informed of the real risk of seizures if they stop taking their AEDs during pregnancy, especially the risk to the fetus.

V. Bone Health

Bone mineral density is often decreased in women and children with epilepsy (Bogliun *et al.*, 1986; Chang and Ahn, 1994; Sheth *et al.*, 1996; Valimaki *et al.*, 1994). AEDs appear to decrease bone mineral density and alter bone mineral metabolism, compromising bone health and producing increased risks for osteo-porosis and fractures (Bogliun *et al.*, 1986; Gough *et al.*, 1986; Valimaki *et al.*, 1994). Women with epilepsy who are taking CYP450 enzyme-inducing AEDs appear to be at especially high risk for osteoporosis. In a study of 93 women with epilepsy between the ages of 18 and 40 years, carbamazepine, valproate, and fosphenytoin were associated with significant reductions in serum calcium concentrations compared to lamotrigine, although serum parathyroid hormone (PTH) and 25-OH vitamin D did not differ among the AED monotherapy groups (Pack *et al.*, 2003, 2005). Bone-specific alkaline phosphatase, a marker of bone formation and turnover, was significantly elevated with phenytoin and not with other AEDs. The biochemical data do suggest that bone turnover is greater in women taking phenyoin than other AEDs (Pack *et al.*, 2003, 2005).

The mechanism of action hypothesized to explain the abnormalities in biochemical indices of bone mineral metabolites is induction of the cytochrome P450 enzyme system. However, the exact mechanism of action is not yet known. Increased bone turnover can produce osteoporosis (Pack *et al.*, 2003, 2005). Women who were taking lamotrigine or gabapentin (non-CYP450 enzyme-inducing AEDs) did not demonstrate any significant changes in the parameters of bone mineral density. Further studies are needed to document these initial findings, clarify the risk of AEDs in the production of osteoporosis, and identify the mechanisms of action that produce the abnormalities in bone mineral metabolism. The importance of this issue in the adolescent population, who are actively growing, must be further explored.

VI. Psychosocial Considerations

A. QUALITY OF LIFE

As their peers begin to explore the myriad of developmental opportunities of the teenage years, adolescents with epilepsy wonder whether their condition will prevent them from driving, working, marrying, having children. These concerns, superimposed on the medical burden of epilepsy, tend to significantly impact on health-related quality of life. While any chronic disorder tends to lower quality of life (QOL) in adolescence (Sawyer *et al.*, 2007), the findings in epilepsy appear worse than other disorders, such as asthma (Austin *et al.*, 1996).

In 1999, Cramer *et al.* reported the development of the QOLIE-48, designed to measure quality of life in epilepsy for adolescents, demonstrating that worsened severity of seizures was significantly associated with poorer QOLIE-48 scores, a finding duplicated in other studies (Benavente-Aguilar *et al.*, 2004). Utilizing this tool in adolescents with epilepsy, Devinsky *et al.* (1999) reported that significant predictors of poorer quality of life (QOL) included older age (14–17), more severe epilepsy, lower socioeconomic status (SES), and medication toxicity. Interestingly, younger adolescents (11–13) reported poorer scores in the social support subscale, implying that social support networks may actually improve as adolescence progresses. Community-dwelling adolescents with epilepsy who are not followed in specialty clinics appear to have better overall QOL scores (Benavente-Aguilar *et al.*, 2004; Stevanovic 2007), reflective of better seizure control.

Gender effects are mixed. Female adolescents appear to do worse than males in overall QOL scores including more self-anxiety, a poorer self-image, and a higher epilepsy-impact (Austin *et al.*, 1996; Benavente-Aguilar *et al.*, 2004; Devinsky *et al.*, 1999; Stevanovic, 2007). However, they may fare better in peer relations (Austin *et al.*, 1996) and have less denial of illness (Devinsky *et al.*, 1999). While teenage females in general appear to have higher emotional distress related to chronic disorders, they do not seek psychiatric help in larger numbers than their male counterparts (Suris *et al.*, 1996).

B. SCHOOL PERFORMANCE

Children and adolescents with epilepsy have a greater risk of educational underachievement than their counterparts without seizures (Aldenkamp *et al.*, 1999, 2005; Austin *et al.*, 1998; Seidenberg *et al.*, 1986). Significant contributing factors have been reported, including localization-related or symptomatic generalized epilepsy syndrome, AED polypharmacy, and frequent epileptiform activity (Aldenkamp *et al.*, 2001, 2005). Increased behavioral problems associated with epilepsy may also play a role (Dunn, 2003). However, most studies have not focused primarily on adolescents, which is an important limitation. Teenagers with epilepsy likely face greater academic hurdles than the challenges posed by cognitive issues related to epilepsy and AED effects. As demonstrated by Adewuya *et al.* (2006) in a Nigerian cohort, psychosocial factors may play a larger role as determinates of school performance in adolescents than seizure type or frequency. Another potentially important feature of school performance may be attendance. School days are lost at a higher rate in the epilepsy population, sometimes directly related to seizure occurrence but also related to "special privileges" granted by parents and teachers, possibly as an overprotective measure (Aguiar *et al.*, 2007).

C. DRIVING

The emerging independence associated with adolescence often includes the ability to start driving. This opportunity is reduced for many young women with epilepsy, and not only in direct relation to seizure-mandated restrictions. Sillanpaa and Shinnar (2005) examined driver's licensing in a cohort of patients with childhood onset of epilepsy. Among patients eligible to obtain a driver's license based on seizure freedom, the number of female patients who obtained a driver's license was significantly less than male patients. This difference was most striking at age 18, where 11% of eligible women with epilepsy had a driver's license, compared to 46% of eligible men with epilepsy. Furthermore, eligible patients of both genders had lower rates of licensing than their counterparts without epilepsy. For patients with epilepsy who do drive, younger age (<25) is associated with a greater risk of accidents and moving violations, however this is more prevalent for males than females (Hansotia and Broste, 1993), and is consistent with higher rates of accidents in younger male patients without medical conditions (Sheth *et al.*, 2004).

D. THE EFFECT OF STIGMA

Stigma presents one of the most difficult challenges in epilepsy, and is felt particularly acutely by teenagers (MacLeod and Austin 2003). Stigma is an important component of health-related quality of life for adolescents with epilepsy (Cramer *et al.*, 1999; Devinsky *et al.*, 1999), and concern about stigma appears to be a major component of poor self-esteem (Westbrook *et al.*, 1992). It is generally accepted that reducing stigma should improve quality of life for adolescents with epilepsy (Epilepsy Foundation), and the World Health Organization "Out of the Shadows" campaign in 1997 highlighted these issues (Reynolds, 2001). Despite these efforts, the problem continues and is very real.

In a large population of high school students, Austin *et al.* (2002) surveyed epilepsy familiarity, knowledge, and perceptions about stigma. The majority of students thought that having epilepsy might "make you unpopular," and might lead to being picked on or bullied in school (Table I). Only one third of respondents would date someone with epilepsy. Although the majority of students said that they would want a friend with epilepsy to tell them about their condition, fewer would in turn reveal this to their friends. In fact, Westbrook *et al.* (1992) demonstrated that

TABLE I
PERCENTAGES FOR STIGMA ITEMS

	Yes	Not sure	No	Do not know
If you had epilepsy, would you tell your friends?	46	31	10	14
Do you think having epilepsy would make you unpopular?	13	31	42	14
Do you think kids with epilepsy are likely to get picked on or bullied more than other kids?	37	26	24	13
If a friend had epilepsy, would you want him or her to tell you?	69	15	5	11
Would you date a person with epilepsy?	31	44	11	14

Reproduced with permission, Austin *et al.* (2002).
Questionnaire administered to a general population of high school students.

70–85% of adolescents with epilepsy do not reveal this fact to their friends, or rarely discuss it. Despite these realities, there are reassuring findings as well. In West-brook's study, most adolescents did not feel stigmatized or perceive that epilepsy affected their ability to have friendships or to date, although many of these subjects were not reporting the epilepsy to their friends, which may have contributed to this lack of perceived stigma (1992). Furthermore, in developing the QOLIE-AD-48, Cramer et al. (1999) reported an overall high quality of life with low levels of stigma in their adolescent cohort. Interestingly, the presence and effect of stigma in adolescence has not generally been associated with gender.

VII. Selected Comorbidities

A. Depression and Suicide

Depressive disorders are the most common psychiatric comorbidity of epilepsy in adolescence (Thome-Souza et al., 2004), with a reported prevalence ranging from 23 to 36% (Dunn et al., 1999; Ettinger et al., 1998; Kanner and Dunn, 2004; Thome-Souza et al., 2004). The first episode of depression in epilepsy often occurs during adolescence (Martinovic et al., 2006). As in all age groups, depression is often unrecognized and untreated (Ott et al., 2003); few or none of the patients in two studies (Dunn et al., 1999; Ettinger et al., 1998) had received psychiatric treatment. Risk factors for depression include a high frequency of seizures and longer duration of epilepsy (Oguz et al., 2002), and a positive family history of depression (Thome-Souza et al., 2004). Antiepileptic drug use may in some cases contribute to depression (Brent et al., 1987; Plioplys, 2003). Gender does not appear to be associated with a differential risk of depression in this age group.

As depression in epilepsy reduces quality of life and is a leading risk factor for suicidality (Jones et al., 2003 see below), the importance of early screening, diagnosis and treatment cannot be overemphasized (Baker, 2006). The mainstays of treatment are psychotherapy and/or pharmacotherapy, preferably with selective serontonin reuptake inhibitors (SSRIs) (Plioplys, 2003) which are typically not proconvulsive. Family education is essential and should include safety counseling and education about suicidal risk. Recently (Martinovic et al., 2006), cognitive behavioral intervention showed an effect in preventing depression in adolescent patients at risk.

Suicide is another important consideration. Epilepsy appears to be one of the few medical disorders that increase the risk of suicide in children and adolescents (Brent et al., 1990), similar to the finding of increased suicide risk in the general epilepsy population (Baker, 2006). While completed suicide in the general population is higher in young males than females (Beautrais, 2002), this finding has not been clearly duplicated in epilepsy. Numerous studies have reported an increased risk of suicide in epilepsy when comorbid Axis 1 disorders, particularly depression are present (Jones *et al.*, 2003; Nilsson *et al.*, 2002). However, the single most prominent seizure-related risk factor for suicide appears to be epilepsy-onset during adolescence (Nilsson *et al.*, 2002).

B. MIGRAINE

Both epilepsy and migraine are common neurologic disorders in adolescence, though migraine is much more common, particularly in females (Haut *et al.*, 2006). In young women, the incidence of migraine with aura peaks between ages 12 and 13 years (14.1 per 1000 person-years), while migraine without aura peaked between ages 14 and 17 years (18.9 per 1000 person-years) (Stang *et al.*, 1992; Stewart *et al.*, 1991). Although young boys have a higher prevalence of migraine than young girls, cyclic hormonal factors are considered to contribute to the excess risk of migraine in females beginning at the age of menarche (Silberstein, 2001), as well as to individual migraine attacks.

Although studies vary, individuals with either migraine or epilepsy are more than twice as likely to have the other disorder (Andermann and Andermann, 1987; Ottman and Lipton, 1996). As there is significant crossover between medications that treat epilepsy and migraine, it is tempting to treat concomitant diagnoses with a single agent, as has been recommended (Pellock, 2004), particularly to reduce the side effects of polypharmacy. Two AEDs, divalproex sodium and topiramate, are approved for both migraine prophylaxis and treatment in epilepsy. While the attempt to treat comorbid conditions with one agent has potential merit, caution must be exercised to avoid undertreating one of the conditions (Haut *et al.*, 2006).

VIII. Patient Management

What advice can we give to health care providers who take care of adolescent women with epilepsy? First and foremost, talking to the adolescent honestly and with compassion will go a long way. In addition, the adolescent needs time to discuss personal issues without a parent present. It may only be at this time that one will learn the adolescents' most distressing concerns—whether it be social/peer relationships, contraception, concerns about AEDs on cognitive or athletic performance, or depression. Specialized teenage clinics have addressed these issues (see below).

Medically, it is very important to perform a careful diagnostic evaluation, including careful history of seizure semiology, EEG, and often, an MRI scan of the brain. Only with a detailed diagnostic evaluation can the appropriate epilepsy syndrome be identified. Knowing the epilepsy syndrome is the single most important step to choosing an appropriate AED and to providing a prognosis.

A. CHOICE OF ANTIEPILEPTIC MEDICATION

Medication choice should be tailored to the epilepsy syndrome, when available. Valproate is relatively contraindicated in young women with epilepsy who are in the reproductive age, given the increased risk of anovulatory cycles, menstrual irregularities, polycystic ovaries, and polycystic ovarian syndrome. In addition, women with epilepsy who are placed on CYP450 enzyme-inducing AEDs appear to be at greater risk for osteoporosis. Furthermore, carbamazepine and valproate increase the risk for fetal neural tube defects. Preliminary evidence also suggests that valproate may produce neurocognitive effects in the fetus (Meador *et al.*, 2006). Unfortunately, the teratogenic risks for the newer AEDs, such as lamotrigine, levetiracetam, oxcarbazepine, and felbamate, are not fully known. There are several active pregnancy registries for women with epilepsy taking AEDs. Hopefully, these registries will provide clearer insights about the relative teratogenicity of these newer AEDs within the next few years. Certainly, these considerations should be fully disclosed to adolescents and their parents when discussing the AED choice—especially when the epilepsy syndrome is known to be a lifelong condition, that is, JME.

B. CHOICE OF CONTRACEPTION

All adolescents should be assumed to be sexually active. Therefore, a discussion about contraception and AED interaction is imperative when discussing new onset epilepsy with a young adolescent woman. Oral contraceptives can be an excellent option for an adolescent who is sexually active, providing that the adolescent can prove herself to be responsible and fully compliant. However, if the adolescent is on a CYP450 enzyme-inducing AED, the oral contraceptive must contain at least 59 μg of estrogen. Other reasonable options include depo-provera and the new copper T intrauterine device. None of these options, however, are protective against sexually transmitted diseases. Only condoms will provide this protection.

C. NUTRITION

Adolescents should be reminded of the importance of good nutrition, particularly during these growth years, with rapid bone mineralization. Adequate calcium intake is 1800 g per day, rarely achieved by the average adolescent. Calcium supplements should be discussed, as well as vitamin supplementation with at least 4 mg of folate.

D. Sports and Safety

Safety precautions are important to review. Sports play an important role in many adolescent's lives. Fortunately, except for swimming restrictions, athletics can be continued. In fact, there is no evidence that athletic competition increases the risk for breakthrough seizures. There is some soft evidence to suggest that regular exercise may actually reduce stress levels and decrease the risk of seizures (Nakken, 1999; Nakken *et al.*, 1990, 1997). It is appropriate, however, to discourage baths, due to increased risk of drowning. Showers are more appropriate. However, a parent should have easy access to the bathroom in case of a seizure. Driving is permitted in all states after a variable period of complete seizure freedom—typically the waiting period is six months to one-year seizure free on AEDs.

E. Compliance

Treatment compliance in epilepsy is a widespread challenge, and all the more so during adolescence. While parents typically administer medication to younger children, at some point, this process undergoes a transition and the responsibility of compliance begins to shift to the teenager. In studies of adolescents with chronic disorders (KyngÄs, 2000; Michaud *et al.*, 2004) including epilepsy (Buck *et al.*, 1997; KyngÄs, 2000), compliance with aspects of medical care is reported to be less than adequate in up to 50% of patients. Compliance in epilepsy is further complicated by the need for strict attention to dosing schedule, as a delay of even a few hours may result in a seizure. This requirement places behavioral demands that may be particularly difficult for teenagers. Conversely however, the perceived benefit to the adolescent of avoiding a seizure is significant, which would tend to increase compliance.

In a large sample of adolescents with epilepsy, KyngÄs (2000) examined factors associated with compliance. By questionnaire, 37% of patients ranked themselves as fully compliant with medication, while 18% reported full compliance with lifestyle (regular bed times and meal times). Longer duration of illness, less exercise, smoking and alcohol use, and more frequent seizures were associated with poorer compliance. Strategies to improve compliance include recognizing and exploring the problem with the patient, and switching to AEDs with more optimal dosing schedules (Nordli, 2001).

F. Sleep Deprivation

Lack of adequate sleep is a growing problem among American teenagers (Smaldone *et al.*, 2007), as teens juggle academic demands, busy social lives, and late nights at the computer. Nowhere is this more relevant than for the adolescent with epilepsy, for whom sleep deprivation may provoke a seizure. The association between sleep deprivation and epilepsy is well documented (Haut *et al.*, 2007; Kotagal, 2001; Mendez and Radtke, 2001), particularly in the setting of the IGE (Beghi *et al.*, 2006) that are prominent during adolescence. Teens must be cautioned to balance the perceived advantages of staying up late with the actual risk of experiencing a seizure the following day.

G. THE ADOLESCENT CLINIC

The topics in this chapter highlight the special issues relevant to treating a teenager with epilepsy. The development of specialized teenage epilepsy clinics was undertaken in response to these issues (Appleton *et al.*, 1997; Smith and Wallace, 2003; Smith *et al.*, 2002). Such clinics address needs specific to adolescence and aid in the transition from the pediatric to the adult service. With the teenage patient as the focus of consultation rather than the parents, the patients are more likely to reveal and discuss concerns (Appleton *et al.*, 1997). As noted by Smith *et al.* (2002), a systematic review of relevant issues may reveal important and unexpected outcomes, such as the discovery that the majority of their female teenage patients had not previously been prescribed folate.

TABLE II

CHECKLIST FOR ADOLESCENT EPILEPSY VISIT

---

1. Epilepsy syndrome diagnosis, prognosis, appropriate AED choices.
2. Seizure control and medication side effects, with special attention to cognitive slowing, weight gain, and mood.
3. The adolescent's concerns about the diagnosis, treatment, and social ramifications. This history may be best obtained by one of the allied health personnel, such as a nurse, social worker, or pediatric nurse practitioner.
4. Contraception and the possible interactions with AEDs. All adolescents should be presumed to be sexually active. If the health provider does not bring up this topic, the adolescent most likely will not.
5. Nutrition. Many adolescent patients have poor nutrition with inadequate sources of calcium, vitamin D, and folate.
6. Safety issues, especially with respect to driving.
7. Exercise. Participation is sports is recommended and should even be encouraged in our adolescent patients with epilepsy. Exercise will not exacerbate their seizures and will assist with weight control and mood.
8. Sleep deprivation and its effects on seizure control.
9. Recreational drugs and alcohol and their effects on seizure control.
10. School performance, attendance, and concerns.
11. Signs of depression and anxiety, important and frequent comorbidities of epilepsy.

AEDs, antiepileptic drugs.

While a specialized adolescent epilepsy clinic may not be feasible in many centers, the strategies employed are applicable to most clinical settings. A checklist of recommended topics is indicated (Table II).

IX. Conclusions

There are many challenges that face an adolescent woman who has been diagnosed with epilepsy. Adolescence is a time of growing independence, physical and emotional change, accompanied by social insecurity. If, in the midst of all of these changes, an adolescent is given the diagnosis of epilepsy, there is an additional burden. She now has to deal with the fact that epilepsy is a chronic disease requiring daily medication and that it may be a lifelong condition. There are frequent comorbidities with this diagnosis, including depression, migraine headaches, and cognitive/behavioral problems. Our role as medical providers is to provide some perspective to the illness and help guide our adolescent patient. We can provide a strong foundation of assistance and emotional support, as well as medical knowledge, particularly in the setting of a specialized adolescent clinic.

References

Adewuya, A. O., Oseni, S. B., and Okeniyi, J. A. (2006). School performance of Nigerian adolescents with epilepsy. *Epilepsia* **47**(2), 415–420.

Aguiar, B. V., Guerreiro, M. M., McBrian, D., and Montenegro, M. A. (2007). Seizure impact on the school attendance in children with epilepsy. *Seizure* **16**(8), 698–702.

Aldenkamp, A. P., Overweg-Plandsoen, W. C., and Arends, J. (1999). An open, nonrandomized clinical comparative study evaluating the effect of epilepsy on learning. *J. Child Neurol.* **14**(12), 795–800.

Aldenkamp, A. P., Arends, J., Overweg-Plandsoen, T. C., van Bronswijk, K. C., Schyns-Soeterboek, A., Linden, I., and Diepman, L. (2001). Acute cognitive effects of nonconvulsive difficult-to-detect epileptic seizures and epileptiform electroencephalographic discharges. *J. Child Neurol.* **16**(2), 119–123.

Aldenkamp, A. P., Weber, B., Overweg-Plandsoen, W. C., Reijs, R., and van Mil, S. (2005). Educational underachievement in children with epilepsy: A model to predict the effects of epilepsy on educational achievement. *J. Child Neurol.* **20**(3), 175–180.

American Academy of Neurology (1998). Quality Standards Subcommitee. Practice parameter: Management issues for women with epilepsy (summary statement). *Neurology* **51,** 944–948.

Andermann, E., and Andermann, F. A. (1987). Migraine-epilepsy relationships: Epidemiological and genetic aspects. *In* "Migraine and Epilepsy" (F. A. Andermann and E. Lugaresi, Eds.), pp. 281–291. Butterworths, Boston.

Appleton, R. E., Chadwick, D., and Sweeney, A. (1997). Managing the teenager with epilepsy: Paediatric to adult care. *Seizure* **6**(1), 27–30.

Austin, J. K., Huster, G. A., Dunn, D. W., and Risinger, M. W. (1996). Adolescents with active or inactive epilepsy or asthma: A comparison of quality of life. *Epilepsia* **37**(12), 1228–1238.

Austin, J. K., Huberty, T. J., Huster, G. A., and Dunn, D. W. (1998). Academic achievement in children with epilepsy or asthma. *Dev. Med. Child Neurol.* **40**(4), 248–255.

Austin, J. K., Shafer, P. O., and Deering, J. B. (2002). Epilepsy familiarity, knowledge, and perceptions of stigma: Report from a survey of adolescents in the general population. *Epilepsy Behav.* **3**(4), 368–375.

Baker, G. A. (2006). Depression and suicide in adolescents with epilepsy. *Neurology* **66**(6 Suppl. 3), S5–S12.

Beautrais, A. L. (2002). Gender issues in youth suicidal behaviour. *Emerg. Med. (Fremantle)* **14**(1), 35–42.

Beghi, M., Beghi, E., Cornaggia, C. M., and Gobbi, G. (2006). Idiopathic generalized epilepsies of adolescence. *Epilepsia* **47**(Suppl. 2), 107–110.

Benavente-Aguilar, I., Morales-Blanquez, C., Rubio, E. A., and Rey, J. M. (2004). Quality of life of adolescents suffering from epilepsy living in the community. *J. Paediatr. Child Health* **40**(3), 110–113.

Blumer, D., and Walker, A. E. (1967). Sexual behavior in temporal lobe epilepsy. *Arch. Neurol.* **16**, 37–43.

Bogliun, G., Beghi, E., Crespi, V., Delodovici, L., and d'Amico, P. (1986). Anticonvulsant drugs and bone metabolism. *Acta Neurol. Scand.* **74**, 284–288.

Brent, D. A., Crumrine, P. K., Varma, R. R., Allan, M., and Allman, C. (1987). Phenobarbital treatment and major depressive disorder in children with epilepsy. *Pediatrics* **80**(6), 909–917.

Brent, D. A., Kolko, D. J., Allan, M. J., and Brown, R. V. (1990). Suicidality in affectively disordered adolescent inpatients. *J. Am. Acad. Child Adolesc. Psychiatry* **29**(4), 586–593.

Buck, D., Jacoby, A., Baker, G. A., and Chadwick, D. W. (1997). Factors influencing compliance with antiepileptic drug regimes. *Seizure* **6**(2), 87–93.

Camfield, C. S., Camfield, P. R., Gordon, K., Wirrell, E., and Dooley, J. M. (1996). Incidence of epilepsy in childhood and adolescence: A population-based study in Nova Scotia from 1977 to 1985. *Epilepsia* **37**(1), 19–23.

Chang, S., and Ahn, C. (1994). Effects of antiepileptic drug therapy on bone mineral density in ambulatory epileptic children. *Brain Dev.* **16**, 382–385.

Christensen, J., Kjeldsen, M. J., Andersen, H., Friis, M. L., and Sidenius, P. (2005). Gender differences in epilepsy. *Epilepsia* **46**(6), 956–960.

Clayton, R. N., Ogden, V., Hodgkinson, J., *et al.* (1992). How common are polycystic ovaries in normal women and what is their significance for the fertility of the population. *Clin. Endocrinol.* **37**, 127–134.

Cramer, J. A., Westbrook, L. E., Devinsky, O., Perrine, K., Glassman, M. B., and Camfield, C. (1999). Development of the Quality of Life in Epilepsy Inventory for Adolescents: The QOLIE-AD-48. *Epilepsia* **40**(8), 1114–1121.

Crawford, P. (2002). Interactions between antiepileptic drugs and hormonal contraception. *CNS Drugs* **16**, 263–272.

Demerdash, A., Shaalon, M., Midori, A., *et al.* (1991). Sexual behavior of a sample of females with epilepsy. *Epilepsia* **32**, 82–85.

Devinsky, O., Westbrook, L., Cramer, J., Glassman, M., Perrine, K., and Camfield, C. (1999). Risk factors for poor health-related quality of life in adolescents with epilepsy. *Epilepsia* **40**(12), 1715–1720.

Drislane, F. W., Coleman, A. E., Schomer, D. L., *et al.* (1994). Altered pulsatile secretion of luteinizing hormone in women with epilepsy. *Neurology* **44**, 306–310.

Dunn, D. W., Austin, J. K., and Huster, G. A. (1999). Symptoms of depression in adolescents with epilepsy. *J. Am. Acad. Child Adolesc. Psychiatry* **38**(9), 1132–1138.

Dunn, D. W., Austin, J. K., Caffrey, H. M., and Perkins, S. M. (2003). A prospective study of teachers' ratings of behavior problems in children with new-onset seizures. *Epilepsy Behav.* **4**(1), 26–35.

Engel, J; International League Against Epilepsy (ILAE). (2001). A proposed diagnostic scheme for people with epileptic seizures and with epilepsy: Report of the ILAE task force on classification and terminology. *Epilepsia* **42**(6), 796–803.

Ettinger, A. B., Weisbrot, D. M., Nolan, E. E., Gadow, K. D., Vitale, S. A., Andriola, M. R., Lenn, N. J., Novak, G. P., and Hermann, B. P. (1998). Symptoms of depression and anxiety in pediatric epilepsy patients. *Epilepsia* **39**(6), 595–599.

Farquhar, C. M., Birdsall, M., Manning, P., *et al.* (1994). The prevalence of polycystic ovaries on ultrasound scanning in a population of randomly selected women. *Aust. N. Z. J. Obstet. Gynaecol.* **34**, 67–72.

Ferin, M., Morrell, M., Xiao, E., *et al.* (2003). Endocrine and metabolic responses to long-term monotherapy with the antiepileptic drug valproate in the normally cycling rhesus monkey. *J. Clin. Endocrinol. Metab.* **88**(6), 2908–2915.

Gough, H., Goggin, T., Bissessar, A., *et al.* (1986). A comparative study of the relative influence of different anticonvulsant drugs, UV exposure and diet on vitamin D and calcium metabolism in outpatients with epilepsy. *QJM (New Series 59)* **230**, 569–577.

Hansotia, P., and Broste, S. K. (1993). Epilepsy and traffic safety. *Epilepsia* **34**(5), 852–858.

Hauser, W. A., Annegers, J. F., and Kurland, L. T. (1993). Incidence of epilepsy and unprovoked seizures in Rochester, Minnesota: 1935–1984. *Epilepsia* **34**(3), 453–468.

Haut, S. R., Bigal, M. E., and Lipton, R. B. (2006). Chronic disorders with episodic manifestations: Focus on epilepsy and migraine. *Lancet Neurol.* **5**, 148–157.

Haut, S. R., Hall, C. B., Masur, J., and Lipton, R. B. (2007). Seizure occurrence: Precipitants and prediction. *Neurology.* Nov 13, **69**(20),1905–1910.

Herzog A. G., Klein P., and Ransil B. (1997). Epilepsia, **38**(10), 1082–1088.

Herzog, A. G., Seibel, M. M., Schomer, D. L., *et al.* (1986). Reproductive endocrine disorders in women with partial seizures of temporal lobe origin. *Arch. Neurol.* **43**, 341–346.

Isojarvi, J. I. T., Laatikainen, T. J., Pakarinen, A. J., *et al.* (1993). Polycystic ovaries and hyperandrogenism in women taking valproate for epilepsy. *N. Eng. J. Med.* **329**, 1383–1388.

Isojarvi, J. I. T., Parakinen, A. J., Rautio, A., *et al.* (1995). Serum sex hormone levels after replacing carbamazepine with oxcarbazepine. *Eur. Clin. Pharmacol.* **47**, 461–464.

Isojarvi, J. I. T., Rattya, J., Myllyla, V. V., *et al.* (1998). Valproate, lamotrigine, and insulin-mediated risks in women with epilepsy. *Ann. Neurol.* **43**, 446–451.

Jensen, S. B. (1992). Sexuality and chronic-illness; biopsychosocial approach. *Semin. Neurol.* **12**, 135–140.

Jones, J. E., Hermann, B. P., Barry, J. J., Gilliam, F. G., Kanner, A. M., and Meador, K. J. (2003). Rates and risk factors for suicide, suicidal ideation, and suicide attempts in chronic epilepsy. *Epilepsy Behav.* **4**(Suppl. 3), S31–S38.

Kanner, A. M., and Dunn, D. W. (2004). Diagnosis and management of depression and psychosis in children and adolescents with epilepsy. *J. Child Neurol.* **19**(Suppl. 1), S65–S72.

Kotagal, P. (2001). The relationship between sleep and epilepsy. *Semin Pediatr. Neurol.* **8**(4), 241–250.

Kotsopoulos, I. A., van Merode, T., Kessels, F. G., de Krom, M. C., and Knottnerus, J. A. (2002). Systematic review and meta-analysis of incidence studies of epilepsy and unprovoked seizures. *Epilepsia* **43**(11), 1402–1409.

Krauss, G. L., Brandt, J., Campbell, M., *et al.* (1996). Antiepileptic medication and oral contraceptive interactions; a national survey of neurologists and obstetricians. *Neurology* **46**, 1534–1539.

KyngÄs, H. (2000). Compliance with health regimens of adolescents with epilepsy. *Seizure* **9**(8), 598–604.

KyngÄs, H. A. (2000). Compliance in adolescents with chronic diseases: A review. *J. Adolesc. Health* **26** (6), 379–388.

Lamictal (package insert) (2004). "Research Triangle Park." GlaxoSmithKline, NC.

Levesque, L. A., Herzog, A. G., and Seibel, M. M. (1986). The effect of phenytoing and carbamazepine on serum dehydroepiandrosterone sulfate in men and women who have partial seizures with temporal lobe involvement. *J. Clin. Endrocrinol. Metab.* **63**, 243–245.

MacLeod, J. S., and Austin, J. K. (2003). Stigma in the lives of adolescents with epilepsy: A review of the literature. *Epilepsy Behav.* **4**(2), 112–117.

Martinovic, Z., Simonovic, P., and Djokic, R. (2006). Preventing depression in adolescents with epilepsy. *Epilepsy Behav.* **9**(4), 619–624. [Epub 2006 Oct 17].

McEwen, B. S. (1998). Multiple ovarian hormone effects on brain structure and function. *J. Gend. Specif. Med.* **1**, 33–41.

Meador, K. J., Baker, G. A., Finnell, R. H., *et al.* (2006). NEAD Study Group. In Utero Antiepileptic Drug Exposure; fetal death and malformations. *Neurology* **67**(3), 407–412.

Mendez, M., and Radtke, R. A. (2001). Interactions between sleep and epilepsy. *J. Clin. Neurophysiol.* **18**(2), 106–127.

Meo, R., Bilo, L., Nappi, C., *et al.* (1993). Derangement of the hypothalamic GnRH pulse generator in women with epilepsy. *Seizure* **2**, 241–252.

Michaud, P. A., Suris, J. C., and Viner, R. (2004). The adolescent with a chronic condition. Part II: Healthcare provision. *Arch. Dis. Child.* **89**(10), 943–949.

Morrell, M. J. (2003). Reproductive and metabolic disorders in women with epilepsy. *Epilepsia* **44**(Suppl. 4), 11–20.

Morrell, M. J., and Guldner, G. T. (1996). Self-reported sexual dysfunction and sexual arousability in women with epilepsy. *Epilepsia* **37**, 1204–1210.

Morrell, M. J., Sarto, G. E., Shafer, P. O., *et al.* (2000). Health issues for women with epilepsy: A descriptive survey to assess knowledge and awareness among healthcare providers. *J. Womens Health Gend. Based Med.* **9**, 959–965.

Morrell, M. J., Flynn, K. L., Seale, C. G., *et al.* (2001). Reproductive dysfunction in women with epilepsy: Antiepileptic drug effects on sex-steroid hormones. *CNS Spectr.* **6**, 771–786.

Morrell, M. J., Giudice, L., Flynn, K. L., *et al.* (2002). Predictors of ovulatory failure in women with epilepsy. *Ann. Neurol.* **52**, 704–711.

Morrell, M. J., Isojarvi, J., Taylor, A. E., *et al.* (2003). Higher androgens and weight gain with valproate compared with lamotrigine for epilepsy. *Epilepsy Res.* **54**(2–3), 189–199.

Murialdo, G., Galimberti, C. A., Gianelli, M. V., *et al.* (1998). Effects of valproate, Phenobarbital and carbamazepine on sex steroid setup in women with epilepsy. *Clin. Neuropharmacol.* **21**, 52–58.

Mullins, G. M., O'sullivan, S. S., Neligan, A., McCarthy, A., McNamara, B., Galvin, R. J., and Sweeney, B. J. (2007). A study of idiopathic generalised epilepsy in an Irish population. *Seizure* **16** (3), 204–210. [Epub 2007 Jan 12].

Nakken, K. O. (1999). Physical exercise in outpatients with epilepsy. *Epilepsia* **40**, 643–651.

Nakken, K. O., Bjorholt, P. G., Johnnessen, S. I., *et al.* (1990). Effect of physical training on aerobic capacity, seizure occurrence and serum level of antiepileptic drugs in adults with epilepsy. *Epilepsia* **31**, 88–94.

Nakken, K. O., Loyning, A., Loyning, T., *et al.* (1997). Does physical exercise influence the occurrence of epileptiform EEG discharges in children? *Epilepsia* **38**, 279–284.

Nilsson, L., Ahlbom, A., Farahmand, B. Y., Asberg, M., and Tomson, T. (2002). Risk factors for suicide in epilepsy: A case control study. *Epilepsia* **43**(6), 644–651.

Nordli, D. R. (2001). Special needs of the adolescent with epilepsy. *Epilepsia* **42**(Suppl. 8), 10–17.

O'Donovan, C., Kusumaker, V., Graves, G. R., *et al.* (2002). Menstrual abnormalities and polycystic ovary syndrome in women taking valproate for bipolar mood disorder. *J. Clin. Psychiatry* **63**, 322–330.

Oguz, A. (2002). Relationship of epilepsy-related factors to anxiety and depression scores in epileptic children. *J. Child Neurol.* **17**(1), 37–40.

Ott, D., Siddarth, P., Gurbani, S., Koh, S., Tournay, A., Shields, W. D., and Caplan, R. (2003). Behavioral disorders in pediatric epilepsy: Unmet psychiatric need. *Epilepsia* **44**(4), 591–597.

Ottman, R., and Lipton, R. B. (1996). Is the comorbidity of epilepsy and migraine due to a shared genetic susceptibility. *Neurology* **47**, 918–924.

Pack, A. M., Morrell, M. J., Randall, A., *et al.* (2003). Markers of general bone function, bone formation, and bone resorption in women with epilepsy on antiepileptic drug monotherapy. (Abstract). *Neurology* **60**(Suppl. 1), A437.

Pack, A. M., Morrell, M. J., Marcus, R., *et al.* (2005). Bone mass and turnover in women with epilepsy on antiepileptic drug monotherapy. *Ann. Neurol.* **57**, 252–257.

Pellock, J. M. (2004). Understanding co-morbidities affecting children with epilepsy. *Neurology* **62**(5 Suppl. 2), S17–S23.

Pfaff, D. W., and McEwen, B. S. (1983). Actions of estrogens and progestins on nerve cells. *Science* **219**, 808–814.

Plioplys, S. (2003). Depression in children and adolescents with epilepsy. *Epilepsy Behav.* **4**(Suppl. 3), S39–S45.

Polson, D. W., Wadsworth, J., Adams, J., *et al.* (1988). Polycystic ovaries-common finding in normal women. *Lancet* **1**, 870–872.

Rasgon, N. L., Altshuler, L. L., Gudeman, D., *et al.* (2000). Medication status and PCO syndrome in women with bipolar disorder: A preliminary report. *J. Clin. Psychiatry* **61**, 173–178.

Reynolds, E. H. (2001). ILAE/IBE/WHO Global Campaign "out of the shadows": Global and regional developments. *Epilepsia* **42**(8), 1094–1100.

Sabers, A., Buchholt, J. M., Uldall, P., *et al.* (2001). Lamotrigine plasma levels reduced by oral contraceptives. *Epilepsy Res.* **47**, 151–154.

Sabers, A., Ohman, I., Christensen, J., *et al.* (2003). Oral contraceptives reduce lamotrigine plasma levels. *Neurology* **61**, 570–571.

Sawyer, S. M., Drew, S., Yeo, M. S., and Britto, M. T. (2007). Adolescents with a chronic condition: Challenges living, challenges treating. *Lancet* **369**(9571), 1481–1489.

Seidenberg, M., Beck, N., Geisser, M., Giordani, B., Sackellares, J. C., Berent, S., Dreifuss, F. E., and Boll, T. J. (1986). Academic achievement of children with epilepsy. *Epilepsia* **27**(6), 753–759.

Sheth, R. D., and Gidal, B. E. (2006). Optimizing epilepsy management in teenagers. *J. Child Neurol.* **21**(4), 273–279.

Sheth, R., Wesolowski, C., Jacob, J., *et al.* (1996). Effect of carbamazepine and valproate on bone mineral density. *J. Pediatr.* **127**, 256–262.

Sheth, S. G., Krauss, G., Krumholz, A., and Li, G. (2004). Mortality in epilepsy: Driving fatalities vs other causes of death in patients with epilepsy. *Neurology* **63**(6), S12–S3.

Silberstein, S. D. (2001). Headache and female hormones: What you need to know. *Curr. Opin. Neurol.* **14**(3), 323–333.

Sillanpaa, M., and Shinnar, S. (2005). Obtaining a driver's license and seizure relapse in patients with childhood-onset epilepsy. *Neurology* **64**(4), 680–686.

Smaldone, A., Honig, J. C., and Byrne, M. W. (2007). Sleepless in America: Inadequate sleep and relationships to health and well-being of our nation's children. *Pediatrics* **119**(Suppl. 1), S29–S37.

Smith, P. E., and Wallace, S. J. (2003). Taking over epilepsy from the paediatric neurologist. *J. Neurol. Neurosurg. Psychiatry* **74**(Suppl. 1), i37–i41.

Smith, P. E., Myson, V., and Gibbon, F. (2002). A teenager epilepsy clinic: Observational study. *Eur. J. Neurol.* **9**(4), 373–376.

Stang, P. E., Yanagihara, T., Swanson, J. W., *et al.* (1992). Incidence of migraine headaches: A population-based study in Olmsted County, Minnesota. *Neurology* **42**, 1657–1662.

Stevanovic, D. (2007). Health-related quality of life in adolescents with well-controlled epilepsy. *Epilepsy Behav.* **10**(4), 571–575.

Stewart, W. F., Linet, M. S., Celentano, D. D., Van Natta, M., and Ziegler, D. (1991). Age and sex-specific incidence rates of migraine with and without visual aura. *Am. J. Epidemiol.* **134,** 1111–1120.

Stoffel-Wagner, B., Bauer, J., Flugel, D., *et al.* (1998). Serum sex hormones are altered in patients with chronic temporal lobe epilepsy receiving anticonvulsant medication. *Epilepsia* **39,** 1164–1173.

Suris, J. C., Parera, N., and Puig, C. (1996). Chronic illness and emotional distress in adolescence. *J. Adolesc. Health* **19**(2), 153–156.

Thome-Souza, S., Kuczynski, E., Assumpcao, F., Rzezak, P., Fuentes, D., Fiore, L., and Valente, K. D. (2004). Which factors may play a pivotal role on determining the type of psychiatric disorder in children and adolescents with epilepsy. *Epilepsy Behav.* **5**(6), 988–994.

Valimaki, M., Tiihonen, M., Laitinen, K., *et al.* (1994). Bone mineral density measured by dual-energy x-ray absorptionmetry and novel markers of bone formation and resorption in patients on antiepileptic drugs. *J. Bone Miner. Res.* **9,** 631–637.

Westbrook, L. E., Bauman, L. J., and Shinnar, S. (1992). Applying stigma theory to epilepsy: A test of a conceptual model. *J. Pediatr. Psychol.* **17**(5), 633–649.

Wheless, J. W., and Kim, H. L. (2002). Adolescent seizures and epilepsy syndromes. *Epilepsia* **43**(Suppl. 3), 33–52.

Woolley, C. S., and Schwartzkroin, P. A. (1998). Hormonal effects on the brain. *Epilepsia* **39**(Suppl. 8), S2–S8.

Zahn, C. A., Morrell, M. J., Collins, S. D., *et al.* (1998). Management issues for women with epilepsy; a review of the literature. American Academy of Neurology Practice Guidelines. *Neurology* **51,** 949–956.

Zupanc, M. L. (2006). Antiepileptic drugs and hormonal contraceptives in adolescent women with epilepsy. *Neurology* **66**(Suppl. 3), S37–S45.

CONTRACEPTION IN WOMEN WITH EPILEPSY: PHARMACOKINETIC INTERACTIONS, CONTRACEPTIVE OPTIONS, AND MANAGEMENT

Caryn Dutton* and Nancy Foldvary-Schaefer[†]

*University of Wisconsin School of Medicine and Public Health,
Madison, Wisconsin 53704, USA
[†]Cleveland Clinic Lerner College of Medicine of Case Western Reserve University,
Cleveland, Ohio 44195, USA

I. Introduction
II. Knowledge of Pregnancy Risk and Practice of Contraception in Women with Epilepsy
III. Pharmacology of Combined Oral Contraceptives
IV. Hormonal Contraceptive–AED Interactions
    A. Cytochrome 3A4 Isoenzyme Inducers
    B. Cytochrome 3A4 Isoenzyme Noninducers
    C. AEDs with Unique or Unanticipated Interactions
    D. Hormonal Contraception and Seizure Control
    E. Other Effects of Oral Contraceptive Interactions with AEDs
V. Other Hormonal Contraceptives and Their Known or Potential Interactions with AEDs
    A. Progestin-Only Oral Contraceptive Pills
    B. Contraceptive Injection
    C. Contraceptive Patch
    D. Contraceptive Vaginal Ring
    E. Contraceptive Implants
    F. Emergency Contraception
VI. Contraceptive Methods Without AED Interaction
    A. Intrauterine Devices
    B. Barrier Methods: Condoms, Contraceptive Sponge, Diaphragm,
       Cervical Cap, and Shield
    C. Sterilization
    D. Other Birth Control Methods Practiced by Women
VII. Counseling and Management of Contraception in Women Requiring
     AED Prescription
    A. Choosing a Contraceptive Method for a Woman with Epilepsy
    B. Women Using Hormonal Contraception Who Require Initiation of
       Antiepileptic Therapy
VIII. Summary
    References

INTERNATIONAL REVIEW OF
NEUROBIOLOGY, VOL. 83
DOI: 10.1016/S0074-7742(08)00006-8

113

Contraceptive counseling is a critical component of the management of the female patient with epilepsy because of the increased risk of pregnancy associated with epilepsy and the multitude of interactions between antiepileptic drugs (AEDs) and hormonal contraception. Steroid hormones and many of the AEDs are substrates for the cytochrome P450 enzyme system, in particular, the 3A4 isoenzyme. As a result, concomitant use of hormonal contraceptives and AEDs may pose a risk for unexpected pregnancy, seizures, and drug-related adverse effects. The risk of combined oral contraceptive (COC) failure is slightly increased in the presence of cytochrome P450 3A4 enzyme-inducing AEDs. Several AEDs induce the production of sex hormone binding globulin (SHBG) to which the progestins are tightly bound, resulting in lower concentrations of free progestin that may also lead to COC failure. There is no increase in the risk of COC failure in women taking nonenzyme-inducing AEDs. Oral contraceptives significantly increase the metabolism of lamotrigine, posing a risk of seizures when hormonal agents are initiated and/or toxicity during pill-free weeks. There is no evidence that COCs increase seizures in women with epilepsy. While higher dose COCs are one contraceptive option for women on enzyme-inducing AEDs, a variety of other options are available. Injectable contraception (depot medroxyprogesterone acetate) appears effective with AED use, but the potential for bone mineral density loss is a concern. Intrauterine devices (IUDs) and barrier methods do not rely on hormonal components for contraceptive efficacy, and are therefore appropriate to recommend for use in women using enzyme-inducing medications. This chapter reviews the evidence regarding the pharmacokinetic interaction between AEDs and oral contraceptive hormones, the known or potential interactions with alternative contraceptive methods, and provides practical advice for management of contraceptive needs in reproductive-age women.

I. Introduction

Epilepsy affects >1% of the population, including approximately one million women of childbearing potential in the United States (AAN Practice Parameter, 1998). Epilepsy increases the risk of abnormal fetal outcome related to intrauterine exposure to antiepileptic drugs (AEDs). Addressing contraception is therefore a critical component of the evaluation and treatment of reproductive-age women with epilepsy.

In recent years, the number of new AEDs and new formulations of older AEDs has increased considerably in the United States and worldwide, offering more therapeutic options for people with epilepsy. In addition, AEDs are increasingly used for conditions other than epilepsy, including psychiatric and sleep disorders and chronic pain. In the United States, nearly 50% of AED prescriptions are written for nonepilepsy indications (Verispan LLC, 2005). For some agents, prescriptions for nonepilepsy indications far exceed those written for epilepsy.

This chapter will review the evidence regarding the pharmacokinetic interaction between AEDs and oral contraceptive hormones, and will apply this understanding to estimate effects between AEDs and the wider variety of hormonal contraceptives now available. The final section provides practical advice for management of contraceptive needs in reproductive-age women requiring AEDs for seizure control or other therapy.

II. Knowledge of Pregnancy Risk and Practice of Contraception in Women with Epilepsy

Despite the known reproductive risks, women with epilepsy are often unaware of the potential for a drug interaction affecting contraception or of the risks of pregnancy. Only rarely do women with epilepsy consult healthcare providers for preconception planning or during the first few weeks of pregnancy (Seale *et al.*, 1998). In a survey by the British Epilepsy Association, 51% of women claimed never to have received advice on contraception or the interaction between oral contraceptive agents and AEDs (Crawford and Lee, 1999).

A more recent U.S. survey confirmed that a high percentage of women with epilepsy were unaware of the potential for drug interactions and side effects. Out of a convenience sample of women presenting for care at an epilepsy clinic, 70% did not know that their prescribed AED might change how well birth control pills work. Women were also poorly informed regarding the consequences of an unplanned pregnancy during AED use. Only 28% of women taking a FDA category C drug and 41% taking a category D drug indicated knowledge of the potential for effects on fetal development (Davis *et al.*, 2007a).

Healthcare providers demonstrate similar gaps in knowledge regarding reproductive risks and contraceptive interactions with AEDs. Among Scottish obstetricians, 51% were unaware of the need for preconception counseling for women with epilepsy (Russell *et al.*, 1996). A survey of U.S. physicians revealed that 4% of the neurologists and none of the obstetricians polled were aware of the interactions between the six most common first-generation AEDs and oral contraceptives, despite the fact that ~25% had reported unexpected pregnancies among patients in their practice (Krauss *et al.*, 1996). In the United Kingdom, a review of prescribing practices reported that 56% of patients coadministered an enzyme-inducing AED and oral contraceptives were on "low-dose" estrogen pills and therefore at risk of contraceptive failure (Shorvon *et al.*, 2002). While more recent surveys suggest that awareness is increasing among neurologists and gynecologists (Foy *et al.*, 2001;

Morrell *et al.*, 2000), these findings underscore the importance of ongoing educational efforts directed to women with epilepsy and their healthcare providers.

Unfortunately, women with epilepsy surveyed at an academic epilepsy clinic report that 50% of their previous pregnancies were unplanned (Davis *et al.*, 2007b). This is similar to the rate of unintended pregnancy for the general U.S. population (Finer and Henshaw, 2006), despite the fact that women with epilepsy represent a high-risk group. Of those who reported using contraception in the previous month, only 53% of women in this clinic population used a highly effective method; 17% reported using withdrawal as their only contraceptive method (Davis *et al.*, 2007b). Current contraceptive use and rates of unintended pregnancy among women with epilepsy likely reflects the inadequate knowledge of patients and providers.

III. Pharmacology of Combined Oral Contraceptives

Exogenous administration of estrogen and progestin suppresses ovulation by inhibition of LH and FSH at the level of the hypothalamic–pituitary axis. This results in prevention of follicular development, and therefore absence of ovulation during most cycles. Initial development of oral contraceptives in the 1950s was focused on providing high doses of progesterone derivatives to mimic pregnancy. The presence of estrogen, discovered to be a contaminant in the "progestin" tablets, resulted in less breakthrough bleeding and improved efficacy (Asbell, 1995). Most formulations are packaged as 21 active pills containing estrogen and progestin followed by 7 placebo pills. During the placebo or pill-free week, a woman experiences withdrawal bleeding to simulate a normal 28-day cycle.

Combined oral contraceptives (COCs) available in the United States primarily contain ethinyl estradiol (EE) as the estrogen component. Mestranol, the alternative estrogen used in the first marketed oral contraceptive in the United States, is partially converted (75–80%) to EE following ingestion. Over time, the dose of EE in oral contraceptives has decreased from 150 mcg to 20–35 mcg daily without any reduction in efficacy and with a significant reduction in cardiovascular risk (Rosenberg *et al.*, 1999).

The progestin component in modern contraceptives varies, both in amount and type of progestin. Progestin doses have been reduced over time as well, or varied during the cycle as with triphasic preparations which have a different dose of progestin in each of the 3 weeks of active tablets to minimize the overall amount of hormone. Progestins also result in thickening of cervical mucus, interfering with sperm activity and penetration. Exogenous administration of both hormones produces effects at the level of the endometrium, though it is unknown if these changes contribute to the overall efficacy (Rivera *et al.*, 1999).

Oral administration of estrogen is significantly effected by first-pass metabolism; EE has a bioavailability of between 40 and 50%, with wide interindividual variation noted. Multiple drug interaction studies in humans and animal models confirm the role of the cytochrome (CYP) P450 system as the primary site for hydroxylation of EE (Crawford, 2002). Hydroxylation and subsequent conjugation with glucuronide or sulfate deactivates EE, which is then excreted in the bile. In humans, a fraction of conjugated EE may be hydrolyzed by bacteria in the colon and then reabsorbed as an active metabolite. There are differences reported between individuals and between ethnic groups, with variation as high as tenfold, in the proportion of EE susceptible to first-pass metabolism, conjugation, and enterohepatic recirculation (Wilbur and Ensom, 2000). This may result in only certain individuals with a clinical effect of a reduction in contraceptive efficacy from a drug interaction, due to the variation in metabolic parameters.

Ethinyl estradiol is primarily bound to serum albumin and increases the production of sex hormone binding globulin (SHBG). Progestins, in contrast, are primarily bound to SHBG in the circulation. The total amount of progestin may vary depending on SHBG levels, and with elevations in SHBG the free concentration of progestin is potentially affected. Progestins are not subject to enterohepatic circulation, but are also susceptible to increased metabolism by the cytochrome (CYP) P450 system (McAuley and Anderson, 2002).

IV. Hormonal Contraceptive–AED Interactions

Kenyon (1972) described the first case of unexpected pregnancy in a woman with epilepsy taking phenytoin several months following initiation of an COC. In the years that followed, similar cases were reported involving phenobarbital, primidone, and carbamazepine. More recently, additional interactions, drug-specific in some cases, have been observed between sex steroids and AEDs.

Many of the currently available AEDs are metabolized primarily by the cytochrome (CYP) P450 mixed function oxidases (Perruca and Richens, 1995). Steroid hormones serve as substrates for the cytochrome P450 enzyme system, in particular, the 3A4 isoenzyme. Enzyme-inducing AEDs increase the metabolism of sex steroids, potentially rendering them less effective. In addition, some AEDs increase the production of SHBG leading to increased capacity to bind to progesterone, ultimately reducing its free concentration. Phenobarbital, primidone, phenytoin, carbamazepine, and oxcarbazepine are operative in this mechanism (Back et al., 1980; Crawford et al., 1990; Klosterskov Jensen et al., 1992). Pharmacokinetic parameters of the currently available AEDs are summarized in Table I.

TABLE I

PHARMACOKINETIC CHARACTERISTICS OF ANTIEPILEPTIC DRUGS (AEDs)[a]

	V_d (l/kg)	Protein binding (%)	$t_{1/2}$ (h)	Elimination route (%)	
				Renal	Liver[b]
(A) Cytochrome 3A4 inducers					
Carbamazepine	0.8	75	9–15	1	99 (oxidation)
Felbamate	0.8	25	13–22	50	50 (oxidation + other)
Oxcarbazepine	0.8	40	9	1	99 (reduction, glucuronidation)
Phenobarbital	0.6	45	75–110	25	75 (oxidation)
Phenytoin	0.8	90	9–36	5	95 (oxidation)
Primidone	0.7	0–20	10–15	40	60 (oxidation)
Topiramate[c]	0.7	15	12–24	65	35 (oxidation)
(B) Cytochrome 3A4 noninducers					
Ethosuximide	0.7	0	30–60	20	80 (oxidation)
Gabapentin	0.7	0	5–7	100	0
Lamotrigine	1.0	55	12–62	10	90 (glucuronidation)
Levetiracetam	0.5–0.7	<10	6–8	100	0
Pregabalin	0.5	0	6–7	100	0
Tiagabine	1.4	96	7–9	2	98 (oxidation)
Valproate	0.2	90	6–18	2	98 (oxidation, glucuronidation
Zonisamide	1.5	40	63	35	65 (conjugation)

[a]Normal values for adults on monotherapy.
[b]Primary mechanism recognized.
[c]Weak inducer. V_d, volume of distribution; $t_{1/2}$, elimination half-life.

A. CYTOCHROME 3A4 ISOENZYME INDUCERS

AEDs that induce the cytochrome 3A4 isoenzyme system accelerate the metabolism of sex steroids, increasing the risk for unexpected pregnancy (Table I, part A). Phenytoin is the most commonly reported in this regard. However, similar findings have been observed with phenobarbital and carbamazepine, both shown to reduce the concentrations of EE and various synthetic progestins by as much as 50% (Back et al., 1980; Crawford et al., 1990). The aforementioned agents are potent inducers of CYP3A4. Among the newer agents, felbamate, topiramate, and oxcarbazepine also induce the CYP3A4 isoenzyme, however to a lesser degree.

B. Cytochrome 3A4 Isoenzyme Noninducers

Ethosuximide, valproic acid, gabapentin, lamotrigine, tiagabine, levetirace-tam, zonisamide, pregabalin, and vigabatrin do not induce the CYP3A4 isoen-zyme system, and as such, do not increase the risk of COC failure (Bartoli *et al.*, 1997; Crawford *et al.*, 1986; Eldon *et al.*, 1998; Griffith and Dai, 2004; Mengel *et al.*, 1994; Molich *et al.*, 1991; Ragueneau-Majlessi *et al.*, 2002) (Table I, part B). However, concomitant use of COCs alters the metabolism of some of these agents, potentially impacting seizure control and drug tolerability. For example, metabolism of lamotrigine is accelerated by COCs which may produce clinically meaningful changes in serum lamotrigine concentrations (see discussion below). In a recent study of nine women on valproic acid monotherapy and a COC, the mean increase in valproic acid apparent clearance was 22% for total and 45% for free fractions as compared to the pill-free period (Galimberti *et al.*, 2006). The proposed mechanism is induction of glucuronosyltransferase by EE. Ethosuxi-mide, tiagabine, and zonisamide undergo hepatic oxidation by CYP3A; inducers of this isoenzyme may increase the clearance and decrease the half-life of these agents, but no reports of this are available.

C. AEDs with Unique or Unanticipated Interactions

1. *Lamotrigine*

Among the AEDs, lamotrigine possesses a unique interaction with hormonal contraceptives. In contrast to most other AEDs, lamotrigine is predominately eliminated by conjugation with glucuronic acid, a reaction catalyzed by the uridine 5′-diphosphate (UDP)-glucuronosyltransferases (UGTs) (Dickens and Chen, 2002). The UGT1A4 isoform is believed to be the major route of metabolism in humans. Estrogenic substrates are also metabolized by glucuronidation, thereby influencing the metabolism of lamotrigine. Findings of several studies demonstrate a significant increase in lamotrigine metabolism with concomitant administration of COCs in women with epilepsy (Browning *et al.*, 2006; Christensen *et al.*, 2007; Sabers *et al.*, 2001, 2003) and normal controls (Sidhu *et al.*, 2004). This effect is likely due to the estrogen component of the combined pill as lamotrigine metabolism is unchanged in the presence of progesterone (Reimers *et al.*, 2005).

The most recent of these studies is a double-blind, placebo-controlled trial in which seven women with epilepsy treated with lamotrigine monotherapy were randomized to an COC containing EE 35 mcg and norgestimate 250 mcg or placebo (Christensen *et al.*, 2007). Dose-corrected plasma lamotrigine concentra-tion and urinary excretion of lamotrigine metabolites after 21 days were com-pared. The mean lamotrigine concentration after placebo was 84% higher than after COC. The majority of this increase occurred within the first week after cessation of COCs, similar to a prior report (Sidhu *et al.*, 2004). The N-2-glucuronide (a lamotrigine metabolite)/lamotrigine ratio in the urine decreased by 31% in the placebo arm compared to active treatment. Three patients experienced seizures during treatment with COCs; none did so while taking placebo. Adverse effects related to lamotrigine were similar between treatment arms, although in another study, the same investigators observed an increase in adverse effects shortly after cessation of COCs. Collectively, findings from this and prior studies suggest that induction of UGT1A4 by EE accounts for the increased metabolism of lamotrigine; de-induction of this metabolic pathway during the pill-free week reverses this effect, increasing lamotrigine serum concentrations by almost 100%.

These findings have important management implications as lamotrigine has become an increasingly popular treatment choice in younger females with epilepsy. The addition of a COC containing EE reduces lamotrigine serum concentrations by an estimated 50% at the onset of therapy. This effect may be enough to produce seizures. Conversely, lamotrigine serum concentrations revert back to baseline during the pill-free week and within 1 week if the pill is discontinued, increasing the likelihood of adverse effects related to lamotrigine. Lamotrigine dosage adjustments may be necessary to maintain a clinical response following the introduction of hormonal contraceptives and to minimize adverse effects following their discontinuation. Monitoring of lamotrigine concentrations during initial introduction of COCs may be warranted. Women with epilepsy taking lamotrigine should be informed of these potential effects as loss of seizure control can have devastating effects, particularly in seizure-free patients, including loss of driving privileges, seizure-related injuries, and even death.

2. *Oxcarbazepine*

In a study involving 13 healthy subjects taking oxcarbazepine 900 mg/day and a triphasic COC (minimum EE dosage of 30 mcg), the area under the plasma concentration–time curve (AUC) decreased by 48% for estradiol and 32% for the progestin compared to baseline (Klosterskov Jensen *et al.*, 1992). Mean SHBG concentration increased by 12%. In another study, 16 healthy female volunteers taking an COC containing EE 50 mcg and levonorgestrel 250 mcg completed a randomized double-blind crossover study comparing oxcarbazepine 1200 mg/day and placebo (Fattore *et al.*, 1999). The AUC decreased by 47% for both components during oxcarbazepine compared to placebo, as did peak plasma concentration and half-life. Although like lamotrigine, oxcarbazepine is metabolized largely through glucuronidation, the proposed mechanism for these findings is stimulation of CYP3A-mediated metabolism in the liver, GI tract, or both.

3. *Topiramate*

Topiramate produced a significant dose-related reduction in EE levels in two studies. In the first study, 12 women with epilepsy taking valproic acid and an COC containing EE 35 mcg and norethindrone 1.0 mg were administered topiramate 200, 400, and 800 mg/day escalating over three consecutive months (Rosenfeld *et al.*, 1997). A significant decline in EE concentration was observed with all topiramate doses with a maximal reduction of 30% at 800 mg/day. Progestin levels remained unchanged. In the second study, healthy female subjects taking a similar COC formulation were administered topiramate 50 , 100, or 200 mg/day, or carbamazepine 600 mg/day (Doose *et al.*, 2003). No significant change in mean AUC of either steroid component was observed with any topiramate dose, while carbamazepine decreased the AUC of estradiol by 42% and norethindrone by 58%. In contrast to the prior study, a dose-related reduction in estradiol was not observed, possibly owing to the weak enzyme-inducing properties of topiramate, particularly at lower doses.

4. *Felbamate*

The effect of felbamate on the pharmacokinetics of a COC containing EE 30 mcg and 75 mcg of the synthetic progestin gestodene was investigated in 24 healthy subjects in a double-blind, placebo-controlled study (Saano *et al.*, 1995). Felbamate 2400 mg/day produced a 42% decline in the AUC of the progestin, whereas, the AUC of estradiol declined by only 13%. No subjects showed evidence of ovulation. Felbamate possesses complex pharmacokinetics. Approximately one half of a dose is excreted in the urine unchanged, while the remainder is metabolized through several hepatic pathways, including CYP3A4. The observed effect on the progesterone component is likely due to CYP3A4 induction, although the lack of a similar effect on estradiol is unexplained.

D. HORMONAL CONTRACEPTION AND SEIZURE CONTROL

The opposing effects of estrogen (proconvulsant) and progesterone (anticonvulsant) on seizure threshold have been well described in both animals and humans. The concentration of female sex steroids fluctuates throughout the menstrual cycle. In up to 30% of women with epilepsy, this fluctuation leads to periods of seizure susceptibility, most typically in the premenstrual period (Herzog *et al.*, 1997). Despite this well-recognized phenomenon, the effect of COCs on seizure control has not been extensively studied. Based on small series (Diamond *et al.*, 1985; Toivakka, 1967) and one placebo-controlled study (Espir *et al.*, 1969), COC agents do not cause seizures in the majority of women with epilepsy.

E. OTHER EFFECTS OF ORAL CONTRACEPTIVE INTERACTIONS WITH AEDs

Many reports of interactions between oral contraceptives and enzyme-inducing AEDs describe breakthrough bleeding in women as evidence of "inadequate" hormone levels. Breakthrough bleeding can be associated with lower hormone levels, but is also common within the first few months after COC initiation. In a study of nonepileptic women administered COCs with doses of EE 35–50 mcg and norethindrone 0.5–1 mg, 20–50% of subjects reported intermenstrual spotting depending on the preparation. Within the first month, the frequency of spotting or unscheduled bleeding was as high as 50–80% (Saleh et al., 1993). In addition, the reduction in serum estrogen and progestin levels with concurrent AED use cannot be assumed to always have a clinically significant effect. Because of the complex metabolism of hormonal contraceptives and the wide variation among individuals, there is no known "mean" serum level of estrogen and/or progesterone to define when a contraceptive will be effective. Studies may cite breakthrough bleeding as evidence of a significant interaction, but this is not an appropriate surrogate marker for contraceptive efficacy.

V. Other Hormonal Contraceptives and Their Known or Potential Interactions with AEDs

A. PROGESTIN-ONLY ORAL CONTRACEPTIVE PILLS

Women should not be prescribed estrogen-containing contraceptives if they are at increased risk for venous thromboembolism, or have heart disease, poorly controlled diabetes, severe migraines with aura, a personal history of breast cancer, or undiagnosed vaginal bleeding. Other relative contraindications include breast-feeding, hypertension, or heavy smoking, particularly if over age 35. These women are often offered progestin-only oral contraceptive pills (POPs) containing norethindrone or levonorgestrel as an alternative oral contraceptive. Since the progestin dose is relatively low, variations in timing of administration can lead to reduced efficacy compared to COCs (Hatcher, 2004). POPs are packaged as a daily, continuous dose with no "placebo week" and more often are associated with irregular bleeding patterns compared to COCs. POPs should not be prescribed to women using enzyme-inducing AEDs since the dose of progesterone is lower than in many COCs, and would likely result in unacceptably higher failure rates.

B. CONTRACEPTIVE INJECTION

DMPA (Depot Medroxyprogesterone Acetate or Depo-Provera®) is administered as a 150 mg IM dose every 3 months to suppress ovulation, and thus far no case reports or studies have documented a reduction in contraceptive efficacy with co-administration of enzyme-inducing agents. This dose of progestin is possibly high enough to be unaffected by any increased metabolism or binding to SHBG. DMPA has been demonstrated to reduce seizure frequency in women with uncontrolled epilepsy, and therefore physicians may specifically recommend use of DMPA to select women with epilepsy (Mattson *et al.*, 1984). Side effects of DMPA use include irregular bleeding or amenorrhea, though troublesome bleeding typically decreases with continued use. Induction of amenorrhea is particularly useful in complicated patients for whom cessation of menses is desired to facilitate personal hygiene and care. Anecdotally, many providers will administer DMPA on a more frequent schedule if bleeding occurs near the end of the 12-week time frame for women using enzyme-inducing AEDs (Wright, 1990).

Disadvantages of DMPA use include a delay in return of spontaneous ovulation (median reported delay = 10 months), and a modest increase in weight averaging less than 5 lb for every year of use (Pfizer, Inc., 2004). A reversible decrease in bone mineral density (BMD) is also associated with long-term DMPA use, which is of particular concern for adolescents who have not yet reached peak bone mass. The United States Food and Drug Administration advises providers to assess risks and benefits of DMPA use for each individual, particularly after 2 years of continuous administration. The World Health Organization Medical Eligibility Criteria for Contraceptive Use advises consideration of alternatives for women less than 18 or over 45 years old, although it states that the benefits of DMPA use generally outweigh the risks (WHO, 2004).

Long-term use of DMPA may be a real concern for women on chronic AEDs, some of which can also result in decreased BMD measurements and associated increased fracture risk (see Chapters 14 and 15 for a detailed discussion). In women without a contraindication to estrogen, low-dose estrogen therapy can be considered for BMD protection though this remains an area of active investigation. Depo-subQ Provera104^{TM}, a 104-mg dose administered subcutaneously every 12 weeks, is also available in the United States for contraception or for therapy of endometriosis-associated pain. There is no available information on the potential for drug interactions with this lower dose of DMPA, therefore the standard 150 mg IM dose is recommended.

C. CONTRACEPTIVE PATCH

Transdermal administration of contraceptive hormones via the contraceptive patch (OrthoEvra®) effectively prevents ovulation by daily release of 20 mcg of EE and 150 mcg of norelgestromin, a metabolite of norgestimate. Advantages include improved compliance by reducing the need for daily recall of contraceptive use and the transdermal absorption of hormones to minimize some hormonal side effects (Audet *et al.*, 2001). No studies have directly evaluated serum hormone levels with contraceptive patch and concurrent AED use. Theoretically, the mechanism for reduction in hormone levels would be similar to COCs, though it is possible that by avoiding the first-pass metabolism the patch may not suffer a clinically relevant reduction in efficacy. Without any pharmacokinetic data or reports available regarding patch efficacy with co-administration of AEDs, use of the contraceptive patch should be subject to the same precaution as COC use.

D. CONTRACEPTIVE VAGINAL RING

The contraceptive vaginal ring (NuvaRing®) suppresses ovulation by continuous release of EE and etonogestrel for 21 days of vaginal ring placement, followed by 7 days with the ring removed. Serum levels of estrogen are 50% lower than seen with oral contraceptive use, but the ring remains effective due to the continuous hormone administration and local effects (Timmer and Mulders, 2000). Contraceptive efficacy is likely to be compromised with concurrent enzyme-inducing AED use, though no specific studies address this potential interaction. The package labeling advises that contraceptive effectiveness may be reduced with co-administration of AEDs based on experience with oral contraceptive pills (Organon USA Inc., 2005).

E. CONTRACEPTIVE IMPLANTS

Contraceptive failures during use of both subdermal levonorgestrel capsules (Norplant®) and the single-rod etonogestrel implant (Implanon™) are documented in women using enzyme-inducing medications (Harrison-Woolrych and Hill, 2005; Odlind and Olsson, 1986; Shane-McWhorter *et al.*, 1998). The etonogestrel implant, which at this time is the only option in the United States for women desiring implantable, progestin-only contraception, is not recommended for women taking enzyme-inducing AEDs. The duration of action for the single-rod etonogestrel implant is 3 years, and it is otherwise a highly effective contraceptive method. Levonorgestrel capsules are not currently available in the United States but are still used in many other countries.

F. EMERGENCY CONTRACEPTION

The only dedicated product marketed in the United States for emergency or postcoital contraception is Plan B® (levonorgestrel, 0.75 mg). The first tablet is taken as soon as possible after unprotected intercourse, and the same dose repeated in 12 h to reduce the rate of unplanned pregnancy by 85% (von Hertzen and Van Look, 1998). Plan B® is available without prescription to women ages 18 and older, and by prescription only to women under 18. Other COCs containing levonorgestrel can be taken postcoitally with similar effect; a table describing dosing of COCs for emergency contraception is available online at www.not-2-late.com.

There is no available data on the efficacy of emergency contraception in women who also use enzyme-inducing AEDs, and no official recommendation in the United States regarding the potential interaction. However, given the significant consequences of unplanned pregnancy for this population and the relative safety of a short course of levonorgestrel, use of emergency contraception should be strongly considered. In the United Kingdom, the Faculty of Family Planning & Reproductive Health Care of the Royal College of Obstetricians & Gynaecologists issued a statement in April 2006 recommending a higher dose of levonorgestrel (2.25 mg orally in a single dose, or 1.5 mg taken once and repeated in 12 h) (FFPRHC, 2006). There have been no studies to evaluate tolerability or efficacy of this increased dose. Women can also be advised of the availability of copper IUD placement within 7 days of unprotected intercourse as a postcoital method that will not interact with AEDs.

VI. Contraceptive Methods Without AED Interaction

With the exception of the levonorgestrel intrauterine system (LNG-IUS), the methods described in this section do not rely on hormonal components for contraceptive efficacy, and are therefore appropriate to recommend for use in women using enzyme-inducing medications. The local hormonal effects of the LNG-IUS do not appear to be compromised by concurrent enzyme-inducing AED use.

A. INTRAUTERINE DEVICES

Use of intrauterine contraception is increasing in the United States, based on escalating evidence of the safety, efficacy, and potential noncontraceptive benefits. IUDs rank as the most effective, reversible option for contraception, and user satisfaction is higher than with other common contraceptive methods (Grimes, 2004). The mechanism of action for IUDs is primarily to interfere with sperm motility and/or fertilization, created by the local inflammatory response to a foreign body in the uterus. Though more than one mechanism of action may contribute to the high efficacy rates, most evidence suggests the action of IUDs occurs pre-fertilization (Rivera *et al.*, 1999). Therefore, there is minimal theoretical risk of any interaction with concurrent use of AEDs.

The Copper T 380A (ParaGard®) and LNG-IUS (Mirena®) are currently available to women in the United States, and the contraceptive effect of both IUDs is immediately reversed after removal. The Copper T 380A IUD is effective for up to 10 years after placement, and has no hormonal activity. The LNG-IUS releases a low dose of levonorgestrel at an initial rate of 20 mcg/day, and is approved for up to 5 years of use. The local endometrial effects of the levonorgestrel result in a significant reduction in menstrual blood loss and contribute to the contraceptive efficacy. Up to 20% of women stop bleeding altogether at 1 year following LNG-IUS placement. This benefit is a highly desirable side effect for many women, and the LNG-IUS has been evaluated extensively for noncontraceptive indications. An observational series of 56 women using the LNG-IUS and enzyme-inducing medications estimated a failure rate of 1.1 per 100 woman-years, more favorable than the estimated failure rate for women using COCs with enzyme-inducing AEDs (Bounds and Guillebaud, 2002). The authors suggest that the LNG-IUS should be considered a first line contraceptive option in women with concurrent use of enzyme-inducing medications.

IUDs can be offered to multiparous and nulliparous women seeking effective, reversible contraception. Previous concerns regarding an increased risk of pelvic inflammatory disease and subsequent infertility have been put to rest by epidemiological and bacteriological evidence relevant to modern IUDs (Darney, 2001). Based on this evidence, the FDA approved a labeling change for the Copper T 380A IUD in September 2005. The previous warning against use of this IUD in nulliparous women has been removed from the package labeling, though precautions still exist against its use in women at risk for pelvic inflammatory disease or ectopic pregnancy. Theoretically, the LNG-IUS should have a similar risk profile and in fact there may be some protective effect from ascending infection due to the progesterone-mediated thickening of the cervical mucus (Jensen, 2005).

B. BARRIER METHODS: CONDOMS, CONTRACEPTIVE SPONGE, DIAPHRAGM, CERVICAL CAP, AND SHIELD

Barriers methods remain an important contraceptive option for many couples, particularly for prevention of sexually transmitted infection (STI). Providers should remind women that most birth control methods do not prevent STI acquisition, and encourage condom use in addition to their primary method. For couples who consistently and correctly use the male condom, only 2% of women will experience unintended pregnancy within the first year of use. Unfortunately, with typical use the failure rate increases to 15% of women reporting unintended pregnancies after 1 year (Trussel, 2004). This difference highlights the importance of accurate and comprehensive education in the correct use of contraceptive methods.

Male condoms have the advantage of being relatively inexpensive and easily accessible, but along with other barrier methods, depend on the couple to remember and initiate use prior to every act of intercourse. Female condoms are not as widely available or known to most patients. The Reality® female condom is approved as a single use device, and should not be used in conjunction with a male condom. Though the cost of each female condom is four to five times that of a male condom, their efficacy is similar to other vaginal barrier methods. The contraceptive sponge has been re-introduced into the United States, and has the advantage of using both a barrier and spermicide to prevent pregnancy. The reported efficacy is higher for nulliparous women compared to multiparous women.

The cervical cap, diaphragm, and a similar method known as Lea's Shield® all require exam and fitting with an experienced provider but can be used repetitively and do not require participation by the male partner. Highly motivated patients who are successful users of these barrier methods report first year unintended pregnancy rates ranging between 5 and 9%. Failure rates are between 20 and 26% in multiparous women, due to the higher risk of displacement during intercourse (Trussel, 2004).

C. STERILIZATION

A new option for female sterilization is a transcervical procedure easily accomplished in the office setting; tubal inserts are placed into the tubal ostia bilaterally with hysteroscopic guidance, and after 3 months tubal scarring and eventual loss of patency are confirmed by fluoroscopy. Following successful placement and tubal blockage, this method (Essure®) is highly effective with only rare reports of unintended pregnancy. The potential for this procedure to be performed as an outpatient (or as an inpatient with minimal sedation) makes it ideal for women with complex medical issues that might otherwise make them poor surgical candidates.

Laparoscopic tubal ligation, postpartum sterilization by mini-laparotomy, and vasectomy remain common and popular procedures in the Unites States. Overall, 27% of women ages 15–44 using a contraceptive method rely on tubal sterilization and it is the leading method for women over age 35. An additional 9.2% of women report relying on vasectomy as their contraceptive method (Mosher et al., 2004). Patients need to clearly understand that the decision to be sterilized is a permanent condition; reversal procedures are available but are costly, generally not covered by insurance, and not always successful. Finally, even sterilization carries the potential risk of method failure, though sterilization and IUDs share status as the most effective birth control methods.

D. Other Birth Control Methods Practiced by Women

The Lactational Amenorrhea Method, relying on ovulation suppression during breastfeeding, can be an effective but temporary method of contraception. Women who exclusively breastfeed and have not menstruated have more than 98% protection from pregnancy within the first 6 months after a birth (Kennedy and Trussell, 2004). Methods involving periodic abstinence (fertility awareness-based methods), depend on the regularity of the woman's menstrual cycle and the ability to identify the fertile days. Highly motivated couples may be quite successful over time; however, the quoted failure rate is as high as 25% within the first year with typical use (Trussel, 2004). Withdrawal is commonly practiced by many couples, but has a similarly high rate of unintended pregnancy.

VII. Counseling and Management of Contraception in Women Requiring AED Prescription

Contraceptive choice is influenced by a variety of factors including convenience, tolerability, life stage, partner preference, and affordability. Perceived side effects or risk, frequency of sexual activity, and ease of use will impact long-term compliance. Women initiating contraception should be counseled extensively regarding accurate method use, as well as potential side effects and risks. Many women fear that hormones will result in excess cancer, blood clots, heart attack, stroke or death, without an adequate understanding of these same risks related to pregnancy, or tobacco use, for example. Time spent counseling women on all these factors will directly impact successful use and continuation rates.

A. Choosing a Contraceptive Method for a Woman with Epilepsy

Contraceptive options that have no known interaction with AEDs include DMPA, IUDs, barrier methods, fertility awareness-based methods, and sterilization. Intrauterine contraception should now be considered a first line option for women who are at low risk of STIs. Women experience first year failure rates of only 0.2% with the LNG-IUS and 0.8% with the Copper T 380A IUD (Trussel, 2004). This high efficacy, combined with minimal need for user involvement, make IUDs a superior choice for a reversible contraceptive method.

If a woman under good seizure control is currently prescribed an AED known to induce cytochrome 3A4, the potential effects of decreased contraceptive hormone levels should be reviewed. The increased failure rate of COCs with enzyme-inducing AEDs has not been quantified, though the serum hormone levels may be decreased 50% or more (O'Brien and Guillebaud, 2006). Oral contraceptives containing 50 mcg of EE will probably inhibit ovulation more reliably than those with 35 mcg or less (ACOG, 2006). However, most case reports of COC failure with enzyme-inducing AEDS were initially reported in women using COCs with at least 50 mcg of EE. Recall that since mestranol is only partially converted to EE, a 50 mcg mestranol pill is not equivalent to 50 mcg of EE. Patients should be reassured that due to the lower serum hormone levels with co-administration of enzyme-inducing AEDs, there should be no significant increase in cardiovascular risk or side effects with prescription of a 50 mcg EE oral contraceptive.

The advantages of oral contraceptive prescription include wide acceptability and broad experience, as up to 82% of women report having used COCs during some point in their life (Mosher et al., 2004). In addition, there are many noncontraceptive benefits of COCs, including a reduction in menorrhagia, dysmenorrhea, irregular menses, functional ovarian cysts, endometrial cancer, ovarian cancer, benign breast disease, premenstrual symptoms, and pelvic inflammatory disease (Mishell, 1993). Prescription of hormonal contraception may alter seizure frequency in a minority of women with epilepsy. Isolated case reports demonstrating an improvement or deterioration in seizure control following the initiation of COCs have been published (Foldvary-Schaefer and Falcone, 2003).

Newer developments in COCs have focused on minimizing the pill-free interval (24/4 formulations), a reduction in number of pill-free intervals (84/7 formulations), or continuous administration of COCs. These extended cycle regimens should more reliably inhibit ovulation by avoiding the potential for early follicular development in the 7-day placebo week. On this basis, O'Brien and Guillebaud (2006) recently recommended a "tri-cycling" regimen of 50–60 mcg EE pills (taken daily for 9 weeks, followed by 4 days off) for women at risk of AED interactions. No studies are yet available to evaluate the contraceptive efficacy or tolerability of this regimen.

As described earlier, women using lamotrigine should be carefully monitored if hormonal contraception is initiated.

B. WOMEN USING HORMONAL CONTRACEPTION WHO REQUIRE INITIATION OF ANTIEPILEPTIC THERAPY

An early consideration in the choice of AED therapy may be a woman's preexisting contraceptive method. If an AED known to be an enzyme inducer is more appropriate, the impact of AED choice on her contraceptive method should be discussed. Offer options for other contraceptive methods if the risk of decreased efficacy is a concern, and advise use of a back-up method such as abstinence or condoms until a contraceptive plan can be finalized. If a woman experiences breakthrough bleeding after enzyme-inducing AED therapy is started, it may indicate lower hormonal levels. The estrogen dose can be increased, if applicable, or an alternative contraceptive method initiated. After discontinuation of an enzyme-inducing AED there may be residual effects of enzyme induction, therefore a woman should be maintained at the higher dose of estrogen for an additional cycle (O'Brien and Guillebaud, 2006).

VIII. Summary

The pharmacokinetics of the interaction between oral contraceptives and AEDs that are inducers of the cytochrome 3A4 system are well defined. The clinical impact of these interactions on hormonal contraceptive efficacy is not as well documented, but is an important area for further investigation. As new therapeutic agents for the treatment of epilepsy and other mood or pain disorders are introduced, it will be crucial to examine the potential for cytochrome 3A4 induction.

Providers for women with epilepsy have an obligation to review each patient's reproductive plan, or to refer her to her primary provider or gynecologist for management. At a minimum, patients need to be informed if the AED prescribed for their epilepsy has the potential to interact with hormonal contraception, or if there are known teratogenic effects. COCs remain a highly effective contraceptive method when compared to many other contraceptive methods. Continuous COC administration or a shortened pill-free interval may be effective at reducing risk of method failure. A variety of new contraceptive hormone delivery systems are now available, but many are likely to have similar reductions in efficacy when taken with enzyme-inducing AEDs. The availability and acceptance of other highly effective contraceptive methods such as DMPA and the intrauterine device (IUD) should assist providers and women with epilepsy in avoiding the AED–hormone interactions.

Acknowledgment

The authors would like to acknowledge Britt Lunde, MD, for her assistance with the literature search for this chapter.

References

American Academy of Neurology. (AAN). (1998). Practice parameter: Management issues for women with epilepsy (summary statement). Report of the Quality Standards Subcommittee of the American Academy of Neurology. *Neurology* **51,** 944–948.

American College of Obstetricians and Gynecologists. (ACOG). (2006). Use of hormonal contraception in women with co-existing medical conditions. ACOG Practice Bulletin no. 73. *Obstet. Gynecol.* **107,** 1453–1472.

Asbell, B. (1995). "The Pill: A Biography of the Drug that Changed the World," Random House, New York, NY.

Audet, M. C., Moreau, M., Koltun, W. D., Waldbaum, A. S., Shangold, G., Fisher, A. C., and Creasy, G. W. (2001). Evaluation of contraceptive efficacy and cycle control of a transdermal contraceptive patch vs. an oral contraceptive. *JAMA* **285,** 2347–2354.

Back, D. J., Bates, M., Bowden, A., Breckenridge, A. M., Hall, M. J., Jones, H., MacIver, M., Orme, M., Perucca, E., Richens, A., Rowe, P. H., and Smith, E. (1980). The interaction of phenobarbital and other anticonvulsants with oral contraceptive steroid therapy. *Contraception* **22,** 495–503.

Bartoli, A., Gatti, G., Cipolla, G., Barzaghi, N., Veliz, G., Fattore, C., Mumford, J., and Perucca, E. (1997). A double-blind, placebo-controlled study on the effect of vigabatrin on *in vivo* parameters of hepatic microsomal enzyme induction and on the kinetics of steroid oral contraceptives in healthy female volunteers. *Epilepsia* **38,** 702–707.

Bounds, W., and Guillebaud, J. (2002). Observational series on women using the contraceptive Mirena concurrently with anti-epileptic and other enzyme-inducing drugs. *J. Fam. Plann. Reprod. Health Care* **28,** 78–80.

Browning, K., Birnbaum, A., Montgomery, J., Newman, M. L., Clements, S. D., and Pennell, P. B. (2006). Lamotrigine clearance is increased by estrogen-containing contraceptives. *Neurology* **66** (Suppl. 2), A273.

Christensen, J., Petrenaite, V., Atterman, J., Sidenius, P., Ohman, I., Tomson, T., and Sabers, A. (2007). Oral contraceptives induce lamotrigine metabolism: Evidence from a double-blind, placebo-controlled trial. *Epilepsia* **48,** 484–489.

Crawford, P. (2002). Interactions between antiepileptic drugs and hormonal contraception. *CNS Drugs* **16,** 263–272.

Crawford, P., and Lee, P. (1999). Gender difference in management of epilepsy—What women are hearing. *Seizure* **8,** 135–139.

Crawford, P., Chadwick, D., Cleland, P., Tjia, J., Cowie, A., Back, D. J., and Orme, M. L. (1986). The lack of effect of sodium valproate on the pharmacokinetics of oral contraceptive steroids. *Contraception* **33,** 23–29.

Crawford, P., Chadwick, D. J., Martin, C., Tjia, J., Back, D. J., and Orme, M. (1990). The interaction of phenytoin and carbamazepine with combined oral contraceptive steroids. *Br. J. Clin. Pharmacol.* **30,** 892–896.

Darney, P. D. (2001). Time to pardon the IUD? *New Engl. J. Med.* **345,** 608–610.

Davis, A. R., Pack, A., Camus, A., Yoon, A., and Krizer, J. (2007a). Patient knowledge of teratogenicity and contraceptive interactions of antiepileptic drugs. *Obstet. Gynecol.* **109,** 60S.

Davis, A. R., Pack, A. M., Kritzer, J., Yoon, A., and Camus, A. (2007b). Reproductive history, sexual behavior, and use of contraception in women with epilepsy. Personal communication to Caryn Dutton. *Contraception* **77,** 405–409. In press.

Diamond, M. P., Greene, J. W., Thompson, J. M., VanHooydonk, J. E., and Wentz, A. C. (1985). Interaction of anticonvulsants and oral contraceptives in epileptic adolescents. *Contraception* **31,** 623–632.

Dickens, M., and Chen, C. (2002). Lamotrigine: Chemistry, biotransformation and pharmacokinetics. *In* "Antiepileptic Drugs" (R. H. Levy *et al.*, Eds.), pp. 370–379. Raven Press, New York, NY.

Doose, D. R., Wang, S. S., Padmanabhan, M., Schwabe, S., Jacobs, D., and Bialer, M. (2003). Effect of topiramate or carbamazepine on the pharmacokinetics of an oral contraceptive containing norethindrone and ethinyl estradiol in healthy obese and nonobese female subjects. *Epilepsia* **44,** 540–549.

Eldon, M. A., Underwood, B. A., Randinitis, E. J., and Sedman, A. J. (1998). Gabapentin does not interact with a contraceptive regimen of norethindrone acetate and ethinyl estradiol. *Neurology* **50**, 1146–1148.

Espir, M., Walker, M., and Lawson, J. (1969). Epilepsy and oral contraception. *Br. Med. J.* **1**, 294–295.

Faculty of Family Planning and Reproductive Health Care Clinical Effectiveness Unit. (FFPRHC). (2006). Faculty statement from the CEU: Levonelle 1500 and the use of liver enzyme inducing drugs. Available at: http://www.ffprhc.org.uk/admin/uploads/563_Levonelle1500 KeyStatement.pdf.

Fattore, C., Cipolla, G., Gatti, G., Limido, G. L., Sturm, Y., Bernasconi, C., and Perucca, E. (1999). Induction of ethinylestradiol and levonorgestrel metabolism by oxcarbazepine in healthy women. *Epilepsia* **40**, 783–787.

Finer, L., and Henshaw, S. K. (2006). Disparities in rates of unintended pregnancy in the United States, 1994 and 2001. *Fam. Plann. Perspect.* **38**, 90–96.

Foldvary-Schaefer, N., and Falcone, T. (2003). Catamenial epilepsy: Pathophysiology, diagnosis, and management. *Neurology* **61**, S2–S15.

Foy, R., Penney, G., and Greer, I. (2001). The impact of national clinical guidelines on obstetricians in Scotland. *Health Bull.* **59**, 364–372.

Galimberti, C., Mazzucchelli, I., Arbasino, C., *et al.* (2006). Increased apparent oral clearance of vaproic acid during intake of combined contraceptive steroids in women with epilepsy. *Epilepsia* **47**, 1569–1572.

Griffith, S. G., and Dai, Y. (2004). Effect of zonisamide on the pharmacokinetics and pharmacodynamics of a combination ethinyl estradiol-norethindrone oral contraceptive in healthy women. *Clin. Ther.* **26**, 2056–2065.

Grimes, D. A. (2004). Intrauterine devices (IUDs). *In* "Contraceptive Technology" (R. A. Hatcher *et al.*, Eds.), pp. 495–502. Ardent Media, Inc., New York, NY.

Harrison-Woolrych, M., and Hill, R. (2005). Unintended pregnancies with the etonogestrel implant (Implanon): A case series from postmarketing experience in Australia. *Contraception* **71**, 306–308.

Hatcher, R. A. (2004). Depo-Provera injections, implants, and progestin-only pills (Minipills). *In* "Contraceptive Technology" (R. A. Hatcher *et al.*, Eds.), pp. 461–494. Ardent Media, Inc., New York, NY.

Herzog, A., Klein, P., and Ransil, B. (1997). Three patterns of catamenial epilepsy. *Epilepsia* **38**, 1082–1088.

Jensen, J. (2005). Contraceptive and therapeutic effects of the levonorgestrel intrauterine system: An overview. *Obstet. Gynecol. Surv.* **60**, 604–612.

Kennedy, K. I., and Trussell, J. (2004). Postpartum contraception and lactation. *In* "Contraceptive Technology" (R. A. Hatcher *et al.*, Eds.), 17th ed., pp. 575–600. Ardent Media, Inc, New York.

Kenyon, I. E. (1972). Unplanned pregnancy in an epileptic. *Br. Med. J.* **1**, 686–687.

Klosterskov Jensen, P., Saano, V., Haring, P., Svenstrup, B., and Menge, G. P. (1992). Possible interaction between oxcarbazepine and an oral contraceptive. *Epilepsia* **33**, 1149–1152.

Krauss, G. L., Brandt, J., Campbell, M., Plate, C., and Summerfield, M. (1996). Antiepileptic medication and oral contraceptive interactions: A national survey of neurologists and obstetricians. *Neurology* **46**, 1534–1539.

Mattson, R., Cramer, J. A., Caldwell, B., and Siconolfi, B. (1984). Treatment of seizures with medroxyprogesterone acetate: Preliminary report. *Neurology* **34**, 1255–1258.

McAuley, J. W., and Anderson, G. D. (2002). Treatment of epilepsy in women of reproductive age: Pharmacokinetic considerations. *Clin. Pharmacokinet.* **41**, 559–579.

Mengel, H. B., Houston, A., and Back, D. J. (1994). An evaluation of the interaction between tiagabine and oral contraceptives in female volunteers. *J. Pharm. Med.* **4**, 141–150.

Mishell, D. R., Jr. (1993). Noncontraceptive benefits of oral contraceptives. *J. Reprod. Med.* **38**, 1021–1029.

Molich, T., Whiteman, P., and Orme, M. (1991). Effect of lamotrigine on the pharmacology of the combined oral contraceptive pill. *Epilepsia* **32,** 96.

Morrell, M., Sarto, G. E., Shafer, P. O., Borda, E. A., Herzog, A., and Callanan, M. (2000). Health issues for women with epilepsy: A descriptive survey to assess knowledge and awareness among healthcare providers. *J. Womens Health Gend. Based Med.* **9,** 959–965.

Mosher, W. D., Martinez, G. M., Chandra, A., Abma, J. C., and Willson, S. J. (2004). Use of contraception and use of family planning services in the United States: 1982–2002. *Adv. Data* 1–36.

O'Brien, M. D., and Guillebaud, J. (2006). Contraception for women with epilepsy. *Epilepsia* **47,** 1419–1422.

Odlind, V., and Olsson, S. E. (1986). Enhanced metabolism of levonorgestrel during phenytoin treatment in a woman with Norplant implants. *Contraception* **33,** 257–261.

Organon USA Inc. (2005). NuvaRing Prescribing Information.

Perruca, E., and Richens, A. (1995). General principles: Biotransformation. *In* "Antiepileptic Drugs" (R. H. Levy *et al.*, Eds.), pp. 31–50. Raven Press, New York, NY.

Pfizer, Inc. (2004). Depo-Provera Contraceptive Injection Product Labeling.

Ragueneau-Majlessi, I., Levy, R. H., and Janik, F. (2002). Levetiracetam does not alter the pharma- cokinetics of an oral contraceptive in healthy women. *Epilepsia* **43,** 697–702.

Reimers, A., Helde, G., and Brodtkorb, E. (2005). Ethinyl estradiol, not progestogens, reduces lamotrigine serum concentration. *Epilepsia* **46**(9): 1414–1417.

Rivera, R., Yacobson, I., and Grimes, D. (1999). The mechanism of action of hormonal contraceptives and intrauterine contraceptive devices. *Am. J. Obstet. Gynecol.* **181,** 1263–1269.

Rosenberg, M. J., Meyers, A., and Roy, V. (1999). Efficacy, cycle control, and side effects of low- and lower-dose oral contraceptives: A randomized trial of 20 micrograms and 35 micrograms estrogen preparations. *Contraception* **60,** 321–329.

Rosenfeld, W. E., Doose, D. R., Walker, S. A., and Nayak, R. K. (1997). Effect of topiramate on the pharmacokinetics of an oral contraceptive containing norethindrone and ethinyl estradiol in patients with epilepsy. *Epilepsia* **38,** 317–323.

Russell, A., Macpherson, H., Cairnie, V., and Brodie, M. J. (1996). The care of pregnant women with epilepsy—A survey of obstetricians in Scotland. *Seizure* **5,** 271–277.

Saano, V., Glue, P., Banfield, C. R., Reidenberg, P., Colucci, R. D., Meehan, J. W., Haring, P., Radwanski, E., Nomeir, A., and Lin, C. C. (1995). Effects of felbamate on the pharmacokinetics of a low-dose combination oral contraceptive. *Clin. Pharmacol. Ther.* **58,** 523–531.

Sabers, A., Buchholt, J. M., Uldall, P., and Hansen, E. L. (2001). Lamotrigine plasma levels reduced by oral contraceptives. *Epilepsy Res.* **47,** 151–154.

Sabers, A., Ohman, I., Christensen, J., and Tomson, T. (2003). Oral contraceptives reduce lamo- trigine plasma levels. *Neurology* **61,** 570–571.

Saleh, W. A., Burkman, R. T., Zacur, H. A., Kimball, A. W., Kwiterovich, P., and Bell, W. K. (1993). A randomized trial of three oral contraceptives: Comparison of bleeding patterns by contraceptive types and steroid levels. *Am. J. Obstet. Gynecol.* **168,** 1740–1745.

Seale, C., Morrell, M. J., Nelson, L., and Druzin, M. L. (1998). Analysis of prenatal and gestational care given to women with epilepsy. *Neurology* **51,** 1039–1045.

Shane-McWhorter, L., Cerveny, J. D., MacFarlane, L. L., and Osborn, C. (1998). Enhanced metabolism of levonorgestrel during phenobarbital treatment and resultant pregnancy. *Pharmaco- therapy* **18,** 1360–1364.

Shorvon, S. D., Tallis, R. C., and Wallace, H. K. (2002). Antiepileptic drugs: Coprescription of proconvulsant drugs and oral contraceptives: A national study of antiepileptic drug prescribing practice. *J. Neurol. Neurosurg. Psychiatry* **72,** 114–115.

Sidhu, J., Bulsara, S., Job, S., and Philipson, R. (2004). A bidirectional pharmacokinetic interaction study of lamotrigine and the combined oral contraceptive pill in healthy subjects. *Epilepsia* **45** (Suppl. 7), 330.

Timmer, C. J., and Mulders, T. M. (2000). Pharmacokinetics of etonogestrel and ethinylestradiol released from a combined contraceptive vaginal ring. *Clin. Pharmacokinet.* **39,** 233–242.

Toivakka, E. (1967). Oral contraception in epileptics. *Arzneimittelforschung* **17,** 1085.

Trussel, J. (2004). The essentials of contraception: Efficacy, safety, and personal considerations. *In* "Contraceptive Technology" (R. A. Hatcher *et al.*, Eds.), pp. 221–252. Ardent Media, Inc., New York, NY.

Verispan LLC. (2005).

von Hertzen, H., and Van Look, P. F. A. (1998). Randomised controlled trial of levonorgestrel versus the Yuzpe regimen of combined oral contraceptives for emergency contraception. *Lancet* **352,** 428–433.

Wilbur, K., and Ensom, M. H. (2000). Pharmacokinetic drug interactions between oral contraceptives and second-generation anticonvulsants. *Clin. Pharmacokinet.* **38,** 355–365.

World Health Organization (WHO). (2004). Medical eligibility criteria for contraceptive use. Available at: http://www.who.int/reproductive-health/publications/mec/pocs.html.

Wright, R. (1990). Drug interaction with enzyme-inducing drugs. *Br. J. Fam. Plann.* **15,** 130.

REPRODUCTIVE DYSFUNCTION IN WOMEN WITH EPILEPSY: MENSTRUAL CYCLE ABNORMALITIES, FERTILITY, AND POLYCYSTIC OVARY SYNDROME

Jürgen Bauer and Déirdre Cooper-Mahkorn

Department of Epileptology, Bonn University Hospital, D-53105 Bonn, Germany

I. Introduction
II. Puberty and Menopause in Women with Epilepsy
III. Fertility of Women with Epilepsy
IV. Evaluation of Women with Epilepsy for Reproductive Endocrine Disorders
V. Polycystic Ovary Syndrome
VI. Final Remarks and Conclusions
References

Epilepsy can be associated with reproductive endocrine disorders. In women these include polycystic ovary syndrome (PCOS), isolated components of this syndrome such as polycystic ovaries or hyperandrogenemia, hypothalamic amenorrhea (HA), or functional hyperprolactinemia (HPRL). The most likely explanations for endocrine disorders related to epilepsy are a direct influence on the endocrine control centers in the brain (the hypothalamic–pituitary axis) or are effects of antiepileptic drugs (AEDs) on peripheral endocrine glands. Furthermore, the effects of AEDs on the metabolism of hormones and binding proteins and secondary endocrine complications of AED-related weight changes or changes of insulin sensitivity must be considered. Therefore, regular monitoring of reproductive function at visits, including questioning about menstrual disorders, fertility, weight, hirsutism and galactorrhea are recommended. Single abnormal laboratory or imaging findings without symptoms may not constitute a clinically relevant endocrine disorder. However, patients with these kinds of abnormalities should be monitored in order to detect the possible development of a symptomatic disorder associated with, for example, menstrual disorders or fertility problems. If a reproductive endocrine disorder is subsequently found, AEDs should be reviewed in terms of their indication for the particular seizure type and their tolerability *vis-à-vis* their potential for contributing to the endocrine problem.

INTERNATIONAL REVIEW OF
NEUROBIOLOGY, VOL. 83
DOI: 10.1016/S0074-7742(08)00007-X

135

I. Introduction

Epilepsy is a neurological disorder which is clinically defined by recurrent seizures. The primary aim in the treatment of patients with epilepsy is therefore the prevention of further seizures. Epilepsy, however, can also be associated with other pathological changes, which may require investigation and treatment. Such changes include endocrine disorders, in particular to those affecting the reproductive system in women (and in men).

Reproductive endocrine disorders observed in women with epilepsy include polycystic ovary syndrome (PCOS), hypothalamic amenorrhea, premature ovarian failure, and functional hyperprolactinemia (HPRL) (Bauer, 2001; Bauer et al., 2002; Herzog, 1997). Such disorders may contribute to infertility among women with epilepsy which is known to be more common than observed in general population studies (Olafsson et al., 1998; Wallace et al., 1998; Webber et al., 1986).

During anovulatory cycles, which are characteristic of reproductive endocrine disorders, seizure frequency may be $\sim$1.5-fold higher than during ovulatory cycles, frequency of generalized tonic–clonic seizures (TCS) may be increased by a factor of 3. An explanation for this, based on reproduction hormone cycling, may be the lack in progesterone elevation during the second phase of the menstrual cycle resulting in a lack in endogenous seizure protection (Herzog, 1997). This relationship was demonstrated in a small study in which anovulatory cycles (with concomitant progesterone deficiency due to lack of progesterone elevation during the luteal phase) were converted to ovulatory cycles (with endogenous progesterone production). This was achieved by means of clomiphene which stimulates the hypothalamic–pituitary axis (Herzog, 1988). Twelve women (nine of which had PCOS) with cyclical disturbances were given clomiphene on days 5–9 of the cycle. The dose was adjusted until ovulatory cycles occurred or side effects were noted. In 10 out of 12 women, the seizure frequency could be halved; in 5 women, the frequency was reduced by more than 90% (Herzog, 1988).

The possible endocrine influence of epilepsy was increasingly noted when postictal elevations in serum concentrations of prolactin were assumed to be a marker for the retrospective evidence of epileptic seizures (Bauer, 1996). This clinical association has lost its relevance in view of the fact that elevated prolactin levels are also possible following syncope or psychogenic seizures (Alving, 1998; Cordingly et al., 1993; Oribe et al., 1996). However, the understanding of endocrine influences of epilepsies in general prevails, particularly as regards those epilepsies which originate in or involve the temporal lobes. In this case, limbic efferents exhibit an impact on the hypothalamic–pituitary axis even in the interictal phase of the disorder (Fig. 1). Postictually elevated prolactin serum

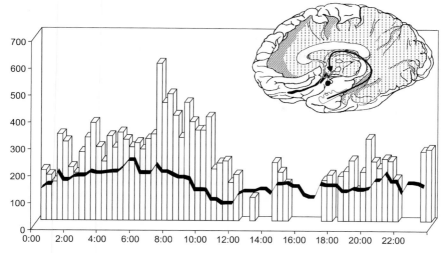

Fig. 1. Increased circadian serum prolactin concentrations, measured interictually in women with epilepsy (bars) and healthy controls (line) (for details see Bauer *et al.*, 1992).

concentrations can be detected following two out of three seizures of temporal or frontal lobe origin (Fig. 2). In correlation with the type of seizure, evidence of elevated prolactin is found in 88% of seizures following generalized TCS, in 78% of seizures following complex partial seizures, and in 22% of seizures following simple partial seizures (Bauer *et al.*, 1989). The epileptic activity in the frontal lobe exhibits a propagation towards the temporal lobe in the majority of cases and thereby influences the hormonal pathway of prolactin and other pituitary hormones which can also show tendencies to postictal elevation (Rao *et al.*, 1989).

The choice of antiepileptic medication for monotherapy in particular gives this understanding a further relevant impact. For instance, antiepileptic drugs (AEDs) can accentuate preexisting, epilepsy-related endocrine disturbances by means of weight gain [as commonly induced by valprote (VPA) or gabapentin].

Contrastingly, serum prolactin levels are not elevated in patients with idiopathic epilepsy with generalized seizures such as absences—neither ictually nor interictually could evidence of elevated serum prolactin levels be found (Bilo *et al.*, 1988). Nevertheless, weight gain may also be of major impact in the development of endocrine disorders in patients with such epilepsies, as is the case in women without epilepsy (Morrell *et al.*, 2002).

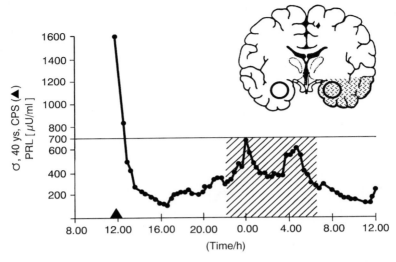

FIG. 2. Postictal increase of serum prolactin following a complex-partial seizure (CPS) from the temporal lobe (for details see Bauer *et al.*, 1992).

II. Puberty and Menopause in Women with Epilepsy

A high incidence of manifestation of epilepsy is found around the event of menarche, thus far, the cause of this remains unknown. Idiopathic epilepsies with generalized seizures often become manifest during this time, further 30% of previously diagnosed epilepsies exacerbate with an increased frequency of focal seizures or even the new occurrence of seizures forms, for example, TCS (Morrell *et al.*, 1998). In an evaluation of 94 women with epilepsy, a retrospective debut of seizure occurrence was established around the time of menarche in 17% of women (statistically expected in 5.5%, $p < 0.001$), and in 38% in the 2 years previous to and following menarche (expected in 22%, $p < 0.001$). Seizure frequency increased in 29% of girls who had epilepsy previous to menarche, in the time of menarche (Klein *et al.*, 2003). Preexisting prepubertal epilepsy did not show negative influence on the development of puberty itself (Morrell *et al.*, 1998).

An external influencing factor on menstrual cycle during puberty is attributed to the treatment with VPA. VPA elevates the serum concentrations of testosterone (T) by inhibition of liver enzymes. In a comparison between 41 girls treated with VPA aged 8–18 years and healthy, untreated controls, the serum concentrations of T in the treated group exceeded the mean of the control group by 2 SD in 38% of prepubertal, 36% of pubertal, and 57% of postpubertal girls with epilepsy

(Vainionpää et al., 1999). Whether this laboratory finding actually causes clinically relevant disorder of the menstrual cycle has not yet been examined, but appears possible.

From a clinical point of view, an approximating comment with regard to ovulatory and anovulatory cycles in women of reproductive age can be made. In a study of 100 women with focal epilepsies, it was shown that a cycle length of 26–32 days was associated with an ovulatory cycle in 73%. This was far more rare with cyclical lengths of 21–25 days (in 45.5%) and 33–35 days (in 50%). Cycles under 21 days and over 35 days (in 0% and 11%, respectively) were not associated with ovulation (Herzog and Friedman, 2001). Monitoring of serum progesterone on day 21, 22, or 23 of the cycle is safer with day 1, being the first day of the menstrual phase. Serum progesterone concentrations above 5 ng/ml give evidence of ovulation (progesterone values very much depend on the laboratory).

Menopause may occur earlier in women with epilepsy than in the general female population. In a series of 50 consecutive women with temporolimbic epilepsy, Herzog et al. (1986) found that two women (i.e., 4%) had primary gonadal failure with amenorrhea and values of follicle stimulating hormone (FSH) above 50 IU/ml in their third decade of life as compared to an expected occurrence of about 1% in the general population. In a recent study, perimenopause or menopause before reaching the age of 40 years was demonstrated in 7 out of 50 (14%) women with epilepsy as compared to 3 out of 82 (4%) of a similarly aged normal control group ($p < 0.05$) (Klein et al., 2001). In another study, a negative correlation between age at menopause and seizure group (women with low, intermediate, or high seizure frequency) was established (Harden et al., 2003). Onset of menopause was earlier in women with a high seizure rate. The authors concluded that seizures may disrupt hypothalamic–pituitary function or alter neurally mediated trophic effects on the ovary.

III. Fertility of Women with Epilepsy

Generally speaking, women with epilepsy show reduced fertility. In the Greater London area, a significantly reduced birth rate was documented in women with epilepsy aged 25–39 years in comparison with women of the general population (Wallace et al., 1998). The reasons for this are manyfold. An elevated rate of anovulatory cycles in women with temporal lobe epilepsy (TLE) can be regarded as an epilepsy-related cofactor. In this type of epilepsy, 25–30% of menstrual cycles are anovulatory, by contrast, in women with idiopathic generalized epilepsy (5%, i.e., in the range of anovulation in women of the general population) (Bauer et al., 1998; Cummings et al., 1995).

The prevalence of PCOS as a possible cause of chronic anovulation is estimated to lie between 15 and 25% in (mostly) untreated women with TLE (Meo and Bilo, 2003). Additionally, an induced increase in weight (particularly by AED, such as VPA) of more than 5 kg or a body mass index (BMI) of >25 kg/m^2 can contribute to an increased incidence of PCOS (Bauer et al., 2002). Not all studies, however, gave evidence of such a profound difference in reproductive functioning in the comparison of healthy women versus women with epilepsy (Duncan et al., 1997; Jensen et al., 1990).

The influence of interictal epileptic activity on cyclical regularity becomes evident on the analyses of menstrual cycles previous to and following the performance of epilepsy surgery on the temporal lobe. Sixteen women were examined preoperatively and followed up to 12 months postoperatively. Eight patients remained seizure-free; in four women, seizure frequency was substantially reduced. On stable medication, a postoperative elevation of serum adrostendione was observed within 6 months. In four women, postoperative menstrual cyclical changes occurred, two seizure-reduced women with previously regular cycles suffered from oligomenorrhea (Bauer et al., 2000b).

Not only a possibly disturbed menstrual cycle, but also reduced libido can influence the fertility of women with epilepsy (Harden, 2005b). Various analyses of disturbed sexual function in women have shown that up to 50% of patients complain of dyspareunia, vaginism, or insufficient vaginal lubrication in the presence of normal sexual appetite (Crawford et al., 1999). In further surveys, sexual dysfunction was found in 17 out of 50 (34%) (Bergen et al., 1992), 126 out of 700 (18%) (Demerdash et al., 1991), 14 out of 30 (47%) (Ndgegwa et al., 1986), and 7 out of 22 (33%) women with epilepsy (Stoffel-Wagner et al., 1998).

In women (and men) with epilepsy, reduced genital blood flow during erotic stimulation via video was found. The examined women with epilepsy showed a reduced elevation of genital blood flow during the presentation of erotic video movies in comparison with healthy controls (11% vs 161%) (Morrell et al., 1994).

Irrespective of gender, sexual questionnaires revealed reduced libido more commonly in right- as opposed to left-sided temporal lobe seizure origin (Daniele et al., 1997). A compelling explanation remains to be found. Possibly, the right-sided temporal lobe disturbance has a more pronounced influence on emotions and therefore indirectly on libido. In a current study, a larger count of patients with hyposexuality (more pronounced in men than in women) showed left-sided TLE. Apart from gender and lateralization of focus, there appears to be a correlation with duration of illness with the existence of disturbance of sexual function or reduced libido (Helmstaedter and Elger, 2004).

These data are supplemented by findings in animal experiments. In one study, the reduction of sexual interest in cats with TLE was demonstrated (Feeney et al., 1998). In a rat model, epileptic foci in the basolateral amygdala lead to self-limiting hypogonadal functional disturbance in a maximal electro-shock model (Edwards et al., 1999).

Following treatment by means of epilepsy surgery in men and women with temporal lobe resection ($N = 58$) and extratemporal resection ($N = 16$), a change in sexual well-being occurred within 3 months of temporal lobe operation in particular (64% vs 25% following extratemporal operation). A right-sided temporal operation seemed to be followed by change in comparison with the left-sided operation, further this occurred more commonly in women than in men. Development towards normo- (22%), hyper- (40%), or hyposexual (38%) activity was observed, findings which remained constant on follow-up (Baird et al., 2003).

Apart from the influence of epileptic activity on sexual steroid hormones and the reduction of libido and arousability, AED can also exert an influence on fertility. The example of PCOS will serve to illustrate this in detail (see below). Additionally, other factors may also be of noticeable impact. In a review, the retrospective analysis of menstrual cycle disturbances in 265 women with epilepsy in comparison with 142 healthy women, a significant difference in the prevalence of menstrual disturbances in women with and without epilepsy (48% vs 30.7%), mono- and polytherapy (45.1% vs 62.2%), >5 seizures per annum oder seizure freedom (66% vs 37.2%) as well as treatment with VPA versus carbamazepine (CBZ) (62% vs 37.2%) was shown (Svalheim et al., 2003). The significance of medication becomes obvious on analysis of cycles in women with idopathic generalized epilepsies which do not show an influence on the menstrual cycle. These patients, too, had increased rates of anovulatory cycles on treatment with VPA (Morrell et al., 2002).

IV. Evaluation of Women with Epilepsy for Reproductive Endocrine Disorders

The possible occurrence of reproductive endocrine disorders in women with epilepsy makes it important for the neurologist to recognize characteristic symptoms and signs. The evaluation of reproductive endocrine disorders typically falls within the domain of the endocrinologist and gynecologist. The investigation of endocrine problems in patients with epilepsy, however, may well require close cooperation between neurologists and endocrinologists or gynecologists since these specialists may not have a detailed understanding of the effects of epilepsy or AEDs on the endocrine system. One should pay attention to menstrual irregularity, infertility, weight gain, hirsutism, and galactorrhea as possible symptoms of a clinically relevant endocrine disorder in women with epilepsy (Table I). Tests include hormonal measurements, pelvic ultrasonography, and pituitary imaging (Table II). Pelvic ultrasonography is indicated if clinical features or

TABLE I

CLINICAL FEATURES OF REPRODUCTIVE ENDOCRINE DISORDERS IN WOMEN WITH EPILEPSY (ADAPTED FROM BAUER ET AL., 2002)

Symptom/sign	Method	Abnormal findings	Comment
Menstrual irregularity	Menstrual chart for at least 6 months	<23 days: polymenorrhea >35 days: oligomenorrhea No bleeding>6 months: amenorrhea	Look for other symptoms of endocrine disorder including thyroid dysfunction, investigate or refer for investigation.
Infertility	Clinical history	Inability to conceive after more than 12 months of regular unprotected intercourse and exclusion of male causes	Assess menstrual regularity. Endocrinologist and/or gynecologist should be consulted to exclude endocrine disorders such as PCOS, hypothalamic amenorrhea, hyperprolactinemia, thyroid dysfunction.
Obesity and weight gain	BMI: Weight (in kg)/ height (in cm) squared	Obese: BMI>25 kg/m^2 Significant weight gain: >5 kg	Assess menstrual regularity. In case of cycle disturbance: investigate or refer.
	WHR: Ratio of supine circumference of waist–hips	Truncal obesity: WHR>0.9	Assess menstrual regularity. In case of cycle disturbance: investigate or refer.
Hirsutism	Inspection or Ferriman–Gallwey score	Male escutcheon	May be genetic or ethnic. Assess menstrual regularity. In case of cycle disturbance: investigate or refer.
Galactorrhea	History	Crusting on nipples; expression of breast milk in nonlactating women	Assess menstrual regularity, look for hirsutism, signs of hypothyroidism. Investigate or refer.

BMI, body mass index; WHR, waist–hip ratio; PCOS, polycystic ovary syndrome.

TABLE II

INVESTIGATION OF WOMEN WITH EPILEPSY AND SYMPTOMS OR SIGNS OF REPRODUCTIVE ENDOCRINE
DISORDER (ADAPTED FROM BAUER *ET AL.*, 2002)

Test	Method	Abnormal findings	Comment
LH, FSH	Measurement of serum levels (calculation based on an average of three estimations taken 20 min apart between days 3 and 6 of the cycle)	LH/FSH ratio>2 FSH>35 IU/l LH>11 IU/l LH<7 mIU/ml	Suggestive of PCOS Suggestive of menopause Suggestive of hypothalamic amenorrhea
Prolactin	Measurement of morning resting serum levels (not postictal!)	>20 μg/l	May be mildly raised in patients with epilepsy. Rule out hypothyroidism or pituitary tumor Drugs may have impact on PRL levels.
Progesterone	Measurement of serum level (blood taken during midluteal phase according to menstrual cycle)	<6 nmol/l	Low levels indicate anovulation. Common cause: PCOS, HA, HPRL.
Testosterone	Measurement of serum level days 3–6 of the cycle	>2.5 nmol/l >4.0 nmol/l	Common cause: PCOS, valproate. Nonclassical adrenal hyperplasia may cause modest elevation of T. Rule out adrenal/ovarian tumor
Androstenedione	Measurement of serum level	>10.0 nmol/l	Rule out nonclassical congenital adrenal hyperplasia
DHEAS	Measurement of serum level	Age 20–29 >3800 ng/ml Age 30–39 >2700 ng/ml	Rule out nonclassical adrenal hyperplasia
Glucose/insulin	Fasting, morning levels glucose/insulin ratio	Fasting glucose >7.8 mmol/l Glucose/insulin ratio>4	Suggestive of diabetes Suggestive of reduced insulin sensitivity. Associated with obesity and PCOS.

(Continued)

TABLE II   *(Continued)*

Test	Method	Abnormal findings	Comment
Pelvic ultrasound	Transvaginal or transabdominal (days 3–9 of the cycle)	>10 peripheral cysts, 2–8 mm diameter in one ultrasound plane, thickening of ovarian stroma	Polycystic ovaries. Associated with PCOS.
		Other structural abnormalities of ovaries	Tumors, atrophy, multifollicular ovaries, etc.

N.B.: Exact values and units of measurement may vary from lab to lab. LH, luteinizing hormone; FSH, follicle stimulating hormone; DHEAS, dehydroepiandrosterone sulfate; PCOS, polycystic ovary syndrome; HPRL, hyperprolactinaemia; HA, hypophyseal adenoma.

hormonal tests raise concern about ovarian pathology. Transvaginal ultrasound is more sensitive than transabdominal ultrasound in the identification of structural abnormalities of the ovaries including tumors and cystic change. Pituitary MRI may be indicated if clinical (e.g., galactorrhea) or laboratory results (e.g., HPRL) suggest an abnormality of the hypothalamic–pituitary axis. However, a small pituitary lactotroph adenoma may not be detected if beyond the resolution of magnetic resonance imaging (Bauer *et al.*, 2002).

Apart from the entity of PCOS described below, evidence of other endocrine disturbances can be found.

Hypothalamic amenorrhea (HA), also called hypogonadotropic hypogonadism, has been found in 6 out of 50 (12%) consecutive women with TLE whereas it is estimated to affect 1.5% of the general population (Herzog *et al.*, 1986). HA is associated with a disturbed secretion of pituitary gonadotropins with low luteinizing hormone (LH) levels. HA causes amenorrhea or oligomenorrhea and infertility in the absence of signs of hyperandrogenemia (Bauer *et al.*, 2002).

The prevalence of functional HPRL may also be increased in women with epilepsy (Bauer *et al.*, 1992; Molaie *et al.*, 1986; Fig. 1). Functional HPRL causes poly-, oligo-, or amenorrhea, subfertility, galactorrhea, and hirsutism.

V. Polycystic Ovary Syndrome

PCOS is a common cause of irregular periods in women. The prevalence of PCOS in patients with TLE has been found to be 10–25% even if they were not receiving AED (Herzog *et al.*, 1984, 1986; Meo and Bilo, 2003). Its high prevalence stands in contrast to evidence of PCOS in 4–6.8% of women of reproductive age (Knochenhauser *et al.*, 1998).

PCOS is a form of hyperandrogenic chronic anovulation. Anovulation may be indicated by low midluteal phase progesterone levels. The pathogenesis of PCOS involves the acceleration of pulsatile gonadotropin releasing hormone (GnRH) secretion, insulin resistance, hyperinsulinemia, and downstream metabolic dysregulation. Abnormalities of the reproductive axis are manifested as hypersecretion of LH, ovarian theca stromal cell hyperactivity, and hypofunction of the FSH granulosa cell axis resulting in hyperandrogenism, hirsutism, follicular arrest, and ovarian acyclicity (Yen, 1999).

PCOS should not be confused with isolated PCO (polycystic change without symptoms, pathological signs, or hormonal abnormality). Isolated PCO is observed in 17–22% of women in the general population although higher frequencies have been reported (Michelmore *et al.*, 1999; Polson *et al.*, 1988). In a population based study, PCO was detected in 74 out of 224 (33%) of women investigated (Michelmore *et al.*, 1999). Two-thirds of these women had menstrual irregularity and four-fifths had at least one feature of PCOS including menstrual irregularity (menstrual irregularity, acne, hirsutism, obesity, raised T or LH). The high number of women with PCOS in this study might result from the low recruitment rate (22% of all women approached) introducing a bias towards women with reproductive endocrine disorders.

Nowadays this diagnosis is founded on the guideline criteria of the National Institute of Health, established in 1990 (Balen, 1999). These define a PCOS as being present in the case of irregular cycles (polymenorrhoea, <23-day cycle or oligomenorrhea, >35-day cycle or amenorrhoea, >6-month or sterility despite sexual intercourse over 12 months or midluteal progesterone, <6 nmol/l as a sign of anovulation) as well as clinical signs (hirsutism) or laboratory (androgen serum concentration >2.5 nmol/l on phlebotomy on day 3, 4, 5, or 6 of the cycle), signs of hyperandrogenemia following exclusion of hormone producing adrenal tumors or adrenal hyperplasia as well as HPRL (postpartum or drug-induced).

Polycystic ovaries show more than 10 (often 20–100) cystic follicles of 2–8 mm in diameter and thickening of the tunica of approximately 50%. The hilus cells reach fourfold volume of a normal ovary with concomitant increase in cortical and subcortical stroma. The impressive structural change of ovaries suggests the cause of PCOS as lying within a primary ovarial disturbance. Many gynecologists would disagree. The structural change of ovaries rather constitutes the end point of hormonal malfunctioning. Causative factors may be entities such as hypothalamic, pituitary, ovarial, or adrenal functional disturbance. The characteristic of polycystic ovary develops following a prolonged anovulatory period (Polson, 2003).

The PCO structure is believed to develop in pubertal women due to a genetic predisposition (Balen, 1999). Only some women with PCO will develop PCOS with chronic oligo- or amenorrhea associated with increased serum androgen levels (Knochenhauser *et al.*, 1998). There are many potential triggers for the development of PCOS; weight gain is one such factor.

The development of PCOS can be explained most plausibly on the grounds of the assumption of a primary functional disturbance of the hypothalamic–pituitary axis. Many, but not all, women with PCOS show an elevated quotient of LH and FSH (>3) due to an elevated level of LH (20–40% do not).

The elevation in amplitude (but not frequency) of LH is probably caused by a changed pulsation of the hypothalamic GnRH (Kazer *et al.*, 1987). Often a change in amplitude and frequency of hypothalamic GnRH is causative of PCOS, that is a central disturbance, which is inducible by the interictal influences of a focal epilepsy. This in turn leads to the initiation of an albeit incomplete follicular development in the ovary (due to the insufficient effect of FSH) which in turn can lead to the structure of a secondary polycystic ovary.

The peripheral hormonal vicious circle also receives its contribution by the various influencing factors of sexual steroid hormones on the hepatic binding of sex hormone-binding globulin (SHBG). T elevates and estrogens reduce the generation of SHBG. By this means, the concentration of SHBG is reduced in women with PCOS and anovulation by 50% which in turn causes elevated amounts of free and hence biologically active estrogen concentrations to exert a negative effect on the pathway of hypothalamic FSH. The consequence of this in turn is an elevated quotient of LH and FSH.

The elevation of androgens thus has a major role in the development of PCOS. Contrasting to male physiology, weight gain is further potential causal aspect for the evaluation of the possible influence of side effects of AED. Being overweight as well as suffering from increased abdominal fat (i.e., suffering from an android fat distribution) in turn causes hyperinsulinemia and imbalance of glucose tolerance.

The effect weight gain exerts on insulin concentration can become an essential factor in the peripheral induction of PCOS. The reason for this is an enhanced formation or availability of androgens. In this case, weight gain is potentially relevant when BMI exceeds 25 kg/m^2, the waist–hip ratio is higher than 0.9 and/or body weight increases by 5 kg (Bauer *et al.*, 2002).

Forty percent of all women with PCOS show elevated rates of insulin resistance, especially, but not exclusively in the case of adipositas and with advanced age (Knuth *et al.*, 2000). The glucose/insulin quotient rises to over four and stimulates insulin formation within the ovaries. This occurs due to ovarial stimulation by means of insulin or indirectly by means of elevated activity of insulin-like growth factor-I. This factor in turn stimulates androgen formation in the ovary (Fig. 3).

The presence of elevated rates of insulin reduces the formation of the binding globulin, insulin-like growth factors which as a result become more biologically active. Simultaneously, the elevated insulin levels inhibit the hepatic production of SHBG and hence elevate the biological impact of T. The majority of

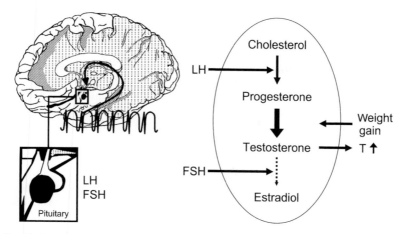

FIG. 3. Increase in the ovarian testosterone (T) production induced by interictal epileptic discharges of the temporal lobe (via hypothalamic–pituitary axis and increase in LH levels) and/or antiepileptic drugs (via weight gain-induced serum insulin level increase). LH, luteinizing hormone; FSH, follicle stimulating hormone.

experimental data suggests that a dysfunctional insulin metabolism precedes a dysfunctional androgen metabolism (Dunaif, 1999).

Jouko Isojärvi and his colleagues from Finland have published studies describing the impact of AED, particularly VPA, on the development of PCOS. In a first study concerning 238 women with epilepsy, 45% of the 29 women on treatment with VPA suffered from cycle irregularities (amenorrhea, oligomenorrhea, prolonged cycles, irregular menstruation), 60% of these women showed a polycystic ovary structure and 30% had an elevated serum T concentration (Isojärvi *et al.*, 1993).

One of the further studies included 65 women with epilepsy. In 14 out of 22 (64%) of patients treated with VPA polycystic ovaries and/or hyperandrogenemia were found—in isolation or combination. Following a change to lamotrigine features such as hyperinsulinemia, hyperandrogenemia, dyslipidemia, and polycystic ovarian structure became significantly normalized in tandem with weight loss over the period of 1 year (Isojärvi *et al.*, 1998).

Meo and Bilo (2003) founded the definition of PCOS of the National Institute of Health on the grounds of these and further studies on PCOS. From published data, they calculated a prevalence of this syndrome in 3%. These results are far below the estimations of the Finnish authors and are in the region of findings in women of the general population (4–6, 8%) as well as those in women with epilepsy without the influence of medication (15–25%).

The investigations of other authors did not assess the endocrinologically negative impact of treatment with VPA (Genton *et al.*, 2001). In our own analyses, we found PCOS in 10–11% of women irrespective of treatment with VPA or CBZ or untreated individuals (Bauer et al., 2000a). Studies in Austria showed identical prevalence of PCOS in women with epilepsy on treatment with VPA (7.7%) or CBZ (7.5%) (Luef et al., 2002).

It must be assumed that the VPA-induced weight gain in some of the women treated with VPA may induce the development of PCOS (Bauer et al., 2002). This is strongly suggested by studies in which VPA was substituted by a different AED (usually LTG) resulting in normalized weight and in studies based on well documented case reports (Isojärvi and Tapanainen, 2000; Isojärvi et al., 1998).

In animal experiments, it was attempted to analyze the influence of VPA as well as the development of PCOS. VPA appeared to exert and influence on steroid genesis and elevated the quotient of T and estradiol in ovary follicle in pigs (Sveberg Røste et al., 2001, 2003; Taubøll et al., 1999). Continuous treatment with VPA elevates the amount of follicular cysts and influences serum concentrations of sexual steroid hormones (reduction of T and estrogen) in rats, while this could not be proven in lamotrigine (Sveberg Røste et al., 2003).

Weight gain aside, VPA is associated with another phenomenon potentially associated with the development of PCOS. VPA is an AED with an inhibitory effect on the hepatic P450 enzyme system. This enzyme system is linked to the metabolism of sexual steroid hormones, for example, T. Following the administration of VPA for 3 months, a significant elevation of serum T can be detected (Morrell, 2003). By contrast, CBZ causes induction of the hepatic P450 enzyme system, leading in turn to a contrary effect on T (i.e., androgens).

Enzyme-inducing AEDs (such as CBZ, phenytoin, or phenobarbital) may exert a protective effect against the development of PCOS. The extent to which a drug-related elevation of T leads to a relevant endocrinopathy, for example, PCOS, is not known in detail. Lowering available free T by means of CBZ may contribute to less evidence/detectability of hyperandrogenous anovulation in women on treatment with CBZ than untreated patients (13% vs 30%) (Herzog et al., 1984).

While normalization of body weight leads to reversibility of PCOS in overweight women, its treatment in women of normal weight is far more complex. As a rule, the only option in these women is the regulation of menstrual cycles by means of oral contraceptive agents without influencing the causal (usually central) process.

VI. Final Remarks and Conclusions

The most likely explanations for endocrine disorders related to epilepsy or AEDs are a direct influence of the epileptogenic lesion, epilepsy, or AED on the endocrine control centers in the brain, the effects of AED on peripheral endocrine glands, the effects of AED on the metabolism of hormones and binding proteins and secondary endocrine complications of AED-related weight changes or changes of insulin sensitivity.

A direct role for epilepsy in the pathogenesis of reproductive endocrine disorders is suggested by acute changes in serum prolactin and gonadotropin levels following seizures (Bauer, 1996), a possible relationship between the laterality of temporolimbic epileptiform discharges and the specific type of reproductive endocrine disorder (i.e., left unilateral temporolimbic epilepsy has been associated with PCOS, right temporolimbic epilepsy with hypothalamic amenorrhea) (Herzog, 1993; Herzog et al., 1986, 2003a,b), and the normalization of menstrual cycles after epilepsy surgery (Bauer et al., 2000b).

AEDs have direct effects on peripheral female endocrine glands in animal models. VPA has been shown to alter steroidogenesis and increase T to estradiol ratios in porcine ovarian follicles (Gregoraszczuk et al., 2000). Long-term use of VPA increased the number of follicular cysts and altered sex steroid hormone levels in rats (Taubøll et al., 1999). VPA but not lamotrigine increased the number of ovarian follicular cysts in rats (Sveberg Røste et al., 2001). All of this experimental work was undertaken in nonepileptic animals. It remains to be proven that direct gonadal AED effects are clinically relevant in humans. Isojärvi et al. (1993, 1996, 2001) found an increased number of ovarian cysts in women on VPA monotherapy. A normalization of such polycystic change was observed after discontinuation of VPA. However, there were corresponding improvements of insulin resistance and it is, therefore, uncertain whether VPA had a direct or insulin-mediated effect on the ovaries (Isojärvi et al., 1998).

AED may decrease or increase biologically active serum sex hormone levels. Many of the older AEDs including CBZ, Phenobarbital, and phenytoin induce hepatic cytochrome P450-dependent steroid hormone breakdown and the production of SHBG, thereby reducing biologically active sex hormone serum concentrations (Bauer et al., 2002; Beastall et al., 1985; Murialdo et al., 1998; Stoffel-Wagner et al., 1998; Victor et al., 1977) (Table III).

Decreases of free serum T levels during CBZ treatment due to an induction of SHBG were documented (Stoffel-Wagner et al., 1998). Free T serum concentration rises when patients are switched from CBZ to oxcarbazepine which causes less hepatic induction (Isojärvi et al., 1995). A reduced rate of PCOS (a condition characterized by a high T) in women treated for epilepsy with enzyme-inducers compared to untreated women with epilepsy (13% vs 30%) was demonstrated (Herzog et al., 1986). Other investigators found that enzyme induction in CBZ treated women with epilepsy causes menstrual disturbance characterized by low estradiol and a low estradiol/SHBG ratio in 25% of cases (Isojärvi et al., 1995).

Conversely, hepatic enzyme inhibitors can increase biologically active sex hormone levels. In a prospective study, an increase in serum androgen concentrations was documented in women with newly diagnosed epilepsy who were

TABLE III

EFFECT OF CARBAMAZEPINE MONOTHERAPY ON HORMONES IN WOMEN WITH EPILEPSY
(STOFFEL-WAGNER *ET AL.*, 1998)

	Women with epilepsy ($N = 22$) median	Healthy women ($N = 60$) median
Testosterone (nM)	0.70	0.90
Free testosterone (pg/ml)	1.00	0.90
SHBG (nM)	95.00[*]	55.10
Cortisol (µg/dl)	9.70	10.20
DHEAS (µg/ml)	812.00[**]	2109.00
17α-Hydroxyprogesterone (µg/l)	0.90	1.25
Androstenedione (µg/l)	1.40	1.50
TSH (µU/ml)	0.48[**]	1.12
Free T4 (ng/dl)	0.99	1.18
Free T3 (pg/ml)	4.31	4.54
hGH (µg/l)	1.05	0.90
IGF-I (µg/l)	209.00	246.00
Prolactin (µg/l)	5.60[***]	3.60

SHBG, sex hormone-binding globulin; DHEAS, dehydroepiandrosterone sulfate; TSH, thyroid stimulating hormone; HGH, human growth hormone; IGF, insulin-like growth factor; T4, thyroxine; T3, triiodothyronine.
[*]$p < 0.01$.
[**]$p < 0.0001$.
[***]$p < 0.02$.

started on VPA (Rättyä *et al.*, 2001). In girls treated with VPA for a mean of 2 years higher serum T levels were found than in untreated controls (Vainionpää *et al.*, 1999). T levels in excess of 2 SD of the mean were found in 38% of prepubertal, 36% of pubertal, and 57% of postpubertal girls on VPA. It should be pointed out that the clinical relevance of an elevated total and/or free T level depends on the presence of symptoms of hyperandrogenism such as cycle disturbance, subfertility, male pattern hair loss, hirsutism, or acne. However, an increase in serum total and/or free T may contribute to altered gonadotropin secretion and lead to the manifestation of reproductive endocrine disorders so that asymptomatic patients with an isolated elevation of total and/or free T should be kept under endocrine review (Eagleson *et al.*, 2000).

Several AEDs may cause weight gain. This adverse effect has been described with VPA, CBZ, vigabatrin, and gabapentin (Biton *et al.*, 2001; Breum *et al.*, 1992; Rättyä *et al.*, 1999). Weight gain and obesity have direct negative effects on many aspects of health and on life expectancy. Weight increase reduces insulin sensitivity and promotes PCOS development in predisposed women who had no previous hormonal abnormality. Thus, AED-related weight increases could trigger the manifestation of a clinically relevant endocrine disorder. Weight-related endocrine problems may be enhanced by the enzyme-inhibiting effects of VPA and masked by enzyme inducers like CBZ. Weight reduction after tapering off VPA has been shown to be associated with a normalization of menstrual cycles and hormonal disturbances (Isojärvi *et al.*, 1998). There are no studies of the effects of weight reduction without change of medication. It should be pointed out that VPA-associated endocrine changes have also been observed in the absence of weight gain (Isojärvi *et al.*, 1996, 2001; Vainionpää *et al.*, 1999).

The treatment of epilepsy aims for complete seizure control with as few side effects as possible. The choice of AED is driven by many considerations including proven efficacy for the particular seizure type, tolerability, the personal experience of the physician, and especially how comfortable the physician and the patient feel using a specific agent. In the treatment of women with epilepsy, a number of additional factors have to be considered. These include the safety of an AED during pregnancy, the compatibility of the AED with hormonal contraception, and the potential impact on reproductive function as outlined above.

Physicians should be aware of reproductive endocrine dysfunction that may occur in women with epilepsy during treatment (Bauer *et al.*, 2002; Harden, 2005a) (Tables I and II). If a reproductive endocrine disorder is found, AEDs should be reviewed in terms of their indication for the particular seizure type and their tolerability *vis-à-vis* their potential for contributing to the endocrine problem. The possible benefits of a change of AED treatment must be balanced against seizure control and cumulative side effect of alternative agents. Many of the newer AEDs have not been studied with regard to (longer term) endocrine reproductive side effects and little is known about their safety in pregnancy. If a patient is seizure-free on an AED, which could be the cause of adverse reproductive endocrine effects, a monotherapy switch is fraught with the risk of seizure relapse and lower dose combination therapy with the risk of additional side effects (Bauer *et al.*, 2002).

References

Alving, J. (1998). Serum prolactin levels are elevated also after pseudo-epileptic seizures. *Seizure* **7**, 85–89.

Baird, A. D., Wilson, S. J., Bladin, P. F., Saling, M. M., and Reutens, D. C. (2003). Sexual outcome after epilepsy surgery. *Epilepsy Behav.* **4**, 268–278.

Balen, A. H. (1999). Pathogenesis of polycystic ovary syndrome—The enigma unravels? *Lancet* **354**, 966–967.

Bauer, J. (1996). Epilepsy and prolactin adults: A clinical review. *Epilepsy Res.* **24**, 1–7.

Bauer, J. (2001). Interactions between hormones and epilepsy in female patients. *Epilepsia* **42**(Suppl. 3), 20–22.

Bauer, J., Stefan, H., Schrell, U., Sappke, U., and Uhlig, B. (1989). Neurophysiologic principles and
  clinical value of postconvulsive serum prolactin determination in epileptic seizures (in German).
  Fortschr. Neurol. Psychiatr. **57,** 457–468.
Bauer, J., Stefan, H., Schrell, U., Uhlig, B., Landgraf, S., Neubauer, U., Neundörfer, B., and Burr, W.
  (1992). Serum prolactin concentrations and epilepsy: A study comparing patients in presurgical
  evaluation with healthy persons and circadian with seizure related variations. *Eur. Arch. Psychiatry
  Clin. Neurosci.* **241,** 365–371.
Bauer, J., Burr, W., and Elger, C. E. (1998). Seizure occurrence during ovulatory and anovulatory
  cycles in patients with temporal lobe epilepsy: A prospective study. *Eur. J. Neurol.* **5,** 83–88.
Bauer, J., Jarre, A., Klingmüller, D., and Elger, C. E. (2000a). Polycystic ovary syndrome in patients
  with focal epilepsy: A study in 93 women. *Epilepsy Res.* **41,** 163–167.
Bauer, J., Stoffel-Wagner, B., Flügel, D., Kluge, M., and Elger, C. E. (2000b). The impact of epilepsy
  surgery on serum sex hormones and menstrual cycles in female patients. *Seizure* **9,** 389–393.
Bauer, J., Isojärvi, J. I. T., Herzog, A. G., Reuber, M., Polson, D., Taubøll, E., Genton, P., van der
  Ven, H., Roesing, B., Luef, G. J., Galimberti, C. A., van Parys, J., et al. (2002). Reproductive
  dysfunction in women with epilepsy: Recommendations for evaluation and management.
  J. Neurol. Neurosurg. Psychiat. **73,** 121–125.
Beastall, G. H., Cowan, R. A., Gray, J. M., and Fogelman, I. (1985). Hormone binding globulins and
  anticonvulsant therapy. *Scott. Med. J.* **30,** 101–105.
Bergen, D., Daugherty, S., and Eckenfels, E. (1992). Reduction of sexual activities in females taking
  antiepileptic drugs. *Psychopathology* **25,** 1–14.
Bilo, L., Meo, R., and Striano, S. (1988). Serum prolactin evaluation after "minor" generalized
  seizures monitored by EEG. *J. Neurol. Neurosurg. Psychiatr.* **51,** 308–309.
Biton, V., Mirza, W., Montouris, G., Vuong, A., Hammer, A. E., and Barrett, P. S. (2001). Weight
  change associated with valproate and lamotrigine monotherapy in patients with epilepsy. *Neurology*
  56, 172–177.
Breum, L., Astrup, A., Gram, L., Andersen, T., Stokholm, K. H., Christensen, N. J., Werdelin, L., and
  Madsen, J. (1992). Metabolic changes during treatment with valproate in humans: Implication for
  untoward weight gain. *Metabolism* **41,** 666–670.
Crawford, P., Appleton, R., Betts, T., Duncan, J., Guthrie, E., and Morrow, J. (1999). The women with
  epilepsy guidelines development group. Best practice guidelines for the management of women
  with epilepsy. *Seizure* **8,** 201–217.
Cordingly, G., Brown, D., Dane, P., Harnish, K., Cadamagnani, P., and O'Hare, T. (1993). Increases
  in serum prolactin levels associated with syncopal attacks. *Am. J. Emerg. Med.* **11,** 251–252.
Cummings, L. N., Giudice, L., and Morrell, M. J. (1995). Ovulatory function in epilepsy. *Epilepsia* **36,**
  355–359.
Daniele, A., Azzoni, A., Bizzi, A., Rossi, A., Gainotti, G., and Mazza, S. (1997). Sexual behavior and
  hemispheric laterality of the focus in patients with temporal lobe epilepsy. *Biol. Psychiatr.* **42,**
  617–624.
Demerdash, A., Shaalan, M., Midani, A., Kamel, F., and Bahri, M. (1991). Sexual behavior of a
  sample of females with epilepsy. *Epilepsia* **32,** 82–85.
Dunaif, A. (1999). Insulin action in the polycystic ovary syndrome. *Endocrinol. Metab. Clin. N. Am.* **28,**
  341–359.
Duncan, S., Blacklaw, J., Beastall, G. H., and Brodie, M. J. (1997). Sexual function in women with
  epilepsy. *Epilepsia* **38,** 1074–1081.
Eagleson, C. A., Gingrich, M. B., and Pastor, C. L. (2000). Polycystic ovarian syndrome: Evidence that
  flutamide restores sensitivity of the gonadotropin-releasing hormone pulse generator to inhibition
  by estradiol and progesterone. *J. Clin. Endocrinol. Metab.* **85,** 4047–4052.
Edwards, H. E., Burnham, W. M., and MacLusky, N. J. (1999). Partial and generalized seizures affect
  reproductive physiology differentially in the male rat. *Epilepsia* **40,** 1490–1498.

Feeney, D. M., Gullotta, F. P., and Gilmore, W. (1998). Hyposexuality produced by temporal lobe epilepsy in the cat. *Epilepsia* **39,** 140–149.

Genton, P., Bauer, J., Duncan, S., Taylor, A. E., Balen, A. H., Eberle, A., Pedersen, B., Salas-Puig, X., and Sauer, M. V. (2001). On the association between valproate and polycystic ovary syndrome. *Epilepsia* **42,** 295–304.

Gregoraszczuk, E., Wojtowicz, A. K., Taubøll, E., and Ropstad, E. (2000). Valproate-induced alterations in T, estradiol and progesterone secretion from porcine follicular cells isolated from small- and medium-sized ovarian follicles. *Seizure* **9,** 480–485.

Harden, C. L. (2005a). Polycystic ovaries and polycystic ovary syndrome in epilepsy: Evidence for neurogonadal disease. *Epilepsy Curr.* **5,** 142–146.

Harden, C. L. (2005b). Sexuality in women with epilepsy. *Epilepsy Behav.* **7,** S2–S6.

Harden, C. L., Koppel, B. S., Herzog, A. G., Nikolov, B. G., and Hauser, W. A. (2003). Seizure frequency is associated with age at menopause in women with epilepsy. *Neurology* **61,** 451–455.

Helmstaedter, C., and Elger, C. E. (2004). The impact of epilepsy on sexual function, behavior, beliefs in, and attitudes toward sexuality. *Epilepsia* **45**(Suppl. 7), 231.

Herzog, A. G. (1988). Clomiphene therapy in epileptic women with menstrual disorders. *Neurology* **38,** 432–434.

Herzog, A. G. (1993). A relationship between particular reproductive endocrine disorders and the laterality of epileptiform discharges in women with epilepsy. *Neurology* **43,** 1907–1910.

Herzog, A. G. (1997). Disorders of reproduction and fertility. *In* "Epilepsy: A Comprehensive Textbook" (J Engel, Jr. and T. A. Pedley, Eds.), pp. 2013–2026. Lippincott-Raven, Philadelphia.

Herzog, A. G., and Friedman, M. N. (2001). Menstrual cycle interval and ovulation in women with localization-related epilepsy. *Neurology* **57,** 2133–2135.

Herzog, A. G., Seibel, M. M., Schomer, D., Vaitukaitis, J., and Geschwind, N. (1984). Temporal lobe epilepsy: An extrahypothalamic pathogenesis for polycystic ovarian syndrome? *Neurology* **34,** 1389–1393.

Herzog, A. G., Seibel, M. M., Schomer, D. L., Vaitikaitis, J. L., and Geschwind, N. (1986). Reproductive endocrine disorders in women with partial seizures of temporal lobe origin. *Arch. Neurol.* **43,** 341–346.

Herzog, A. G., Coleman, A. E., Jacobs, A. R., Klein, P., Friedman, M. N., Drislane, F. W., and Schomer, D. L. (2003a). Relationship of sexual dysfunction to epilepsy laterality and reproductive hormone levels in women. *Epilepsy Behav.* **4,** 407–413.

Herzog, A. G., Coleman, A. E., Jacobs, A. R., Klein, P., Friedman, M. N., Drislane, F. W., Ransil, B. J., and Schomer, D. L. (2003b). Interictal EEG discharges, reproductive hormones, and menstrual disorders in epilepsy. *Ann. Neurol.* **54,** 625–637.

Isojärvi, J. I. T., and Tapanainen, J. S. (2000). Valproate, hyperandrogenism, and polycystic ovaries: A report of 3 cases. *Arch. Neurol.* **57,** 1064–1068.

Isojärvi, J. I. T., Laatikainen, T. J., Knip, M., Pakarinen, A. J., Juntunen, K. T., and Myllylä, V. V. (1993). Polycystic ovaries and hyperandrogenism in women taking valproate for epilepsy. *N. Engl. J. Med.* **329,** 1383–1388.

Isojärvi, J. I. T., Laatikainen, T. J., Pakarinen, A. J., Juntunen, K. T., and Myllylä, V. V. (1995). Menstrual disorders in women with epilepsy receiving carbamazepine. *Epilepsia* **36,** 676–681.

Isojärvi, J. I. T., Laatikainen, T. J., Knip, M., Pakarinen, A. J., Juntunen, K. T., and Myllylä, V. V. (1996). Obesity and endocrine disorders in women taking valproate for epilepsy. *Ann. Neurol.* **39,** 579–584.

Isojärvi, J. I. T., Rättyä, J., Myllylä, V. V., Knip, M., Koivunen, R., Pakarinen, A. J., Tekay, A., and Tapanainen, J. S. (1998). Valproate, lamotrigine, and insulin-mediated risks in women with epilepsy. *Ann. Neurol.* **43,** 446–451.

Isojärvi, J. I. T., Taubøll, E., Pakarinen, A. J., van Parys, J., Rättyä, J., Harbo, H. F., Dale, P. O., Fauser, B. C., Gjerstad, L., Koivunen, R., Knip, M., and Tapanainen, J. S. (2001). Altered ovarian function and cardiovascular risk factors in valproate treated women. *Am. J. Med.* **111,** 290–296.

Jensen, P., Jensen, S. B., and Sorensen, P. S. (1990). Sexual dysfunction in male and female patients with epilepsy: A study of 86 outpatients. *Arch. Sex Behav.* **19,** 1–14.

Kazer, R. R., Kessel, B., and Yen, S. S. C. (1987). Circulating luteinizing hormone pulse frequency in women with polycystic ovary syndrome. *J. Clin. Endocrinol. Metab.* **65,** 233–236.

Klein, P., Serje, A., and Pezzullo, J. C. (2001). Premature ovarian failure in women with epilepsy. *Epilepsia* **42,** 1584–1589.

Klein, P., van Passel-Clark, L. M. A., and Pezzullo, J. C. (2003). Onset of epilepsy at the time of menarche. *Neurology* **60,** 495–497.

Knochenhauser, E. S., Key, T. J., Kashar-Miller, M., Waggoner, W., Boots, L. R., and Azziz, R. (1998). Prevalence of polycystic ovary syndrome in unselected black and white women of the southeastern United States: A prospective study. *J. Clin. Endocrinol. Metab.* **83,** 3078–3082.

Knuth, U. A., Schneider, H. P. G., and Behre, H. M. (2000). Andrologierelevante Gynäkologie. *In* "Andrologie" (E. Nieschlag and H. M. Behre, Eds.), pp. 301–348. Springer, Heidelberg.

Luef, G., Abraham, I., Trinka, E., Alge, A., Windisch, J., Daxenbichler, G., Unterberger, I., Seppi, K., Lechleitner, M., Krämer, G., and Bauer, G. (2002). Hyperandrogenism, postprandial hyperinsulism and the risk of PCOS in a cross sectional study of women with epilepsy treated with valproate. *Epilepsy Res.* **48,** 91–102.

Meo, R., and Bilo, L. (2003). Polycystic ovary syndrome and epilepsy. A review of the evidence. *Drugs* **63,** 1185–1227.

Michelmore, K. F., Balen, A. H., Dunger, D. B., and Vessey, M. P. (1999). Polycystic ovaries and associated biochemical features in young women. *Clin. Endocrinol.* **51,** 779–786.

Molaie, M., Culebras, A., and Miller, M. (1986). Effect of interictal epileptiform discharges on nocturnal plasma prolactin concentrations in epileptic patients with complex partial seizures. *Epilepsia* **27,** 724–728.

Morrell, M. J. (2003). Reproductive and metabolic disorders in women with epilepsy. *Epilepsia* **44** (Suppl. 4), 11–20.

Morrell, M. J., Sperling, M. R., Stecker, M., and Dichter, M. A. (1994). Sexual dysfunction in partial epilepsy: A deficit in physiologic sexual arousal. *Neurology* **44,** 243–247.

Morrell, M. J., Hamdy, S. F., Seale, C. G., and Springer, E. A. (1998). Self-reported reproductive history in women with epilepsy: Puberty onset and effects of menarche and menstrual cycle on seizures. *Neurology* **50,** A558.

Morrell, M. J., Giudice, L., Flynn, K. L., Seale, C. G., Paulson, A. J., Done, S., Flaster, E., Ferin, M., and Sauer, M. V. (2002). Predictors of ovulatory failure in women with epilepsy. *Ann. Neurol.* **52,** 704–711.

Murialdo, G., Galimberti, C. A., Gianelli, M. V., Manni, R., Ferrri, E., Polleri, A., and Tartara, A. (1998). Effects of valproate, phenobarbital and carbamazepine on sex steroid setup in women with epilepsy. *Clin. Neuropharmacol.* **21,** 52–58.

Ndgegwa, D., Rust, J., Golombok, S., and Fenwick, P. (1986). Sexual problems in epileptic women. *Sex Marital Ther.* **1,** 175–177.

Olafsson, E., Hauser, W. A., and Gudmundsson, G. (1998). Fertility in patients with epilepsy: A population-based study. *Neurology* **51,** 71–73.

Oribe, E., Amini, R., Nissenbaum, E., and Boal, B. (1996). Serum prolactin concentrations are elevated after syncope. *Neurology* **47,** 60–62.

Polson, D. W. (2003). Polycystic ovary syndrome and epilepsy—A gynaecological perspective. *Seizure* **12,** 397–402.

Polson, D. W., Adams, J., Wadsworth, J., and Franks, S. (1988). Polycystic ovaries. A common finding in normal women. *Lancet* **1,** 870–872.

Rao, M. L., Stefan, H., and Bauer, J. (1989). Epileptic but not psychogenic seizures are accompanied by simultaneous elevation of serum pituitary hormones and cortisol levels. *Neuroendocrinology* **49,** 33–39.

Rättyä, J., Vainionpaa, L., Knip, M., Lanning, P., and Isojärvi, J. I. T. (1999). The effects of valproate, carbamazepine, and oxcarbazepine on growth and sexual maturation in girls with epilepsy. *Pediatrics* **3,** 588–593.

Rättyä, J., Pakarinen, A. J., Repo, M., Myllylä, V. V., and Isojärvi, J. I. T. (2001). Early hormonal changes during valproate or carbamazepine treatment—A 3 months study. *Neurology* **57,** 440–441.

Stoffel-Wagner, B., Bauer, J., Flügel, D., Brennemann, W., Klingmüller, D., and Elger, C. E. (1998). Serum sex hormones are altered in patients with chronic temporal lobe epilepsy receiving anticonvulsant medication. *Epilepsia* **39,** 1164–1173.

Svalheim, S., Taubøll, E., Bjornenak, T., Sveberg Røste, L., Morland, T., Saetre, E. R., and Gjerstad, L. (2003). Do women with epilepsy have increased frequency of menstrual disturbances? *Seizure* **12,** 529–533.

Sveberg Røste, L., Taubøll, E., Berner, A., Isojärvi, J. I. T., and Gjerstad, L. (2001). Valproate, but not lamotrigine, induces ovarian morphological changes in Wistar rats. *Exp. Toxicol. Pathol.* **52,** 545–552.

Sveberg Røste, L., Taubøll, E., Isojärvi, J. I. T., Berner, A., Berg, K. A., Pakarinen, A. J., Huhtaniemi, I. T., Knip, M., and Gjerstad, L. (2003). Gonadal morphology and sex hormones in male and female Wistar rats after long-term lamotrigine treatment. *Seizure* **12,** 621–627.

Taubøll, E., Isojärvi, J. I. T., Flinstad Harbo, H., Pakarinen, A. J., and Gjerstad, L. (1999). Long-term valproate treatment induces changes in ovarian morphology and serum sex steroid hormone levels in female Wistar rats. *Seizure* **8,** 490–493.

Vainionpää, L. K., Rättyä, J., Knip, M., Tapanainen, J. S., Pakarinen, A. J., Lanning, P., Tekay, A., Myllylä, V. V., and Isojärvi, J. I. T. (1999). Valproate-induced hyperandrogenism during pubertal maturation in girls with epilepsy. *Ann. Neurol.* **45,** 444–450.

Victor, A., Lundberg, P. O., and Johansson, E. D. (1977). Induction of sex hormone binding globulin by phenytoin. *Br. Med. J.* **2**(6092), 934–935.

Wallace, H., Shorvon, S., and Tallis, R. (1998). Age-specific incidence and prevalence rates of treated epilepsy in an unselected population of 2,052,922 and age-specific fertility rates of women with epilepsy. *Lancet* **352,** 1970–1973.

Webber, M. P., Hauser, W. A., Ottman, R., and Annegers, J. F. (1986). Fertility in persons with epilepsy: 1935–1974. *Epilepsia* **27,** 746–752.

Yen, S. S. C. (1999). Polycystic ovary syndrome (hyperandrogenic chronic anovulation). *In* "Reproductive Endocrinology" (S. S. C. Yen, R. B. Jaffe, and R. L. Barbieri, Eds.), 4th ed., pp. 436–478. WB Saunders, Philadelphia.

SEXUAL DYSFUNCTION IN WOMEN WITH EPILEPSY: ROLE OF ANTIEPILEPTIC DRUGS AND PSYCHOTROPIC MEDICATIONS

Mary A. Gutierrez,* Romila Mushtaq,[†] and Glen Stimmel[‡]

*Department of Pharmacology and Outcomes Sciences, Loma Linda University School of Pharmacy, Loma Linda, California 92350, USA
[†]Medical College of Wisconin, Milwaukee, Wisconin 53226, USA
[‡]University of Southern California Schools of Pharmacy and Medicine, Los Angeles, California 90089, USA

I. Effect of Psychotropic and Antiepileptic Drugs on Sexual Function
  A. Antiepileptic Drugs
  B. Antidepressant Drugs
  C. Antipsychotic Drugs
II. Treatment Strategies for Female Sexual Dysfunction
  A. Hypoactive Sexual Desire Disorder
  B. Female Sexual Arousal Disorder
  C. Female Orgasmic Disorder
  References

Sexual dysfunction is a frequently encountered comorbid disorder in patients with neurological and psychiatric disorders. Importantly, sexual dysfunction can also occur as a treatment emergent adverse effect of a number of commonly used psychotropic and antiepileptic medications, and can include decreased libido, erectile dysfunction, disordered arousal, delayed orgasm, and anorgasmia. These effects can occur in both men and women, and can be seen across age groups. Understanding the neurobiology of normal sexual response, as well as the pharmacologic mechanisms of these commonly used medications can enable the clinician to predict how medication use may impact different phases of sexual response. Discussion of the current treatment strategies for female sexual dysfunction is also elucidated in this chapter.

I. Effect of Psychotropic and Antiepileptic Drugs on Sexual Function

The two classes of psychotropic drugs most commonly associated with causing sexual dysfunction in women are antidepressant and antipsychotic drugs, while there is very limited literature regarding antiepileptic drugs (AEDs) (Gitlin, 2003). Sexual dysfunction can have many causes, and medication should not be too quickly blamed for preexisting dysfunction or other etiologies. A differential

157

diagnosis of drug-induced sexual dysfunction requires that the problem starts after drug therapy begins or after a dose increase, the problem is not situation or partner specific but tends to be present in all sexual situations, it is not explained by ongoing disease or environmental stress, and the effect dissipates with drug discontinuation (Graziottin, 2006; Seagraves, 1997).

A. ANTIEPILEPTIC DRUGS

Assessing AED-induced sexual dysfunction is difficult because seizure disorders have been associated with sexual dysfunction, and AEDs have not been systematically studied for their effect on sexual function (Crenshaw and Goldberg, 1996; Gitlin, 2003). Furthermore, epilepsy and AEDs can alter sex hormone levels that lead to both reproductive disorders and sexual dysfunction (Morrell *et al.*, 2005). Disorders of both sexual desire and arousal affect 30–60% of women with epilepsy. Sexual dysfunction is more common in women with localization-related epilepsy (LRE), in women receiving phenytoin, and in women with low levels of estradiol and dehydroepiandrosterone sulfate (Morrell *et al.*, 2005). In a series of reviews in the 1980s, hyposexuality among patients with epilepsy was commonly reported (Crenshaw and Goldberg, 1996). The incidence of decreased sexual desire and responsiveness among men and women with temporal lobe epilepsy ranges from 31% to 67%. The relative role of epilepsy versus AEDs in causing sexual dysfunction is difficult to establish. The enzyme-inducing AEDs (phenobarbital, phenytoin, carbamazapine, topiramate, and oxcarbazepine) increase hepatic synthesis of sex hormone binding globulin (SHBG) which reduces testosterone availability, and they also increase the metabolism of sex hormones and contraceptive hormones not seen with nonenzyme-inducing drugs (lamotrigine, valproate, gabapentin, and vigabatrin) (Penovich, 2000). A consistent finding is that more sexual dysfunction occurs in patients taking carbamazepine and phenytoin compared to patients taking lamotrigine or valproate (Herzog *et al.*, 2005; Morrell, 2003). Women treated with valproate for bipolar disorder, however, have been reported to have severely decreased libido and anorgasmia, while there are case reports of gabapentin-associated anorgasmia in women with epilepsy (Harden, 2005). A recent comprehensive review of pregabalin efficacy and tolerability makes no mention of sexual dysfunction as an observed adverse effect (Tassone *et al.*, 2007). No specific treatment strategies have been formulated for AED-induced sexual dysfunction beyond switching from enzyme-inducing drugs to drugs like valproate or lamotrigine if clinically appropriate.

B. ANTIDEPRESSANT DRUGS

1. *Incidence of Sexual Dysfunction*

Antidepressant drugs, among all psychotropic drugs, are most likely to cause sexual dysfunction, with delayed ejaculation and anorgasmia the most common disturbance (Labbate *et al.*, 1998). In most antidepressant clinical trials, orgasmic dysfunction is underestimated because of short study duration and reliance on patient self-report to detect sexual dysfunction. In one large prospective study, the incidence of SSRI-induced sexual dysfunction as given by self-report was 14%, while use of a questionnaire with direct inquiry about sexual functioning yielded an overall incidence of 58% (Montejo-Gonzalez et al., 1997).

2. Differences Among Antidepressant Drugs

Tricyclic antidepressants (TCAs) (e.g., amitriptyline, imipramine) and mono-amine oxidase inhibitors (MAOIs) (e.g., phenelzine) are commonly associated with sexual dysfunction. Very few studies were conducted in the past regarding these drugs, so it is difficult to compare their relative incidence of sexual dysfunction to SSRIs. A 6-week placebo-controlled trial that compared imipramine (200–300 mg) and phenelzine (60–90 mg) reported delayed orgasm in 27% of women with imipra-mine, while phenelzine was associated with orgasmic delay in 36% of women (Harrison et al., 1986). Orgasmic delay was noted in 11% of women on placebo.

The SSRIs are the best studied antidepressants in relation to their likelihood of causing sexual dysfunction. SSRIs can adversely affect all three phases of sexual function, though their most prominent effect is causing delayed ejaculation in men and anorgasmia in men and women (Labbate et al., 1998; Seagraves, 1998). SSRIs have been reported to cause decreased libido (Montejo et al., 2001; Rosen et al., 1999). SSRI-induced decreased libido may be understood through a mechanism of increased serotonin causing decreased dopaminergic activity (Stahl, 2001a,b). The association of antidepressant drugs and decreased libido must be viewed cautiously, however, since 50–90% of untreated depressed patients experience decreased libido as part of their depression (Rosen et al., 1999). Most depressed patients actually experience increased libido from their antidepressant drug once the depression is successfully treated. SSRIs have also been reported to cause arousal disturbances, primarily decreased vaginal lubrication in women (Montejo et al., 2001; Rosen et al., 1999). The difficulty in establishing a causal relationship of SSRIs to either de-creased libido or arousal disorder reinforces the need for a careful baseline of assessment of sexual functioning prior to initiation of SSRI drug therapy.

The most common sexual dysfunction caused by drugs with serotonin agonist activity in women is anorgasmia (Labbate et al., 1998; Rosen et al., 1999; Seagraves, 1998). Table I lists the observed frequency of anorgasmia seen in two studies (Montejo et al., 2001; Montejo-Gonzalez et al., 1997). As can be seen, SSRIs and venlafaxine cause anorgasmia in one-third to one-half of patients. Venlafaxine, while it has a different mechanism as a serotonin and norepinephrine reuptake inhibitor, is still a potent serotonin agonist that will commonly cause sexual dysfunction. Mirtazapine and nefazodone, though sero-tonin (5-HT) agonists, have an additional mechanism of postsynaptic blockade of the 5-HT-2 receptor that blocks the orgasmic dysfunction (Stahl, 1998; Stimmel and Gutierrez, 2006). Bupropion, not included in these studies, has no direct serotonin agonist activity, and also has a very low likelihood of causing sexual

TABLE I

OBSERVED FREQUENCY (%) OF ANTIDEPRESSANT-INDUCED ANORGASMIA IN MEN AND WOMEN

	$N = 1022^a$	$N = 344^b$
Fluoxetine	39	34
Paroxetine	53	48
Sertraline	47	37
Citalopram	52	nr
Fluvoxamine	38	31
Venlafaxine	42	nr
Mirtazapine	8	nr
Nefazodone	2	nr

[a]Adapted from Montejo *et al.* (2001).
[b]Adapted from Montejo-Gonzalez *et al.* (1997).
nr, not reported.

dysfunction (Stahl, 1998; Stimmel and Gutierrez, 2006). In a more recent study, there were no statistically significant differences between citalopram and paroxetine in women with decreased desire (35% vs 26%, respectively) and orgasmic dysfunction (29% vs 11%, respectively) (Landen *et al.*, 2005). Two newer antidepressants, escitalopram and duloxetine, have not been compared in head-to-head clinical trials with SSRIs for their relative sexual dysfunction adverse effects. Their premarketing clinical efficacy trials show relatively low incidence of sexual dysfunction, but these trials suffer from the same difficulties of reliance on patient self-report and brief duration of clinical trials. Based upon both drugs being potent serotonin agonists, it would be predicted that the likelihood of escitalopram and duloxetine causing orgasmic dysfunction would be similar to other SSRIs.

3. *Treatment Strategies for Antidepressant Drug-Induced Sexual Dysfunction*

Both the identification and management of antidepressant-induced sexual dysfunction are crucial. Sexual dysfunction has been cited as one of the most common reasons for patients discontinuing treatment with antidepressants (Montejo *et al.*, 2001). Patients should be counseled about the potential for antidepressant-induced changes in their sexual function, but if it occurs, they need not discontinue treatment since it can be managed (Stimmel and Gutierrez, 2006). Possible options to manage and treat antidepressant-induced sexual dysfunction include waiting for tolerance to develop, decreasing the dose, giving drug holidays, augmenting with an additional drug, or switching to an alternative antidepressant drug less likely to cause sexual dysfunction (Zajecka, 2001). The first two options have not been shown to be effective. Few patients actually experience less sexual dysfunction due to drug adaptation, and most find that the sexual dysfunction persists for as long as the drug is continued (Boyarsky and Hirschfeld, 2000). Antidepressant-induced sexual dysfunction seems to be a dose-related effect, so dose reduction might seem an attractive strategy. However, all depression treatment guidelines suggest that both continuation and maintenance therapy with antidepressants be given in the same dose that was effective for the acute depressive episode. While dose reduction will likely decrease the severity of the sexual dysfunction, it will also increase the risk of relapse (Rothschild, 2000). Antidepressant drug holidays are an effective strategy for some patients. Stopping either sertraline or paroxetine for 2 days of a weekend for 1 month was shown to improve sexual functioning in 50% of patients during the weekend (Rothschild, 1995). Drug holidays are not recommended for patients with a history of noncompliance, for patients whose depressive symptoms are not in remission, or for patients taking higher doses of SSRIs (Boyarsky and Hirschfeld, 2000; Zajecka, 2001).

A number of augmentation strategies have been tried in an attempt to treat antidepressant-induced sexual dysfunction. Augmentation with a second drug is most appropriate when the patient's depression has been successfully treated, but the sexual dysfunction persists and threatens compliance. Augmentation drugs that are no longer recommended include cyproheptadine, yohimbine, and nefazodone. Augmentation drugs that have only anecdotal reports of benefit, but lack sufficient clinical evidence of efficacy, include *Ginkgo biloba*, amantadine, and buspirone. The most viable augmenting drug treatment options include bupropion, mirtazapine, and sildenafil (Boyarsky and Hirschfeld, 2000; Zajecka, 2001). Bupropion is an antidepressant virtually devoid of sexual dysfunction and devoid of direct activity on serotonin, but with mixed reports of efficacy (Rosen *et al.*, 1999; Zajecka, 2001). Addition of bupropion SR 150 mg daily for 6 weeks to patients experiencing sexual dysfunction from SSRIs found no difference versus placebo on any measure of sexual functioning (DeBattista *et al.*, 2005). A placebo-controlled trial of adding bupropion SR 150 mg twice daily to an SSRI found no difference in global sexual functioning, orgasm, or arousal, but a significant difference in improved feelings of desire and frequency of sexual activity (Clayton *et al.*, 2004). Mirtazapine represents a more logical augmenting agent since its mechanism of postsynaptic 5-HT-2 blockade will directly block the orgasmic dysfunction caused by serotonin agonist antidepressants (Stimmel and Gutierrez, 2006; Zajecka, 2001). Open label addition of mirtazapine to SSRIs for 6 weeks was found to restore normal sexual function in 11/19 (58%) of patients, with another two patients experiencing significant improvement in sexual function (Gelenberg *et al.*, 2000). Sildenafil has the best evidence as an effective augmenting agent to SSRIs, though it is more effective in men than women. Sildenafil is effective on an as needed dosing basis, 50–100 mg given 30–60 min before sexual activity (Zajecka, 2001). Though indicated only for treatment of erectile dysfunction, sildenafil has shown efficacy in improving antidepressant-induced difficulties in libido, arousal, and orgasm delay. It is believed that sildenafil is effective for other phases of sexual function due to indirect effects of increasing blood flow to improve and sustain arousal. Possible disadvantages of sildenafil include the lack of proven efficacy for women, unclear benefits for libido, and its usual contraindications with nitrates and significant cardiovascular disease. In a study in 98 women, sildenafil augmentation resulted in significantly improved sexual function rating scales compared to placebo (71% vs 35%, $p < 0.001$), while desire, lubrication, arousal, orgasm, and satisfaction were improved with sildenafil but not statistically significantly different from placebo (Nurnberg *et al.*, 2006).

The final treatment option for antidepressant-induced sexual dysfunction is to switch from the offending drug and substitute either bupropion or mirtazapine (Stimmel *et al.*, 1997; Walker *et al.*, 1993; Zajecka, 2001). Switching antidepressants is a reasonable first-line approach for those patients who are not responding adequately to the initial antidepressant, or for patients refusing to continue taking an antidepressant because of sexual dysfunction.

C. Antipsychotic Drugs

1. *Differences Among Antipsychotic Drugs*

The most common effect of antipsychotic drugs on sexual function is decreased libido, due to dopamine antagonism. Increased prolactin levels caused by dopamine blockade also contributes to decreased libido (Smith *et al.*, 2002). The older antipsychotic drugs (e.g., haloperidol, fluphenazine, and chlorpromazine) decrease libido very commonly since they are potent dopamine blockers, with 30–60% of patients experiencing disturbances in sexual function (Boyarsky and Hirschfeld, 2000). There is limited data regarding sexual dysfunction associated with the newer atypical antipsychotic drugs (e.g., risperidone, olanzapine, quetiapine). A study of 636 patients receiving a single antipsychotic compared overall sexual dysfunction. Frequency of sexual dysfunction was 38% with haloperidol, 43% with risperidone, 35% with olanzapine, and 18% with quetiapine (Bobes *et al.*, 2003). In an open 6-week trial, sexual functioning in patients taking either risperidone or quetiapine was compared (Knegtering *et al.*, 2004). Sexual dysfunction, based upon the Antipsychotics and Sexual Functioning Questionnaire (ASFQ), was found in 16% of quetiapine-treated patients and 50% of risperidone-treated patients ($p = 0.006$). High rates of sexual dysfunction and hypogonadism were also demonstrated in 50 women being treated with antipsychotic drugs (Howes *et al.*, 2007). Sixty-eight percent of female patients reported sexual dysfunction compared to 14% of healthy controls ($p < 0.001$), and in the premenopausal women taking antipsychotic drugs, 79% had hypoestrogenism and 92% had low progesterone levels.

2. *Treatment Strategies for Antipsychotic Drug-Induced Sexual Dysfunction*

Management of antipsychotic drug-induced sexual dysfunction is primarily directed toward avoiding the underlying mechanism of the adverse effect—dopamine blockade, elevated prolactin levels, or alpha-adrenergic blockade.

Since these are dose-related effects, a lower dose can be tried if clinically appropriate, or change to a different atypical antipsychotic drug (Seagraves, 1997). An open trial that switched from risperidone or haloperidol to quetiapine demonstrated reduced prolactin levels and improved sexual dysfunction (Byerly *et al.*, 2004).

II. Treatment Strategies for Female Sexual Dysfunction

The most common female sexual dysfunction disorders, not related to drug-induced causes, include lack of sexual desire and difficulty in achieving orgasm. There are no approved pharmacologic treatments for female hypoactive sexual desire disorder (HSDD) or female orgasmic disorder (FOD); female sexual arousal disorder (FSAD) is treated with estrogen replacement therapy when indicated, or vaginal lubricants.

A. HYPOACTIVE SEXUAL DESIRE DISORDER

There are no approved pharmacological treatments for HSDD in women. In premenopausal women, any medical problem should be treated that might be contributing to decreased desire (e.g., hypothyroidism, depression), and drug-induced causes need to be managed. In postmenopausal women, in addition to the above, signs and symptoms of estrogen deficiency can be treated with estrogen replacement, and signs and symptoms of androgen deficiency can be treated with androgen replacement. Testosterone replacement is more helpful in women after oophorectomy or in women receiving estrogen replacement therapy. Use of testosterone treatment in the absence of oophorectomy or ERT remains controversial and further investigation is needed in women with normal testosterone levels before testosterone treatment can be recommended (Shepherd, 2002). Side effects of testosterone occur in 5–35% of women and include decreased levels of HDL, acne, hirsutism, clitorimegaly, and voice deepening (Phillips, 2000). Several studies have demonstrated that testosterone can significantly increase sexual desire, as well as arousal and orgasm, in women who have undergone surgical menopause (Ragucci and Culhane, 2003). In a 24-week trial, a 300 μg testosterone patch was given to 533 surgically menopausal women on concomitant estrogen therapy (Buster *et al.*, 2005). Compared to baseline, the patch significantly increased sexual desire and sexual activity ($p < 0.05$). Androgenic side effects were rated as mild and well tolerated. Bupropion was studied in premenopausal women with HSDD with mixed results (Segraves *et al.*, 2004). Changes in sexual desire scores were not significantly different than placebo, though total sexual function and orgasm scores with bupropion were significantly greater than with placebo.

B. Female Sexual Arousal Disorder

Current treatment of FSAD is limited to ERT and water-based vaginal lubricants. Hypoestrogenism is the most common physiologic condition associated with FSAD, which leads to urogenital atrophy and a decrease in vaginal lubrication. Lack of lubrication can then contribute to dyspareunia and the development of hyposexual desire disorder (Ragucci and Culhane, 2003). Long-term use of estrogen vaginal creams is considered unopposed estrogen treatment in women with an intact uterus, meaning progesterone is also required. Premenopausal women with arousal disorders, women who do not respond to estrogen therapy or who are unwilling to take estrogen represent difficult patient groups since so few treatment options are available (Phillips, 2000).

There was hope that, similar to erectile dysfunction in men, the phosphodiesterase inhibitor drugs (e.g., sildenafil) would be effective in women with arousal disorders. Clinical studies thus far have reported mixed results, and PDE-5 inhibitors are not indicated in women for FSAD. Sildenafil 50 mg given to postmenopausal women in an uncontrolled trial resulted in modest, statistically insignificant improvement in lubrication, clitoral sensation, and orgasm frequency, but no effect on sexual desire or satisfaction with intercourse (Kaplan *et al.*, 1999). Seven of 33 patients experienced clitoral discomfort and oversensitivity. One controlled trial of sildenafil 25 mg, 50 mg, or placebo in 51 premenopausal women found more positive results (Caruso *et al.*, 2001). Both doses of sildenafil resulted in greater arousal, more frequent orgasms, and greater sexual satisfaction compared to placebo. The equivocal efficacy results with sildenafil in women have caused the manufacturer to terminate further studies.

C. Female Orgasmic Disorder

There are no pharmacological treatments for anorgasmia (Meston *et al.*, 2004). A careful history is most important for FOD, however, since it is often secondary to disorders of desire or arousal, or may be medication induced. While up to 70% of women may not be able to achieve orgasm with intercourse, only 4% are not able to achieve orgasm with masturbation. Thus, FOD can be very responsive to therapy techniques that focus on maximizing stimulation and minimizing inhibition (Phillips, 2000; Ragucci and Culhane, 2003).

References

Bobes, J., Garc A-Portilla, M. P., Rejas, J., Hern Ndez, G., Garcia-Garcia, M, Rico-Villademoros, F., and Porras, A. (2003). Frequency of sexual dysfunction and other reproductive side-effects in patients with schizophrenia treated with risperidone, olanzapine, quetiapine, or haloperidol: The results of the EIRE study. *J. Sex Marital Ther.* **29**(2), 125–147.

Boyarsky, B. K., and Hirschfeld, R. M. (2000). The management of medication-induced sexual dysfunction. *Essent. Psychopharmacol.* **3**(2), 151–170.

Buster, J. E., Kingsberg, S. A., Aguirre, O., Brown, C., Breaux, J. G., Buch, A., Rodenberg, C. A., Wekselman, K., and Casson, P. (2005). Testosterone patch for low sexual desire in surgically menopausal women: A randomized trial. *Obstet. Gynecol.* **105,** 944–952.

Byerly, M. J., Lescouflair, E., Weber, M. T., Bugno, R. M., Fisher, R., Carmody, T., Varghese, F, and Rush, A. J. (2004). An open-label trial of quetiapine for antipsychotic-induced sexual dysfunction. *J. Sex Marital Ther.* **30**(5), 325–332.

Caruso, S., Intelisano, G., Lupo, L., and Agnello, C. (2001). Premenopausal women affected by sexual arousal disorder treated with sildenafil: A double-blind, cross-over, placebo-controlled study. *Br. J. Obstet. Gynecol.* **108,** 623–628.

Clayton, A. H., Warnock, J. K., Kornstein, S. G., Pinkerton, R., Sheldon-Keller, A., and McGarvey, E. L. (2004). A placebo-controlled trial of bupropion SR as an antidote for selective serotonin reuptake inhibitor-induced sexual dysfunction. *J. Clin. Psychiatry* **65**(1), 62–67.

Crenshaw, T. L., and Goldberg, J. P. (1996). "Sexual Pharmacology: Drugs that Affect Sexual Function." W.W. Norton & Company, New York.

DeBattista, C., Solvason, B., Poirier, J., Kendrick, E., and Loraas, E. (2005). A placebo-controlled, randomized, double-blind study of adjunctive bupropion sustained release in the treatment of SSRI-induced sexual dysfunction. *J. Clin. Psychiatry* **66**, 844–848.

Gelenberg, A. J., Laukes, C., McGahuey, C., Okayli, G., Moreno, F., Zentner, L., and Delgado, P. (2000). Mirtazapine substitution in SSRI-induced sexual dysfunction. *J. Clin. Psychiatry* **61**(5), 356–360.

Gitlin, M. (2003). Sexual dysfunction with psychotropic drugs. *Expert Opin. Pharmacother.* **4**(12), 2259–2269.

Graziottin, A. (2006). "Iatrogenic and Post-Traumatic Female Sexual Disorder in Standard Practice in Sexual Medicine" (H. Porst and J. Buvat, Eds.), pp. 351–361. Blackwell Publishing, Malden, Massachusetts.

Harden, C. L. (2005). Sexuality in women with epilepsy. *Epilepsy Behav.* **7,** S2–S6.

Harrison, W. M., Rabkin, J. G., Ehrhardt, A. A., *et al.* (1986). Effects of antidepressant medication on sexual function: A controlled study. *J. Clin. Psychopharmacol.* **6,** 144–149.

Herzog, A. G., Drislane, F. W., Schomer, D. L., Pennell, P. B., Bromfield, E. B., Dworetzky, B. A., Farina, E. L., and Frye, C. A. (2005). Differential effects of antiepileptic drugs on sexual function and hormones in men with epilepsy. *Neurology* **65**(10), 1016–1020.

Howes, O. D., Wheeler, M. J., Pilowsky, L. S., Landau, S., Murray, R. M., and Smith, S. (2007). Sexual function and gonadal hormones in patients taking antipsychotic treatment for schizophrenia or schizoaffective disorder. *J. Clin. Psychiatry* **68**(3), 361–367.

Kaplan, S. A., Reis, R. B., Kohn, I. J., Ikeguchi, E. F., Laor, E., Te, A. E., and Martins, A. C. (1999). Safety and efficacy of sildenafil in postmenopausal women with sexual dysfunction. *Urology* **53**(3), 481–486.

Knegtering, R., Castelein, S., Bous, H., Van Der Linde, J., Bruggeman, R., Kluiter, H., and van den Bosch, R. J. (2004). A randomized, open-label study of the impact of quetiapine versus risperidone on sexual functioning. *J. Clin. Psychopharmacol.* **24**(1), 56–61.

Labbate, L. A., Grimes, J., Hines, A., Oleshansky, M. A., and Arana, G. W. (1998). Sexual dysfunction induced by serotonin reuptake antidepressants. *J. Sex Marital Ther.* **24,** 3–12.

Landen, M., Hogberg, P., and Thase, M. E. (2005). Incidence of sexual side effects in refractory depression during treatment with citalopram or paroxetine. *J. Clin. Psychiatry* **66**(1), 100–106.

Meston, C. M., Hull, E., Levin, R. J., and Sipski, M. (2004). Disorders of orgasm in women. *J. Sex Med.* **1**(1), 66–68.

Montejo, A. L., Llorca, G., Izquierdo, J. A., and Rico-Villademoros, F. (2001). Incidence of sexual dysfunction associated with antidepressant agents: A prospective multicenter study of 1022 outpatients. *J. Clin. Psychiatry* **62**(Suppl. 3), 10–21.

Montejo-Gonzalez, A. L., Liorca, G., Izquierdo, J. A., Ledesma, A., Bousoño, M., Calcedo, A., Carrasco, J. L., Ciudad, J., Daniel, E., De la Gandara, J., Derecho, J., Franco, M., *et al.* (1997). SSRI-induced sexual dysfunction: Fluoxetine, paroxetine, sertraline, and fluvoxamine in a prospective, multicenter, and descriptive clinical study of 344 patients. *J. Sex Marital Ther.* **23,** 176–194.

Morrell, M. J. (2003). Reproductive and metabolic disorders in women with epilepsy. *Epilepsia* **44**(Suppl. 4), 11–20.

Morrell, M. J., Flynn, K. L., Doñe, S., Flaster, E., Kalayjian, L., and Pack, A. M. (2005). Sexual dysfunction, sex steroid hormone abnormalities, and depression in women with epilepsy treated with antiepileptic drugs. *Epilepsy Behav.* **6**(3), 360–365.

Nurnberg, H. G., and Hensley, P. (2006). Randomized, double-blind, placebo-controlled trial of sildenafil for serotonergic antidepressant-associated sexual dysfunction in women with major depressive disorder in remission. Presented at the Sexual Medicine Society of North America, November 2–5, Las Vegas, Nevada.

Penovich, P. E. (2000). The effects of epilepsy and its treatment on sexual and reproductive function. *Epilepsia* **41**(Suppl. 2), S53–S61.

Phillips, N. A. (2000). Female sexual dysfunction: Evaluation and treatment. *Am. Fam. Physician* **62**(1), 127–136, 141–142.

Ragucci, K. R., and Culhane, N. S. (2003). Treatment of female sexual dysfunction. *Ann. Pharmacother.* **37**(4), 546–555.

Rosen, R. C., Lane, R. M., and Menza, M. (1999). Effects of SSRIs on sexual function: A critical review. *J. Clin. Psychopharmacol.* **19**(1), 67–85.

Rothschild, A. J. (1995). Selective serotonin reuptake inhibitor-induced sexual dysfunction: Efficacy of a drug holiday. *Am. J. Psychiatry* **152,** 1514–1516.

Rothschild, A. J. (2000). Sexual side effects of antidepressants. *J. Clin. Psychiatry* **61**(Suppl. 11), 28–36.

Seagraves, R. T. (1997). The effects of minor tranquilizers, mood stabilizers, and antipsychotics on sexual function. *Prim. Psychiatry* **4,** 46–48.

Seagraves, R. T. (1998). Antidepressant-induced sexual dysfunction. *J. Clin. Psychiatry* **59**(Suppl. 4), 48–54.

Segraves, R. T., Clayton, A., Croft, H., Wolf, A., and Warnock, J. (2004). Bupropion sustained release for the treatment of hypoactive sexual desire disorder in premenopausal women. *J. Clin. Psychopharmacol.* **24**(3), 339–342.

Shepherd, J. E. (2002). Therapeutic options in female sexual dysfunction. *J. Am. Pharm. Assoc.* **42**(3), 479–488.

Smith, S. M., O'Keane, V., and Murray, R. (2002). Sexual dysfunction in patients taking conventional antipsychotic medication. *Br. J. Psychiatry* **181,** 49–55.

Stahl, S. M. (1998). Selecting an antidepressant by using mechanism of action to enhance efficacy and avoid side effects. *J. Clin. Psychiatry* **59**(Suppl. 18), 23–29.

Stahl, S. M. (2001a). The psychopharmacology of sex Part 1: Neurotransmitters and the 3 phases of the human sexual response. *J. Clin. Psychiatry* **62**(2), 80–81.

Stahl, S. M. (2001b). The psychopharmacology of sex Part 2: Effects of drugs and disease on the 3 phases of the human sexual response. *J. Clin. Psychiatry* **62**(3), 147–148.

Stimmel, G. L., and Gutierrez, M. A. (2006). Counseling patients about sexual issues. *Pharmacotherapy* **26**(11), 1608–1615.

Stimmel, G. L., Dopheide, J. A., and Stahl, S. M. (1997). Mirtazapine: An antidepressant with noradrenergic and specific serotonergic effects. *Pharmacotherapy* **17**(1), 10–21.

Tassone, D. M., Boyce, E., Guyer, J., and Nuzum, D. (2007). Pregabalin: A novel gamma-aminobutyric acid analogue in the treatment of neuropathic pain, partial-onset seizures, and anxiety disorders. *Clin. Ther.* **29**(1), 26–48.

Walker, P. W., Cole, J. O., Gardner, E. A., *et al.* (1993). Improvement in fluoxetine-associated sexual dysfunction in patients switched to bupropion. *J. Clin. Psychiatry* **54,** 43459–43465.

Zajecka, J. (2001). Strategies for the treatment of antidepressant-induced sexual dysfunction. *J. Clin. Psychiatry* **62**(Suppl. 3), 35–43.

PREGNANCY IN EPILEPSY: ISSUES OF CONCERN

John DeToledo

Wake Forest University, School of Medicine, Medical Center Boulevard,
Winston Salem, NC, 27157

I. Approach to Assessment
   A. Is Anything Entirely "Safe" in Pregnancy in Patients with Epilepsy?
   B. The Experiment
   C. Is It Epilepsy?
   D. Will the Baby be Normal?
   E. Normal and Abnormal—The Individual Variability
   F. Seizures in the Mother
   G. Positive Family History for Malformations and AEDs
   H. Other Maternal Factors
   I. The Timing of Exposure
   J. Late Exposure
   K. The Serum Level and Exposure to the Fetus
   L. Safety of Newer Drugs During Pregnancy
II. Conclusion
   References

Every pregnancy, even under the best of circumstances, carries risks with it. Having epilepsy and taking medications to treat seizures further increase these risks and not all patients are willing to accept risks. The issues related to pregnancy, epilepsy, and antiepileptic drugs and pregnancy are fraught with confusion and misperceptions. Lay publications may misinform the public by assigning risks to drugs not known to be teratogenic in humans. Women report that their physicians have encouraged them to terminate otherwise wanted pregnancies "just to be on the safe side" which is clearly an excess of caution. In this chapter, we review the most common risk factors and divide them in two broad categories: (a) avoidable or modifiable risk factors and (b) unavoidable or non modifiable risk factors. Physicians counseling women with epilepsy who are pregnant or are planning a pregnancy should make every effort to understand the nature and magnitude of the risks associated with epilepsy and antiepileptic drugs in order to ensure the best possible outcomes in these cases. We discuss preventive measures that, when properly followed, can minimize risks and allow the vast majority of women with epilepsy to give birth to normal children.

INTERNATIONAL REVIEW OF
NEUROBIOLOGY, VOL. 83
DOI: 10.1016/S0074-7742(08)00009-3

169

I. Approach to Assessment

A. Is Anything Entirely "Safe" in Pregnancy in Patients with Epilepsy?

Every pregnancy, even under the best of circumstances, carries risks with it. Having epilepsy and taking medications to treat seizures further increase these risks. For the woman with epilepsy, the decision to become pregnant has to be made taking into consideration the possibility of an adverse outcome. Not all patients are willing to accept risks. If that is the case, this patient should be advised not to become pregnant. Although there is always risk, it is helpful to remind the patient that many risk factors can be reduced and more than 90% of patients with epilepsy will have a healthy baby.

B. The Experiment

Definitions of the word "experiment" in the Webster dictionary include: (1) a test under controlled conditions that is made to determine the efficacy of something previously untried, (2) to try something new, especially in order to gain experience, and (3) to examine the validity of a hypothesis. These definitions are a reasonably accurate description of what takes place during the treatment of epilepsy in pregnancy. Ultimately, the treatment of epilepsy in pregnancy is an experiment and the hypothesis is that one can do good to the patient without doing harm to the fetus. Like any other experiment in humans, this "experiment" requires an informed consenting on the part of the patient.

As the patient consents to adhere to the treatment recommended for her seizures, she should only agree to do so, based on adequate knowledge of the relevant facts. It is the responsibility of the physician, therefore, to thoroughly discuss the issues so that the patient has the necessary information to make the decision that suits her best. Conversely, it is the responsibility of the patient to make the decision to voluntarily follow the physician's recommendation (i.e., to participate in the "experiment"). The decision to become pregnant, to keep the pregnancy and to accept the risks involved with drug treatments must be made by the patient. If either the physician or the patient is uncomfortable with the terms they see before them, a second opinion should be sought.

The assessment consists of a review of preventive measures and of risk factors involved in a particular case. These risk factors fall within two broad categories: (a) avoidable or modifiable risk factors and (b) unavoidable or non modifiable risk factors.

C. Is It Epilepsy?

Conditions that mimic epilepsy such as syncope and nonepileptic seizures are common in women of child-bearing age and should be considered whenever one encounters new onset of seizures or worsening of seizures in the setting of pregnancy. Patients may either develop nonepileptic seizures or have a worsening of preexisting nonepileptic seizures in situations of unwanted pregnancy (DeToledo *et al.*, 2000). Every effort should be made to confirm the diagnosis of epilepsy prior to initiating or continuing AED therapy in these cases.

D. Will the Baby be Normal?

It is estimated that 1 in 33 babies are born each year with congenital malformations in the United States [Centers for Disease Control and Prevention (CDC), 2006]. Some of these malformations have genetic or environmental causes but in about 70% of the cases, both parents are "normal" and the cause of the birth defects are unknown [Centers for Disease Control and Prevention (CDC), 2006]. Families should be counseled that having had a normal child is no guaranty that the next pregnancy will be normal.

E. Normal and Abnormal—The Individual Variability

No two individuals are exactly identical. As discussed in previous chapter (8), differences between individuals are determined by their genetic make-up and external factors present during their development. By averaging individual variations among all members of a group one can define a "norm." Individuals whose features fall within this perceived norm, are classified as "normal" and those who fall outside of these limits are "abnormal." Since these structural congenital abnormalities occur within a spectrum ranging from minimally abnormal to maximally abnormal, there are as many definitions as there are disagreements of what constitutes a congenital malformation (Table I).

The definition that major malformations are "gross structural defects present at birth which requires corrective intervention" used by Strickler (Strickler *et al.*, 1985) is a simplification but permits a comparison of cases in different published series. Regardless of the definition used, in the eyes of parents, any deviation from the norm is abnormal and quickly become a source of anxiety and concern. Physicians should tell families that even the best studies do not discuss each and

TABLE I

VARIOUS DEFINITIONS OF CONGENITAL MALFORMATIONS

Congenital malformations [are] abnormalities of structure present at birth and attributable to faulty development (Carter, 1963)

... a major anomaly is one which has an adverse effect on either the function or the social acceptability of the individual; a minor defect [on the other hand] is one which is neither of medical nor cosmetic consequence to the patient (Marden *et al.*, 1964)

A malformation is an abnormality in size, shape, location, or structure of any part caused by antenatal disturbances in development (Potter, 1964)

... a defect of structure or form present at birth and noted at routine inspection within the first 10 days of life ... (Nelson and Forfar, 1969)

Even the slightest abnormality ... (Endl and Schaller, 1973)

... a gross physical or anatomic developmental anomaly ... present at birth or

... detected during the first year of life (Myrianthopoulos and Chung, 1974)

... conditions thought to be of prenatal origin whether or not they were manifest at birth [including] structural defects, functional abnormalities, inborn errors of metabolism, and chromosomal aberrations (Christianson *et al.*, 1981)

... malformations are all-or-none traits, that is, they are not graded ... and at their mild end do not shade into normality (Opitz and Gilbert, 1982)

A major congenital anomaly [is] one that is incompatible with survival, is life threatening, or seriously compromises an individual's capacity to function normally in society (Otake *et al.*, 1990).

every malformation occurring with each drug and that we only have an imperfect knowledge about the occurrence of more discrete structural defects with these various drugs.

F. SEIZURES IN THE MOTHER

Patients must be informed that epileptic seizures by themselves may increase the risk of birth defects. This was demonstrated by two studies that separated the effects of AEDs from those of seizures during pregnancy (Annegers *et al.*, 1978; Nakane *et al.*, 1980). Parents should be made aware of the fact that under the best of circumstances, any pregnancy may carry a 1–2% risk of having an offspring with a malformation and that, the fact that the mother has seizures may double that risk (Annegers *et al.*, 1978).

Many patients are aware of the fact that the use of AEDs during pregnancy increases the risk of malformations and it is not uncommon for patients to entertain the idea of stopping AED treatment as they plan for pregnancy. Clinical experience and circumstantial evidence suggest that women with epilepsy who have uncontrolled seizures during pregnancy have a significantly increased (up to tenfold) morbidity and mortality as compared to the general population (Adab *et al.*, 2004). Patients should be advised that stopping AED treatment prior to pregnancy is not an option for those cases with active seizure disorder.

G. Positive Family History for Malformations and AEDs

Birth defects associated with use of medications often result from a combination of genetic make-up and environmental exposure, a "multi-factorial inheritance." In these cases, the individual may inherit one or more genes that increase the predisposition to birth defects if there is exposure to certain environmental substances (such as AEDs). These individuals have the genetic predisposition to a birth defect but may not develop it unless there is exposure to that substance during its early development. Having a previous case of congenital malformation in the family is a red flag for this type of genetic susceptibility. These patients should be advised that their risk of having another child with malformation may be substantially increased. The treating physician should take a careful family history in order to uncover these cases and to properly counsel the patient.

H. Other Maternal Factors

There are a number of maternal factors, including genetic, endocrine, infectious, dietary, and use of medications or illicit drugs that can independently add to the risk of birth defects in patients with epilepsy.

1. Endocrine

Maternal obesity by itself may increase the risk for birth defects, particularly neural tube defects (Werler et al., 1996). Some endocrine conditions that are common in overweight women may carry an added risk of birth defects, specifically diabetes, polycystic ovary syndrome, and gastric bypass surgery. These three conditions are not uncommon in patients with epilepsy and each of them may add to the risk. In the case of obesity and diabetes, the two conditions may act synergistically in the pathogenesis of congenital anomalies (Moore et al., 2000). Two other factors contribute to the difficulty of managing these patients: (1) the recommended daily dose of 400 mcg of folic acid does not seem to reduce the risk of neural tube defect among these women (Werler et al., 1996) and (2) prenatal diagnosis of neural tube defects with ultrasound and alpha fetoprotein testing is less accurate in overweight women.

2. Folic Acid Deficiency

Studies show that women of child-bearing age may not remember being told about topics which are significant for their own health and that of their children. A survey in the UK showed that less than half of the patients taking AEDs remembered being told that they should also take folic acid supplementation (Bell et al., 2002). A written prescription of folic acid given to the patient following the discussion of this topic may improve compliance. In addition to inadequate intake, a number of conditions can be associated with decreased serum levels of folic acid and may increase the risk of defects. Virtually all weight loss diets are deficient in folic acid (Table II). Overweight patients engaged in these diets would be at greater risk. Patients with gastric bypass surgery (Madan, *et al.*, 2006), pernicious anemia, and on proton pump inhibitors (Russell *et al.*, 1988) and oral contraceptives (Barone *et al.*, 1979) are also at risk of developing folic acid deficiency.

Another cause for folic acid deficiency is genetic defects of the enzyme that catalyzes the conversion of an inactive precursor into the active folic acid in the body (MTHFR) (van der Put *et al.*, 1995). The prevalence of these enzymatic defects varies among different ethnic groups and mothers who are homozygous for the defect may have a two-to sevenfold increased risk of having a child with neural tube defect (Ou *et al.*, 1996). In the presence of any of these risk factors, high dose supplementation with 4–5 mg/day of folic acid is recommended (Wilson *et al.*, 2003). This supplementation should be taken as folic acid alone, not in a multivitamin format due to risk of excessive intake of other vitamins such as vitamin A.

3. *Tobacco, Alcohol, and Illicit Drugs*

More than 90% of pregnant women take prescription or nonprescription drugs or use tobacco and alcohol at some time during pregnancy. Nearly 4% of pregnant women admit using illicit drugs such as marijuana, cocaine, amphetamines, and heroin, according to a 2005 U.S. government survey (Substance Abuse and Mental Health Administration, 2006). Pregnant women with epilepsy who use illicit drugs are a high risk group for malformations and other complications during pregnancy. The fact that most of these patients also use alcohol and tobacco adds to their overall risk of malformations.

4. *Other Medications with Teratogenic Potential*

The experience with isotretinoin is informative. The Retinoid Pregnancy Prevention Program includes explicit and detailed printed warnings requires the patient to sign a consent form indicating that they agree to use two effective

TABLE II
VITAMIN CONTENT OF FIVE WEIGHT LOSS DIETS: PERCENT U.S.
RDA-RECOMMENDED DAILY ALLOWANCE

Vitamin	Set point	Fit for life	Immune power	Family circle	Eat to succeed
Vitamin D	33	0	0	24	76
Vitamin E	30	83	18	99	117
Vitamin B6	75	151	103	124	135
Folate	74	130	65	79	81
Vitamin B12	51	6	42	33	82

methods of contraception before therapy is started (Pastuszak *et al.*, 1994). Since the program was implemented in 1989, a substantial number of fetuses have been exposed to the drug. As many as 30% of the women with exposed fetuses did not use any mode of contraception, even though they were cognizant of the high risk for the fetus. Many of these women explained that they did not believe they were fertile, since they had not conceived during periods of months or years when they had not used contraceptive methods (Koren, 1997). This type of observation underscores the risks of assumptions. Is may be naive to assume that the patient understands each aspect of their complex decisions. Fewer assumptions are more likely to produce better decisions and outcomes; time should be taken to address these issues as many times as necessary.

I. THE TIMING OF EXPOSURE

The occurrence and degree of an abnormality (i.e., deviation from the norm) bear close relationship with the time of exposure, the "critical period." Insults at very early stages of development (first few hours or days) are more likely to affect primordial cell lines responsible for organ formation and result in significant abnormalities or absence of all its subordinate structures. These are often lethal defects. It is estimated that 40% of all pregnancies miscarry so early that women do not realize they were pregnant as menstruation is on time or only minimally disrupted. It is not known how often AEDs contribute to these very early losses. Most of the recognized malformations associated with the use AED seem to affect organs that anatomically develop between 2 and 5 weeks of development but this may be misleading (Fig. 1).

The period during which a given abnormality can be induced in the developing organism is known as the critical period. The "timing" of this critical period varies depending on the method used to assess the abnormality. The critical period for the molecular biologist occurs much earlier that the critical period as defined by the histologist or anatomist (Kretchmer, 1982). In neurological parlance, the "anatomic critical period" is the time of occurrence of a given malformation (i.e., neural tube defects occur between 30 and 31 days). This is not accurate in most instances. In the case of the neural tube for example, the critical period for disruption of pluripotent neural crest cells as detected by the molecular biologist certainly occurs before the anatomic occurrence of the spina bifida. The practice of stopping AEDs by the second or third weeks of pregnancy hoping to prevent early malformations is probably not be warranted, as irreversible AED induced changes may already have taken place at the molecular level. For this reason, patients should be made aware of these facts and any concerns about AED-induced malformations should be addressed prior to pregnancy.

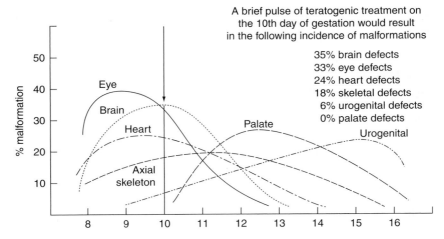

FIG. 1. Hypothetical representation of how the syndrome of malformations produced by a given agent might be expected to change when treatment is given at different times (Wilson, 1965).

J. LATE EXPOSURE

Susceptibility to developmental abnormalities is not limited to the first trimester of pregnancy. The central nervous system continues to grow and change during pregnancy. Agents that interfere with neurocognitive development can do so throughout that period. In some cases, the neurocognitive disorders can be as devastating as a malformation on children and families. Valproic acid, phenobarbital, and primidone (Neri *et al.*, 1983) can have adverse effects on CNS development (Adab *et al.*, 2004; Meador *et al.*, 2006). The mechanism of these adverse CNS effects has not been elucidated. Clinically, they are manifested as small head circumference and various forms of attentional and learning deficits that may go undetected until school years. Given the potentially serious cognitive implications and the uncertainties in ascertaining causation, the use of valproic acid phenobarbital, and primidone should, if at all possible, be avoided throughout the duration of pregnancy.

K. THE SERUM LEVEL AND EXPOSURE TO THE FETUS

In experimental models of teratogenesis, the risk of a given agent to cause a malformation often depends on the concentration of the agent. Although evidence of this dose/effect has been slow to come by in humans, classic teratology showed more than 70 years ago that by manipulating the concentration of a teratogen, one can alter the degree of fusion of midline structures during development (Weiss, 1939). Data from pregnancy registries have suggested this to be the case in humans as well (Fig. 2) (Morrow *et al.*, 2006). To the physician and the patient, this should be a reminder that at the time of conception one should use the smallest dose of AED that is sufficient to control seizures in a given patient. Because pregnancy can alter the disposition of AEDs, continuous monitoring and dose adjustments are needed during the pregnancy in these cases.

Some of the congenital malformations reported with the use of different AEDs are remarkably similar and include congenital heart defects, cleft lip/palate, spina bifida, anencephaly, and genitourinary malformations. These observations show that the same type of malformation can be associated with the use of various agents, and that various types of malformations can be associated with the use of a same agent. The physician's discussion with the patient who is considering becoming pregnant should include all these abnormalities because unusual outcomes can and do occur from time to time.

L. SAFETY OF NEWER DRUGS DURING PREGNANCY

Whereas it is true that much is known about the use of older AEDs and of some of the newer AEDs in pregnancy (i.e., lamotrigine), this is clearly not the case for some of the others (see previous chapters in this book). New drugs are never tested in pregnant women prior to marketing in order to determine their effects on the fetus. Consequently, new drugs are not labeled for use during pregnancy. Typically, the package inserts contain the statement, "Use in

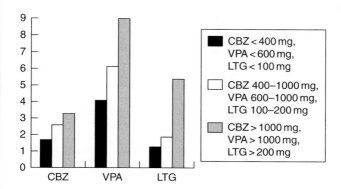

FIG. 2. Major congenital malformation role (%) by drug dose. CBZ, carbamazepine; LTG, lamotrigine; and VPA, valproate (Meador *et al.*, 2006).

178 JOHN DETOLEDO

pregnancy is not recommended unless the potential benefits justify the potential risks to the fetus" and it may take years before the safety of some compounds is established. The association between the use of phenytoin and malformations was first described in 1976, almost 40 years after the drug was introduced to clinical use. The potential adverse effects of phenobarbital to the fetus were first identified more than 60 years after its introduction in 1912. Patients should be reminded that absence of evidence can not be construed as evidence of absence.

II. Conclusion

The issues related to pregnancy, epilepsy, and antiepileptic drugs and pregnancy are fraught with confusion and misperceptions. Lay publications may misinform the public by assigning risks to drugs not known to be teratogenic in humans. Women report that their physicians have encouraged them to terminate otherwise wanted pregnancies "just to be on the safe side" which is clearly an excess of caution.

As it has been discussed throughout this book, if the proper recommendations are followed, the vast majority of women with epilepsy will give birth to normal children.

Physicians counseling women with epilepsy who are pregnant or are planning a pregnancy should make every effort to understand the nature and magnitude of the risks associated with epilepsy and antiepileptic drugs in order to ensure the best possible outcomes in these cases.

References

Adab, N., Kini, U., Vinten, J., Ayres, J., Baker, G., Clayton-Smith, J., Coyle, H., Fryer, A., Gorry, J., Gregg, J., Mawer, G., Nicolaides, P., *et al.* (2004). The longer term outcome of children born to mothers with epilepsy. *J. Neurol. Neurosurg. Psychiatry* **75**(11), 1575–1583.

Annegers, J. F., Hauser, W. A., Elveback, L. R., Nakane, Y., Okuma, T., Takahashi, R., Sato, Y., Wada, T., Sato, T., Fukushima, Y., Kumashiro, H., Ono, T., *et al.* (1978). Congenital malformations and seizure disorders among offspring of parents with epilepsy. *Int. J. Epidemiol.* **7**, 241–247.

Barone, C., Bartoloni, C., Ghirlanda, G., and Gentiloni, N. (1979). Megaloblastic anemia due to folic acid deficiency after oral contraceptives. *Haematologica* **64**(2), 190–195.

Bell, G. S., Nashef, L., Kendall, S., Solomon, J., Poole, K., Johnson, A. L., Moran, N. F., McCarthy, M., McCormick, D., Shorvon, S. D., and Sander, J. W. (2002). Information recalled by women taking anti-epileptic drugs for epilepsy: A questionnaire study. *Epilepsy Res.* **52**(2), 139–146.

Carter, C. O. (1963). Chromosomes and congenital malformations. *Practitioner* **191**, 129–135.

Centers for Disease Control and Prevention (CDC). (2006). Birth Defects: Frequently Asked Questions. *March* **21**2006.

Christianson, R. E., van den Berg, B. J., Milkovich, L., and Oechsli, F. W. (1981). Incidence of congenital anomalies among white and black live births with long-term follow-up. *Am. J. Public Health* **71**(12), 1333–1341.

DeToledo, J. C., Lowe, M. R., and Puig, A. (2000). Nonepileptic seizures in pregnancy. *Neurology* **55**(1), 120–121.

Endl, J., and Schaller, A. (1973). Malformation rate in newborn infants of foreign workers. *Wien. Klin. Wochenschr.* **85**(42), 718–720.

Koren, G. (1997). The children of neverland: The silent human disaster The Kid in us Publications, Toronto, 1997.

Kretchmer, N. (1982). Advances in theratogenesis. *Acta Paediatr. Jpn.* **1,** 46–50.

Madan, A. K., Orth, W. S., Tichansky, D. S., and Ternovits, C. A. (2006). Vitamin and trace mineral levels after laparoscopic gastric bypass. *Obes. Surg.* **16**(5), 603–606.

Marden, P. M., Smith, D. W., and Mcdonald, M. J. (1964). Congenital anomalies in the newborn infant, including minor variations. A study of 4,412 babies by surface examination for anomalies and buccal smear for sex chromatin. *J. Pediatr.* **64,** 357–371.

Meador, K. J., Baker, G. A., Finnell, R. H., Kalayjian, L. A., Liporace, J. D., Loring, D. W., Mawer, G., Pennell, P. B., Smith, J. C., Wolff, M. C., and NEAD Study Group. (2006). In utero antiepileptic drug exposure: Fetal death and malformations. *Neurology* **67**(3), 407–412.

Moore, L. L., Singer, M. R., Bradlee, M. L., Rothman, K. J., and Milunsky, A. (2000). A prospective study of the risk of congenital defects associated with maternal obesity and diabetes mellitus. *Epidemiology* **11**(6), 689–694.

Morrow, J., Russell, A., Guthrie, E., Parsons, L., Robertson, I., Waddell, R., Irwin, B., McGivern, R. C., Morrison, P. J., and Craig, J. (2006). Malformation risks of antiepileptic drugs in pregnancy: A prospective study from the UK Epilepsy and Pregnancy Register. *J. Neurol. Neurosurg. Psychiatry* **77**(2), 193–198.

Myrianthopoulos, N. C., and Chung, C. S. (1974). Congenital malformations in singletons: Epidemiologic survey. Report from the Collaborative Perinatal project. *Birth Defects. Orig. Artic. Ser.* **10**(11), 1–58.

Nakane, Y., Okuma, T., Takahasi, R., Sato, Y., Wada, T., Sato, T., Fukushima, Y., Kumashiro, H., Ono, T., Takahashi, T., Aoki, Y., Kazamatsuri, H., *et al.* (1980). Multi institutional study on the teratogenicity and fetal toxicity of antiepileptic drugs: A report of a collaborative study group in Japan. *Epilepsia* **21,** 663–680.

Nelson, M. M., and Forfar, J. O. (1969). Congenital abnormalities at birth: Their association in the same patient. *Dev. Med. Child Neurol.* **11**(1), 3–16.

Neri, A., Heifetz, L., Nitke, S., and Ovadia, J. (1983). Neonatal outcome in infants of epileptic mothers. *Eur. J. Obstet. Gynecol. Reprod. Biol.* **16**(4), 263–268.

Opitz, J. M., and Gilbert, E. F. (1982). CNS anomalies and the midline as a "developmental field." *Am. J. Med. Genet.* **12**(4), 443–455.

Otake, M., Schull, W. J., and Neel, J. V. (1990). Congenital malformations, stillbirths, and early mortality among the children of atomic bomb survivors: A reanalysis. *Radiat. Res.* **122**(1), 1–11.

Ou, C. Y., Stevenson, R. E., Brown, V. K., Schwartz, C. E., Allen, W. P., Khoury, M. J., Rozen, R., Oakley, G. P., Jr., and Adams, M. J., Jr. (1996). 5,10 Methylenetetrahydrofolate reductase genetic polymorphism as a risk factor for neural tube defects. *Am. J. Med. Genet.* **63**, 610–614.

Pastuszak, A. L., Koren, G., and Rieder, M. J. (1994). Use of the retinoid pregnancy prevention program in Canada: Patterns of contraception use in women treated with isotretinoin and etretinate. *Reprod. Toxicol.* **8,** 63–68.

Potter, E. L. (1964). Classification and pathology of congenital anomalies. *Am. J. Obstet. Gynecol.* **90** (Suppl), 985–993.

Russell, R. M., Golner, B. B., Krasinski, S. D., Sadowski, J. A., Suter, P. M., and Braun, C. L. (1988). Effect of antacid and H2 receptor antagonists on the intestinal absorption of folic acid. *J. Lab. Clin. Med.* **112**(4), 458–463.

Strickler, S. M., Dansky, L. V., Miller, M. A., Seni, M. H., Andermann, E., and Spielberg, S. P. (1985). Genetic predisposition to phenytoin-induced birth defects. *Lancet* **2**(8458), 746–749.

Substance Abuse Mental Health Administration (2006). Results from the 2005 National Survey on Drug Use and Health: National Findings. Office of Applied Studies, NSDUH Series H-30, DHHS, Publication No. SMA 06–4194, Rockville, MD, 2006.

van der Put, N. M., Steegers-Theunissen, R. P., Frosst, P., Trijbels, F. J., Eskes, T. K., van den Heuvel, L. P., Mariman, E. C., den Heyer, M., Rozen, R., and Blom, H. J. (1995). Mutated methylenetetrahydrofolate reductase as a risk factor for spina bifida. *Lancet* **346,** 1070–1071.

Weiss, P. (1939). *In* "Principles of Development: Malformations," pp. 481–483. Henry Holt and Company, New York.

Werler, M. M., Louik, C., Shapiro, S., and Mitchell, A. A. (1996). Prepregnant weight in relation to risk of neural tube defects. *JAMA* **275**(14), 1089–1092.

Wilson, J. G. (1965). Embryologic considerations in teratology. *In* "Teratology: Principles and Techniques" (J. G. Wilson and J. Warkany, Eds.), pp. 251–261. University of Chicago Press, Chicago.

Wilson, R. D., Davies, G., Désilets, V., Reid, G. J., Summers, A., Wyatt, P., and Young, D. Genetics Committee and Executive and Council of the Society of Obstetricians and Gynaecologists of Canada (2003). The use of folic acid for the prevention of neural tube defects and other congenital anomalies. *J. Obstet. Gynaecol. Can.* **25**(11), 959–973.

TERATOGENICITY AND ANTIEPILEPTIC DRUGS: POTENTIAL MECHANISMS

Mark S. Yerby

North Pacific Epilepsy Research, Portland, Oregon 97210, USA

I. Introduction
II. Historical Aspects
III. Is Increased Fetal Risk Related to Maternal Epilepsy or to AED Exposure?
IV. The Role of Maternal Epilepsy as a Confounder for Teratogenic Risk
V. Type and Pattern of AED-Related Malformations
VI. Potential Mechanisms of AED-Related Teratogenicity
   A. Epoxide Metabolites of AEDs and Teratogenicity
   B. Free Radical Intermediates of AEDs and Teratogenicity
   C. Hypoxia/Reoxygenation Hypothesis
   D. Phenytoin Teratogenicity and Glucocorticoid Receptors
   E. Potential Role of Homeobox (HOX) Genes
   F. Potential AED-Related Teratogenic Mechanisms
VII. Folate Deficiency as a Potential Mechanism of AED-Induced Teratogenicity
VIII. NTDs and VPA Exposure
   A. NTDs: Epidemiology and Pathogenesis
   B. The Association of NTDs with Valproate
   C. Possible Mechanisms of Valproate Teratogenicity
IX. Carbamazepine and NTDs
X. Phenobarbital Teratogenicity
XI. Conclusions
   References

Congenital malformations often the most concerning risk of taking antiepileptic drugs (AEDs) during pregnancy for both the patient and the physician. This chapter reviews aspects of the association between AEDs and congenital malformations, including a historical perspective, type and patterns of congenital malformations, possible confounding factors, and potential mechanisms of teratogenicity. The role of folic acid in preventing birth defects in the general population and in setting of taking AEDs is also presented. One of the most serious congenital malformations, spina bifida (SB), and its association with intrauterine valproate exposure, is discussed in depth.

INTERNATIONAL REVIEW OF
NEUROBIOLOGY, VOL. 83
DOI: 10.1016/S0074-7742(08)00010-X

181

I. Introduction

Congenital malformations remain the most widely reported and clinically dramatic adverse outcomes of pregnancy. Congenital malformations are defined as a physical defect requiring medical or surgical intervention and causing major functional disturbance. In North America, malformations account for 2–3% of all live births. For infants of mothers with epilepsy (IME) exposed to antiepileptic drugs (AEDs) *in utero*, the risks of malformations is doubled (Canger *et al.*, 1999; Fedrick, 1973; Speidel and Meadow, 1972; Thomas *et al.*, 2001; Vajda *et al.*, 2003; Wide *et al.*, 2004).

II. Historical Aspects

The first report of a malformation associated with AEDs described a child exposed to mephenytoin *in utero* who developed microcephaly, cleft palate, malrotation of the intestine, a speech defect, and an IQ of 60 (Mullers-Kupper, 1963). The pregnancy was also complicated by vaginal bleeding. In 1964, Janz and Fuchs (1964) performed a retrospective survey of AED-associated malformations at the University of Heidelberg. Four hundred twenty-six pregnancies in 246 mothers with epilepsy were studied. The rates of miscarriages and stillbirths were increased, but the malformation rate was only 2.2%, not significantly different from that of the general population of what was then known as West Germany. The authors therefore concluded that AEDs were not associated with an increased risk of malformations.

Though now recognized as the most common malformation seen with AED exposure, Centa and Rasore-Quartino (1965) were the first to report a case of congenital heart disease with *in utero* exposure to phenytoin and phenobarbital. Melchior *et al.* (1967) provided one of the first descriptions of orofacial clefts with exposure to primidone or phenobarbital.

In a letter to Lancet in 1968, S.R. Meadow reported six cases of children with orofacial clefts, four of whom had additional abnormalities of the heart and dysmorphic facial features. All of these children had been exposed to AEDs *in utero*. He noted that similar abnormalities had been reported following the unsuccessful use of abortifactant folic acid antagonists. Since some AEDs acted as folic acid antagonists, he postulated that this might account for AED teratogenicity and asked for other clinicians to inform him of similar cases (Meadow, 1968).

In the first report of a malformation associated with a specific AED, trimethadione was implicated as a teratogen in 8 of 14 patients who took it in the first trimester (German *et al.*, 1970).

Dr. Meadow's 1968 request for information on other AED-associated malformations resulted in the collection of 30 additional cases. This prompted a retrospective survey in which 427 pregnancies in 186 women with epilepsy were identified. For the first time, a clear increase in the malformation rates for IMEs was demonstrated (Speidel and Meadow, 1972). From this information, it was concluded that:

congenital malformations are twice as common in IMEs exposed to AEDs;
no single abnormality was specific for AED exposure; and
a group of these children would have a characteristic pattern of anomalies, which at its fullest expression consisted of trigonocephaly, microcephaly, hypertelorism, low set ears, short neck, transverse palmer creases, and minor skeletal abnormalities.

These early observations have for the most part been borne out by subsequent studies, although the exact increased risk with each AED is still under investigation.

III. Is Increased Fetal Risk Related to Maternal Epilepsy or to AED Exposure?

The increased rate of malformations in the offspring of mothers with epilepsy appears to be related to AED exposure *in utero*. Evidence to support this association comes from four observations.

1. Comparisons of the malformation rates in the offspring of mothers with epilepsy treated with AEDs as opposed to those with no AED treatment reveal consistently higher rates in the children of the treated group (Annegers *et al.*, 1978; Jick and Terris, 1997; Lowe, 1973; Monson *et al.*, 1973; South, 1972).
2. Mean plasma AED concentrations are higher in mothers with malformed infants than mothers with healthy children (Dansky *et al.*, 1980).
3. Infants of mothers taking multiple AEDs have higher malformation rates than those exposed to monotherapy (Lindhout *et al.*, 1984; Nakane, 1979).
4. Maternal seizures during pregnancy do not appear to increase the risk of congenital malformations (Fedrick, 1973).

Further elaboration of point 4 is merited, due to conflicting evidence. Most investigators have found that maternal seizures during pregnancy had no impact on the frequency of malformations, development of epilepsy or febrile convulsions (Annegers *et al.*, 1978; Morrow *et al.*, 2005). However, Majewski *et al.* (1980) described increased malformation rates and central nervous system injury in IMEs exposed to maternal seizures, more recently, Lindhout and Omtzigt (1992) described a marked increase in malformations amongst infants exposed to first trimester seizures (12.3%) compared to fetuses that were not subjected to any maternal seizures (4.0%). Malformations were more often observed in infants exposed to partial seizures than to generalized tonic clonic seizures. The contribution of maternal epilepsy itself (discussed in the following section) and other lifestyle factors cannot be completely accounted for in these reports, and therefore seizures themselves are not clearly an independent factor for increasing risk of malformations.

IV. The Role of Maternal Epilepsy as a Confounder for Teratogenic Risk

While a strong relationship between anticonvulsant use in maternal epilepsy and the development of congenital malformations has been established, the degree of increased risk from AEDs may confounded by that imparted by the genetic factors associated with epilepsy itself (Battino, 2001; Sankar, 2007). A genetic susceptibility to the AED teratogenic effect has been suggested by family studies (Duncan et al., 2001; Erickson, 1974; Gardner et al., 2001; Karpathios et al., 1989; Kozma, 2001; Lindhout et al., 1992; Malm et al., 2002). Several case-control studies reported a higher proportion of relatives with epilepsy in patients with cleft palate or lip (Abrishamchian et al., 1994; Erickson and Oakley, 1974; Friis, 1979; Kelly et al., 1984b) or neural tube defects (NTDs) (Lindhout and Meinardi, 1984; Robert and Guibaud, 1982). A number of cohort studies evaluating pregnancy outcomes in maternal epilepsy identified a familial occurrence of fetal abnormalities (Annegers and Hauser, 1982; Annegers et al., 1974; Canger et al., 1999; Dansky, 1989; Dean et al., 2002; Elshove and van Eck, 1971; Kaneko et al., 1999; Moore et al., 2000; Nakane, 1982; Nakane et al., 1980; Starreveld-Zimmerman et al., 1973; Weber et al., 1977), but the majority of the studies reported conflicting findings (Beck-Mannagetta and Drees, 1982; Holmes et al., 2001; Kaaja et al., 2003; Lindhout and Meinardi, 1984; Oguni et al., 1992; Omtzigt et al., 1992; Sabers et al., 2004).

The issue of parental epilepsy increasing the risk of congenital malformations was first raised by a prospective American and Finnish study (Shapiro et al., 1976) reporting higher rates of malformations in children of treated epileptic mothers and epileptic fathers. Later studies confirmed these findings and added that even untreated epileptic mothers had a higher risk of having a child with birth defects (Beck-Mannagetta and Drees, 1982; Fried et al., 2004; Friis and Hauge, 1985; Koch et al., 1982, 1992; Meyer, 1973; Rating et al., 1987).

Interpretation of results should be cautious due to differences in ascertaining cases and controls, since a meta-analysis has suggested that the malformation rate among the offspring of women with untreated epilepsy was similar to that of nonepileptic controls. An epilepsy and pregnancy registry from the United Kingdom, demonstrated similar malformation rates for infants of women with epilepsy who had not taken AEDs during pregnancy (3.3%) and AED monotherapy exposures (3.7%) (Morrow et al., 2005). In the aggregate data support the observation that AED treatment increases the risk of birth defects but also suggests that the increased risk cannot be entirely ascribed to AEDs alone.

V. Type and Pattern of AED-Related Malformations

A wide variety of congenital malformations have been reported in children of mothers with epilepsy, and every anticonvulsant medication (with the exception of pregabalin, a recently approved AED for which we have no data), has been implicated in the development of congenital malformations. Cleft lip and/or palate and congenital heart disease account for a majority of all reported cases (Annegers et al., 1978; Elshove and van Eck, 1971; Holmes et al., 2004).

Orofacial clefts are relatively common malformations in the general population, occurring with a frequency of 1.5/1000 live births. IME have a rate of orofacial clefting of 13.8/1000, a ninefold increase in risk (Kallen, 1986; Kelly et al., 1984b). Early observations that persons with clefting of the lip or palate were twice as likely to have family members with epilepsy as controls suggested that orofacial clefts were associated with epilepsy (Friis, 1979). Subsequent studies of the prevalence of facial clefts in the siblings and children of 2072 persons with epilepsy found observed/expected ratios increased only for maternal epilepsy. The risk was greater if AEDs were taken during pregnancy than if no AED treatment was used. The authors concluded that there was no evidence that epilepsy itself contributed to the development of orofacial clefts (Friis et al., 1986). Israeli researchers have found that children with cleft lip/palate are four times as likely to have a mother with epilepsy as the general population, and mothers with epilepsy are six times as likely to bear a child with an orofacial cleft as nonepileptic women (Gadoth et al., 1987). Hungarian investigators have demonstrated an increase in posterior cleft palate in children of mothers with epilepsy (Metneki et al., 2005). Orofacial clefts account for 30% of the excess of congenital malformations in IMEs.

Congenital heart defects primarily midline defects are the most frequently reported teratogenic abnormality associated with AEDs (Holmes and Wyszynski, 2004). IME have a 1.5–2% prevalence of congenital heart disease, a relative risk (RR) of threefold over the general population (Kallen, 1986). Anderson prospectively studied maternal epilepsy and AED use in 3000 children with heart defects at the University of Minnesota. Eighteen IMEs were identified. Twelve of these had ventricular septal defects; 9 of the 18 children had additional noncardiac defects, 8 of which were orofacial clefts (Anderson, 1976).

No AED can be considered absolutely safe in pregnancy, but for the vast majority of drugs no specific pattern of major malformations has been identified. The lack of a characteristic pattern of defects has been cited as evidence that AEDs are not teratogenic. When phenobarbital was given during pregnancy for conditions other than epilepsy, no increase in malformation rates has been demonstrated (Shapiro *et al.*, 1976). The preponderance of evidence, however, supports an effect of AED on the development of malformations.

VI. Potential Mechanisms of AED-Related Teratogenicity

A body of evidence has accumulated supporting the hypotheses that an arene oxide metabolite of phenytoin or other AED is the ultimate teratogen (Speidel and Meadow, 1972), a genetic defect in epoxide hydrolase (arene oxide detoxifying enzyme system) increases the risk of fetal toxicity (Fedrick, 1973), free radicals produced by AED metabolism are cytotoxic (Canger *et al.*, 1999), and a genetic defect in free radical scavenging enzyme activity (FRSEA) increases the risk of fetal toxicity (Thomas *et al.*, 2001). Folate efficiency as a potential mechanism of AED-induced teratogenicity will be discussed in Section VI. Other less established but potential teratogenic mechanisms such as fetal hypoxic/reoxygenation injury and glucocorticoid receptor-mediated injury in relation to phenytoin teratogenicity are also discussed herein.

A. EPOXIDE METABOLITES OF AEDs AND TERATOGENICITY

A large number of chemicals are converted into epoxide intermediates by reactions, reactions that are catalyzed by the microsomal monoxygenase system (Jerina and Daly, 1974; Sims and Grover, 1974). Arene oxides are unstable epoxides formed by aromatic compounds. Various epoxides are electrophilic and may elicit carcinogenic, mutagenic, and other toxic effects by covalent binding to critical cell macromolecules (Nebert and Jensen, 1979; Shum *et al.*, 1979). Epoxides are detoxified by two types of processes: conversion to dihydro-diols catalyzed by epoxide hydrolase in the cytoplasm (Speidel and Meadow, 1972) and conjugation with glutathione in the microsomes (spontaneously or mediated by glutathione transferase) (Fedrick, 1973). Epoxide hydrolase activity has been found in the cytosol and the microsomal subcellular fraction of adult and fetal human hepatocytes. Interestingly, epoxide hydrolase activity in fetal livers is much lower than that of adults (Pacifici *et al.*, 1983). One-third to one-half of fetal circulation bypasses the liver, resulting in higher direct exposure of extrahepatic fetal organs to potential toxic metabolites (Pacifici and Rane, 1982).

Arene oxides are obligatory intermediates in the metabolism of aromatic compounds to *trans*-dihydrodiols. Phenytoin forms a *trans*-dihydrodiol metabolite in several species (Chang *et al.*, 1970). This metabolite is also formed by neonates exposed to phenytoin *in utero* (Horning *et al.*, 1974). *In vitro* studies have shown that an oxidative (NADPH/02-dependent) metabolite of phenytoin binds irreversibly to rat liver microsomes by a process that is reduced nicotinamide-adenine nucleotide phosphate and oxygen dependent (Martz *et al.*, 1977). This binding is increased by trichloroponene oxide, an inhibitor of epoxide hydrolase (TCPO) and decreased by glutathione (Martz *et al.*, 1977; Pantarotto *et al.*, 1982; Wells and Harbison, 1980). Using a mouse hepatic microsomal system to produce phenytoin metabolites, and human lymphocytes to assess cell defense mechanisms against toxicity, Spielberg *et al.* (1981) showed that cytotoxicity was enhanced by inhibitors of epoxide hydrolase.

Using a mouse model, Martz *et al.* (1977) showed that treatment with an inhibitor of epoxide hydrolase was associated with an increased in the rate of orofacial anomalies in fetal animals exposed to phenytoin. Furthermore, there was a correlation between the teratogenic effect correlated with and the amount of covalently bound material in fetal tissue.

Strickler and coworkers examined lymphocytes from 24 children exposed to phenytoin during gestation and lymphocytes from their families using the Spielberg test of cytotoxicity in order to elucidate the teratogenic mechanisms (Spielberg *et al.*, 1981; Strickler *et al.*, 1985). In this system, a positive response was highly correlated with major birth defects. Lymphocytes were incubated with phenytoin in a mouse microsomal system. A positive response was defined as increase in cell death over baseline. Cells from 15 children gave a positive response, and each positive child had a positive parent. A positive *in vitro* response was highly correlated with major birth defects. The authors concluded that a genetic defect in arene oxide detoxification increased the risk of the child having major birth defects (Strickler *et al.*, 1985). However, no measurement of epoxide hydrolase activity was included in this study.

The evidence that epoxide metabolites of phenytoin are teratogenic can be summarized as follows: Phenytoin is metabolized to an epoxide metabolite that binds to tissues. Inhibition of the detoxifying enzyme, epoxide hydrolase, increases lymphocyte cytotoxicity, and increases the binding of epoxide metabolite to liver microsomes and increases the rate of orofacial clefts in experimental animals.

These facts cannot completely explain the teratogenicity seen in phenytoin or other AEDs. The lymphocyte cytotoxicity mediated by epoxide metabolites correlates with major but not minor malformations (Dansky *et al.*, 1987b). Dysmorphic abnormalities have been described in siblings exposed to ethotoin *in utero* even though ethotoin is not metabolized through an arene oxide intermediate (Finnell and DiLiberti, 1983). Embryopathies have been described with exposure to mephytoin, which does not form an arene oxide intermediate (Wells *et al.*, 1982). Trimethadione is clearly teratogenic but has no phenyl rings and thus cannot form an arene oxide metabolite. Therefore, alternate mechanisms must exist.

B. Free Radical Intermediates of AEDs and Teratogenicity

Some drugs are metabolized or bioactivated by co-oxidation during prostaglandin synthesis. Such drugs serve as electron donors to peroxidases, resulting in an electron deficient drug molecule, which by definition, is called a free radical. In the search for additional electrons to complete their outer ring, free radicals can covalently bind to macromolecules, including nucleic acids (DNA, RNA), proteins, cell membranes, and lipoproteins resulting in cytotoxicity.

Phenytoin is co-oxidized by prostaglandin synthetase (PGS), thyroid peroxidase, and horseradish peroxidase producing reactive free radical intermediates that bind to proteins (Kubow and Wells, 1989). Phenytoin teratogenicity can be modulated by substances that reduce the formation of phenytoin free radicals. Acetylsalicylic acid (ASA) irreversibly inhibits PGS, caffeic acid is an antioxidant, and alpha-phenyl-butylnitrone (PBN) is a free radical spin trapping agent. Pretreatment of pregnant mice with these compounds reduces the number of cleft lip and palates secondary to phenytoin in their offspring (Wells *et al.*, 1989).

Glutathione is believed to detoxify free radical intermediates by forming a nonreactive conjugate. *N*-acetylcysteine, a glutathione precursor, decreases phenytoin induced orofacial clefts and fetal weight loss in rodents (Wong and Wells, 1988). BCNU (carmustine) inhibits glutathione reductase, an enzyme necessary to maintain adequate cellular glutathione concentrations, and increases phenytoin embryopathy at doses at which BCNU alone has no embryopathic effect (Wong and Wells, 1989). The metabolism of phenytoin or other AEDs to free radical intermediates may be responsible for the teratogenicity seen in IMEs.

C. Hypoxia/Reoxygenation Hypothesis

A group of European researchers have demonstrated fetal injury in *in vitro* rodent models. In these systems, antiarrhythmic drugs inhibit potassium channels resulting in fetal bradycardia and cardiac arrest. The fetal hypoxia is then followed by reoxygenation and generation of reactive oxygen species The resulting reduction in oxygen saturation causes fetal injury. Low doses of phenytoin in association with brief periods of clamping the uterine artery result in distal digital hypoplasia in animal models. Thus an alternate mechanism of anticonvulsant teratogenicity has been proposed (Danielsson et al., 2001; Leist and Grauwiler, 1974; Webster et al., 1987). It may well be that a variety of mechanism may operate on an individual fetus at any one time.

D. PHENYTOIN TERATOGENICITY AND GLUCOCORTICOID RECEPTORS

It has been proposed that the glucocorticoid receptor mediates the teratogenicity of phenytoin. Arachidonic acid reverses clefting induced by glucocorticoids in rats. Phospholipase inhibitory proteins (PLIPs) inhibit arachidonic acid release. Glucocorticoid receptors mediate the induction of PLIPs. IME exposed to phenytoin with the stigmata of fetal hydantoin syndrome have increased levels of glucocorticoid receptors (Goldman et al., 1987).

E. POTENTIAL ROLE OF HOMEOBOX (HOX) GENES

Recently, mechanisms involving homeobox (HOX) genes have been proposed to explain teratogenicity of AEDs (Nau et al., 1995). Retinoic acid signaling regulates the transcription of these genes that are critical to early brain development, and may respond to teratogens (Rodier, 2004). Such mechanisms include alteration of the expression of retinoic acid receptor (Gelineau-van Waes et al., 1999) or valproate inhibition of histone deacetylases (Bertollini et al., 1987; Duncan et al., 2001; Gottlicher et al., 2001; Gurvich et al., 2005; Phiel et al., 2001). This is considered to be a key element in regulating many genes, playing an important role in cellular proliferation and differentiation (Faiella et al., 2000; Kawanishi et al., 2003; Massa et al., 2005).

F. POTENTIAL AED-RELATED TERATOGENIC MECHANISMS

Other postulated mechanisms are tissue damage due to fetal hemorrhage, possibly involving vitamin K deficiency (Howe et al., 1999) or interference with placental carnitine transport (Wu et al., 2004).

Phosphodiesterase-mediated inhibition of cyclic adenosine monophosphate (Gallagher et al., 2004), increase of reactive oxygen species levels (Na et al., 2003), disruption of normal pH within the embryonic milieu (Scott et al., 1997), or inhibition of the detoxifying epoxide hydrolase could also be relevant to the teratogenic effect of valproic acid (VPA) (Ingram et al., 2000).

VII. Folate Deficiency as a Potential Mechanism of AED-Induced Teratogenicity

Maternal folate supplementation has been shown to reduce the risk of spina bifida (SB) in the general population. This has led to a recommendation by the Centers for Disease Control (CDC) for folate supplementation in all women of child bearing age. In deriving this recommendation, the CDC reviewed eight studies, four observational and four interventional. The interventional studies randomly assigned women with a previous history of bearing a child with a NTD to either 0.36, 4.0, 5.0 mg of folate daily or placebo. The observational studies compared SB defect rates in children with or without *in utero* folate exposure. In 7 of the 8 studies, the risks of NTDs were reduced by 60–100% (Table I). The CDC therefore recommended that all women of childbearing age take 0.4 mg of folate/day (MMWR, 1992). These recommendations are not specific for WWE taking AEDs, however.

In animal models, the effect of folate on mitigating the risk of AED-related birth defects has been variable. Co-treatment of mice with folate, with or without vitamins and amino acids, reduced malformation rates and increased fetal weight and length in mice pups exposed to phenytoin *in utero* (Zhu and Zhou, 1989). However in other studies, folate administration failed to reduce NTDs and embryotoxicity in rodent models (Hansen and Grafton, 1991; Hansen *et al.*, 1995).

In the offsping of women with epilepsy, the possibility of folate deficiency as a potential mechanism for AED-induced teratogenicity was first postulated in 1968 (Meadow, 1968). Other investigators have found evidence for the role of folate in AED-related teratogenicity. Dansky *et al.* (1987a) found significantly lower blood folate concentrations in women with epilepsy with abnormal pregnancy outcomes. Biale and Lewenthal (1984) reported a 15% malformation rate in IMEs with no folate supplementation, whereas none of 33 folate supplemented children had congenital abnormalities.

Unfortunately preconceptual folate supplementation may not consistently prevent NTDs in children born to women with epilepsy. Craig *et al.* (1999) reported a young woman whose seizures were controlled for 4 years by 2000 mg of VPA a day. Although she took 4.0 mg of folic acid a day for 18 months prior to her pregnancy, she delivered a child with a lumbosacral NTD, a ventricular and atrial septal defect, cleft palate and bilateral talipes equinovarus. Two Canadian women delivered children with NTDs despite folate supplementation. One taking 3.5 mg folic acid for 3 months prior to conception and 1250 mg of VPA aborted a child with lumbosacral SB, Arnold Chiari malformation and hydrocephalus. A second woman who took 5.0 mg of folic acid had one spontaneous abortion of a fetus with an encephalocele and two therapeutic abortions of fetuses with lumbosacral SB (Duncan *et al.*, 2001). These cases might have been predicted given the demonstrated failure of folate to reduce

TABLE I
PRECONCEPTUAL FOLATE, AFTER LEWIS *ET AL.*

Authors	Study type	N	Dose of folate	Results
Smithells *et al.* (1983)	Non-randomized, controlled	Fully supplemented = 454 Partially supplemented = 519 Unsupplemented = 114	0.36 mg	86% risk reduction
Seller and Nevin (1984)	Non-randomized	Unsupplemented = 543 Supplemented = 421	0.36 mg	Risk reduction
Mulinare *et al.* (1988)	Case-control	Case = 181 Control = 1480	Multivitamins with folate	60% risk reduction
Milinsky *et al.* (1989)	Cohort	23,491	"	71% risk reduction
MRC (1991)	Randomized, double blind, controlled	1195	4.0 mg	72% risk reduction
Czeizel and Dudas (1992)	Randomized, controlled	Case = 2420 Control = 2333	0.8 mg	No defects with folate supplementation
Werler *et al.* (1993)	Case-control	Case = 436 Control = 2615	?	60% risk reduction
Werler *et al.* (1996)	Case-control	Case = 604 Control = 1658	Folate supplements	Folate did not decrease rates in women >70 kg

NTD and embryotoxicity in *in vitro* and *in vivo* rodent models (Hansen and Grafton, 1991; Hansen *et al.*, 1995). In fact not all research supports the association with folate deficiency and malformations. Mills *et al.* (1992) found no difference between serum folate levels in mothers of children with NTDs and controls. A number of other studies reports also failed to demonstrate a protective effect of preconceptual folate (Bower and Stanley, 1992; Freil *et al.*, 1995; Kirke *et al.*, 1992; Laurence *et al.*, 1981; Vergel *et al.*, 1990; Winship *et al.*, 1984). These studies are problematic due to small sample sizes, failure to document folate supplementation and recall bias in the retrospective investigation.

The protective effect of folate may be variable simply because women with similar folate intake may have different serum concentrations due to differences in folate metabolism. Absorption does not account for the difference in plasma concentration between cases and controls (Davis *et al.*, 1995). Whether women with epilepsy taking AED will have their risk of congenital malformations reduced is unclear. The recommended daily allowances (RDA) of folate have been increased to 400 μg/day for nonpregnant, 600 μg/day for pregnant, and 500 μg/day for lactating women. The increased folate catabolism during pregnancy coupled with the variation of requirements by individual women has led some authorities to call for recommend higher folate supplementation doses on the order of 500–600 μg/day (Oakley, 1998). Women with epilepsy like all other women of childbearing age should take folate supplementation. However, the dose recommended by the CDC of 400 μg/day may not be high enough for many women who do not metabolize folate effectively (CDC, 1992), or who are taking AEDs with antifolate actions; many physicians recommend 1–5 mg/day of folate for women taking AEDs although the evidence for the usefulness of this dose is based more on speculation than fact.

VIII. NTDs and VPA Exposure

A. NTDs: Epidemiology and Pathogenesis

NTDs are uncommon malformations occurring in 6/10,000 pregnancies. SB and anencephaly are the most commonly reported NTD and affect approximately 4000 pregnancies annually resulting in 2500–3000 births in the United States each year (Hernandez-Diaz *et al.*, 2000; Mulinare and Erickson, 1997). The types of NTD associated with AED exposure are primarily myelomeningocele and anencephaly which are the result of abnormal neural tube closure between the third and fourth weeks of gestational age.

Previous thinking about NTD visualized the fusion of the neural tube as one in which the lateral edges met in the middle and fused both rostrally and caudally similar to a bidirectional zipper. Recent studies have suggested there are multiple sites for neural tube closure (Rosa, 1991; VanAllen *et al.*, 1993) and that different etiologies may result in different types of abnormality.

There are four separate sites along the neural tube where neuralation develops. The first is midcervical. The second is at the cranial junction of the prosencephalon and mesencephalon. The third at the site of the future mouth or stomadeum. This region fuses in a caudal direction only. The fourth is the region over the rhombencephalon between the second and third regions (VanAllen *et al.*, 1993).

There are differences in the specific sites and timing of the closure of each individual region. The majority of human NTD can be explained by failure of one or more closure sites. Anencephaly with frontal and parietal defects is due to failure at closure site two. Holocrania which also involves defects of the posterior cranium to the foramen magnum is due to failure of closure of areas two and four. Lumbar spinal bifida results from failure of closure one. The development of closure sites appears to be under genetic control and is also affected by environmental factors. In twins, concordance rates are only 56% for anencephaly but 71% for SB. In Great Britain, there is a male preponderance of lumbar SB and female preponderance of holocrania and anencephaly. Even VPA appears to have species differential effects being associated with SB in humans and exencephaly in mice (Seller, 1995).

The risk of potential association of valproate with NTDs is further complicated because a number of risk factors are associated with NTDs. A previous pregnancy with a NTD has the strongest predictive value with a RR of 20. There are strong ethnic/geographic associations with NTDs. Rates per 1000 are 0.22 for Caucasians, 0.58 for persons of Hispanic descent, and 0.08 for persons of African descent. The incidence of NTDs in Mexico is 3.26/1000, for Mexican-born persons living in California 1.6/1000 and for United States born persons of Mexican descent 0.68/1000 (Webster et al., 1987). Diabetic mothers with diabetes have 7.9 times the rates of NTDs in their offspring (Becerra et al., 1990). Deficiencies of glutathione, folate, vitamin C, riboflavin, zinc, cyanocobalamin, selenium, and excessive exposure to Vitamin A have been associated with NTDs. Higher rates are seen in children of farmers, cleaning women, and nurses (Blatter et al., 1996; Matte et al., 1993). Prepregnancy weight has also been demonstrated to be a factor. Werler and colleagues compared RR for NTDs in control women weighing 50–59 kg and found the RR increased to 1.9 in women weighing 80–8 kg and 4.0 for those weighing over 110 kg. Therefore, AED exposure may be a necessary but not sufficient risk factor for the development of NTDs (Werler et al., 1996).

B. The Association of NTDs with Valproate

It has been argued that for a substance to be classified as a teratogen a specific clinical defect must consistently be demonstrated. Phocomelia associated with exposure to thalidomide is an example. Although orofacial clefts and midline heart defects are the most commonly reported malformations associated with AED exposure, they are clearly not the majority of malformations. This has led some investigators to contend that true teratogenicity is not associated with AEDs.

Experience with VPA has modified our thinking in this regard. Dysmorphism has been associated with in utero exposure to VPA. The first such case was reported by Dalens *et al.* (1980), who described an infant exposed to VPA *in utero* who was born with low birth weight, hypoplastic nose and fronto-orbital ridges, and levocardia. The baby died at 19 days of life. Subsequent reports of dysmorphism followed by Clay *et al.* (1981) and a child with lumbosacral meningocele was described by Gomez (1981). Dickinson *et al.* (1979) had previously demonstrated the ability of VPA to cross the placenta. Kaneko *et al.* (1988) found VPA to result in the highest malformation rate of any AED utilized in 172 pregnancies. As already noted, a fetal valproate syndrome has been described (DiLiberti *et al.*, 1984) and several additional cases were reported (Jeavons, 1984; Tein and MacGregor, 1985).

A report in Morbidity and Mortality Weekly Report (MMWR) in October 1982 made the first association of VPA with a specific malformation, NTDs. The Institute European de Genomutations in Lyon, France, has developed a system of birth defect surveillance and registered 145 cases of SB between 1976 and 1982. They noted that of IME exposed to VPA, 34% had malformations, and 5 of 9 exposed to VPA monotherapy had SB, a rate 20 times that expected (MMWR, 1982).

Subsequent reports confirmed the linkage between intrauterine VPA exposure and SB. Robert and colleagues sent questionnaires to 646 women with epilepsy, aged 15–45 years. Of 280 responses they collected 74 deliveries, to which they added 74 additional cases collected from women delivering in Lyon, France. The malformation rate of the entire group was 13%, with a higher than expected rate of NTDs in children exposed to VPA (Robert *et al.*, 1986).

Stanley and Chambers (1982) reported an infant exposed to VPA *in utero* with SB whose two normal siblings were not exposed to the drug. Lindhout and Schmidt (1986) surveyed 18 epilepsy groups and collected 12 cases of infants and epileptic mothers with NTDs. A higher rate was seen in children exposed to VPA monotherapy (2.5%) than polytherapy (1.5%). The increased risk appears to be limited to SB rather than other NTDs with an overall risk of an infant exposed to VPA *in utero* of 1.5%.

Other reports have also implicated carbamazepine as a cause of SB apperta. Further evaluations of these exposures have determined that it is SB apperta, which is specifically associated with this exposure as opposed to other NTDs (Kallen, 1994; Lindhout *et al.*, 1992; Rosa, 1991). Methodological difficulties make prevalence estimates imprecise, because most of the data published is are in the form of case reports, case series, or very small cohorts from registries which were not designed to evaluate pregnancy outcomes.

It has been estimated that the prevalence of SB following valproate exposure is 1–2% (Wells *et al.*, 1982), and with following carbamazepine 0.5% (Rosa, 1991). A prospective study in Holland, however, demonstrated a prevalence rate of SB with valproate exposure of 5.4%. This increased rate was associated with higher average daily doses (1640+136 mg/day) of valproate in the affected than in the unaffected IME (941+48 mg/day). The authors therefore suggest that the dose reduction be reduced practiced whenever valproate must be used in pregnancy (Omtzigt *et al.*, 1992). An Australian pregnancy and epilepsy registry has also found a dose-dependent response of valproate and malformations with higher rates (30.2%) at doses over 1100 mg daily than doses of less than 1100 mg (3.2%) (Vajda *et al.*, 2004).

C. Possible Mechanisms of Valproate Teratogenicity

The actual mechanism of VPA teratogenicity is unknown. A combination of valpromide and carbamazepine results in an increase in carbamazepine 10–11 epoxide (Pacifici *et al.*, 1985). Valpromide and valproate inhibit epoxide hydrolase (Kerr *et al.*, 1989). Epoxides have been implicated as teratogens, but carbamazepine's epoxide is quite stable, and there appears to be a greater risk of SB with VPA monotherapy than polytherapy. VPA appears to be embryotoxic to cultured whole rat embryos, but none of the hydroxylated metabolites have exhibited a significant embryotoxicity (Rettie *et al.*, 1986). This implies a direct teratogenic effect of the parent drug. Weak acids are frequently teratogenic. The intracellular pH of mouse and rat embryos is higher than maternal plasma. Valproate and its 4en metabolite accumulate in embryonic tissue. Alterations in intracellular pH may explain the teratogenicity of VPA (Nau and Scott, 1986). Lindhout (1989) has proposed different mechanisms, such as interference with lipid metabolism, alterations in zinc concentrations, or disruption of folate utilization.

IX. Carbamazepine and NTDs

An association of carbamazepine and SB has been proposed. Data from Michigan Medicaid Registry revealed four cases of SB in 1490 births to women with epilepsy between 1980 and 1988 or 0.2%. Of the four cases, three were exposed to carbamazepine, but all three were also exposed to VPA, phenytoin, or a barbiturate (Rosa, 1991). A Danish study described 6 of 9 IME exposed to carbamazepine *in utero* developed SB. This out of a cohort of 3635 children (Kallen, 1994). All cases were identified between 1984 and 1986. No new NTD and carbamazepine cases being described subsequently. While there is a suggestion that carbamazepine may be associated with SB, the data is sparse and lacks statistical significance. Improved prenatal diagnostic techniques make determination of associations more difficult now than ever before. More recent registry reports from Sweden and the United Kingdom suggest that carbamazepine's risks of developing malformations may be much less than previously thought ranging from 2.1% to 4% lower than with other commonly used AEDs (Morrow *et al.*, 2006; Wide *et al.*, 2004).

X. Phenobarbital Teratogenicity

The North American pregnancy and epilepsy registry established in 1996 has prospectively enrolled over 5000 women, 2970 of whom were on monotherapy. Higher than expected risk of malformations have been identified with phenobarbital; 5 of 72 monotherapy exposed children or 6.3% had major congenital malformations (95% C.I. 1.9–9.6) (Holmes *et al.*, 2004). Others have found lower malformation rates with phenobarbital; in one study 5 of 172 children had congenital malformations, resulting in a rate of 2.6% (95% C.I. 0.8–5.3) (Samren *et al.*, 1999) Using case-control methods, the same investigators found a higher rate of 1 of 17 phenobarbital or 16.6%, however; this result is not significant as evidenced by a wide confidence interval of 0.3–23% (Samren *et al.*, 1997).

XI. Conclusions

Reports of malformation rates in various populations of IMEs range from 1.25% to 11.5% (Canger *et al.*, 1999; Fedrick, 1973; Kelly *et al.*, 1984a; Morrow *et al.*, 2005; Nakane *et al.*, 1980; Philbert and Dam, 1982; Speidel and Meadow, 1972; Steegers-Theunissen *et al.*, 1994; Thomas *et al.*, 2001; Vajda *et al.*, 2003; Wide *et al.*, 2004). These combined estimates yield a risk of malformations in an individual pregnancy of a woman with epilepsy of 4–6%.

AEDs are associated with an increased risk of malformations in exposed offspring of mothers with epilepsy. The most commonly reported are midline heart defects and oral facial clefts. There is convincing evidence of an association between NTDs and valproic acid. Though data is limited on all AED, there are case reports of malformations for all of the commonly used medications with the exception of pregabalin, which has been marketed only recently. One should interpret this information cautiously, however. Epilepsy remains a serious condition with significant morbidity and mortality. While uncontrolled seizures do not increase the risk of malformations, they do increase the risk of maternal and fetal injury, developmental delay, and death. Clinicians must proceed carefully when managing women with epilepsy in the childbearing years, but none of the data would support discontinuation of AED unless it was clear that it was not medically necessary for seizure control.

References

Abrishamchian, A. R., Khoury, M. J., and Calle, E. E. (1994). The contribution of maternal epilepsy and its treatment to the etiology of oral clefts: A population based case-control study. *Genet. Epidemiol.* **11**(4), 343–351.

Anderson, R. C. (1976). Cardiac defects in children of mothers receiving anticonvulsant therapy during pregnancy. *J. Pediatr.* **89**, 318–319.

Annegers, J. F., and Hauser, I. (1982). The frequency of malformations in relative of patients with epilepsy. *In* "Epilepsy, Pregnancy, and the Child" (D. Janz, M. Dam, L. Bossi, H. Helge, A. Richens, and D. Schmidt, Eds.), pp. 263–267. Raven Press, New York.

Annegers, J. F., Elveback, L. R., Hauser, W. A., *et al.* (1974). Do anticonvulsants have a teratogenic effect? *Arch. Neurol.* **31**(6), 364–373.

Annegers, J. F., Hauser, W. A., Elveback, L. R., *et al.* (1978). Congenital malformations and seizure disorders in the offspring of parents with epilepsy. *Int. J. Epidemiol.* **7**(3), 241–247.

Battino, D. (2001). Assessment of teratogenic risk. *Epilepsy Res.* **45**(1–3), 171–173.

Becerra, J. E., Khoury, M. J., Cordero, J. F., and Erickson, J. D. (1990). Diabetes mellitus during pregnancy and the risks for specific birth defects: A population based case control study. *Pediatrics* **85,** 1–9.

Beck-Mannagetta, G., and Drees, G. D. J. (1982). Malformations and minor anomalies in the offspring of epileptic parents: A retrospective study. *In* "Epilepsy, Pregnancy, and the Child" (D. Janz, M. Dam, L. Bossi, H. Helge, A. Richens, and D. Schmidt, Eds.), pp. 317–323. New York, Raven Press.

Bertollini, R., Kallen, B., Mastroiacovo, P., *et al.* (1987). Anticonvulsant drugs in monotherapy. Effect on the fetus. *Eur. J. Epidemiol.* **3**(2), 164–171.

Biale, Y., and Lewenthal, H. (1984). Effect of folic acid supplementation on congenital malformations due to anticonvulsive drugs. *Eur. J. Obstet. Gynecol. Reprod. Biol.* **18**(4), 211–216.

Blatter, B. M., Roeleveld, N., Zielhuis, G. A., Mullaart, R. A., and Gabreels, F. J. M. (1996). Spina bifida and prenatal occupation. *Epidemiology* **7,** 188–193.

Bower, C., and Stanley, F. J. (1992). Periconceptual vitamin supplementation and neural tube defects: Evidence form a case control study in Western Australia and a review of recent publications. *J. Epidemiol. Community Health* **46,** 157–161.

Canger, R., Battino, D., Canevini, M. P., *et al.* (1999). Malformations in offspring of women with epilepsy: A prospective study. *Epilepsia* **40**(9), 1231–1236.

Centa, A., and Rasore-Quartino, A. (1965). The "digito-cardiac" malformative syndrome (Holt-Oram): Genetic forms and phenocopy. Probable teratogenic action of antiepileptic drugs]. *Pathologica* **57**(853), 227–232.

Centers for Disease Control (CDC). (1982). Valproic acid and spina bifida: A preliminary report—France. *MMWR Morbid. Mortal. Wkly. Rep.* **31**(42), 565–566.

Chang, T., Savory, A., and Glazko, A. J. (1970). A new metabolite of 5,5-diphenylhydantoin (Dilantin). *Biochem. Biophys. Res. Commun.* **38**, 444–449.

Clay, S. A., McVie, R., and Chen, H. C. (1981). Possible teratogenic effect of valproic acid. *J. Pediatr.* **98,** 828.

Craig, J., Morrison, P., Morrow, J., and Patteerson, V. (1999). Failure of preconceptual folic acid to prevent a neural tube defect in the offspring of a mother taking sodium valproate. *Seizure* **8,** 253–254.

Czeizel, A. E., and Dudas, I. (1992). Prevention of the first occurrence of neural tube defects by preconceptional vitamin supplementation. *N. Engl. J. Med.* **327**, 1832–1835.

Dalens, B., Raynaud, E. J., and Gaulme, J. (1980). Teratogenicity of valproic acid. *J. Pediatr.* **97**(2), 332–333.

Danielsson, B. R., Skold, A. C., and Azarbayjani, F. (2001). Class III antiarrhythmics and phenytoin: Teratogenicity due to embryonic cardiac dysrhythmia and reoxygenation damage. *Curr. Pharm. Des.* **7**(9), 787–802.

Dansky, L. (1989). "Outcome of Pregnancy in Epileptic Women." PhD thesis, Mc Gill University, Montreal.

Dansky, L., Andermann, E., Sherwin, A. L., *et al.* (1980). Maternal epilepsy and congenital malformations: A prospective study with monitoring of plasma anticonvulsant levels during pregnancy. *Neurology* **3**, 15.

Dansky, L. V., Andermann, E., Rosenblatt, D., *et al.* (1987a). Anticonvulsants, folate levels, and pregnancy outcome: A prospective study. *Ann. Neurol.* **21**(2), 176–182.

Dansky, L. V., Strickler, S. M., Andermann, E., Miller, M. A., Seni, M. H., and Spielberg, S. P. (1987b). Pharmacogenetic susceptibility to phenytoin teratogenesis. *In* "The XIIth Epilepsy International Symposium", (P. Wolf, M. Dam, D. Janz, and F. E. Dreifuss, Eds.) (Advances in Epileptology; Vol. 16), pp. 555–559. Raven Press, New York.

Davis, B. A., Bailey, L. B., Gregory, J. F., Toth, J. P., Dean, J., and Stevenson, R. E. (1995). Folic acid absorption in women with a history of pregnancy with neural tube defect. *Am. J. Clin. Nutr.* **62**, 782–784.

Dean, J. C., Hailey, H., Moore, S. J., *et al.* (2002). Long term health and neurodevelopment in children exposed to antiepileptic drugs before birth. *J. Med. Genet.* **39**(4), 251–259.

Dickinson, R. G., Harland, R. C., Lynn, R. K., BrewsterSmith, W., and Gerber, N. (1979). Transmission of valproic acid (Depakene) across the placenta: Half-life of the drug in mother and baby. *J. Pediatr.* **94**, 832–835.

DiLiberti, J. H., Farndon, P. A., Dennis, N. R., and Curry, C. J. R. (1984). The fetal valproate syndrome. *Am. J. Med. Genet.* **19**, 473–481.

Duncan, S., Mercho, S., Lopes-Cendes, I., Seni, M. H., Benjamin, A., Dubeau, F., Andermann, F., and Andermann, E. (2001). Repeated neural tube defects and valproate monotherapy suggest a pharmacogenetic abnormality. *Epilepsia* **42**(6), 750–753.

Elshove, J., and van Eck, J. H. (1971). Congenital abnormalities, cleft lip and cleft palate in particular, in children of epileptic mothers. *Ned. Tijdschr. Geneeskd.* **115**(33), 1371–1375.

Erickson, J. D. (1974). Facial and oral form in sibs of children with cleft lip with or without cleft palate. *Ann. Hum. Genet.* **38**(1), 77–88.

Erickson, J. D., and Oakley, G. P. (1974). Seizure disorder in mothers of children with orofacial clefts: A case-control study. *J. Pediatr.* **84**(2), 244–246.

Faiella, A., Wernig, M., Consalez, G. G., *et al.* (2000). A mouse model for valproate teratogenicity: Parental effects, homeotic transformations, and altered HOX expression. *Hum. Mol. Genet.* **9**(2), 227–236.

Fedrick, J. (1973). Epilepsy and pregnancy: A report from the Oxford record linkage study. *Br. Med. J.* **2**(5864), 442–448.

Finnell, R. H., and DiLiberti, J. H. (1983). Hydantoin-induced teratogenesis: Are arene oxide intermediates really responsible? *Helv. Paediatr. Acta* **38**(2), 171–177.

Freil, J. K., Frecker, M., and Fraser, F. C. (1995). Nutritional patterns of mothers of children with neural tube defects in Newfoundland. *Am. J. Med. Genet.* **55**, 195–199.

Fried, S., Kozer, E., Nulman, I., *et al.* (2004). Malformation rates in children of women with untreated epilepsy: A meta-analysis. *Drug Saf.* **27**(3), 197–202.

Friis, M. L. (1979). Epilepsy among parents of children with facial clefts. *Epilepsia* **20**(1), 69–76.

Friis, M. L., and Hauge, M. (1985). Congenital heart defects in live-born children of epileptic parents. *Arch. Neurol.* **42**(4), 374–376.

Friis, M. L., Holm, N. V., Sindrup, E. H., *et al.* (1986). Facial clefts in sibs and children of epileptic patients. *Neurology* **36**(3), 346–350.

Gadoth, N., Millo, Y., Taube, E., and Bechar, M. (1987). Epilepsy among parents of children with cleft lip and palate. *Brain Dev.* **9**(3), 296–299.

Gallagher, H. C., Bacon, C. L., Odumeru, O. A., *et al.* (2004). Valproate activates phosphodiesterase-mediated cAMP degradation: Relevance to C6 glioma G1 phase progression. *Neurotoxicol. Teratol.* **26**(1), 73–81.

Gardner, R. J., Savarirayan, R., Dunne, K. B., *et al.* (2001). Microlissencephaly with cardiac, spinal and urogenital defects. *Clin. Dysmorphol.* **10**(3), 203–208.

Gelineau-van Waes, J., Bennett, G. D., and Finnell, R. H. (1999). Phenytoin-induced alterations in craniofacial gene expression. *Teratology* **59**(1), 23–34.

German, J., Ehlers, K. H., Kowal, A., *et al.* (1970). Possible teratogenicity of trimethadione and paramethadione. *Lancet* **2**(7666), 261–262.

Goldman, A. S., Van Dyke, D. C., Gupta, C., and Katsumata, M. (1987). Elevated glucocorticoid receptor levels in lymphocytes of children with the fetal hydantoin syndrome. *Am. J. Med. Genet.* **28,** 607–618.

Gomez, M. R. (1981). Possible teratogenicity of valproic acid. *J. Pediatr.* **9,** 508.

Gottlicher, M., Minucci, S., Zhu, P., *et al.* (2001). Valproic acid defines a novel class of HDAC inhibitors inducing differentiation of transformed cells. *Embo J.* **20**(24), 6969–6978.

Gurvich, N., Berman, M. G., Wittner, B. S., *et al.* (2005). Association of valproate-induced teratogenesis with histone deacetylase inhibition *in vivo. Faseb J.* **19**(9), 1166–1168.

Hansen, D. K., and Grafton, T. F. (1991). Lack of attenuation of valproic acid induced effects by folinic acid in rat embryos *in vitro. Teratology* **43,** 575–582.

Hansen, D. K., Grafton, T. F., Dial, S. L., Gehring, T. A., and Siitonen, P. H. (1995). Effect of supplemental folic acid on valproic acid induced embryotoxicity and tissue zinc levels *in vivo. Teratology* **52,** 277–285.

Hernandez-Diaz, S., Werler, M. M., Walker, A. M., *et al.* (2000). Folic acid antagonists during pregnancy and the risk of birth defects. *N. Engl. J. Med.* **343**(22), 1608–1614.

Holmes, L. B., and Wyszynski, D. F. (2004). North American antiepileptic drug pregnancy registry. *Epilepsia* **45**(11), 1465.

Holmes, L. B., Harvey, E. A., Coull, B. A., *et al.* (2001). The teratogenicity of anticonvulsant drugs. *N. Engl. J. Med.* **344**(15), 1132–1138.

Holmes, L. B., Wyszynzki, D. F., and Lieberman, E. (2004). The AED (antiepileptic drug) Pregnancy Registry: A 6-year experience. *Arch. Neurol.* **61**(5), 673–678.

Horning, M. G., Stratton, C., Wilson, A., Horning, E. C., and Hill, R. M. (1974). Detection of 5~3,4} diphenylhydantoin in the newborn human. *Anal. Lett.* **4,** 537–582.

Howe, A. M., Oakes, D. J., Woodman, P. D., *et al.* (1999). Prothrombin and PIVKA-II levels in cord blood from newborn exposed to anticonvulsants during pregnancy. *Epilepsia* **40**(7), 980–984.

Ingram, J. L., Peckham, S. M., Tisdale, B., *et al.* (2000). Prenatal exposure of rats to valproic acid reproduces the cerebellar anomalies associated with autism. *Neurotoxicol. Teratol.* **22**(3), 319–324.

Janz, D., and Fuchs, U. (1964). Sind antiepileptische Medikamente waehrend der Schwangerschaft schaedlich? *Dtsch. Med. Wochenschr.* **89,** 241–243.

Jeavons, P. M. (1984). Non dose related side effects of valproate. *Epilepsia* **25**(Suppl. 1), 550–555.

Jerina, D. M., and Daly, J. W. (1974). Arene oxides: A new aspect of drug metabolism. *Science* **185,** 573.

Jick, S. S., and Terris, B. Z. (1997). Anticonvulsants and congenital malformations. *Pharmacotherapy* **17**(3), 561–564.

Kaaja, E., Kaaja, R., and Hiilesmaa, V. (2003). Major malformations in offspring of women with epilepsy. *Neurology* **60**(4), 575–579.

Kallen, B. (1986). A register study of maternal epilepsy and delivery outcome with special reference to drug use. *Acta Neurol. Scand.* **73**(3), 253–259.

Kallen, B. (1994). Maternal carbamazepine and infant spina bifida. *Reprod. Toxicol.* **8,** 203–205.

Kaneko, S., Otani K Fukushima, Y., Ogawa, Y., Nomura, Y., Ono, T., Nakane, Y., Teranishi, T., and Goto, M. (1988). Teratogenicity of antiepileptic drugs: Analysis of possible risk factors. *Epilepsia* **29,** 459–467.

Kaneko, S., Battino, D., Andermann, E., *et al.* (1999). Congenital malformations due to antiepileptic drugs. *Epilepsy Res.* **33**(2–3), 145–158.

Karpathios, T., Zervoudakis, A., Venieris, F., *et al.* (1989). Genetics and fetal hydantoin syndrome. *Acta Paediatr. Scand.* **78**(1), 125–126.

Kawanishi, C. Y., Hartig, P., Bobseine, K. L., *et al.* (2003). Axial skeletal and Hox expression domain alterations induced by retinoic acid, valproic acid, and bromoxynil during murine development. *J. Biochem. Mol. Toxicol.* **17**(6), 346–356.

Kelly, T. E., Edwards, P., Rein, M., *et al.* (1984a). Teratogenicity of anticonvulsant drugs. II: A prospective study. *Am. J. Med. Genet.* **19**(3), 435–443.

Kelly, T. E., Rein, M., and Edwards, P. (1984b). Teratogenicity of anticonvulsant drugs. IV: The association of clefting and epilepsy. *Am. J. Med. Genet.* **19**(3), 451–458.

Kerr, B. M., Rettie, A. E., and Eddy, A. C. (1989). Inhibition of human microsomal epoxide hydrolase by valproate and valpromide: *In vitro/in vivo* correlation. *Clin. Pharmacol. Ther.* **46,** 82–93.

Kirke, P. N., Daly, L. E., and Elwood, J. H. (1992). A randomized trial of low dose folic acid to prevent neural tube defects. *Arch. Dis. Child* **67,** 1442–1446.

Koch, S., Hartmann, A., and Jager, E. (1982). "Major Malformation in Children of Epileptic Mothers—Due to Epilepsy or Its Therapy? Epilepsy, Pregnancy and the Child." Raven Press, New York.

Koch, S., Losche, G., Jager-Roman, E., *et al.* (1992). Major and minor birth malformations and antiepileptic drugs. *Neurology* **42**(4 Suppl. 5), 83–88.

Kozma, C. (2001). Valproic acid embryopathy: Report of two siblings with further expansion of the phenotypic abnormalities and a review of the literature. *Am. J. Med. Genet.* **98**(2), 168–175.

Kubow, S., and Wells, P. G. (1989). *In vitro* bioactivation of phenytoin to a reactive free radical intermediate by prostaglandin synthetase, horseradish peroxidase, and thyroid peroxidase. *Mol. Pharmacol.* **35,** 504–511.

Laurence, K. M., James, J., Miller, M. H., Tennant, G. B., and Campbell, H. (1981). Double blind randomized controlled trial of folate treatment before conception to prevent recurrence of neural tube defects. *BMJ* **282,** 1509–1511.

Leist, K. H., and Grauwiler, J. (1974). Fetal pathology in rats following uterine vessel clamping on day 14 of gestation. *Teratology* **10,** 55–68.

Lindhout, D. (1989). Commission reviews teratogenesis and genetics in epilepsy. *World Neurol.* **4,** 3–7.

Lindhout, D., and Meinardi, H. (1984). Spina bifida and in-utero exposure to valproate. *Lancet* **2** (8399), 396.

Lindhout, D., and Omtzigt, J. G. (1992). Pregnancy and the risk of teratogenicity. *Epilepsia* **33** (Suppl. 4), S41–S48.

Lindhout, D., and Schmidt, D. (1986). In-utero exposure to valproate and neural tube defects. *Lancet* **1** (8494), 1392–1393.

Lindhout, D., Hoppener, R. J., and Meinardi, H. (1984). Teratogenicity of antiepileptic drug combinations with special emphasis on epoxidation (of carbamazepine). *Epilepsia* **25**(1), 77–83.

Lindhout, D., Omtzigt, J. G., and Cornel, M. C. (1992). Spectrum of neural-tube defects in 34 infants prenatally exposed to antiepileptic drugs. *Neurology* **42**(4 Suppl. 5), 111–118.

Lowe, C. R. (1973). Congenital malformations among infants born to epileptic women. *Lancet* **1**(7793), 9–10.

Majewski, F., Raff, W., Fischer, P., *et al.* (1980). Teratogenicity of anticonvulsant drugs (author's transl.)]. *Dtsch. Med. Wochenschr.* **105**(20), 719–723.

Malm, H., Kajantie, E., Kivirikko, S., et al. (2002). Valproate embryopathy in three sets of siblings: Further proof of hereditary susceptibility. *Neurology* **59**(4), 630–633.

Martz, F., Failinger, C., 3rd, and Blake, D. A. (1977). Phenytoin teratogenesis: Correlation between embryopathic effect and covalent binding of putative arene oxide metabolite in gestational tissue. *J. Pharmacol. Exp. Ther.* **203**(1), 231–239.

Massa, V., Cabrera, R. M., Menegola, E., et al. (2005). Valproic acid-induced skeletal malformations: Associated gene expression cascades. *Pharmacogenet. Genomics* **15**(11), 787–800.

Matte, T. D., Mulinare, J., and Erickson, J. D. (1993). Case-control study of congenital defects and parental employment in health care. *Am. J. Ind. Med.* **24**, 11–23.

Meadow, S. R. (1968). Anticonvulsant drugs and congenital abnormalities. *Lancet* **2**(7581), 1296.

Melchior, JC, Svensmark, O, and Trolle, D (1967). Placental transfer of phenobarbitone in epileptic women, and elimination in newborns. *Lancet.* **2**(7521), 860–861.

Metneki, J., Puho, E., and Czeizel, A. E. (2005). Maternal diseases and isolated orofacial clefts in Hungary. *Birth Defects Res. A Clin. Mol. Teratol.* **73**(9), 617–623.

Meyer, J. G. (1973). The teratological effects of anticonvulsants and the effects on pregnancy and birth. *Eur. Neurol.* **10**(3), 179–190.

Milinsky, A., Jick, H., Jick, S. S., Bruell, C. L., MacLaughlin, D. S., and Rothman, K. J. (1989). Multivitamin/folic acid supplementation in early pregnancy reduces the prevalence of neural tube defects. *JAMA* **262**, 2847–2852.

Mills, J. L., Tuomileho, J., Yu, K. F., Colman, N., Blaner, W. S., and Koskela, P. (1992). Maternal vitamin levels during pregnancies producing infants with neural tube defects. *J. Pediatr.* **120**, 863–871.

MMWR Recomm. Rep. 1992, Sep. 11:41 (RR–14):1–7. Review. Recommendations for the use of folic acid to reduce the number of cases of Spina bifida and other neural tube defects.

Monson, R. R., Rosenberg, L., Hartz, S. C., et al. (1973). Diphenylhydantoin and selected congenital malformations. *N. Engl. J. Med.* **289**(20), 1049–1052.

Moore, S. J., Turnpenny, P., Quinn, A., et al. (2000). A clinical study of 57 children with fetal anticonvulsant syndromes. *J. Med. Genet.* **37**(7), 489–497.

Morrow, J. I., Russell, A., Gutherie, E., et al. (2005). Malformations risks of anti-epileptic drugs in pregnancy: A prospective study from the UK Epilepsy and Pregnancy Register. *J. Neurol. Neurosurg. Psychiatr* .

Morrow, J., Russell, A., Guthrie, E., Parsons, L., Robertson, I., Waddell, R., Irwin, B., McGivern, R. C., Morrison, P. J., and Craig, J. (2006). Malformation risks of antiepileptic drugs in pregnancy: A prospective study from the UK Epilepsy and Pregnancy Register. *J. Neurol. Neurosurg. Psychiatr.* **77**(2), 193–198.

MRC Vitamin Study Group. (1991). Prevention of neural tube defects: Results of the medical research council vitamin study. *Lancet* **2**(131), 432.

Mulinare, J., and Erickson, J. D. (1997). Prevention of neural tube defects. *Teratology* **56**(1–2), 17–18.

Mulinare, J., Cordero, J. F., Erickson, J. D., and Berry, R. J. (1988). Periconceptional use of multi-vitamins and the occurrence of neural tube defects. *JAMA.* **260**(21), 3141–5.

Mullers-Kupper, V. M. (1963). Embryopathy during pregnancy caused by taking anticonvulsants. *Acta Paeddopsychiatr.* **30**, 401–405.

Na, L., Wartenberg, M., Nau, H., et al. (2003). Anticonvulsant valproic acid inhibits cardiomyocyte differentiation of embryonic stem cells by increasing intracellular levels of reactive oxygen species. *Birth Defects Res. Part A Clin. Mol. Teratol.* **67**(3), 174–180.

Nakane, Y. (1979). Congenital malformations among infants of epileptic mothers treated during pregnancy. *Folia Psychiatr. Neurol. Jpn.* **33**, 363–369.

Nakane, Y. (1982). Factors influencing the risk of malformations among infants born to epileptic mothers. *In* "Epilepsy, Pregnancy, and the Child" (D. Janz, M. Dam, L. Bossi, H. Helge, A. Richens, and D. Schmidt, Eds.), Raven Press, New York.

Nakane, Y., Okuma, T., Takahashi, R., *et al.* (1980). Multi-institutional study on the teratogenicity and fetal toxicity of antiepileptic drugs: A report of a collaborative study group in Japan. *Epilepsia.* **21** (6), 663–680.

Nau, H., and Scott, W. J. (1986). Weak acids may act as teratogens by accumulating in the basic milieu of the early mammalian embryo. *Nature* **323,** 276–278.

Nau, H., Tzimas, G., Mondry, M., *et al.* (1995). Antiepileptic drugs alter endogenous retinoid concentrations: A possible mechanism of teratogenesis of anticonvulsant therapy. *Life Sci.* **57**(1), 53–60.

Nebert, D. W., and Jensen, N. M. (1979). The Ah locus: Genetic regulation of the metabolism of carcinogens, drugs, and other environmental chemicals by cytochrome P-450 mediated mono-oxygenases. *CRC Crit. Rev. Biochem.* **6,** 401–437.

Oakley, G. P. (1998). Folic acid preventable spina bifida and anencephaly. *Bull World Health Organ.* **76** (Suppl. 2), 116–117.

Oguni, M., Dansky, L., Andermann, E., *et al.* (1992). Improved pregnancy outcome in epileptic women in the last decade: Relationship to maternal anticonvulsant therapy. *Brain Dev.* **14**(6), 371–380.

Omtzigt, J. G., Los, F. J., Grobbee, D. E., *et al.* (1992). The risk of spina bifida aperta after first-trimester exposure to valproate in a prenatal cohort. *Neurology* **42**(4 Suppl. 5), 119–125.

Pacifici, G. M., and Rane, A. (1982). Metabolism of styrene oxide in different human fetal tissues. *Drug Metab. Dispos.* **10,** 302–305.

Pacifici, G. M., Colizzi, C., Giuliani, L., and Rane, A. (1983). Cytosolic epoxide hydrolase in fetal and adult human liver. *Arch. Toxicol.* **54,** 331.

Pacifici, G. M., Tomson, T., Beatilsson, L., and Rane, A. (1985). Valpromide/carbamazepine and the risk of teratogenicity. *Lancet* **1,** 397–398.

Pantarotto, C., Arboix, M., Sezzano, P., *et al.* (1982). Studies on 5,5-diphenylhydantoin irreversible binding to rat liver microsomal proteins. *Biochem. Pharmacol.* **31**(8), 1501–1507.

Phiel, C. J., Zhang, F., Huang, E. Y., *et al.* (2001). Histone deacetylase is a direct target of valproic acid, a potent anticonvulsant, mood stabilizer, and teratogen. *J. Biol. Chem.* **276**(39), 36734–36741.

Philbert, A., and Dam, M. (1982). The epileptic mother and her child. *Epilepsia.* **23,** 85–99.

Rating, D., Jager-Roman, E., Koch, S., *et al.* (1987). "Major Malformations and Minor Anomalies in the Offspring of Epileptic Parents: The Role of Antiepileptic Drugs. Pharmacokinetics in Teratogenesis." pp. 205–224. CRC Press, Boca Raton, Florida.

Rettie, A. K., Rettenmeir, A. W., Beyer, B. K., Baile, T. A., and Juchau, M. R. (1986). Valproate hydroxylation by human fetal tissues and embryotoxicity of metabolites. *Clin. Pharmacol. Ther.* **40,** 172–177.

Robert, E., and Guibaud, P. (1982). Maternal valproic acid and congenital neural tube defects. *Lancet* **2**(8304), 937.

Robert, E., Lofkvist, E., Mauguiere, F., *et al.* (1986). Evaluation of drug therapy and teratogenic risk in a Rhone-Alpes district population of pregnant epileptic women. *Eur. Neurol.* **25**(6), 436–443.

Rodier, P. M. (2004). Environmental causes of central nervous system maldevelopment. *Pediatrics* **113** (4 Suppl.), 1076–1083.

Rosa, F. W. (1991). Spina bifida in infants of women treated with carbamazepine during pregnancy. *N. Engl. J. Med.* **324**(10), 674–677.

Sabers, A., Dam, M. A., Rogvi-Hansen, B., *et al.* (2004). Epilepsy and pregnancy: Lamotrigine as main drug used. *Acta Neurol. Scand.* **109**(1), 9–13.

Samren, E. B., van Duijn, C. M., Koch, S., Hiilesmaa, V. K., Klepel, H., Bardy, A. H., Beck Mannagetta, G., Deichl, A. W., Gaily, E., Granstrom, M. L., Meinardi, H., Grobbee, D. E., *et al.* (1997). Maternal use of antiepileptic drugs and the risk of major congenital malformations: A joint European prospective study of human teratogenesis. *Epilepsia* **38**(9), 981–990.

Samren,, E. B., van Duijn,, C.M, Christiaens,, G. C., Hofman, A., and Lindhout, D. (1999). Antiepileptic drug regimens and major congenital abnormalities in the offspring. *Ann. Neurol.* **46** (5), 739–746.

Sankar, R. (2007). Teratogenicity of antiepileptic drugs: Role of drug metabolism and pharmacogenomics. *Acta Neurol. Scand.* **116**(1), 65–71.

Scott, W. J., Jr., Schreiner, C. M., Nau, H., *et al.* (1997). Valproate-induced limb malformations in mice associated with reduction of intracellular pH. *Reprod. Toxicol.* **11**(4), 483–493.

Seller, M. J. (1995). Recent developments in the understanding of the aetiology of neural tube defects. *Clin. Dysmorphol.* **4,** 93–104.

Seller, M. J., and Nevin, N. C. (1984). Periconceptional vitamin supplementation and the prevention of neural tube defects in south-east England and Northern Ireland. *J. Med. Genet.* **21** (5), 325–330.

Shapiro, S., Hartz, S. C., Siskind, V., *et al.* (1976). Anticonvulsants and parental epilepsy in the development of birth defects (prospective study). *Lancet* **1**(7954), 272–275.

Shum, S., Jensen, N. M., and Nebert, D. W. (1979). The murine Ah locus: *In utero* toxicity and teratogenesis associated with genetic differences in benzo[a]pyrene metabolism. *Teratology* **20**(3), 365–376.

Sims, P., and Grover, P. L. (1974). Epoxides in polycyclic aromatic hydrocarbon metabolism and carcinogenesis. *Adv. Cancer Res.* **20,** 165.

Smithells, R. W., Nevin, N. C., and Seller, M. J. (1983). Further experience of vitamin supplementation for prevention of neural tube defect recurrences. *Lancet* **I,** 1027–1031.

South, J. (1972). Teratogenic effect of anticonvulsants. *Lancet* **2**(7787), 1154.

Speidel, B. D., and Meadow, S. R. (1972). Maternal epilepsy and abnormalities of fetus and the newborn. *Lancet* **2**(7782), 839–43.

Spielberg, S. P., Gordon, G. B., Blake, D. A., MeUits, E. D., and Bross, D. S. (1981). Anticonvulsant toxicity *in vitro*: Possible role of arene oxides. *J. Pharmacol. Exp. Ther.* **217,** 386–389.

Stanley, O. H., and Chambers, T. L. (1982). Sodium valproate and neural tube defects. *Lancet* **2,** 1282–1283.

Starreveld-Zimmerman, A. A., Kolk, W. J. V. D., Meinardi, H., *et al.* (1973). Are anticonvulsants teratogenic? *Lancet* **2**(819), 48–49.

Steegers-Theunissen, R. P., Renier, W. O., Borm, G. F., *et al.* (1994). Factors influencing the risk of abnormal pregnancy outcome in epileptic women: A multi-centre prospective study. *Epilepsy Res.* **18**(3), 261–269.

Strickler, S. M., Dansky, L. V., Miller, M. A., *et al.* (1985). Genetic predisposition to phenytoin-induced birth defects. *Lancet* **2**(8458), 746–749.

Tein, I., and MacGregor, D. L. (1985). Possible valproate toxicity. *Arch. Neurol.* **42,** 291–293.

Thomas, S. V., Indrani, L., Devi, G. C., Jacob, S., Beegum, J., Jacob, P. P., Kesavadas, K., Radhakrishnan, K., and Sarma, P. S. (2001). Pregnancy in women with epilepsy: Preliminary results of Kerela registry of epilepsy and pregnancy. *Neurol. India* **49,** 60–66.

Vajda, F. J., O'Brien, T. J., Hitchcock, A., *et al.* (2003). The Australian registry of anti-epileptic drugs in pregnancy: Experience after 30 months. *J. Clin. Neurosci.* **10**(5), 543–549.

Vajda, F. J., O'brien, T. J., Hitchcock, A., Graham, J., Cook, M., Lander, C., and Eadie, M. J. (2004). Critical relationship between sodium valproate dose and human teratogenicity: Results of the Australian register of anti-epileptic drugs in pregnancy. *J. Clin. Neurosci.* **11**(8), 854–858.

VanAllen, M. I., Kalousek, D. K., Chernoff, G. F., Juriloff, D., Harris, M., and McGillivray, B. C. (1993). Evidence for multi-site closure of the neural tube in humans. *Am. J. Genet.* **47,** 723–743.

Vergel, R. G., Sanchez, L. R., Heredero, B. L., Rodrigez, P. L., and Martinez, A. J. (1990). Primary prevention of neural tube defects with folic acid supplementation: Cuban experience. *Prenat. Diagn.* **10**(3), 149–152.

Weber, M., Schweitzer, M., Andre, J. M., *et al.* (1977). Epilepsy, anticonvulsants and pregnancy. *Arch. Fr. Pediatr.* **34**(4), 374–383.

Webster, W. S., Lipson, A. H., and Brown-Woodman, P. D. C. (1987). Uterine trauma and limb defects. *Teratology* **28**, 1–8.

Wells, P. G., and Harbison, R. D. (1980). Significance of the phenytoin reactive arene oxide intermediate, its oxepin tautomer, and clinical factors modifying their roles in phenytoin-induced teratology. *In* "Phenytoin-Induced Teratology and Gingival Pathology" (T. M. Hassell, M. C. Johnston, and K. H. Dudley, Eds.), pp. 83–108. Raven Press, New York.

Wells, P. G., Kuper, A., Lawson, J. A., and Harbison, R. D. (1982). Relahon of *in vivo* drug metabolism to stereoselective fetal hydantoin toxicology in mouse: Evaluation of mephenytoin and its metabolite, nirvanol. *J. Pharmacol. Exp. Ther.* **221**, 228–234.

Wells, P. G., Zubovits, J. T., Wong, S. T., *et al.* (1989). Modulation of phenytoin teratogenicity and embryonic covalent binding by acetylsalicylic acid, caffeic acid, and alpha-phenyl-N-t-butylnitrone: Implications for bioactivation by prostaglandin synthetase. *Toxicol. Appl. Pharmacol.* **97**(2), 192–202.

Werler, M. M., Shapiro, S., and Mitchell, A. A. (1993). Periconceptual folic acid exposure and risk of occuring neural tube defects. *JAMA* **269**, 1257–1261.

Werler, M. M., Louik, C., Shapiro, S., and Mitchell, A. A. (1996). Prepregnant weight in relation to risk of neural tube defects. *JAMA* **275**, 1089–1092.

Wide, K., Winbladh, B., and Kallen, B. (2004). Major malformations in infants exposed to antiepileptic drugs *in utero*, with emphasis on carbamazepine and valproic acid: A nation-wide, population-based register study. *Acta Paediatr.* **93**(2), 174–176.

Winship, K. A., Cahal, D. A., Weber, J. C. P., and Griffin, J. P. (1984). Maternal drug histories and central nervous system anomalies. *Arch. Dis. Child* **59**, 1052–1060.

Wong, M., and Wells, P. G. (1988). Effects of N-acetylcysteine on fetal development and on phenytoin teratogenicity in mice. *Teratog. Carcinog Mutagen.* **8**, 65–79.

Wong, M., and Wells, P. G. (1989). Modulation of embryonic glutathione reductase and phenytoin teratogenicity by 1,3-bis(2-chloroethyl i 1-nitrosurea (BCNU). *J. Pharmacol. Exp. Ther.* **250**, 336–342.

Wu, S. P., Shyu, M. K., Liou, H. H., *et al.* (2004). Interaction between anticonvulsants and human placental carnitine transporter. *Epilepsia* **45**(3), 204–210.

Zhu, M., and Zhou, S. (1989). Reduction of the teratogenic effects of phenytoin by folic acid and a mixture of folic acid, vitamins, and amino acids: A preliminary trial. *Epilepsia* **30**, 246–251.

ANTIEPILEPTIC DRUG TERATOGENESIS: WHAT ARE THE RISKS FOR CONGENITAL MALFORMATIONS AND ADVERSE COGNITIVE OUTCOMES?

Cynthia L. Harden

Department of Neurology, Leonard M. Miller School of Medicine,
University of Miami, Miami, Florida, USA

I. Introduction
II. Criteria for High-Quality Studies that Assess AED-Related Teratogenesis
III. The Risk of MCMs with AEDs Overall Among WWE
IV. Are Some AEDs Associated with More Risk of MCMs than Others?
V. Polytherapy Versus Monotherapy MCM Risk
VI. Relationship of Dose to Malformations
VII. AED-Specific MCMs
VIII. AED-Related Cognitive Teratogenesis
IX. Minor Malformations
X. Conclusions
References

Antiepileptic drug (AED) exposure *in utero* has been associated with major congenital malformations (MCMs) and adverse cognitive outcomes in the offspring of women with epilepsy (WWE). However, determining the exact risk and the relative risks of AEDs for these outcomes has been challenging, and only in recent years has improved study designs enabled us to get a clearer picture of the risks. Still, there is a startling lack of information for many of the newer and widely used AEDs. At this point of time, studies clearly show that valproate (VPA) as a part of polytherapy or when used as a monotherapy is associated with an increased risk of MCMs, and that it poses about threefold the risk of carbamazepine (CBZ). It is unclear if any other AEDs studied pose an increased risk of MCM occurrence; in the best available large study the absolute rates of MCMs with other several other AEDs were not different from untreated WWE. The absolute risks have been reported as CBZ 2.2%, lamotrigine (LTG) 3.2%, phenytoin (PHT) 3.7%, untreated WWE 3.5%, with VPA as the outlier at 6.2%. *In utero* VPA exposure is also associated with a risk of lower verbal intelligence quotient (IQ) in children, at ~10 points lower than controls. CBZ appears to pose no risk to cognitive outcome, and there is some evidence that PHT and phenobarbital (PB) may be associated with risk of reduced cognitive outcome. Polytherapy is associated with greater risk than monotherapy for both MCMs and cognitive outcome.

Although more information is needed and hopefully will be obtained from ongoing prospective studies, it is clear that WWE taking VPA and planning pregnancy should have a discussion with their physician about considering changing to another AED before pregnancy, if possible.

I. Introduction

The magnitude of teratogenic risks due to antiepileptic drugs (AEDs) has been a moving target since the association was first put forth in 1964 (Janz and Fuchs, 1964). Since then, hundreds of reports have emerged associating every available AED with minor and major congenital malformations (MCMs). With all this data, how can the absolute magnitude of risk and the relative risks of AED-related teratogenesis can be determined when many articles are confined to retrospective series from one hospital or even from a single neurologic practice? Further, it remains a frustrating and unsatisfying phenomenon that human AED-related teratogenic information is gathered only well after AEDs are marketed; this has been the case in the United States and in other countries as well. This situation cannot help but give the impression that the outcome of pregnancies to women with epilepsy (WWE) is a low priority, although there are many highly vested groups involved, including patients, physicians, economists, the pharmaceutical industry, and the American Food and Drug Administration. Most disconcerting is that some of the most widely used of the newer generation of AEDs have been used worldwide for 8–12 years and there is still little information available with which to advise our female patients of child-bearing potential.

Fortunately, AED-pregnancy outcome registries have been established across the globe over the past 10–15 years, and the valiant efforts of these investigators are bringing us closer to the true picture of AED-related teratogenic risks. The data discussed in this chapter will be confined to those registries and prospective studies that comprise some of the most scientifically rigorous, peer-reviewed evidence on this topic; it is hoped that this information is improving both the precision and accuracy of the "moving target" of AED-related teratogenesis.

II. Criteria for High-Quality Studies that Assess AED-Related Teratogenesis

The most scientifically rigorous studies evaluating causative factors choose subjects to enroll in the most unbiased manner possible and follow subjects prospectively. For AED-related teratogenesis, this means that women should be enrolled before knowing any information regarding the progress of their pregnancy, basically before the first ultrasound is performed. The studies should be population based or population representative, which are sometimes the most difficult research criteria to achieve. However, it is more easily accomplished in countries when health care is provided from a national system and much less easily accomplished in the United States. Known and accepted confounders should be taken into account in the statistical analysis. For the analyses under consideration here, the confounders would include maternal age and socioeconomic status, and in particular maternal intelligence quotient (IQ) for cognitive teratogenesis, since this is the single most important influence on the child's IQ in group studies (Sattler, 1992). Although the outcome for MCMs is so objective as to not require blinding as to AED exposure, the cognitive outcomes are more subtle and high-quality studies would include a blinded or masked assessment. Neither evaluation (MCMs or cognitive outcomes) is amenable to a randomized paradigm, in that the AED treatment for the mother's seizures is already determined and randomization would be unethical. The studies discussed herein generally meet or approach these rigorous criteria. For clarification, MCMs are defined as structural abnormalities with surgical, medical, or cosmetic importance according to the definition of Holmes *et al.* (2001).

III. The Risk of MCMs with AEDs Overall Among WWE

Comparing the outcomes in the offspring of WWE taking AEDs to those not taking AEDs is a strategy that attempts to control for a confounding factor that still has not been well sorted out, that of the contribution of maternal epilepsy. It is thought that the risk imparted by epilepsy itself is minimal (Fried *et al.*, 2004), but there are confounding factors that cannot be equal between these two groups, with seizure frequency and severity being the most obvious. Therefore, even when using WWE not taking AEDs as a comparator group for WWE taking AEDs, the confounding factor of epilepsy itself cannot be completely eliminated.

That being stated, when using the single available rigorous study with large numbers of treated ($n = 3186$) and untreated WWE ($n = 227$) (Morrow *et al.*, 2006), it is actually difficult to find evidence that taking AEDs in general increases the risk of MCMs. In this study, the relative risk was 1.19 (0.59–2.40) and the results are not significant as shown by wide confidence intervals. Two smaller retrospective studies, however, found significantly increased risks of MCMs with maternal AED exposure compared to an untreated group of WWE (Holmes *et al.*, 2001) [OR 3.92 (1.29–11.90)], and Artama *et al.* (2005) [OR 1.70 (1.07–2.68)].

When analyzing the data further, valproate (VPA) exposure was responsible for the overall increased risk in the study by Artama *et al.* (2005). When VPA was excluded from the analysis, the risk became nonsignificant and the overall risk estimate became less than one. This effect was also present when the same type of analysis was performed using the data by Morrow et al. (2006). VPA, whether used in polytherapy or as monotherapy contributed to an increased risk of MCMs in the exposed offspring, and no significant risk was imparted by the other AEDs as either polytherapy or monotherapy. The absolute risk of MCMs in the VPA exposed offspring was 6.2% in Morrow et al. (2006).

These analyses give us a clearer picture that VPA is teratogenic and further provide little evidence that other AEDs are significantly teratogenic. It should be kept in mind, however, that none of these studies include significant numbers of the newer AEDs.

These data also raise the question as to whether these studies found any nonteratogenic AEDs. Morrow et al. (2006), is the only study with substantial numbers of WWE treated with specific AEDs. The findings suggest no increased risk of MCMs for carbamazepine (CBZ) [RR 0.63 (0.28–1.41)] and for lamotrigine (LTG) [RR 0.92 (0.41–2.05] exposure, although wide confidence intervals indicate that possibility of some increased risk cannot be excluded. The absolute rate of MCMs for CBZ was 2.2% and for LTG was 3.2%, both of which are lower that the rate in untreated WWE of 3.5%.

IV. Are Some AEDs Associated with More Risk of MCMs than Others?

It follows from the previous discussion that VPA likely poses more risk than other AEDs. Indeed, two large, prospective, population-representative studies that VPA is associated with a greater risk for MCMs than CBZ, with ~2.5 to 3-fold greater risk with VPA than CBZ (Morrow et al., 2006; Wide et al., 2004) Further, VPA as a part of polytherapy was associated with 2.5-fold greater risk than polytherapy without VPA (Morrow et al., 2006). In the study by Artama et al. (2005), there is negligible difference in risk between VPA as a part of polytherapy versus VPA as monotherapy [OR 0.85 (0.63–1.13]. Other studies showed that VPA is associated with a ninefold greater risk than phenytoin (PHT) (Samren et al., 1999), a sixfold greater risk than LTG (Vajda et al., 2006) and a sixfold greater risk than phenobarbital (PB) (Canger et al., 1999).

Therefore, although much information is lacking regarding the newer AEDs, there is clear evidence that VPA carries more teratogenic risk than CBZ and when used as part of polytherapy, and likely carries more risk than LTG, PHT, and PB. Little difference in the absolute risk between LTG, PHT, and CBZ is present in Morrow et al. (2006); the absolute risk for PHT was 3.7% in this data set. Overall, no significant differences between the risks of AEDs other than with VPA can be discerned.

V. Polytherapy Versus Monotherapy MCM Risk

In the most rigorous study addressing the question of polytherapy versus monotherapy, Morrow *et al.* (2006) showed an increased risk with polytherapy versus monotherapy [RR 1.62 (1.14–2.31)]. Many other studies, which were usually not population representative, prospective, or assessing large numbers of subjects, showed an increased risk as well, but did not reach significance. Importantly, no study showed a decreased risk with polytherapy versus Monotherapy; therefore, this is a situation in which a large, carefully performed study was needed to prove what was strongly suggested in previous work.

VI. Relationship of Dose to Malformations

Many studies have found a relationship between VPA dose and MCMs (Artama *et al.*, 2005; Canger *et al.*, 1999; Mawer *et al.*, 2002; Meador *et al.*, 2006; Omtzigt *et al.*, 1992; Samren *et al.*, 1997, 1999; Vajda *et al.*, 2006). The cutoff point for VPA dose above which MCMs were significantly more likely to occur was not consistent, but was ~1000 mg per day in five studies (Mawer *et al.*, 2002; Omtzigt *et al.*, 1992; Samren *et al.*, 1997, 1999; Vajda *et al.*, 2006). In Morrow *et al.* (2006), a relationship between AED dose and MCMs was reported for LTG but not for VPA, however, a relationship between dose and MCMs for LTG was not found in the Lamotrigine Pregnancy Registry, which has assessed several thousand LTG-exposed pregnancies (Cunnington and Tennis, 2005). Therefore, at this time, there is a body of evidence suggesting a dose-malformation relationship with VPA, and emerging evidence regarding LTG; whether this dose-malformation relationship for LTG is borne out in other studies remains to be seen.

VII. AED-Specific MCMs

AED-related MCMs fit into a pattern of teratogenicity, therefore all of the outcomes discussed herein have been reported with each AED. However, some MCMs occur more frequently in relationship to a single AED. There is strong evidence from multiple studies that VPA is associated with neural tube defects including *spina bifida*, as well as midline defects of *hypospadias*, and facial clefts (Arpino *et al.*, 2000; Bertollini *et al.*, 1985; Morrow *et al.*, 2006; Samren *et al.*, 1999). There is also evidence for an increased risk for cleft palate with PHT and posterior cleft palate with CBZ (Puho *et al.*, 2007). Cardiac malformations appear to be specifically associated with PB (Arpino *et al.*, 2000; Canger *et al.*, 1999). More information about specific malformations in relationship to other AEDs, particularly for facial clefts with LTG, will be forthcoming as more data from pregnancy registries emerge.

VIII. AED-Related Cognitive Teratogenesis

The assessment for cognitive teratogenesis is quite different than for MCMs. The studies must be blinded or masked due to the relative subjectivity of the outcome. Confounders, such as social environment and maternal IQ, must be accounted for in the analysis. Further, the intellectual assessment of young children begins to be reliable only after the age of 2 years, therefore the studies must be long term in design. Another consideration is the timing of exposure for cognitive versus structural teratogenesis. MCMs develop within the first 13 weeks of gestation; however, there is evidence that perhaps later exposure during pregnancy has a impact on cognitive outcomes (Reinisch *et al.*, 1995). Given these considerations, there are several well-performed studies that shed light on this important concern for WWE. Firstly, similar to the risks for MCMs, several studies indicate that AED polytherapy exposure during pregnancy poses an increased risk for adverse cognitive outcome compared to monotherapy (Gaily *et al.*, 2004; Koch *et al.*, 1999; Lösche *et al.*, 1994).

There is some information regarding the risks of specific AEDS. VPA is associated with reduced cognitive outcomes in children exposed *in utero* (Adab *et al.*, 2004; Gaily *et al.*, 2004). In both studies, the risks for VPA were dose dependent and were greater for children exposed to CBZ and than nonexposed controls. Both studies also found that verbal IQ was specifically affected and that it was ~10 points lower than controls or CBZ-treated patients. In one of these reports, the risk was also greater for VPA than for PHT exposure (Adab *et al.*, 2004).

However, five studies show that CBZ does not increase the risk of reduced cognitive outcome compared to unexposed controls (Adab *et al.*, 2004; Eriksson *et al.*, 2005; Gaily *et al.*, 2004; Scolnik *et al.*, 1994; Wide *et al.*, 2002). Three studies also suggest an increased risk of PHT exposure for reduced cognitive outcomes (Scolnik *et al.*, 1994; Vanoverloop *et al.*, 1992; Wide *et al.*, 2002).

One interesting report indicates that *in utero* exposure to PB is associated with reduced cognitive abilities, specifically verbal IQ, when subjects were tested as adults; this study was only performed in men, which potentially limits its general-izability (Reinisch *et al.*, 1995).

A reassuring finding in this realm is that cognitive outcome appears not to be reduced in children of WWE unexposed to AEDs (Gaily *et al.*, 2004; Holmes *et al.*, 2000). However, VPA is associated with a risk of adverse cognitive outcome. Lesser evidence suggests that PHT and PB may pose some risk to cognition for children exposed *in utero*, but it is reassuring that CBZ does not appear to be associated with risk to cognitive outcome.

IX. Minor Malformations

Minor malformations have not been addressed herein and are in general a difficult outcome to assess. Because of the subtlety of the findings, examiners must be blind to any exposures and these findings require long-term follow-up, since they can change over time. In general, hypoplasia of the midface and fingers are thought to be minor malformations that could be related to *in utero* AED exposure. The significance of these minor malformations has also been unclear. However, one recent report indicated that the presence of these specific minor anomalies can be associated with cognitive developmental delay later in life (Holmes *et al.*, 2005). Seventy-six children whose mothers took AEDs in pregnancy underwent systematic evaluation of physical features and of intelligence using the Wechsler Intelligence Scale for Children scores. Midface or digit hypoplasia correlated significantly with deficits in verbal IQ, performance IQ, and full-scale IQ. Interestingly, there was no decrease in IQ in association with major malforma-tions. The authors concluded that minor malformations should prompt cognitive evaluation in such children.

X. Conclusions

The important risks associated with AEDs during pregnancy are slowly becoming clearer. Much information still remains to be discerned, particularly how to mitigate risks, safe alternatives to VPA, the risks or safety of polyther-apeutic AED combinations that exclude VPA. VPA is clearly associated with more risk for MCMs and adverse cognitive outcomes, and appears to have about threefold the risk for MCMs compared to CBZ, PHT, and LTG for MCMs. The absolute risk of MCMs with VPA is ~6% from the best available data. It is unclear whether there is any increased risk of MCMs with CBZ, LTG, or PHT either as monotherapy or polytherapy; there appears to be a possibility that there is actually no increased risk with these AEDs. Reliable estimates of risks associated with other AEDs are still outstanding.

WWE taking AED should be advised to discuss reasonable options to VPA with their physicians before becoming pregnant and should use effective birth control until a course of action is determined. LTG, topiramate, and levetiracetam may all be appropriate AEDs to maintain seizure control for WWE with primary generalized epilepsy in particular, but as yet there is little information regarding the safety of topiramate and levetiracetam during pregnancy. It is hoped that information from multiple pregnancy registries will soon be forthcoming and to help us further guide our patient. Ongoing long-term studies such as the NEAD study (neurodevelopmental effects of antiepileptic drugs) will help to clarify the relative risks to cognitive outcome of VPA, CBZ, LTG, and PHT.

References

Adab, N., Kini, U., Vinten, J., Ayres, J., Baker, G., Clayton-Smith, J., Coyle, H., Fryer, A., Gorry, J., Gregg, J., Mawer, G., Nicolaides, P., et al. (2004). The longer term outcome of children born to mothers with epilepsy. *J. Neurol. Neurosurg. Psychiatry* **75**(11), 1575–1583.

Arpino, C., Brescianini, S., Robert, E., et al. (2000). Teratogenic effects of antiepileptic drugs: Use of an international database on malformations and drug exposure (MADRE). *Epilepsia* **41**(11), 1436–1443.

Artama, M., Auvinen, A., Raudaskoski, T., Isojarvi, I., and Isojarvi, J. (2005). Antiepileptic drug use of women with epilepsy and congenital malformations in offspring. *Neurology* **64**, 1874–1878.

Bertollini, R., Mastoiacovo, P., and Segni, G. (1985). Maternal epilepsy and birth defects: A case-control study in the Italian Multicenter Registry of Birth Defects (IPIMC). *Eur. J. Epidemiol.* **1**(1), 67–72.

Canger, R., Battino, D., Canevini, M. P., et al. (1999). Malformations in offspring of women with epilepsy: A prospective study. *Epilepsia* **40**(9), 1231–1236.

Cunnington, M., and Tennis, P. and the International Lamotrigine Pregnancy Registry Scientific Advisory Committee (2005). Lamotrigine and the risk of malformations in pregnancy. *Neurology* **64**, 955–960.

Eriksson, K., Viinikainen, K., Mönkkönen, A., Äikiä, M., Nieminen, P., Heinonen, S., and Kälviäinen, R. (2005). Children exposed to valproate in utero—Population based evaluation of risks and confounding factors for long-term neurocognitive development. *Epilepsy Res.* **65**, 189–200.

Fried, S., Kozer, E., Nulman, I., Einarson, T. R., and Koren, G. (2004). Malformation rates in children of women with untreated epilepsy: A meta-analysis. *Drug Saf.* **27**(3), 197–202.

Gaily, E., Kantola-Sorsa, E., Hiilesmaa, V., Isoaho, M., Matila, R., Kotila, M., Nylund, T., Bardy, A., Kaaja, E., and Granstrom, M. L. (2004). Normal intelligence in children with prenatal exposure to carbamazepine. *Neurology* **62**(1), 28–32.

Holmes, L. B., Coull, B. A., Dorfman, J., and Rosenberger, P. B. (2005). The correlation of deficits in IQ with midface and digit hypoplasia in children exposed *in utero* to anticonvulsant drugs. *J. Pediatr.* **146**, 118–122.

Holmes, L. B., Harvey, E. A., Coull, B. A., *et al.* (2001). The teratogenicity of anticonvulsant drugs. *N. Eng. J. Med.* **344**(15), 1132–1138.

Holmes, L. B., Rosenberger, P. B., Harvey, E. A., Khoshbin, S., and Ryan, L. (2000). Intelligence and physical features of children of women with epilepsy. *Teratology* **61**(3), 196–202.

Janz, D., and Fuchs, M. (1964). Are antiepileptic drugs harmful when given during pregnancy? *Ger. Med. Mon.* **9**, 20–22.

Koch, S., Titze, K., Zimmermann, R. B., Schröder, M., Lehmkuhl, U., and Rauh, H. (1999). Long-term neuropsychological consequences of maternal epilepsy and anticonvulsant treatment during pregnancy for school-age children and adolescents. *Epilepsia* **40**(9), 1237–1243.

Lösche, G., Steinhausen, H. C., Koch, S., and Helge, H. (1994). The psychological development of children of epileptic parents. II. The differential impact of intrauterine exposure to anticonvulsant drugs and further influential factors. *Acta Paediatr.* **83**(9), 961–966.

Mawer, G., Clayton-Smith, J., Coyle, H., and Kini, U. (2002). Outcome of pregnancy in women attending an outpatient epilepsy clinic; adverse features associated with higher doses of sodium valproate. *Seizure* **11**, 512–518.

Meador, K. J., Baker, G. A., Finnell, R. H., *et al.* (2006). *In utero* antiepileptic drug exposure: Fetal death and malformations. *Neurology* **67**, 407–412.

Morrow, J., Russell, A., Guthrie, E., *et al.* (2006). Malformations risks of antiepileptic drugs in pregnancy: A prospective study from the UK Epilepsy and Pregnancy Register. *J. Neurol. Neurosurg. Psychiatry* **77**, 193–198.

Omtzigt, J. G. C., Los, F. J., Grobbee, D. E., *et al.* (1992). The risk of spina bifida aperta after first-trimester exposure to valproate in a prenatal cohort. *Neurology* **42**(Suppl. 5), 119–125.

Puho, E. H., Szunyogh, M., Metneki, J., and Czeizel, A. E. (2007). Drug treatment during pregnancy and isolated orofacial clefts in Hungary. *Cleft Palate-Craniofac. J.* **4**(2), 194–202.

Reinisch, J. M., Sanders, S. A., Mortensen, E. L., and Rubin, D. B. (1995). *In utero* exposure to phenobarbital and intelligence deficits in adult men. *JAMA* **274**(19), 1518–1525.

Samren, E. B., van Duijn, C. M., Christiaens, G. C. M. L., Hofman, A., and Lindhout, E. (1999). Antiepileptic drug regimens and major congenital abnormalities in the offspring. *Ann. Neurol.* **46**, 739–746.

Samren, E. B., van Duijn, C. M., Koch, S., *et al.* (1997). Maternal use of antiepileptic drugs and the risk of major congenital malformations: A joint European prospective study of human teratogenesis associated with maternal epilepsy. *Epilepsia* **38**(9), 981–990.

Sattler, J. M. (1992). "Assessment of Children revd/updated," 3rd ed. Jerome M. Sattler, San Diego.

Scolnik, D., Nulman, I., Rovet, J., Gladstone, D., Czuchta, D., Gardner, H. A., Gladstone, R., Ashby, P., Weksberg, R., Einarson, T., *et al.* (1994). Neurodevelopment of children exposed *in utero* to phenytoin and carbamazepine monotherapy. *JAMA* **271**(10), 767–770.

Vajda, F. J. E., Hitchcock, A., Graham, J., *et al.* (2006). Foetal malformations and seizurescontrol:52 months data of the Australian Pregnancy Registry. *Eur. J. Neurol.* **13**, 645–654.

Vanoverloop, D., Schnell, R. R., Harvey, E. A., and Holmes, L. B. (1992). The effects of prenatal exposure to phenytoin and other anticonvulsants on intellectual function at 4 to 8 years of age. *Neurotoxicol. Teratol.* **14**(5), 329–335.

Wide, K., Henning, E., Tomson, T., and Winbladh, B. (2002). Psychomotor development in preschool children exposed to antiepileptic drugs *in utero*. *Acta Paediatr.* **91**(4), 409–414.

Wide, K., Winbladh, B., and Kallen, B. (2004). Major malformations in infants exposed to antiepileptic drugs *in utero*, with emphasis on carbamazepine and valproic acid: A nation-wide, population-based register study. *Acta Paediatr.* **93**, 1774–176.

TERATOGENICITY OF ANTIEPILEPTIC DRUGS: ROLE OF PHARMACOGENOMICS

Raman Sankar and Jason T. Lerner

David Geffen School of Medicine at UCLA, Mattel Children's Hospital at UCLA, Los Angeles, California 90095-1752, USA

I. Introduction
II. Drug Metabolism
III. Genetics
IV. Conclusion
   References

The teratogenic potential of an antiepileptic drug is determined by the chemical attributes of the molecule under discussion and the genetic attributes of the host. The role of the hepatic mixed function oxidase system may be especially important in conferring teratogenic risk. However, systems such as epoxide hydrolase, glutathione reductase, and superoxide dismutase and other toxin scavenging systems may be important modifiers that lower the risk. Genetic variability in these systems is important in determining the type and severity of the final outcome. While our knowledge of these factors is incomplete, progress can be achieved by beginning to include these concepts in our discussion on the topic and by promoting research that may improve our ability to *individualize* the analysis of risk for a specific patient with regard to specific antiepileptic drugs. Such an approach will most likely involve DNA microchip technology and has the potential to overcome some of the limitations of pregnancy registries. Such an approach may also lead to novel interventions and therapeutics design to lower the teratogenic potential of pharmacologic treatment of epilepsy during conception.

I. Introduction

One of the greatest concerns of women with epilepsy is having a successful pregnancy and delivering a healthy baby. Through clinical experience and pregnancy registries, it is known that there is an increased risk of birth defects

INTERNATIONAL REVIEW OF
NEUROBIOLOGY, VOL. 83
DOI: 10.1016/S0074-7742(08)00012-3

215

while taking certain antiepileptic drugs (AEDs) during pregnancy. While these registries are successful at documenting rates and types of birth defects they fail to evaluate the underlying cause and pathophysiology. The registries are simply designed to monitor the number of pregnancies, AEDs being taken and the outcomes of the pregnancies. It is much more likely that to accurately predict occurrence rates and even help prevent defects in the future we must undertake evaluations at the molecular level, specifically at the interaction between the AED and organ morphogenesis. The mechanisms of metabolism of the medications and the underlying genetic makeup of each individual person are key elements in this interaction (Sankar, 2007). This interaction is determined by the chemical nature of the AED as well as the genetic endowment of the individual host. Nutrition and environmental exposures also have a role in modifying the actions of metabolism and possible teratogenicity.

Drug metabolism plays an important role in teratogenesis. One of the most prominent enzyme systems that has evolved to tackle the detoxification and excretion of foreign compounds (xenobiotics) is the cytochrome P-450 (cyt P-450) family of enzymes. The role of the cyt P-450 family is to oxidize (adding functional group such as a hydorxyl group suitable for conjugation) foreign compounds such as medications to make them water soluble for excretion. This reaction can be summarized as

$$RH + NADPH + H^+ + O_2 \rightarrow R - OH + NADP^+ + H_2O$$

Most central nervous system (CNS)-active drugs possess high lipid solubility and require conjugation to a water-soluble moiety such as glucuronic acid to allow them to be excreted. This mechanism is used during the metabolism of many of the AEDs, including phenytoin (PHT) and carbamazepine (CBZ), and is completed in two phases. The phase 1 reaction (Fig. 1) is actually a two-step process catalyzed by cyt P-450 that produces an intermediate. These intermediate structures are frequently chemically reactive electrophiles and are often susceptible to a nucleophilic attack by biomolecules, including nucleic acid bases, which can contribute to teratogenesis. They can also interact with proteins to modify gene expression and influence morphogenesis. Interaction with proteins that result in covalent binding is also an important step in the generation of haptens that elicit hypersensitivity reactions (Leeder, 1998). The final product of the phase 1 reaction is converted to a glucuronide by the transfer of the glucuronide moiety from UDP-glucuronic acid (UDPGA). This step is catalyzed by UDP-glucuronyl-transferase (Fig. 2).

Drugs that contain an aromatic ring, such as CBZ and lamotrigine (LTG), produce a highly reactive epoxide or arene oxide with great potential which interact with other biological macromolecules with a variety of outcomes. In the

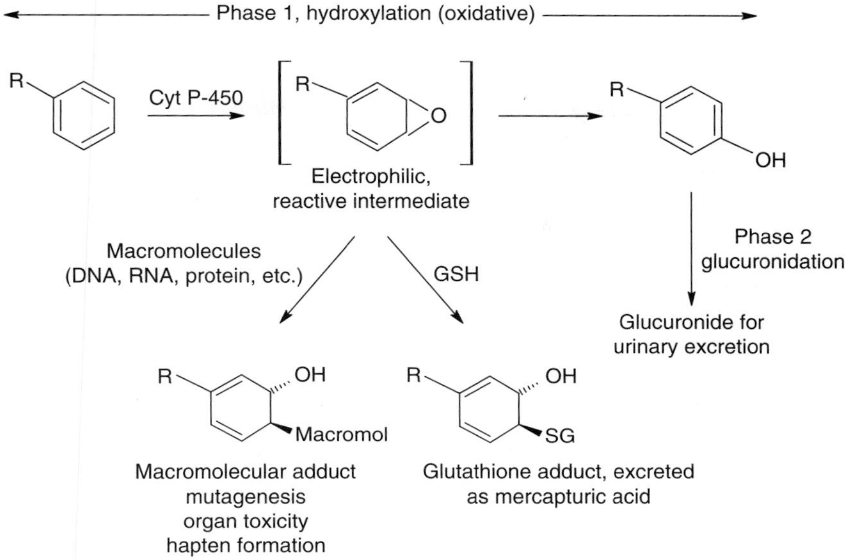

FIG. 1. Formation of electrophilic reactive intermediate by cytochrome P-450 (cyt P-450) can lead to toxicity or be harmlessly excreted as a glucuronide or as a mercapturic acid derivative. Reaction with a protein can lead to hapten generation, while interaction with a nucleic acid can lead to teratogenicity.

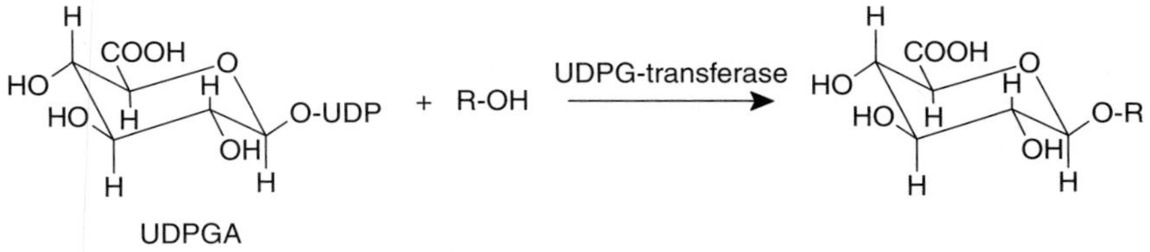

FIG. 2. Phase 2 reaction involving glucuronidation. The drug molecule R-H was oxidized to R-OH by Phase 1 reaction involving cytochrome P-450 (cyt P-450). The final product of Phase 2 reaction is a highly water-soluble glucuronide derivative of the original drug.

majority of cases, this intermediate is made innocuous through a variety of mechanisms, including conversion to a phenolic hydroxyl group (easily glucuronidated for urinary excretion) or reacting with glutathione (containing a neucleophilic sulfhydryl group that reacts with the electrophilic site of the molecule). Other enzyme systems that could play a critical part in the scavenging of reactive intermediates capable of lipid peroxidation include catalase and superoxide dismutase. In the case of PHT, the CYP2C9 and CYP2C19 types of cyt P-450 are involved. The interaction between teratogenic exposure of PHT and relevant tissues (maternal liver and placenta) has been studied in mice, and the results support the notion that the activity of reactive intermediate-scavenging systems such as glutathione reductase, superoxide dismutase, catalase, and others may play a role in teratogenesis (Amicarelli *et al.*, 2000). Interaction of the arene oxide with a protein can form a hapten capable of eliciting an immunological reaction. This can increase the probability of Stevens-Johnson syndrome (SJS) when a severe and sometimes fatal rash is caused by a cutaneous reaction involving a hapten produced in this manner (Leeder , 1998). If the arene oxide reacts with a nucleic acid, this can alter transcription which may be a major cause of teratogenicity. The primary goal is to get the intermediate to Phase 2 reaction (glucuronidation) which is catalyzed by UDP-glucuronyltransferase and produces a highly water-soluble product for urinary excretion.

II. Drug Metabolism

The metabolism of CBZ (briefly discussed above, Fig. 3), PHT, LTG (Fig. 4), and valproic acid (VPA, Fig. 5) provide excellent examples of the mechanisms and theories discussed. The structure of CBZ consists of two aromatic rings linked by a double bond. Phase 1 is catalyzed by the CYP3A4 form of cyt P-450. The intermediate structure formed is a highly reactive epoxide. CYP3A4 is a highly inducible enzyme by many drugs including many of the AEDs. Phase 2 is catalyzed by microsomal epoxide hydrolase (mEH, gene symbol EPHX1) which is known to exhibit polymorphisms (Hassett *et al.*, 1997) which result in a large variation in how individuals hydrolyze epoxide intermediates.

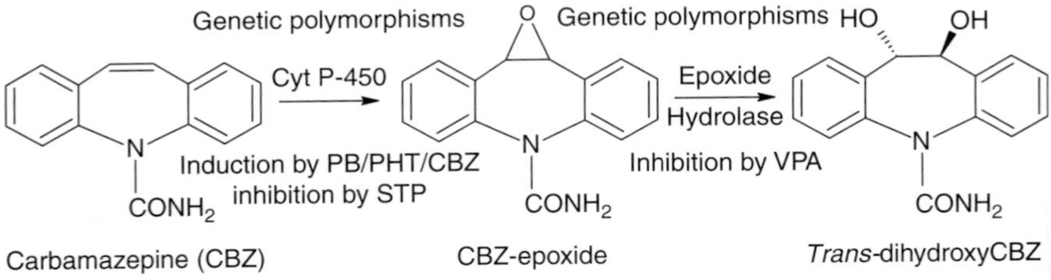

FIG. 3. Carbamazepine (CBZ) is converted to a reactive epoxide that can interact with macromolecules to produce toxicity. This epoxide is rendered harmless by epoxide hydrolase and the resulting product (Phase 1 metabolite) can be glucuronidated (Phase 2 reaction) to facilitate urinary excretion. Genetic and environmental (drug interaction) factors can modify all steps of these processes.

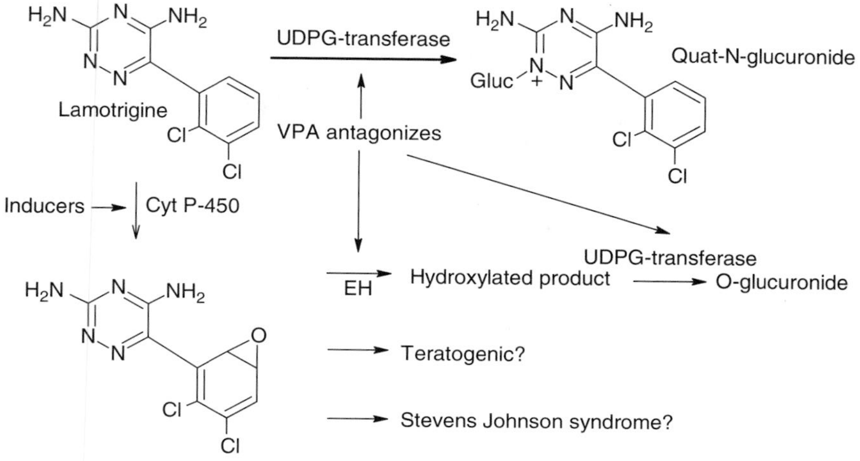

FIG. 4. Metabolism of lamotrigine (LTG) illustrating several steps where drug interactions can modify the teratogenicity as well as the potential for cutaneous toxicity of this antiepileptic drug (AED).

PHT metabolism produces an arene oxide intermediate in the process of conversion to a hydroxylated product. Animal studies (Martz *et al.*, 1977) have shown that mice exposed to PHT in addition to a mEH inhibitor (trichloropropene oxide) displayed an increased incidence of cleft lip and cleft palate in their offspring as well as embryo demise. On further examination increased covalent binding attributed to the arene oxide intermediate metabolite was seen in placental and fetal tissues. Buehler *et al.* (1990) monitored pregnant females taking PHT and found that the 4/19 infants had findings consistent with fetal hydantoin syndrome also had much lower levels of mEH activity compared to the unaffected infants.

During the metabolism of LTG, a quaternary ammonium-linked glucuronide is created as one of the metabolites (Fig. 4). This occurs when the LTG molecule interacts with a UDPG-transferase. If, however, cyt P-450 acts on the LTG structure, an arene oxide is formed which can interact with a protein forming a hapten and possibly causing SJS. This is not typically favored since the two chlorine substituents on the ring make the ring less active. However, with very high doses of LTG or a second medication that induces metabolism, the cyt P-450 pathway may be favored. This is also the case when VPA or another enzyme inducer is given along with the LTG. VPA not only antagonizes UDPG-transferase, but also inhibits mEH which normally would act as a "rescue" system and decrease the levels of the arene oxide produced. Combining this with the inherent high levels of cyt P-450 in children may explain the increased incidence of SJS in this age group. An examination of this pathway also provides a plausible

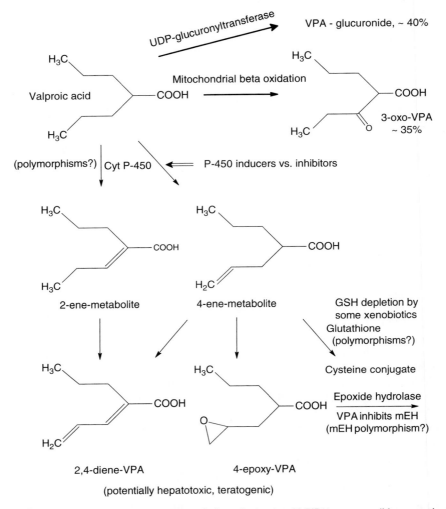

FIG. 5. Several steps involved in the metabolism of valproic acid (VPA) are susceptible to genetic influences as well as induction or inhibition by other agents.

explanation for the observation by Morrow *et al.* (2006), as well as the observation that VPA may exacerbate both the cutaneous toxicity (Schlienger *et al.*, 1998) and teratogenicity (Cunnington and Tennis, 2005) of VPA.

VPA is typically metabolized by three different pathways (Fig. 5): mitochondrial β-oxidation, glucuronidation with UDP-glucuronyltransferase, and through the microsomal cyt P-450 pathway. However, if there is excess VPA, there may be a spill over pushing metabolism toward microsomal oxidation and the cyt P-450 pathway (Anderson *et al.*, 1992). Inducers of cyt P-450 subspecies may also make this probability of microsomal activation of VPA higher (Levy *et al.*, 1990). This pathway produces 2-ene and 4-ene intermediates. The production of the 4-ene intermediate may involve specific isoforms of cyt P-450 (CYP2C9 and CYP2A6) in the human (Sadeque *et al.*, 1997). The 2-ene intermediate is considered nontoxic; however, the 4-ene metabolite may be hepatotoxic. Both may be further converted to problematic derivatives. Levy *et al.* (1990) found that coadministration of stiripentol (STP) with VPA decreased the formation of the 4-ene metabolite. Both mEH and the glutathione system could modify the toxicity of these derivatives, but are subject to the influences of genetic polymorphisms as well the presence of xenobiotics.

In reviewing the mechanisms of metabolism, it is apparent that the classical thinking that the best pregnancy outcomes occur with monotherapy may not always be entirely correct. Even though the results from the different pregnancy registries appear to conclude that one medication is better, the available data is generally confounded by a high incidence of polypharmacy involving enzyme inducers. The Lamictal Pregnancy Registry reevaluated the rate of major congenital malformations (MCM) which, in the LTG monotherapy population was 2.9% while the MCM in polytherapy (not including VPA) was not elevated (2.7%) (Cunnington and Tennis, 2005). This supports the idea that polytherapy is not always inferior to monotherapy and it is likely that the patients taking multiple medications may have been on lower doses of each. It is also essential to evaluate all other medications prescribed along with an AED like LTG. The minimal enzyme inducing activity of the newer AEDs on the market may be their greatest advantage.

Inhibition of cyt P-450-mediated activation may also influence the teratogenicity of certain AEDs (Finnell *et al.*, 1992, 1994, 1995, 1999). Mice given PHT with STP, an AED that is also a cyt P-450 inhibitor, were found to have lower rates of malformations in their offsprings, including cleft lip and cleft palate (Finnell *et al.*, 1999). Indeed, the teratogenicity of CBZ could be increased by phenobarbital pretreatment while STP cotreatment was protective (Finnell *et al.*, 1995). Thus, the guidelines that advocate against polypharmacy on an absolute basis can be challenged, in principle. Unfortunately, we do not have the clinical data at the present time to demonstrate clearly that certain combinations may be safer.

III. Genetics

The role of polymorphisms in cyt P-450 genes such as CYP1A1 and glutathione-S-transferase (GST) in modifying the interactions of xenobiotics with the biological system to produce malformations is beginning to receive attention (Kurahashi *et al.*, 2005). A detailed discussion of cyt P-450 isoforms, their role in AED metabolism, and known human polymorphisms of each isoform are beyond the scope of this chapter. The role of genetics is one possible explanation for the variance between the benign outcome reported by Morrow *et al.* (2006) pertaining to pregnancies with exposure to CBZ and the results of a study in Israel (Ornoy and Cohen, 1996) that reported a significantly poorer pregnancy outcome with CBZ monotherapy in terms of dysmorpholoy and cognitive functioning compared to those that did not involve that AED.

The concept that genetics may play a very important role is supported by the variability seen in the susceptibility of individuals to a variety of adverse events and teratogenicity. A recent study from Taiwan (Yang *et al.*, 2007) reported that a subpopulation of the Han Chinese had HLA-B(*)1502 which predisposed them to CBZ-associated SJS and toxic epidermal necrolysis (TEN). However, Lonjou *et al.* (2008), in a study of SJS and TEN associated with several high risk drugs, found that an HLA-B association was insufficient to explain the risk. This suggests that the determinants for risk for SJS and TEN are likely to be related to multiple genes and more specifically to complex interactions among those genes in an individual. Indeed, knowledge about the polymorphisms associated with the various cyt P-450 isoforms has not led to clear understanding of their relationship to adverse drug reactions (Pirmohamed and Park, 2003). This is likely because other genetic attributes (glutathione system, for example) may modify the risk.

The teratogenic effects of VPA may involve numerous genes, but the expression of many of those may be regulated by histone deacytelase (HDAC) (Kultima *et al.*, 2004). VPA by itself, and some of the metabolites, like the 4-ene, can mediate teratogenesis by inhibition of HDACs (Eikel *et al.*, 2006). The difficulty inherent in attempting a correlation with any one molecular function is highlighted by a recent study (Eyal *et al.*, 2004) of the effects of various AEDs on HDAC and histone acetylation. The authors confirmed a high rate of acetylation in the presence of VPA, but little effect by some of the known teratogens such as CBZ and PHT. They also noted that topiramate had an effect on HDAC that was quantitatively less than that of VPA, and that levetiracetam exhibited no effect on its own, but its metabolite 2-pyrrolidinone-*n*-butyric acid showed a modest effect. VPA itself as well as its metabolite 4-ene can inhibit HDACs, which may be a factor in teratogenicity.

Peroxisome proliferator-activated receptor delta (PPAR-δ) is activated by VPA and the known teratogenic analogues of VPA (Lampen *et al.*, 1999, 2001). That PPAR-δ may be involved in the teratogenicity of VPA in particular, neural tube toxicity, is suggested by the high levels of the receptor expressed during tube development. PPAR-δ may serve as a specific marker for the teratogenic effects of VPA. VPA and its teratogenic derivatives but not the non-teratogenic derivatives induce expression of other molecules possibly involved in teratogenesis, including neural cell adhesion molecule (NCAM) and polysialyltransferase (PST), the roles of which are being actively evaluated (Skladchikova *et al.*, 1998). Also, a blocking agent of PPAR-δ has been shown to prevent the increased expression of NCAM.

IV. Conclusion

As pharmacogenomics evolves, we anticipate improving capability in the hands of the clinician to screen patients for vulnerabilities related to a large number of genetic polymorphisms with DNA microchip technology. The challenges in linking genetic polymorphism to fetal phenotype as expressed by birth defects have been reviewed by Van Dyke *et al.* (2000). At the time of their review in 2000, insufficient correlations between polymorphism and phenotype were available. However, phenotypic correlations with a specific polymorphism may not be readily discerned due to possible coexistence of polymorphisms in other genes that may modify the risk.

We anticipate that research in pharmacogenomics and bioinformatics will evolve to the point that clinicians are given the tools to screen patients for genetic polymorphisms with DNA microchip technology. This would be the first step to determining a pharmacological plan when treating patients, and the risk for a particular patient may based on that patient's genetic endowments, play a more important role in decision making than population-based data. The future may well accommodate "rational polypharmacy" where "rational" requires taking into account not only the pharmacodynamic and pharmacokinetic aspects of the AED to enhance anticonvulsant (and perhaps, antiepileptogenic) efficacy, but also the pharmacogenomically determined propensity of a particular patient to experience significant adverse events or sustain injury to her offspring. The possibility exists that we can develop nontoxic supplements to mitigate teratogenicity in a manner analogous to the use of N-acetyl cysteine to rescue patients form acetaminophen-induced hepatotoxicity. Even nutritional interventions similar to folic acid, to not only prevent teratogenesis but also to alleviate idiosyncratic side effects, may emerge.

References

Amicarelli, F., Tiboni, G. M., Colafarina, S., Bonfigli, A., Iammarrone, E., Miranda, M., and Di Ilio, C. (2000). Antioxidant and GSH-related enzyme response to a single teratogenic exposure to the anticonvulsant phenytoin: Temporospatial evaluation. *Teratology* **62,** 100–107.

Anderson, G. D., Acheampong, A. A., Wilensky, A. J., and Levy, R. H. (1992). Effect of valproate dose on formation of hepatotoxic metabolites. *Epilepsia* **33,** 736–742.

Buehler, B. A., Delimont, D., van Waes, M., and Finnell, R. H. (1990). Prenatal prediction of risk of the fetal hydantoin syndrome. *N. Engl. J. Med.* **322,** 1567–1572.

Cunnington, M., and Tennis, P. International Lamotrigine Pregnancy Registry Scientific Advisory Committee (2005). Lamotrigine and the risk of malformations in pregnancy. *Neurology* **64,** 955–960.

Eikel, D., Lampen, A., and Nau, H. (2006). Teratogenic effects mediated by inhibition of histone deacetylases: Evidence from quantitative structure activity relationships of 20 valproic acid derivatives. *Chem. Res. Toxicol.* **19,** 272–278.

Eyal, S., Yagen, B., Sobol, E., Altschuler, Y., Shmuel, M., and Bialer, M. (2004). The activity of antiepileptic drugs as histone deacetylase inhibitors. *Epilepsia* **45,** 737–744.

Finnell, R. H., Buehler, B. A., Kerr, B. M., Ager, P. L., and Levy, R. H. (1992). Clinical and experimental studies linking oxidative metabolism to phenytoin-induced teratogenesis. *Neurology* **42**(Suppl. 5), 25–31.

Finnell, R. H., Kerr, B. M., van Waes, M., Steward, R. L., and Levy, R. H. (1994). Protection from phenytoin-induced congenital malformations by coadministration of the antiepileptic drug stiripentol in a mouse model. *Epilepsia* **35,** 141–148.

Finnell, R. H., Bennett, G. D., Slattery, J. T., Amore, B. M., Bajpai, M., and Levy, R. H. (1995). Effect of treatment with phenobarbital and stiripentol on carbamazepine-induced teratogenicity and reactive metabolite formation. *Teratology* **52,** 324–332.

Finnell, R. H., Bennett, G. D., Mather, G. G., Wlodarczyk, B., Bajpai, M., and Levy, R. H. (1999). Effect of stiripentol dose on phenytoin-induced teratogenesis in a mouse model. *Reprod. Toxicol.* **13,** 85–91.

Hassett, C., Lin, J., Carty, C. L., Laurenzana, E. M., and Omiecinski, C. J. (1997). Human hepatic microsomal epoxide hydrolase: Comparative analysis of polymorphic expression. *Arch. Biochem. Biophys.* **337,** 275–283.

Kultima, K., Nystrom, A. M., Scholz, B., Gustafson, A. L., Dencker, L., and Stigson, M. (2004). Valproic acid teratogenicity: A toxicogenomics approach. *Environ. Health Perspect.* **112,** 1225–1235.

Kurahashi, N., Sata, F., Kasai, S., Shibata, T., Moriya, K., Yamada, H., Kakizaki, H., Minakami, H., Nonomura, K., and Kishi, R. (2005). Maternal genetic polymorphisms in CYP1A1, GSTM1 and GSTT1 and the risk of hypospadias. *Mol. Hum. Reprod.* **11,** 93–98.

Lampen, A., Siehler, S., Ellerbeck, U., Gottlicher, M., and Nau, H. (1999). New molecular bioassays for the estimation of the teratogenic potency of valproic acid derivatives *in vitro*: Activation of the peroxisomal proliferator-activated receptor (PPARdelta). *Toxicol. Appl. Pharmacol.* **160,** 238–249.

Lampen, A., Carlberg, C., and Nau, H. (2001). Peroxisome proliferator-activated receptor delta is a specific sensor for teratogenic valproic acid derivatives. *Eur. J. Pharmacol.* **431,** 25–33.

Leeder, J. S. (1998). Mechanisms of idiosyncratic hypersensitivity reactions to antiepileptic drugs. *Epilepsia* **39**(Suppl. 7), S8–S16.

Levy, R. H., Rettenmeier, A. W., Anderson, G. D., Wilensky, A. J., Friel, P. N., Baillie, T. A., Acheampong, A., Tor, J., Guyot, M., and Loiseau, P. (1990). Effects of polytherapy with phenytoin, carbamazepine, and stiripentol on formation of 4-ene-valproate, a hepatotoxic metabolite of valproic acid. *Clin. Pharmacol. Ther.* **48,** 225–235.

Lonjou, C., Borot, N., Sekula, P., Ledger, N., Thomas, L., Halevy, S., Naldi, L., Bouwes-Bavinck, J. N., Sidoroff, A., de Toma, C., Schumacher, M., Roujeau, J. C., *et al.* RegiSCAR study group (2008). A European study of HLA-B in Stevens-Johnson syndrome and toxic epidermal necrolysis related to five high-risk drugs. *Pharmacogenet. Genomics* **18,** 99–107.

Martz, F., Failinger, C. 3rd, and Blake, D. A. (1977). Phenytoin teratogenesis: Correlation between embryopathic effect and covalent binding of putative arene oxide metabolite in gestational tissue. *J. Pharmacol. Exp. Ther.* **203,** 231–239.

Morrow, J., Russell, A., Guthrie, E., Parsons, L., Robertson, I., Waddell, R., Irwin, B., McGivern, R. C., Morrison, P. J., and Craig, J. (2006). Malformation risks of antiepileptic drugs in pregnancy: A prospective study from the UK epilepsy and pregnancy register. *J. Neurol. Neurosurg. Psychiatr.* **77,** 193–198.

Ornoy, A., and Cohen, E. (1996). Outcome of children born to epileptic mothers treated with carbamazepine during pregnancy. *Arch. Dis. Child.* **75,** 517–520.

Pirmohamed, M., and Park, B. K. (2003). Cytochrome P450 enzyme polymorphisms and adverse drug reactions. *Toxicology* **192,** 23–32.

Sadeque, A. J., Fisher, M. B., Korzekwa, K. R., Gonzalez, F. J., and Rettie, A. E. (1997). Human CYP2C9 and CYP2A6 mediate formation of the hepatotoxin 4-ene-valproic acid. *J. Pharmacol. Exp. Ther.* **283,** 698–703.

Sankar, R. (2007). Teratogenicity of antiepileptic drugs: Role of drug metabolism and pharmacogenomics. *Acta Neurol. Scand.* **116,** 65–71.

Schlienger, R. G., Shapiro, L. E., and Shear, N. H. (1998). Lamotrigine-induced severe cutaneous adverse reactions. *Epilepsia* **39**(Suppl. 7), S22–S26.

Skladchikova, G., Berezin, V., and Bock, E. (1998). Valproic acid, but not its non-teratogenic analogue 2-isopropylpentanoic acid, affects proliferation, viability and neuronal differentiation of the human teratocarcinoma cell line NTera-2. *Neurotoxicology* **19,** 357–370.

Van Dyke, D. C., Ellingrod, V. L., Berg, M. J., Niebyl, J. R., Sherbondy, A. L., and Trembath, D. G. (2000). Pharmacogenetic screening for susceptibility to fetal malformations in women. *Ann. Pharmacother.* **34,** 639–645.

Yang, C. W., Hung, S. I., Juo, C. G., Lin, Y. P., Fang, W. H., Lu, I. H., Chen, S. T., and Chen, Y. T. (2007). HLA-B*1502-bound peptides: Implications for the pathogenesis of carbamazepine-induced Stevens-Johnson syndrome. *J. Allergy Clin. Immunol.* **120,** 870–877.

ANTIEPILEPTIC DRUG THERAPY IN PREGNANCY I: GESTATION-INDUCED EFFECTS ON AED PHARMACOKINETICS

Page B. Pennell[*] and Collin A. Hovinga[†]

[*]Emory Epilepsy Program, Emory University School of Medicine, Atlanta, Georgia 30322, USA
[†]Departments of Clinical Pharmacy and Pediatrics, University of Tennessee Health Science Center, LeBonheur Children's Medical Center, Memphis, Tennessee 38105, USA

I. Introduction
II. Seizure Frequency and AED Concentrations
III. AEDs During Pregnancy
    A. Phenytoin
    B. Carbamazepine
    C. Phenobarbital
    D. Primidone
    E. Valproic Acid
    F. Ethosuximide
    G. Lamotrigine
    H. Oxcarbazepine
    I. Levetiracetam
IV. Summary
    References

The ideal management of women with epilepsy during pregnancy involves achieving an optimal balance between minimizing fetal exposure to the deleterious influences of both antiepileptic drugs (AEDs) and of seizures. Women with increased seizures during pregnancy tend to have subtherapeutic AED concentrations. Multiple physiological changes during pregnancy influence drug disposition, including increased volume of distribution, increased renal elimination, altered hepatic enzyme activity, and a decline in plasma protein concentrations. Many of the AEDs are characterized by significant increases in clearance during pregnancy. Studies performed thus far provide convincing findings for significant increases in the clearance of lamotrigine and phenytoin during pregnancy; other studies support that phenobarbital, oxcarbazepine, and levetiracetam clearances also most likely increase during pregnancy. Therapeutic drug monitoring of lamotrigine with adjustment of dosages during pregnancy to maintain that individual's target concentration has been shown to decrease the risk for increased seizure frequency. Reports of seizure worsening with decreased concentrations of

INTERNATIONAL REVIEW OF
NEUROBIOLOGY, VOL. 83
DOI: 10.1016/S0074-7742(08)00013-5

other AEDs have been reported but not studied in similar formal protocols. Future studies of formal pharmacokinetic modeling of AEDs during pregnancy, with assessment of maternal and fetal/newborn consequences, could provide an important step toward achieving effective drug dosing to maintain therapeutic objectives for the mother but at the same time minimize fetal drug exposure.

I. Introduction

Approximately 1.1 million women with epilepsy are of child-bearing age in the United States and give birth to over 20,000 babies each year (Yerby, 2000). Pregnancy in women with epilepsy is accompanied by increased maternal risks and increased adverse neonatal outcomes compared to the general population, not only due to antiepileptic drugs (AEDs) but also due to seizure occurrence. Over the past decade, consensus guidelines have emphasized minimizing the associated risks by optimizing a woman's AED regimen and initiating supplemental folic acid prior to conception (Report of the Quality Standards Subcommittee of the American Academy of Neurology, 1998). However, there are no guidelines regarding the best management once a woman with epilepsy is pregnant. It is generally agreed that avoidance of generalized tonic-clonic seizures during pregnancy is paramount, and that avoidance of all seizure types is desirable for psychosocial and socioeconomic reasons as well as for the physical well-being of the mother and the fetus (Zahn et al., 1998). Maintaining seizure control during pregnancy requires an understanding of the time course and magnitude of gestation-induced alterations in AED pharmacokinetics. Clinical decisions regarding management of AEDs during pregnancy also need to consider the potential effects of fetal exposure through transplacental transfer. After birth, the newborn may continue to receive exposure to an AED through ingestion of breast milk. Fetal and neonatal exposure to AEDs through transplacental and breast milk passage is discussed in detail in the following chapter.

II. Seizure Frequency and AED Concentrations

Some studies have examined the correlation of AED concentrations during pregnancy and seizure occurrence. Although reduction of the AED concentration is not always accompanied by an increase in seizure frequency, it is remarkable that many of these studies report that the women with increased seizures tended to have subtherapeutic AED concentrations (Dansky et al., 1980, 1982;

Janz, 1982; Otani, 1985; Pennell, 2003; Schmidt *et al.*, 1982, 1983). A study by Dansky *et al.* (1980) of women on phenytoin (PHT) during pregnancy reported that approximately half of the women who had at least a 25% decrease in their total PHT level/dose ratio demonstrated an increase in seizure frequency. Krishnamurthy *et al.* (2002) followed 23 pregnancies of women on monotherapy with phenobarbital (PB), PHT, carbamazepine (CBZ), or valproic acid (VPA). Half of these pregnant women on PB, PHT, or CBZ were associated with breakthrough seizures when the drug levels fell below the patient's therapeutic range. A more recent detailed prospective study of lamotrigine (LTG) and seizure frequency in women with epilepsy during pregnancy reported that the risk for seizure worsening occurred when the serum LTG concentration fell to less than 65% of the target concentration, determined for each individual based on prepregnancy information (Pennell *et al.*, 2008).

In addition to the direct effects of pregnancy on AED concentrations, non-compliance may play a major role in women with increased seizures (Otani, 1985; Schmidt *et al.*, 1983). Pregnancy is also associated with other physiologic and psychological factors that can alter seizure control, including marked increases in sex steroid hormone concentrations, anxiety and stress, and sleep deprivation.

III. AEDs During Pregnancy

Multiple physiologic changes occur during the course of pregnancy that influence drug disposition (DeVane *et al.*, 2006; Leppik and Rask, 1988; McAuley and Anderson, 2002; Pennell, 2003; Tomson and Battino, 2007). These are summarized in Table I. The expansion of plasma volume alters the volume of distribution and therefore the elimination half-life of drugs. Increased

TABLE I
PHYSIOLOGIC CHANGES DURING PREGNANCY: EFFECTS ON DRUG DISPOSITION

Parameter	Consequences
↑ Total body water, extracellular fluid	Altered drug distribution
↑ Fat stores	↓ Elimination of lipid soluble drugs
↑ Cardiac output	↑ Hepatic blood flow leading to ↑ elimination
↑ Renal blood flow and glomerular flow rate	↑ Renal clearance of unchanged drug
Altered CYP450 activity and UGT activity	Altered systemic absorption & hepatic elimination
↓ Maternal albumin	Altered free fraction; increased availability of drug for hepatic extraction

UGT, UDP-glucuronosyltransferase. CYP450, cytochrome P450.

cardiac output and renal blood flow often leads to enhanced renal drug elimination. Hepatic microsomal enzyme activity can be induced by increased endogenous steroids but competitive inhibition may also occur. A decrease occurs in the
concentrations of the main plasma proteins albumin and alpha 1-acid glycoprotein (α-AGP) that are responsible for the binding of many acidic and basic drugs,
respectively. These changes will affect the free (unbound) fraction that determines
the amount of drug in plasma that is available for therapeutic and adverse effects
at the site of action, tissue distribution, metabolism, and elimination. Albumin
concentration falls from 35 g/liter to 25–30 g/liter during the first half of pregnancy (Krauer et al., 1980), and the free fraction of the AEDs with high protein
binding increases during pregnancy (Perucca and Crema, 1982).

Yerby et al. (1990, 1992) investigated the discrepancy between total AED
concentrations and free AED concentrations of four AEDs that are highly protein
bound: PHT, CBZ, PB, and VPA. They performed prospective, cohort studies of
51 women with epilepsy who were enrolled prior to their second trimester. AED
concentrations at 8 weeks postpartum were used as patient baseline values.
Approximately 80% of the women were on AED monotherapy. AED (total and
free) concentrations were measured monthly at clinic visits until 8 weeks postpartum. Data were organized into subgroups by stage of pregnancy and mean
measures were compared with baseline measures. Although these studies were
limited by lack of correction for dosage and weight changes, this large data set
does provide information on many of the older AEDs. They reported that the free
concentrations did not change as dramatically as the total concentrations, but
were lower than baseline during at least one stage of pregnancy.

Almost all studies of AED levels during pregnancy demonstrate that plasma
concentrations decrease even in the face of constant and, in some cases, increasing
doses, and plasma concentrations tend to increase postpartum (McAuley and
Anderson, 2002; Pennell, 2003; Tomson and Battino, 2007). But the dynamic
changes during pregnancy that influence drug disposition result in varying and
often unpredictable drug dosage requirements in the individual patient. The
different routes of metabolism for individual AEDs are a major factor in the
alterations that occur during pregnancy (Table II). The primary route of metabolism for most of the older AEDs involves the cytochrome P450 (CYP450) pathway, with the exception that VPA is metabolized by β-oxidation (40%) and
glucuronide conjugation (30–50%) (Faught, 2001). LTG is extensively hepatically
metabolized by an isozyme of the UDP-glucuronosyltransferase (UGT) family of
enzymes to the 5N and 2N glucuronide metabolites (Green et al., 1995). The
active metabolite of oxcarbazepine (OXC), the monohydroxy derivative (MHD),
also undergoes significant glucuronidation. Renal elimination is a major pathway
for many of the other newer AEDs.

Several small to moderate-sized studies have investigated the changes in specific
AED concentrations during pregnancy and the puerperium. However, details of

TABLE II

PHARMACOKINETIC CHARACTERISTICS OF THE MAJOR AEDs

AED	Major route of metabolism	Protein binding
PHT	CYP2C9 major; CYP2C19 minor; saturable metabolism	High
PB	30% CYP2C9/CYP2C19; 25% renal; 30% N-glucoside	
CBZ	85% CYPs (CYP3A4 major); 15% glucuronidation; 10,11-epoxide metabolite	High
VPA	50% by glucuronide conjugation; 40% by beta-oxidation; 10% by CYP	High, but saturable binding
PB	CYP2C9 and 2C19	High
PRM	Hepatic biotransformation to PB; renal excretion of parent drug	<20%
LTG	70–90% glucuronidation by UGT1A4 and UGT1A3; Increases/decreases in presence of other meds	55%
TPM	60–80% excreted unchanged; 20–40% CYP; clearance increases in presence of CYP inducers	15%
OXC	Keto-reduction to MHD, then 50% glucuronide conjugation; 27% renal excretion; minor CYP	40%
LEV	66% renal excretion; 24% extrahepatic hydrolysis	0%
ZNS	50% CYP 3A4; 15% N-acetylation, oxidation; 35% renal excretion	60%
PGB	Renal excretion	0%

AED = antiepileptic drug; PHT = phenytoin; CBZ = carbamazepine; VPA = valproic acid; PB = phenobarbital; PRM = primidone; LTG = lamotrigine; TPM = topiramate; OXC = oxcarbazepine; MHD = monohydroxy derivative of oxcarbazepine; LEV = levetiracetam; ZNS = zonisamide; PGB = pregabalin.

concomitant influential factors on AED concentrations such as weight, polytherapy with other AEDs, other medications and illnesses, time of sampling relative to dose, and even dosage changes were often lacking. Even fewer studies reported on free levels for the AEDs that are highly protein bound. These studies of AED metabolism during pregnancy use different measures and varying terminology. The term "clearance" is often used to represent the ratio of "daily dose/steady-state concentration" and may include adjustments for weight. This term allows for comparisons when the dosing has been changed during pregnancy for an individual patient.

A. PHENYTOIN

Previous studies of PHT suggest that apparent clearance increases during pregnancy by 20–150% and is often associated with increased seizures (Bossi *et al.*, 1980; Chen *et al.*, 1982; Dansky *et al.*, 1982; Lander *et al.*, 1980; Tomson *et al.*, 1994). PHT clearance decreases again to pregestational levels over the first 12 weeks postpartum. One case report described a substantial decrease in PHT absorption that led to status epilepticus during pregnancy (Ramsey et al., 1978). Malabsorption may sometimes be related to use of antacids, which can form insoluble complexes with PHT. However, the most common factor responsible for the decrease in PHT concentrations during pregnancy is likely the increased hepatic metabolism by the CYP450 system.

Although the ratio of free PHT to total plasma drug concentration increases during pregnancy, most studies have reported that the actual free-drug concentration still declines significantly (Chen et al., 1982; Perucca and Crema, 1982; Tomson et al., 1994).

Tomson et al. (1994) performed a population-based prospective study of 93 pregnancies in 70 women with epilepsy. The vast majority were on AED monotherapy, with 29 patients on PHT monotherapy and 7 on polytherapy. Dosages were kept constant unless poor seizure control occurred. Total PHT levels decreased steadily throughout pregnancy and by 61% at the end, but free levels only dropped by 16% compared to baseline.

Yerby et al. (1990) reported that the mean concentration of PHT declined by 56% (p 0.005) with the sharpest decline occurring during the first trimester. Although the free concentrations did not change as dramatically, the free concentrations of PHT during all three trimesters were significantly different from baseline ($p < 0.05$), with an overall decrease in free concentration of 31%.

Dickinson et al. (1989) performed an elegant study with use of stable isotope-labeled PHT given intravenously to five women during different time points in pregnancy and postpartum (nonpregnant baseline), for a total of 14 pharmacokinetic studies (Table III). Use of this compound eliminated the impact of bioavailability. The mean ± SD half-life for PHT was significantly shorter in pregnancy than postpartum (31 ± 14 vs 39 ± 28 h). The mean ± SD for whole plasma clearance was also significantly greater (0.025 ± 0.012 vs 0.021 ± 0.013 kg^{-1} h^{-1}), and the mean ± SD Vmax for PHT elimination was significantly greater in pregnancy (1170 ± 600 mg/day) than postpartum (780 ± 470 mg/day).

Lander et al. (1981) prospectively studied 30 women on PHT monthly during pregnancy. The mean ratio of the plasma PHT clearance in the third trimester to that in the pre- or postpregnancy state was 2.5:1 ($p < 0.001$), although the limitations of using plasma clearance calculations for PHT, which is eliminated primarily by Michealis–Minten kinetic mechanisms, was noted by the authors.

B. CARBAMAZEPINE

A prospective study by Tomson et al. (1994) was fairly large with 50 pregnancies including 35 on CBZ monotherapy without a change in dosage. Despite this, results were mixed. Total CBZ concentrations were only slightly lower during the

TABLE III

ALTERATIONS OF AED CLEARANCE AND/OR CONCENTRATIONS DURING PREGNANCY: SUMMARY OF CLASS I, II, AND III STUDIES

AED	Reported increases in clearance	Reported decreases in total concentrations	Reported changes in free AED or metabolites	References
PHT	19–150%	60–70%	Free PHT clearance increased in TM3 by 25%, free PHT concentration decreased by 16–40% in TM3.	Bardy et al. (1987), Dickinson et al. (1989), Lander et al. (1980), Tomson et al. (1994), Yerby et al. (1990), Chen et al. (1982)
CBZ	–11% to +27%	0–12%	No change	Battino et al. (1985), Tomson et al. (1994), Yerby et al. (1985), Yerby et al. (1992)
PB	60%	55%	Decrease in free PB concentration by 50%	Battino et al. (1984), Lander et al. (1981), Yerby et al. (1990)
PRM	Inconsistent	Inconsistent	Decrease in derived PB concentrations, with lower PB/PRM ratios.	Battino et al. (1984), Rating et al. (1982)
VPA	Increased by TM2 and TM3.		No change in clearance of free VPA. Free fraction increased by TM2 and TM3.	Koerner et al. (1989)
ESX	Inconsistent	Inconsistent		Kuhnz et al. (1984), Tomson et al. (1990)
LTG	65–230%, substantial interindividual variability		89% increase in clearance of free LTG	de Haan et al. (2004), Ohman et al. (2000), Pennell et al. (2004), Pennell et al. (2008), Petrenaite et al. (2005), Tran et al. (2002)
OXC		MHD & active moiety decreased by 36–61%.		Christensen et al. (2006), Mazzucchelli et al. (2006)
LEV	243%	60% by TM3		Tomson et al. (2007)

AED, antiepileptic drug; TM, trimester; PHT, phenytoin; CBZ, carbamazepine; PRM, primidone; PB, phenobarbital; VPA, valproic acid; ESX, ethosuximide; LTG, lamotrigine; OXC, oxcarbazepine; MHD, monohydroxy derivative of oxcarbazepine; LEV, levetiracetam.

third trimester and the free CBZ concentrations were unchanged. Plasma clearance of both total and free CBZ actually decreased during pregnancy compared to baseline. Other studies have supported little (<15%) to no change in CBZ clearance during pregnancy (Battino *et al.*, 1985; Yerby *et al.*, 1985, 1992). Findings for free CBZ and CBZ-epoxide concentrations are inconsistent, although some studies indicate that the ratios of these to CBZ tend to increase during pregnancy (Battino *et al.*, 1985; Yerby *et al.*, 1992). CBZ binds to both albumin and α-AGP, which may work together to resist changes in protein binding during pregnancy (Perucca and Crema, 1982).

C. Phenobarbital

Limited studies of PB during pregnancy suggest that clearance increases throughout pregnancy (Battino *et al.*, 1984; Lander *et al.*, 1981; Yerby *et al.*, 1990). Yerby *et al.* (1990) reported that the mean concentrations of total PB declined by 55% as pregnancy progressed ($p < 0.005$), with the sharpest decline during the first trimester. Free concentration decreases of PB were statistically significant ($p < 0.005$), with a decrease of 50%. Despite prospectively studying only seven women on PB monthly during pregnancy, Lander *et al.* (1981) were able to determine that the mean ratio of PB plasma clearance in the third trimester to clearance in the pre- or postpregnancy state was 1.6:1 ($p < 0.001$).

D. Primidone

A study of primidone (PRM) in nine women demonstrated that PRM concentrations tended to increase during the second quarter of pregnancy, but with a lower concentration of derived PB (Battino *et al.*, 1984). Another prospective study in 14 women suggested that both PRM and PB levels decrease, but still with an overall lower PB/PRM ratio (Rating *et al.*, 1982).

E. Valproic Acid

Koerner *et al.* (1989) reported on nine women on VPA with prospective monthly visits. VPA clearance increased in the second trimester and later, but free VPA clearance did not change, consistent with an increase in the free fraction.

F. Ethosuximide

Studies of ethosuximide (ESX) metabolism demonstrate inconsistent changes during pregnancy (Kuhnz *et al.*, 1984; Tomson *et al.*, 1990).

G. LAMOTRIGINE

The magnitude of the reported increases in LTG clearance during pregnancy exceeds that described for AEDs that are primarily eliminated via the cytochrome P450 system. Greater than 90% of LTG is glucuronidated and is controlled primarily by UGT1A4 and to a lesser extent by UGT1A3 (Chen *et al.*, 2005; Green *et al.*, 1998; Green and Tephly, 1996). One theory is that the rising sex steroid hormone concentrations enhance expression of UGTs (Chen *et al.*, 2005). An early retrospective study reported an ~150% increase in LTG Cl in the second and third trimesters of pregnancy ($n = 11$)(Petrenaite *et al.*, 2005), associated with seizure worsening in 45% of the pregnancies and specifically occurring in women that had >60% change in level/dose ratio. Other studies also noted up to 75% of women experienced seizure worsening during pregnancies on LTG or complications of convulsive seizures, status epilepticus, and even fetal loss (de Haan *et al.*, 2004; Tran *et al.*, 2002; Vajda *et al.*, 2006).

Two Class II studies showed an increase in the LTG clearance (Pennell *et al.*, 2004; Tran *et al.*, 2002). The first study by Tran *et al.* (2002) showed >65% increase in clearance between prepregnancy baseline and second and third trimesters, although women on interacting AEDs were included. The second study by Pennell *et al.* (2004) reported that LTG clearance increased until 32 weeks of gestational age, with a peak of 230% above prepregnancy baseline.

A more recent Class I study by Pennell *et al.* (2008) of 53 pregnancies in 53 women, using 305 samples throughout preconception baseline, pregnancy and postpartum reported that both LTG free and total clearance were increased during all three trimesters, with peaks of 94% (total) and 89% (free) in the third trimester. Clearance of free LTG was significantly higher in whites compared to black patients. These studies noted substantial interindividual variability, which may be related to UGT polymorphism variants (Ehmer *et al.*, 2004).

This study also examined therapeutic drug monitoring and seizure frequency, and changes in LTG dosing to avoid postpartum toxicity. The authors reported that seizure frequency significantly increased when the LTG level decreased to 65% of the preconceptional individualized target LTG concentration. This finding supports the recommendation to monitor levels of LTG and possibly other AEDs for which the levels decrease during pregnancy.

Previous studies on LTG noted a rapid decrease in LTG Cl during the early postpartum period with reports of symptomatic toxicity (de Haan *et al.*, 2004; Tran *et al.*, 2002). Pennell *et al.* (2007) also examined the effectiveness of using an empiric postpartum taper schedule for LTG, with steady decreases in dosing at postpartum days 3, 7, and 10, with return to preconception dose or preconception dose plus 50 mg to help counteract the effects of sleep deprivation. Patients were assessed for symptoms of LTG toxicity (dizziness, imbalance, and blurred or double vision). Nonadherence to the standard taper schedule was associated with significantly higher risk of experiencing postpartum toxicity ($p = 0.04$).

H. OXCARBAZEPINE

OXC undergoes keto-reduction to the active MHD. Approximately 50% of MHD undergoes glucuronidation, and the remainder is eliminated via renal excretion and CYP450 metabolism. Not surprisingly, seizure worsening during pregnancy has also been reported for women on OXC. The international EURAP Epilepsy Pregnancy Registry reported on 1956 pregnancies in 1,882 women with epilepsy (2006). Seizure frequency remained unchanged throughout pregnancy in 63.6%, was increased in 17.3%, and decreased in 15.9%. Factors that were associated with an increased risk for occurrence of all seizures were localization-related epilepsy (OR: 2.5; 1.7–3.9) and polytherapy (OR: 9.0; 5.6–14.8). OXC monotherapy was associated with a greater risk for occurrence of convulsive seizures (OR: 5.4; 1.6–17.1). The number or dosage of AEDs were more often increased in pregnancies with seizures (OR: 3.6; 2.8–4.7) or pregnancies treated with OXC monotherapy (OR: 3.7; 1.1–12.9) or LTG monotherapy (OR: 3.8; 2.1–6.9).

Two Class III studies have examined OXC concentrations during pregnancy. Christensen *et al.* (2006) reported retrospectively on nine pregnancies in seven women. The mean dose-corrected concentrations of MHD were decreased during pregnancy ($p = 0.0016$), and were 72% (SD = 13%) in the first trimester, 74% (SD = 17%) in the second trimester, and 64% (SD = 6%) in the third trimester, versus dose-corrected concentration before pregnancy. Mazzucchelli *et al.* (2006) reported on five pregnancies, with measurements of OXC, its active R-(−)- and S-(+)-MHD, and the metabolite CBZ-10,11-trans-dihydrodiol (DHD) at regular intervals. The active moiety was defined as the molar sum of OXC, R-(−)-MHD, and S-(+)-MHD. Alterations were significant for R-(−)-MHD ($p < 0.02$) and borderline for the active moiety ($p = 0.086$). The mean concentration/100 mg dose was 45% lower in the second trimester compared to the puerperium.

I. LEVETIRACETAM

Levetiracetam (LEV) is primarily eliminated via renal excretion (66%), with the remaineder via extrahepatic hydrolysis. One Class II study prospectively examined LEV trough concentrations in 15 pregnancies in 14 women every trimester and at least 1 month postpartum (Tomson *et al.*, 2007). Tomson *et al.* (2007) reported that in the seven women without dosage changes, plasma LEV concentrations during the third trimester were only 40% of baseline concentrations outside pregnancy ($p < 0.001$). For all 12 pregnancies, clearance of

LEV was significantly higher during the third trimester, with an increase from 124.7 $\pm$ 57.9 (mean $\pm$ SD) liter/day at baseline to 427.3 $\pm$ 211.3 ($p < 0.0001$), an increase of 243%.

IV. Summary

The ideal management of women with epilepsy during pregnancy and the postpartum state involves achieving an optimal balance between minimizing fetal and neonatal exposure to the deleterious influences of both AEDs and seizures. Effectiveness of therapeutic drug monitoring has been demonstrated for LTG (Pennell *et al.*, 2008), but future studies should be performed to determine if it is possible to reduce the percentage of women who experience seizure worsening by aggressive AED concentration monitoring and dosage adjustments for each of the AEDs. The evidence for gestational-induced alterations in clearance is most convincing for PHT and LTG, moderately convincing for PB, OXC, and LEV, and contradictory or lacking for CBZ, VPA, ESX, and PRM. However, because of the myriad of factors that can contribute to the decrease in all AED concentrations during pregnancy (including noncompliance, enhanced metabolism, and excretion) and large intraindividual and interindividual variability, some authors have recommended at least monthly monitoring of all AED concentrations, with obtaining free (unbound) measurements for those medications that are highly protein bound (Krishnamurthy *et al.*, 2002; Levy and Yerby, 1985; Pennell, 2003; Yerby, 2000). For each individual patient, the ideal AED (free) level should be established for each patient prior to conception, and should be the level at which seizure control is the best possible for that patient without debilitating side effects. Future studies with formal pharmacokinetic modeling of each of the AEDs during pregnancy in women with epilepsy could be very helpful in achieving maternal seizure control while minimizing fetal AED exposure. With identification of additional pharmacogenetic factors, these models can be adapted for critical individualization for each woman with epilepsy.

References

EURAP Study Gorup. (2006). Seizure control and treatment in pregnancy: Observations from the EURAP epilepsy pregnancy registry. *Neurology* **66,** 354–360.

Bardy, A. H., Hiilesmaa, V. K., and Teramo, K. A. (1987). Serum phenytoin during pregnancy, labor and puerperium. *Acta Neurol. Scand.* **75,** 374–375.

Battino, D., Binelli, S., Bossi, L., Como, M. L., Croci, D., Cusi, C., and Avanzini, G. (1984). Changes in primidone/phenobarbitone ratio during pregnancy and the puerperium. *Clin. Pharmacokinet.* **9,** 252–260.

Battino, D., Binelli, S., Bossi, L., Canger, R., Croci, D., Cusi, C., De Giambattista, M., and Avanzini, G. (1985). Plasma concentrations of carbamazepine and carbamazepine 10,11-epoxide during pregnancy and after delivery. *Clin. Pharmacokinet.* **10,** 279–284.

Bossi, L., Assael, B. M., Avanzini, G., Battino, D., Caccamo, M. L., Canger, R., Como, M. L., Pifarotti, G., de Giambattista, M., Franceschetti, S., Marini, A., Pardi, G., *et al.* (1980). Plasma levels and clinical effects of antiepileptic drugs in pregnant epileptic patients and their newborns. *In* "Antiepileptic Therapy: Advances in Drug Monitoring" (S. I. Johannessen, P. L. Morselli, C. E. Pippenger, A. Richens, D. Schmidt, and H. Meinardi, Eds.), pp. 9–14. Raven Press, New York.

Chen, S. S., Perucca, E., Lee, J. N., and Richens, A. (1982). Serum protein binding and free concentration of phenytoin and phenobarbitone in pregnancy. *Br. J. Clin. Pharmacol.* **13,** 547–552.

Chen, S., Beaton, D., Nguyen, N., Senekeo-Effenberger, K., Brace-Sinnokrak, E., Argikar, U., Remmel, R. P., Trottier, J., Barbier, O., Ritter, J. K., and Tukey, R. H. (2005). Tissue-specific, inducible, and hormonal control of the human UDP-glucuronosyltransferase-1 (UGT1) locus. *J. Biol. Chem.* **280,** 37547–37557.

Christensen, J., Sabers, A., and Sidenius, P. (2006). Oxcarbazepine concentrations during pregnancy: A retrospective study in patients with epilepsy. *Neurology* **67,** 1497–1499.

Dansky, L., Andermann, E., Sherwin, A. L., Anderman, F., and Kinch, R. A. (1980). Maternal epilepsy and congenital malformations: A prospective study with monitoring of plasma anticonvulsant levels during pregnancy. *Neurology* **3,** 15.

Dansky, L., Andermann, E., Sherwin, A. L., and Andermann, F. (1982). Plasma levels of phenytoin during pregnancy and the puerperium. *In* "Epilepsy, Pregnancy, and the Child" (D. Janz, L. Bossi, M. Dam, H. Helge, A. Richens, and D. Schmidt, Eds.), pp. 155–162. Raven Press, New York.

de Haan, G. J., Edelbroek, P., Segers, J., Engelsman, M., Lindhout, D., Devile-Notschaele, M., and Augustijn, P. (2004). Gestation-induced changes in lamotrigine pharmacokinetics: A monotherapy study. *Neurology* **63,** 571–573.

DeVane, C. L., Stowe, Z. N., Donovan, J. L., Newport, D. J., Pennell, P. B., Ritchie, J. C., Owens, M. J., and Wang, J. S. (2006). Therapeutic drug monitoring of psychoactive drugs during pregnancy in the genomic era: Challenges and opportunities. *J. Psychopharmacol.* **20,** 54–59.

Dickinson, R. G., Hooper, W. D., Wood, B., Lander, C. M., and Eadie, M. J. (1989). The effect of pregnancy in humans on the pharmacokinetics of stable isotope labelled phenytoin. *Br. J. Clin. Pharmacol.* **28,** 17–27.

Ehmer, U., Vogel, A., Schutte, J. K., Krone, B., Manns, M. P., and Strassburg, C. P. (2004). Variation of hepatic glucuronidation: Novel functional polymorphisms of the UDP-glucuronosyltransferase UGT1A4. *Hepatology* **39,** 970–977.

Faught, E. (2001). Pharmacokinetic considerations in prescribing antiepileptic drugs. *Epilepsia* **42,** 19–23.

Green, M. D., and Tephly, T. R. (1996). Glucuronidation of amines and hydroxylated xenobiotics and endobiotics catalyzed by expressed human UGT1.4 protein. *Drug Metab. Dispos.* **24,** 356–363.

Green, M. D., Bishop, W. P., and Tephly, T. R. (1995). Expressed human UGT1.4 protein catalyzes the formation of quaternary ammonium-linked glucuronides. *Drug Metab. Dispos.* **23,** 299–302.

Green, M. D., King, C. D., Mojarrabi, B., Mackenzie, P. I., and Tephly, T. R. (1998). Glucuronidation of amines and other xenobiotics catalyzed by expressed human UDP-glucuronosyltransferase 1A3. *Drug Metab. Disp.* **26,** 507–512.

Janz, D. (1982). Antiepileptic drugs and pregnancy; altered utilization patterns and teratogenesis. *Epilepsia* **23,** 53–63.

Koerner, M., Yerby, M., Friel, P., and McCormick, K. (1989). Valproic acid disposition and protein binding in pregnancy. *Ther. Drug Monit.* **11,** 228–230.

Krauer, B., Krauer, F., and Hytten, F. E. (1980). Drug disposition and pharmacokinetics in the maternal-placental-fetal unit. *Pharmacol. Ther.* **10,** 301–328.

Krishnamurthy, K., Sundstrom, D., Beaudoin, J., and Kiriakopoulos, E. (2002). Pregnant women with epilepsy taking older anticonvulsants must have drug levels checked frequently to avoid seizures. *Epilepsia* **43**, 232–233.

Kuhnz, W., Koch, S., Jakob, S., Hartmann, A., Helge, H., and Nau, H. (1984). Ethosuximide in epileptic women during pregnancy and lactation period. Placental transfer, serum concentrations in nursed infants and clinical status. *Br. J. Clin. Pharmacol.* **18**, 671–677.

Lander, C. M., Livingstone, I., Tyrer, J. H., and Eadie, M. J. (1980). The clearance of anticonvulsant drugs in pregnancy. *Clin. Exp. Neurol.* **17**, 71–78.

Lander, C. M., Livingstone, I., Tyrer, J. H., and Eadie, M. J. (1981). The clearance of anticonvulsant drugs in pregnancy. *Clin. Exp. Neurol.* **17**, 71–78.

Leppik, I., and Rask, C. (1988). Pharmacokinetics of antiepileptic drugs during pregnancy. *Semin. Neurol.* **8**, 240–246.

Levy, R. H., and Yerby, M. S. (1985). Effects of pregnancy on antiepileptic drug utilization. *Epilepsia* **26**, 52–57.

Mazzucchelli, I., Onat, F. Y., Ozkara, C., Atakli, D., Specchio, L. M., Neve, A. L., Gatti, G., and Perucca, E. (2006). Changes in the disposition of oxcarbazepine and its metabolites during pregnancy and the puerperium. *Epilepsia* **47**, 504–509.

McAuley, J. W., and Anderson, G. D. (2002). Treatment of epilepsy in women of reproductive age: Pharmacokinetic considerations. *Clin. Pharmacokinet.* **41**, 559–579.

Ohman, I., Vitols, S., and Tomson, T. (2000). Lamotrigine in pregnancy: Pharmacokinetics during delivery, in the neonate, and during lactation. *Epilepsia* **41**, 709–713.

Otani, K. (1985). Risk factors for the increased seizure frequency during pregnancy and puerperium. *Folia Psychiatr. Neurol. Jpn.* **39**, 33–41.

Pennell, P. B. (2003). Antiepileptic drug pharmacokinetics during pregnancy and lactation. *Neurology* **61**, S35–S42.

Pennell, P. B., Newport, D. J., Stowe, Z. N., Helmers, S. L., Montgomery, J. Q., and Henry, T. R. (2004). The impact of pregnancy and childbirth on the metabolism of lamotrigine. *Neurology* **62**, 292–295.

Pennell, P. B., Peng, L., Newport, D. J., Ritchie, J. R., Koganti, A., Holley, D. K., Newman, M., and Stowe, Z. N. (2007). Lamotrigine in pregnancy: Clearance, therapeutic drug monitoring, and seizure frequency. *Neurology* **70**, 2130–2136.

Perucca, E., and Crema, A. (1982). Plasma protein binding of drugs in pregnancy. *Clin. Pharmacokinet.* **7**, 336–352.

Petrenaite, V., Sabers, A., and Hansen-Schwartz, J. (2005). Individual changes in lamotrigine plasma concentrations during pregnancy. *Epilepsy Res.* **65**, 185–188.

Ramsey, R. E., Wilder, B. J., Strauss, R., and Willmore, L. J. (1978). Status epilepticus during pregnancy: Effects of gastrointestinal malabsorption on phenytoin kinetics and seizure control. *Neurology* **28**, 85–89.

Rating, D., Nau, H., Jager-Roman, E., Gopfert-Geyer, I., Koch, S., Beck-Mannagetta, G., Schmidt, D., and Helge, H. (1982). Teratogenic and pharmacokinetic studies of primidone during pregnancy and in the offspring of epileptic women. *Acta Paediatr. Scand.* **71**, 301–311.

Report of the Quality Standards Subcommittee of the American Academy of Neurology (1998). Practice parameter: Management issues for women with epilepsy (summary statement). *Neurology* **51**, 944–948.

Schmidt, D., Beck-Mannagetta, G., Janz, D., and Koch, S. (1982). The effect of pregnancy on the course of epilepsy: A prospective study. *In* "Epilepsy, Pregnancy, and the Child" (D. Janz, L. Bossi, M. Dam, H. Helge, A. Richens, and D. Schmidt, Eds.), pp. 39–49. Raven Press, New York.

Schmidt, D., Canger, R., Avanzini, G., Battino, D., Cusi, C., Beck-Mannagetta, G., Koch, S., Rating, D., and Janz, D. (1983). Change of seizure frequency in pregnant epileptic women. *J. Neurol. Neurosurg. Psychiatry* **46**, 751–755.

Tomson, T., and Battino, D. (2007). Pharmacokinetics and therapeutic drug monitoring of newer antiepileptic drugs during pregnancy and the puerperium. *Clin. Pharmacokinet.* **46,** 209–219.

Tomson, T., Lindbom, U., and Hasselstrom, J. (1990). Plasma concentrations of ethosiximide and clonazepam during pregnancy. *J. Epilepsy* **3,** 91–95.

Tomson, T., Lindbom, U., Ekqvist, B., and Sundqvist, A. (1994). Disposition of carbamazepine and phenytoin in pregnancy. *Epilepsia* **35,** 131–135.

Tomson, T., Palm, R., Källén, K., Ben-Menachem, E., Söderfeldt, B., Danielsson, B., Johansson, R., Luef, G., and Ohman, I. (2007). Pharmacokinetics of levetiracetam during pregnancy, delivery, in the neonatal period, and lactation. *Epilepsia* **48,** 1111–1116.

Tran, T. A., Leppik, I. E., Blesi, K., Sathanandan, S. T., and Remmel, R. (2002). Lamotrigine clearance during pregnancy. *Neurology* **59,** 251–255.

Vajda, F. J., Hitchcock, A., Graham, J., Solinas, C., O'Brien, T. J., Lander, C. M., and Eadie, M. J. (2006). Foetal malformations and seizure control: 52 months data of the Australian Pregnancy Registry. *Eur. J. Neurol.* **13,** 645–654.

Yerby, M. S. (2000). Quality of life, epilepsy advances, and the evolving role of anticonvulsants in women with epilepsy. *Neurology* **55,** 21–31.

Yerby, M. S., Friel, P. N., and Miller, D. Q. (1985). Carbamazepine protein binding and disposition in pregnancy. *Ther. Drug Monit.* **7,** 269–273.

Yerby, M. S., Friel, P. N., McCormick, K., Koerner, M., Van Allen, M., Leavitt, A. M., Sells, C. J., and Yerby, J. A. (1990). Pharmacokinetics of anticonvulsants in pregnancy: Alterations in plasma protein binding. *Epilepsy Res.* **5,** 223–228.

Yerby, M. S., Friel, P. N., and McCormick, K. (1992). Antiepileptic drug disposition during pregnancy. *Neurology* **42,** 12–16.

Zahn, C. A., Morrell, M. J., Collins, S. D., Labiner, D. M., and Yerby, M. S. (1998). Management issues for women with epilepsy: A review of the literature. *Neurology* **51,** 949–956.

ANTIEPILEPTIC DRUG THERAPY IN PREGNANCY II: FETAL AND NEONATAL EXPOSURE

Collin A. Hovinga* and Page B. Pennell[†]

*Departments of Clinical Pharmacy and Pediatrics, University of Tennessee Health Science Center, LeBonheur Children's Medical Center, Memphis, Tennessee 38105, USA
[†]Emory Epilepsy Program, Emory University School of Medicine, Atlanta, Georgia 30322, USA

I. Introduction
II. Factors Influencing Anticonvulsant Distribution to the Neonate
   A. Anticonvulsant Properties
   B. Placental Factors
   C. Neonatal Pharmacokinetics
III. Quantifying AED Exposures
IV. Review of AEDs and Transplacental and Lactation Exposures
   A. Carbamazepine (CBZ)
   B. Ethosuximide (ESX)
   C. Phenobarbital/Primidone (PB/PRM)
   D. Phenytoin (PHT)
   E. Valproate (VPA)
   F. Gabapentin (GBP)
   G. Levetiracetam (LEV)
   H. Lamotrigine (LTG)
   I. Oxcarbazepine (OXC)
   J. Topiramate (TPM)
   K. Zonisamide (ZNS)
V. Summary
   References

The issue of how much an antiepileptic drug (AED) crosses the placenta and relative safety of lactation in mothers receiving AEDs are common clinical questions. Educating potential mothers with epilepsy regarding available information is warranted so that informed decisions and any needed neonatal monitoring is performed. Unfortunately, there is still limited data regarding the degree in which anticonvulsants cross the placenta and penetrate into breast milk. There is a greater appreciation of the factors that influence AED passive transfer across the placenta and into breast milk, as well as factors that ultimately influence neonatal AED distribution. In general, women with epilepsy can have healthy babies even with significant placental exposure and can breast-feed their babies safely with some cautions. Phenobarbital and primidone should be avoided in parents wishing to breast-feed. For the AEDs ethosuximide, levetiracetam, lamotrigine, topiramate, and zonisamide, there is a potential for significant breast milk concentrations; however, there are no firm guidelines on whether lactation is safe. In all cases, parents should be counseled to monitor their child for side effects and the need for routine monitoring.

I. Introduction

Indirect neonatal anticonvulsant exposure comes from two situations. First, involuntary exposure occurs *in utero* through placental transfer in mothers receiving anticonvulsants. The second is through ingestion of milk containing anticonvulsants in mothers with epilepsy. The latter is elective and dependent upon caregivers' knowledge and wishes regarding the benefits of breastfeeding and the potential risk of drug exposure in the neonate. The positive effects of breastfeeding are well recognized and make it an increasingly attractive practice for parents with newborns. This is also true of mothers who happen to have epilepsy. The question as to whether breastfeeding is safe in this population is a common clinical question to those who treat women with epilepsy and in pediatricians who follow the newborn. Perinatal counseling of families with available information is warranted so that informed decisions and any needed monitoring is performed. Unfortunately, there still is limited data regarding the degree in which antiepileptic drugs (AEDs) cross the placenta and penetrate into breast milk. Available studies tend to be limited, in that they are small in sample size, lack complete sampling, and few have long-term follow-up. Polytherapy is still common in these studies and adverse effects, particularly cognitive ones are not systematically evaluated. This chapter will review factors that influence anticonvulsant transfer across the placenta and into breast milk. It will also discuss neonatal factors that influence the relative risk of exposure in the neonate. Lastly, it will review individual anticonvulsants and what is known regarding exposure through placental and lactation exposures.

II. Factors Influencing Anticonvulsant Distribution to the Neonate

A. ANTICONVULSANT PROPERTIES

Many of the factors that determine placental and milk transfer are similar. Passive diffusion is the most common means by which drugs reach the neonate. In such instances, the amount of drug that crosses a membrane per unit of time is dependent on the difference in concentration of drug in the maternal and fetal or neonatal circulations, its physiochemical properties, and the rapidity of maternal drug clearance. Lipid soluble, un-ionized drugs with low molecular weights

(<500 Daltons) tend to diffuse more readily. It is important to remember that it is the sum of all these drug properties that results in the extent of transfer, not simply one. In some cases, this makes precise estimates of anticonvulsant drug exposure difficult. Because only free anticonvulsants can cross biological membranes, the percentage of drug unbound affects the extent a drug passes to the neonate. This is an inverse relationship with the drugs possessing a higher degree of protein binding resulting in less drug passive exposure. The relative concentration and affinity of maternal as compared to fetal or neonatal albumin can also affect neonate anticonvulsant exposure transplacentally. Ionized (charged) drugs do not readily cross membranes, and pH is an important regulatory of the degree of drug polarity. As a general rule, anticonvulsants with salt forms ending in an anion (e.g., chloride) tend to be weak bases and those with a cation (sodium) tend to be weak acids. Most AEDs tend to be either weak acids or weak bases; therefore, the drug's pK_a and maternal/neonatal blood pH ratio affects its relative ionization. Because fetal pH tends to be slightly lower than maternal pH, basic drugs can be expected to pass more easily across the placenta than do acidic ones (Syme *et al.*, 2004). In cases of neonatal acidosis, the degree of neonatal transfer can significantly increase. Breast milk is also slightly more acidic (pH 7.2) as compared to plasma (pH 7.4), and it is also expected that weak acids would transfer less readily in to milk than anticonvulsants that are weak bases (Hibberd *et al.*, 1982; Neville 2001). Weak bases once transferred into milk remain ionized and are trapped and concentrate in breast milk.

Differences in lipid solubility can significantly affect the degree of neonatal AED exposure via breast milk (Hägg and Spigset, 2000). Many AED passive drug exposure studies are performed during the first few days postnatally and fail to describe from which milk fraction the sample is obtained. There are dramatic changes in milk composition during the first month of life with maternal milk being mostly comprised of protein (colostrums) initially and triglyceride content gradually increasing during the following weeks (Hibberd *et al.*, 1982; Neville 2001). The amount of triglyceride also varies in each milk fraction (foremilk vs hindmilk), as well as the maturity of lactation. Because it depends on maternal diet, the extent of transfer can vary across the course of a day or between days. AEDs with greater lipid solubility tend to distribute more readily into breast milk. However, distribution may not be uniform across milk fractions. This is particularly true for mature milk, hindmilk, and postfeed milk which tend to be of higher triglyceride content, and therefore may contain higher concentrations of lipophilic AEDs.

B. PLACENTAL FACTORS

In the case of placental transfer, there is an increasing appreciation of drug transporters or efflux proteins that regulate AED passage into the fetal circulation. Many of the drug transporters are located at the blood–brain barrier [P-glycoprotein aka. MDR1 (Atkinson *et al.*, 2007; Syme *et al.*, 2004)].

Although the placenta expresses many CYP450 (including CYP1A1, 2E1, 3A4, 3A7, 4B1) and uridine diphosphate glucuronosyltransferase (UGT) isoenzymes, it is felt that AED metabolism through this route has a relatively minor impact on neonatal drug concentrations; however, this is an area of continued research. Recently, more attention is being paid to placental drug transporters and efflux proteins. Attention within the area of epilepsy first arose from the discovery that these drug transporters have increased blood–brain barrier expression in those with refractory epilepsy. Transporters like MDR1, multidrug resistance protein 1 and 2 (MRP1, MRP2), and monocarboxylate transports are located at the apical membrane of the syncytiotrophoblast where they extrude drugs from the fetal circulation back into the maternal one (Atkinson et al., 2007; Syme et al., 2004). Most of the currently available AEDs are substrates for one of more of these transporters, and therefore are of clinical importance. There are also less commonly known transporters that may be active in transporting AEDs [e.g., carbamazepine (CBZ) and primidone (PRM)] to the fetus as well such as sodium/multivitamin transporter (SMVT).

C. Neonatal Pharmacokinetics

It is important to understand that the same quantity of AED delivered to the neonate does not necessarily result in a similar concentration in different neonates. In predicting the relative magnitude of AED drug exposure in the neonate, an appreciation of developmental pharmacokinetics is important. Both the gestational age and postnatal age affect the pharmacokinetics of AEDs (Battino et al.,1995a,b; Hines and McCarver, 2002; McCarver and Hines, 2002). Body composition and maturity of elimination pathways varies dramatically over the first weeks and months of life (Kearns et al., 2003). Neonates have decreased bioavailability of many drugs secondary to erratic absorption and alkaline gastrointestinal pH. AED distribution may be affected both because total body water and adipose stores are different in neonates and adults. Fetal and neonatal albumin may be decreased and have decreased affinity for certain specific drugs. This means the unbound fraction of drugs may be increased. Hepatic and renal elimination pathways are relatively immature, making neonates prone to drug accumulation. Irrespective of gestational age, hepatic metabolism begins to mature at birth. Certain CYP450 enzymes are particularly relevant to antiepileptic medications, namely, CYP3A4/5/7 and CYP2C9/19. CYP3A4/5/7 is responsible for the metabolism of many antiepileptic medications, including CBZ, ESX, felbamate, tiagabine, and ZNS (Battino et al., 1995a, b; Perucca, 2006). While CYP2C9/ is involved in the elimination of phenytoin (PHT), CYP2C19 metabolizes both PHT and phenobarbital (PB). Although there are subtle differences, examination of the ontogeny of these enzyme subfamilies reveals that expression is reduced or nonexistent in early fetal development and in neonates and increases during infancy (Hines and McCarver, 2002; McCarver and Hines, 2002). The Phase II reactions relevant to epilepsy are catalyzed by the UGTs. Lamotrigine (UGT1A4), valproate (VPA) (UGT2B1), and oxcarbazepine (OXC) all are metabolized in various degrees by UGT isoenzyme enzymes. In contrast to the CYP450 systems, substrate specificity is less well defined for UGT isoenzymes. Interestingly, maturation of UGT isoenzymes occurs much more slowly than the CYP450 system with some isoenzymes not reaching maturation until early adolescence (DeWildt *et al.*, 1999). In some instances, *in utero* exposure to hepatic enzyme inducing AEDs, clearance maturation pathways may be more rapid. This immaturity has been implicated in some of the severe idiosyncratic drug reactions that have been observed in pediatric patients receiving certain medications including LTG and VPA (Anderson, 2002).

Renal maturation is highly dependent upon gestational age and tends to develop more slowly in the preterm neonate (Kearns *et al.*, 2003). However, in the preterm and term neonate elimination is reduced because of a decrease in the number of functioning nephrons. Regardless of gestational age in both groups, there is significant maturation of renal function during the first 2 weeks of life. This is due to redistribution of renal blood flow which permits the recruitment of additional functional nephrons. However, renal function at this stage is still reduced and is ~25% of that observed in the adult. This is believed to contribute to the prolonged half-life of PB observed in this group because unlike in the adult and older child this medication is eliminated primarily renally. By 6 months renal function is 50–75% of that observed in the adult and by 2–3 years of age renal function approximates that in the adult. If one examines filtration and secretion separately, a discrepancy in functional maturation is observed. Specifically, for up to 6 months of age glomerular filtration matures more rapidly than tubular function, so drugs in which tubular secretion is involved are eliminated much more slowly in those younger than 6 months of age. This suggests that renally eliminated AEDs [particularly LEV, gabapentin (GBP), pregabalin] may have prolonged elimination in neonates (Perucca, 2006).

III. Quantifying AED Exposures

There is no universally accepted threshold concentration that defines significant placental- or lactation-associated exposure. Various methods have been put forth reflecting the relative amount of placental/maternal plasma concentrations at birth or milk/maternal plasma concentrations (M/P) (Begg and Atkinson, 1993). Because of the wide variability of drug concentrations in each phase across a dosing interval, multiple milk and blood samples are recommended so that a larger estimate of exposure can be made [i.e., calculation of the area under curve (AUC) for the milk or plasma ratio MAUC/PAUC]. Unfortunately, this is rarely done and lessens the sensitivity of this calculation. Intuitively, ratios of 1 would signify significant transfer; however, this fails to be sensitive to the absolute amount of drug received by the neonate and it does not consider the adverse effect potential of the drug. Calculating the relative infant dose (RID) is another method of normalizing the quantity of drug the neonate is exposed to the mother's dose, U.S. Department of Health and Human Services, FDA, Guidance for industry. First the infant's dose (D_{infant}) is estimated (1). Then the infant dose is normalized to that received by the mother and is expressed as a percentage (2).

$$D_{infant}(mg/kg/day) = C_{maternal}(mg/l) \times \frac{MAUC}{PAUC} \times V_{infant}(l/kg/day) \qquad (1)$$

where $C_{maternal}$ (drug concentration in mother) and V_{infant} (volume of milk ingested by infant) can be measured and estimated to be 0.150 l/kg/day in term neonates.

$$RID = \frac{D_{infant}}{D_{maternal}} \times 100 \qquad (2)$$

In cases in which the drug is used in children, the infant dose can also be normalized to the commonly used pediatric dose. An RID of 10% has been used as an arbitrary cut off, with concentrations less than 10% being considered relatively safe. However, there are many medications that have been found to violate this rule. For example, many immunosuppressant and isotretinoin have RIDs less than 10%, yet their risk for toxicity makes them contraindicated or not recommended in breastfeeding. Most of the literature involving mothers with epilepsy focusing on lactation contains women receiving polytherapy. The potential for drug interactions and pharmacodynamically associated side effects makes the RID less sensitive in this population. Another method of identifying significant AED exposure that may pose a significant risk to the neonate is to define a threshold proportion for the observed placental or breast milk transfer. This assessment has the advantage that it is independent of maternal dose and pharmacokinetic confounders. A transfer rate (umbilical or neonatal: maternal plasma concentration ratio or a milk: maternal concentration ratio) of greater than 0.6 is a reasonable estimate of a threshold for clinical significance. To assess neonatal accumulation, a change in the neonatal plasma concentration following lactation can be used. In such instances, a reasonable threshold would be a trend of increasing neonatal AED plasma concentrations (>25%) over the evaluated period (generally over 3 days to up to 1 month). Such methodology has the potential advantage of examining the affects of maturation on passively acquired drug clearance.

IV. Review of AEDs and Transplacental and Lactation Exposures

With the exception of felbamate, pregabalin, and tiagabine, most AEDs have some data regarding the degree of placental transfer and extent of milk penetration. The available data for each AED will be discussed (Table I).

A. CARBAMAZEPINE (CBZ)

Approximately 69–78% of total CBZ and 75% of CBZ-epoxide crosses the placenta (Kuhnz et al., 1983; Niebyl, J. R. et al., 1979; Pynnonen and Sillanpaa,1975; Pynnonen et al., 1977; Takeda et al., 1992; Yerby et al., 1990). These are significantly less than observed in the mother. In contrast, free CBZ concentrations tend to be comparable or exceed that found in the mother (100–140%). These values are consistent whether CBZ is given as mono- or polytherapy. In breast-fed neonates, M/P ratios for CBZ and the epoxide are 0.36–0.41 and 0.49–0.53, respectively (Froescher et al., 1984; Kuhnz et al., 1983, Niebyl, J. R. et al., 1979). CBZ concentrations in breast-fed neonates are below the normal therapeutic range, with most being ~1–2 mg/l (range 4–12 mg/l) or less than 20% of maternal concentrations. In breast-fed infants, concentrations generally decrease in the infant over time. Across all studies, the RID ranges from 0.4% to 8% even when the epoxide is included in the estimation. CBZ elimination is prolonged in these neonates (half-life of 8–36 h); however, there is no accumulation even with continued lactation (Froescher et al., 1984; Kuhnz et al., 1983; Niebyl, J. R. et al., 1979; Rane et al., 1975). A case report of a woman receiving CBZ 1 g/day showed CBZ distributes more readily into nonfat portion (skimmed 2.3 mg/l) when compared to the fat-containing portion (1.4 mg/l). The incidence of side effects in neonates exposed to CBZ through lactation is relatively low and most neonates experience no problems with lactation. However, there have been reports of sedation, poor suckling, vomiting with poor weight gain, withdrawal reactions, and rare cases of hepatic dysfunction (Frey et al., 1990, 2002; Froescher et al., 1984; Kuhnz et al., 1983; Wisner and Perel, 1998). These seem to be uncorrelated with maternal CBZ dose or neonatal plasma concentrations. The American Academy of Pediatrics (AAP) guidelines states that CBZ is potentially safe with breastfeeding (AAP, 2001).

B. ETHOSUXIMIDE (ESX)

ESX almost completely crosses the placenta (97%), with many exposed neonates achieving plasma concentrations within the therapeutic range (Kuhnz et al., 1984). Half-life in exposed neonates at 4 days of life has been 32–38 h.

TABLE I

Summary of Antiepleptic Drug Exposure Across the Placenta and in Lactation

Antiepileptic drugs	Umbilical cord (UC)/Maternal plasma concentration (M/P)	Concentrations crossing placenta significant (UC/P>0.6)	Breast milk/ Maternal plasma concentration (M/P)	Relative infant dose (RID, %)	Concentrations in milk significant (M/P>0.6 or RID>10%)	AAP compatibility with lactation[a]	Neonatal half-life (h)	Adult half-life (h)	Possible neonatal side effects
Carbamazepine	Total CBZ	Yes	CBZ	0.4–8	No	Potentially safe	8–36	8–25	Sedation, poor suckling, vomiting, lack of weight gain, withdrawal reactions, hepatic dysfunction
	0.69–0.78 Free CBZ		0.36–0.41 CBZ-epoxide 0.49–0.53						
	1.0–1.4 CBZ-epoxide 0.75								
Ethosuximide	0.97	Yes	0.86–1.36	32–115	Yes	Usually compatible	32–38	32–60	Sedation, poor feeding, hyperactivity, and withdrawal symptoms
Phenobarbital	Total 0.7–1.0	Yes	0.36–0.46	<350	Yes	Use with caution	100–500	75–25	Poor feeding, jitteriness, sedation, tremor, unmotivated crying, and withdrawal symptoms have been described in neonates exposed to PB
Primidone	PRM 0.88–0.99	Yes	PRM 0.72	18	Yes	Use with caution	7–60	4–12	
	Free 0.98								
	PEMA 0.97–1.05		PEMA 0.64–0.76						
	PB 0.84–1.0		PB 0.36–0.41						

(Continued)

TABLE I (*Continued*)

Antiepileptic drugs	Umbilical cord (UC)/Maternal plasma concentration (M/P)	Concentrations crossing placenta significant (UC/P>0.6)	Breast milk/Maternal plasma concentration (M/P)	Relative infant dose (RID, %)	Concentrations in milk significant (M/P>0.6 or RID>10%)	AAP compatibility with lactation[a]	Neonatal half-life (h)	Adult half-life (h)	Possible neonatal side effects
Phenytoin	Total 0.86–1.0 Free 1.1–1.25	Yes	0.06–0.19	<10	No	Usually compatible	15–105	12–15	Drowsiness, poor feeding, irritability, and rare instances of methehemoglobinemia
Valproate	Total 1.59–1.71 Free 0.5–0.82	Yes	0.01–0.1	<7	No	Usually compatible	30–60	6–20	Hypotonia, excitability, and sleepiness shortly after birth but in many instances patients were also on phenobarbital or primidone, rare thrombocytopenia, anemia, and petechiae
Gabapentin	1.74 (1.3–2.1)	Yes	0.7–1.3	1.3–3.8	Yes	NA	14	7–9	Reversible hypotonia
Levetiracetam	1.14 (0.56–2.0)	Yes	1.0–3.09	8	Yes	NA	16–18	6–8	None reported
Lamotrigine	0.9 (0.6–1.3)	Yes	0.61 (0.5–0.77)	2–20	Yes	NA	NA	30	None reported
Oxcarbazepine	0.92–1.0	Yes	0.5–0.65	NA	No	NA	17–22	19.3 ± 6.2	None reported
Topiramate	0.95 (0.85–1.06)	Yes	0.86 (0.67–1.1)	3–23	Yes	NA	24	21	Rare hypocalcemic seizures
Zonisamide	0.92	Yes	0.41–0.93	23–28	Yes	NA	61–109	63	None reported

AAP, American Academy of Pediatrics Guidelines; CBZ, Carbamazepine; PRM, Primidone; PB, Phenobarbital; NA, Not addressed

[a]Recommendation from the American Academy of Pediatrics.

Milk penetration is significant ($M/P = 0.86$–1.36) and results in neonatal plasma concentrations in the range of 25–75% of ESX maternal concentrations (Koup *et al.*, 1978; Kuhnz *et al.*, 1984; Rane and Tunell, 1981; Soderman and Rane, 1986; Tomson, 1994). The M/P in colostrum is comparable to that in whole milk (0.79–1.0) (Soderman and Rane, 1986). It is estimated that the RID for ESX-exposed neonates is in the range of 32–115%, which also supports extensive passive exposure. Sedation, poor feeding, hyperactivity, and withdrawal symptoms have been observed in ESX-exposed infants; however, the interpretation of this is complex, in that these patients were also exposed to PB, PRM, or clonazepam. In spite of extensive exposure, the AAP currently states that ESX is usually compatible with lactation (AAP, 2001).

C. PHENOBARBITAL/PRIMIDONE (PB/PRM)

PB significantly crosses the placental with the proportion of total and free PB transferring ranging from 0.7 to 1.0 and 0.98, respectively (Gomita *et al.*, 1995; Ishizaki *et al.*, 1981; Takeda *et al.* , 1992; Yerby *et al.*, 1990). PRM distribution is similar with a PRM umbilical cord/maternal concentration of 0.88–0.99, for phenylethylmalonamide (PEMA) (0.97–1.05) and for PRM-derived PB (0.84–1.0) (Kuhnz *et al.*, 1988; Nau, 1980). PB's penetration into breast milk is slightly less than is PRM (M/F PB = 0.36–0.46, PRM = 0.72, PEMA = 0.64–0.76, PRM-derived PB = 0.36–0.41) (Kaneko *et al.*, 1979; Kuhnz *et al.*, 1988; Nau, 1980). Elimination for both PB and PRM is significantly prolonged in the neonate even with prenatal hepatic induction of metabolism (half-life neonate/adult: PB 100–500 h/75–125 h; PRM 7–60 h/4–12 h). The reported RDIs for PB and PRM are considered significant (PB up to 350%; PRM 18%) (Kaneko *et al.*, 1979; Nau, 1980). Unfortunately, many of the available studies for these AEDs fail to report maternal doses and RID calculations are not possible. Poor feeding, jitteriness, sedation, tremor, unmotivated crying, and withdrawal symptoms have been described in neonates exposed to PB. This can be observed in up to 50% of exposed neonates (Gomita *et al.*, 1995; Ishizaki *et al.*, 1981; Nau, 1980). The risk for adverse effects in the neonate is concerning and has made the AAP classify PB and PRM as a drug that should be used with caution in mothers wishing to breast-feed (AAP, 2001).

D. PHENYTOIN (PHT)

Total and free PHT readily distribute across the placenta with a umbilical cord/maternal concentration of 0.86–1.0 and 1.1–1.25, respectively (Ishizaki *et al.*, 1981; Mirkin, 1971; Takeda *et al.*, 1992; Yerby *et al.*, 1990). PHT excretion into breast milk is minimal, with M/P ratios 0.06–0.19 in most women, and has rarely been as high as 0.69 (Kaneko *et al.*, 1979, Mirkin, 1971, Shimoyama *et al.*, 1998, Steen *et al.*, 1982). The RDI is generally less than 10% in breast-fed neonates. PHT's estimated half-life in neonates (15–105 h) is markedly variable and pro-longed when compared to that in adults (12–15 h). In breast-fed neonates, PHT concentrations rarely are greater than 2 mg/l and well below those used clinically. Studies examining PHT during lactation have been confounded largely because they have been in women receiving polytherapy. Drowsiness, poor feeding, irritability, and rare instances of methehemoglobinemia have been described in Finch and Lorber (1954). It is difficult to draw a definite causal relationship for these adverse effects given PHT's low potential for exposure. The AAP currently classifies PHT as usually compatible with breastfeeding (AAP, 2001).

E. Valproate (VPA)

Total VPA concentrations cross the placenta and are greater in the neonate than in the maternal plasma [umbilical cord/maternal concentration = 1.59–1.71 (Ishizaki *et al.*, 1981; Nau *et al.*, 1981, 1984; Takeda *et al.*, 1992)]. In contrast, free VPA concentrations are markedly less in the cord blood (umbilical cord/maternal concentration = 0.5–0.82) and suggest the interpretation of total VPA concentrations may be misleading in assessing active drug (i.e., free VPA) exposure. VPA concentrations decrease more slowly in neonates than in adults. Estimated half-life in neonates (30–60 h) are significantly longer than those observed in adults (6–20 h) (Nau *et al.*, 1981). Because of VPA's high degree of protein binding, its penetration into breast milk is limited, with M/P ratios of 0.01–0.10 (Nau *et al.*, 1981, 1984; Von Unruh *et al.*, 1984). The RID is less than 7% and neonatal plasma concentrations following breastfeeding are well below that observed in mothers receiving VPA for epilepsy (<8%). Rarely there have been reports of hypotonia, excitability, and sleepiness shortly after birth, but in many instances patients were also on PB or PRM. There have also been instances of blood dyscrasias (thrombocytopenia, anemia) and petechiae in neonates exposed to VPA through lactation (Stahl *et al.*, 1997). The risk of these side effects is considered low because of the small percentage of VPA that reaches the neonate from lactation. Therefore, the AAP currently considers VPA usually compatible with breastfeeding (AAP, 2001).

F. Gabapentin (GBP)

A study with six women showed that the transplacental transfer of GBP is extensive, with mean (range) umbilical/maternal concentrations of 1.74% (1.3–2.1) (Ohman *et al.*, 2005). After 24 h, mean GBP concentrations in exposed neonates were 27% (12–36) of umbilical cord concentrations. GBP's half-life is 14 h, which is prolonged when comparing older children (5.5 ± 0.8 h) and adults (7–9 h) (Tallian et al., 2004). At 2 weeks to 3 months, GBP's M/P ratio is 1.0% (0.7–1.3) and the RID is 1.3–3.8% (Ohman et al., 2005). GBP plasma concentrations in breast-fed neonates are <12% of maternal concentrations. One neonate exposed to GBP had reversible hypotonia which resolved quickly. Another case report in neonates born to women receiving GBP for other indications are consistent with this finding, with neonatal plasma concentrations <7% (following an RID of 2.3%) than maternal concentration (Kristensen, 2006). The AAP guidelines do not address GBP; however, existing studies fail to show any clear side effect risks following passive exposure with GBP.

G. Levetiracetam (LEV)

LEV placental transfer is complete with cord samples in the equivalent to that found in the mother, with the mean (range) in two studies 1.14 (0.97–1.45) and 1.15 (0.56–2.0) (Johannessen et al., 2005; Thomson et al., 2007). In spite of extensive transfer, LEV concentrations decrease fairly rapidly with a half-life of 16–18 h in exposed neonates (Allegaert et al., 2006; Thomson et al., 2007). This is significantly longer than that observed in infants/children (2–46 months, $t_{1/2} =$ 5.3±1.3 h) and adults ($t_{1/2} = 7±1$ h) (Glauser et al., 2007). Mean breast milk penetration (M/P) is also extensive, 1.0–1.05 (up to 3.09) (Johannessen et al., 2005; Kramer et al., 2002; Thomson et al., 2007). However, the RID is ~8% and there is little accumulation in breast-fed neonates. The infant/maternal plasma concentration is low following lactation (0.13, range 0.07–0.22). By 36 h, concentrations in neonates irrespective of whether breastfeeding or not decline to minimal levels (20% of cord values at birth) and are significantly below maternal values (Thomson et al., 2007). This is interesting given the immaturity of the kidney and the fact that LEV is primarily renally eliminated. There is little change in concentrations in M/P ratio in up to 10 months of follow-up, suggesting accumulation is unlikely (Johannessen et al., 2005). Although no formal assessments have been performed, routine monitoring of neonates exposed to LEV transplacentally and/or through lactation has shown no acute adverse effects. The AAP guidelines do not include LEV (AAP, 2001).

H. Lamotrigine (LTG)

LTG efficiently crosses the placenta with an umbilical cord blood/maternal median LTG concentration ratio was 0.9 (range 0.6–1.3) (Ohman et al., 2000). Over the next 72 h, neonatal LTG concentrations only decrease 25% when compared to cord. At 2–3 weeks, median breast M/P ratio is 0.61 (range 0.5–0.77), giving neonatal plasma concentration ~30% (range 23–60%) of that measured in the mother. It is estimated that neonates receive a minimum of 0.2–1 mg/kg/day when breast-fed or a median RID of 9% (2–20%). Other studies show comparable neonatal exposure through lactation with RID of 5.7–9.9% (Page-Sharp et al., 2006). It has been reported that LTG concentrations in breast-fed infants do not decrease as rapidly other AEDs and can remain at 22–23% of that found in maternal plasma for periods of at least 2 months. This is likely due to immaturity in UGT transferases when compared to other hepatic and renal elimination pathways. No adverse effects including rash have been reported in LTG-exposed neonates. However, the immediate lack of decay in LTG concentrations has made some question as to whether women electing to breast-feed should also use formula supplements and/or defer lactation in their infants (Liporance, J. et al., 2004). The AAP has not evaluated the relative risk of LTG in lactation (AAP, 2001).

I. Oxcarbazepine (OXC)

Both OXC and the 10-OH-OXC (MHD) cross the placenta to a great extent (umbilical cord/plasma = 0.92–1.0) (Bülau et al., 1988; Myllynen et al., 2001). Both OXC and 10-OH-OXC are eliminated without accumulation regardless of intake through breast milk. By 5 days, 7–12% of OXC and 10-OH-OXC remain in the neonatal plasma. It is estimated that in exposed neonates, OXC and 10-OH-OXC have a half-life of 22 and 17 h, respectively. This is in the range found in adults receiving OXC (10-OH-OXC = 19.3 ± 6.2 h) (Kristensen et al., 1983). The milk concentration of OXC and 10-OH-OXC is approximately half of that found in the maternal plasma (M/P = 0.5–0.65) (Bülau et al., 1988). No acute side effects have been noted in these neonates. Currently, the AAP guidelines do not address OXC; however, the available information does not suggest significant risk to the neonate (AAP, 2001).

J. Topiramate (TPM)

A series of five women receiving TPM suggests its mean placental transfer is extensive (umbilical cord/maternal concentrations = 0.95, 0.85–1.06) (Ohman et al., 2002). In the three neonates studied at 3 h, TPM plasma concentrations had decreased to 40% of that measured in the cord sample and a concentration 54% lower than that found in maternal plasma. The observed neonatal half-life of 24 h is comparable to that found in healthy adults receiving TPM monotherapy (Johannessen 1997). In neonates not undergoing breastfeeding, TPM concentrations were undetectable by 48 h. After 3 weeks following delivery, the TPM M/P ratio was 0.86 (0.67–1.1) and an estimated RID of 3–23% or neonatal dose of 0.1–0.7 mg/kg/day. All mothers were receiving TPM in combination with either CBZ or VPA. At this time, neonates who were breast-fed had TPM concentrations ~10–20% of maternal concentrations. No side effects were reported in these neonates. Recently, there has been a case of neonatal hypocalcemic seizures in two separate neonates born from a mother receiving TPM during pregnancy (Gorman and Soul, 2007). It is hypothesized that *in utero* exposure caused a transient hypoparathyroidism in these neonates. The AAP guidelines do not include TPM; however, the available data TPM does not accumulate or commonly lead to acute side effects in neonates indirectly exposed to TPM (AAP, 2001).

K. ZONISAMIDE (ZNS)

Information regarding ZNS transfer comes in many cases. In one of two neonates born to a mother receiving ZNS, the umbilical/maternal plasma concentration ratio was 0.92 (Kawada *et al.*, 2002). The M/P ratio ranged from 0.41 to 0.57 during the first 10 days after delivery. Whey and maternal-free ZNS concentrations were similar (10.7–13.3 mg/l). In the neonates, ZNS half-life is 61 and 109 h, which is comparable or prolonged compared to the average half-life of 63 h in adults (Kawada *et al.*, 2002; Sills and Brodie, 2007). In the first week following delivery, the ZNS concentration in these infants was 11–14 mg/l; subsequently it decreased at 24 days to 3.9 mg/l even with breastfeeding. This represented ~15% of the maternal concentration. In another case, the M/P was ~0.93 ± 0.09 and the RID in these studies was ~23–28% (Kawada *et al.*, 2002; Shimoyama and Ohkubo, 1999). No side effects were noted in these cases and no conclusions can be drawn from these cases regarding the risk to the neonate. The AAP guidelines do not include ZNS (AAP, 2001).

V. Summary

The ideal counseling of women with epilepsy during pregnancy and in making the decisions regarding lactation necessitates communicating the currently available information regarding potential neonatal exposure secondary to placental transmission and through breastfeeding. Many of the available AEDs cross the placenta and are available in the breast milk (Table I). In general, women with epilepsy can have healthy babies and can breast-feed their babies, safely. Parents should be counseled on the available information and possible side effects. PB and PRM should be avoided in parents wishing to breast-feed. For the AEDs ESX,

LEV, LTG, TPM, and ZNS there is a potential for significant breast milk concentrations; however, there are no firm guidelines on whether lactation is safe. In general, the lowest effective dose to achieve seizure control in the mother should be used and in these instances, parents should be advised to report any excessive, sedation, irritability, feeding difficulty, or failure to gain weight. If this occurs, supplementation with formula or discontinuation of lactation may be needed. Future studies of AEDs during pregnancy and lactation should be designed to provide accurate pharmacokinetic and pharmacogenetic models to predict relative neonatal drug exposure and the long-term effects of passive drug exposure on neurological development.

References

Allegaert, K., Lewis, L., Naulaer, G., and Lagae, L. (2006). Levetiracetam Pharmacokinetics in Neonates at Birth. *Epilepsia* **47,** 1068–1069.

American Academy of Pediatrics, and Committee on Drug. (2001). The transfer of drugs and other chemicals into human milk. *Pediatrics* **108,** 776–789.

Anderson, G. D. (2002). Children versus adults: Pharmacokinetic and adverse-effect differences. *Epilepsia* **43**(Suppl 3), 53–59.

Atkinson, D. E., Brice-Bennett, S., and D'Souza, S. W. (2007). Antiepileptic medication during pregnancy: Does fetal genotype affect outcome? *Pediatr. Res.* **62,** 120–127.

Battino, D., Estienne, M., and Avanzini, G. (1995). Clinical pharmacokinetics of antiepileptic drugs in pediatric patients. Part I: Phenobarbital, primidone, valproic acid, ethosuximide and mesuximide. *Clin. Pharmacokinet.* **29,** 257–286.

Battino, D., Estienne, M., and Avanzini, G. (1995). Clinical pharmacokinetics of antiepileptic drugs in pediatric patients. Part II: Phenytoin, carbamazepine, sulthiame, lamotrigine, vigabatrin, oxcarbazepine and felbamate. *Clin. Pharmacokinet.* **29,** 341–369.

Begg, E. J., and Atkinson, H. C. (1993). Modelling of the passage of drugs intro milk. *Pharmacol. Ther.* **59,** 301–310.

Bülau, P., Paar, W. D., and von Unruh, G. E. (1988). Pharmacokinetics of oxcarbazepine and 10-hydroxycarbamazepine in the newborn child of an oxcarbazepine-treated mother. *Eur. J. Clin. Pharmacol.* **34,** 311–313.

DeWildt, S. N., Kearns, G. L., Leeder, J. S., and van den Anker, J. N. (1999). Glucuronidation in humans. Pharmacogenetic and developmental aspects. *Clin. Pharmacokinet.* **36,** 439–452.

Finch, E., and Lorber, J. (1954). Methaemoglobinaemia in the newborn. Probably due to phenytoin excreted in human milk. *J. Obstet. Gynaecol. Br. Emp.* **61,** 833–834.

Frey, B., Schubiger, G., and Musy, J. P. (1990). Transient cholestatic hepatitis in a neonate associated with carbamazepine exposure during pregnancy and breast-feeding. *Eur. J. Pediatr.* **150,** 136–138.

Frey, B., Braegger, C. P., and Ghelfi, D. (2002). Neonatal cholestatic hepatitis from carbamazepine exposure during pregnancy and breast feeding. *Ann. Pharmacother.* **36,** 644–647.

Froescher, W., Eichelbaum, M., Niesen, M., Niesen Dietrich, K., and Rausch, P. (1984). Carbamazepine levels in breast milk. *Ther. Drug. Monit.* **6,** 266–271.

Glauser, T. A., Mitchell, W. G., Weinstock, A., Bebin, M., Chen, D., Coupez, R., Stockis, A., and Lu, Z. S. (2007). Pharmacokinetics of levetiracetam in infants and young children with epilepsy. *Epilepsia* **48,** 1117–1122.

Gomita, Y., Furuno, K., Araki, Y., Yamatogi, Y., and Ohtahara, S. (1995). Phenobarbital in sera of epileptic mothers and their infants. *Am. J. Ther.* **2**, 968–971.

Gorman, M. P., and Soul, J. S. (2007). Neonatal hypocalcemic seizures in neonates exposed to topiramate in utero. *Pediatr. Neurol.* **36**, 274–276.

Hägg, S., and Spigset, O. (2000). Anticonvulsant use during lactation. *Drug Safety* **22**, 425–440.

Hibberd, C. M., Brooke, O. G., Carter, N. D., Haug, M., and Harzer, G. (1982). Variation in the composition of breast milk during the first 5 weeks of lactation: Implications for the feeding of preterm infants. *Arch. Dis. Child.* **57**, 658–662.

Hines, R. N., and McCarver, D. G. (2002). The ontogeny of human drug-metabolizing enzymes: Phase I oxidative enzymes. *J. Pharmacol. Exp. Ther.* **300**, 355–359.

Ishizaki, T., Yokochi, K., Chiba, K., Tabuchi, T., and Wagatsuma, T. (1981). Placental transfer of anticonvulsants (phenobarbital, phenytoin, valproic acid) and elimination from neonates. *Pediatr. Pharmacol.* **1**, 291–303.

Johannessen, S. I. (1997). Pharmacokinetics and interaction profile of topiramate: Review comparison with newer antiepileptic drugs. *Epilepsia* **38**(Suppl. 1), S18–23.

Johannessen, S. I., Helde, G., and Brodtkorb, E. (2005). Levetiracetam Concentrations in Serum in Breast Milk at Birth and during Lactation. *Epilepsia* **46**, 775–777.

Kaneko, S., Sato, T., and Suzuki, K. (1979). The levels of anticonvulsants in breast milk. *Br. J. Clin. Pharmacol.* **7**, 624–627.

Kawada, K., Itoh, S., Kusaka, T., Isobe, K., and Ishii, M. (2002). Pharmacokinetics of zonisamide in perinatal period. *Brain Dev.* **24**, 95–97.

Kearns, G. L., Abdel-Rahman, S. M., Alander, S. W., Blowey, D. L., Leeder, J. S., and Kauffman, R. E. (2003). developmental Pharmacology-Drug Disposition, Action, and Therapy in Infants and Children. *NEJM* **349**, 1157–1167.

Koup, J. R., Rose, J. Q., and Cohen, M. E. (1978). Ethosuximide pharmacokinetics in a pregnant patient and her newborn. *Epilepsia* **19**, 535–539.

Kramer, G., Hösli, I., Glanzmann, R., and Holzgreve, W. (2002). Levetiracetam accumulation in breast milk. *Epilepsia* **43**(Suppl. 7), 105.

Kristensen, O., Klitgaard, N. A., Jönsson, B., and Sindrup, S. (1983). Pharmacokinetics of 10-OH-carbazepine, the main metabolite of the antiepileptic oxcarbazepine, from serum saliva and concentrations. *Acta. Neurol. Scand.* **68**, 145–150.

Kristensen, J. H., Llett, K. F., Hackett, P. L., and Kohan, R. (2006). Gabapentin and breastfeeding: A case report. *J. Hum. Lact.* **22**, 426–428.

Kuhnz, W., Jäger-Roman, E., Rating, D., Deichl, A., Kunze, J., Helge, H., and Nau, H. (1983). Carbamazepine and carbamazepine-10, 11-epoxide during pregnancy and postnatal period in epileptic mother and their nursed infants: Clinical and pharmacokinetic effects. *Pediatr. Pharmacol.* **3**, 199–208.

Kuhnz, W., Koch, S., Jakob, S., Hartmann, A., Helge, H., and Nau, H. (1984). Ethosuximide in Epileptic Women during Pregnancy and Lactation Period. Placental Transfer, Serum Concentrations in Nursed Infants and Clinical Status. *Br. J. Clin. Pharmacol.* **18**, 671–677.

Kuhnz, W., Koch, S., Helge, H., and Nau, H. (1988). Primidone and phenobarbital during lactation period in epileptic women: Total and free drug levels in the nursed infants and their effects on neonatal behavior. *Dev. Pharmacol. Ther.* **11**, 147–154.

Liporace, J., Kao, A., and D'Abreu, A. (2004). Concerns regarding lamotrigine and breast-feeding. *Epilepsy Behav.* **5**, 102–105.

McCarver, D. G., and Hines, R. N. (2002). The ontogeny of human drug-metabolizing enzymes: Phase II oxidative enzymes. *J. Pharmacol. Exp. Ther.* **300**, 361–365.

Mirkin, B. L. (1971). Diphenylhydantoin: Placental transfer, fetal localization, neonatal metabolism and possible tetratogenic effects. *J. Pediatr.* **78**, 329–337.

Myllynen, P., Pienimäki, P., and Vähäkangas, K. (2001). Transplacental passage of oxcarbazepine and Its metabolites *in vivo*. *Epilepsia* **42,** 1482–1485.

Nau, H., Helge, H., and Luck, W. (1984). Valproic acid in the perinatal period: Decreased maternal serum protein binding results in fetal accumulation and neonatal displacement of the drug and some metabolites. *J. Pediatr.* **104,** 627–634.

Nau, H., Rating, D., Häuser, I., Jäger, E., Koch, S., and Helge, H. (1980). Placental transfer and pharmacokinetics of primidone and its metabolites, Phenobarbital, PEMA and hydroxypheno-barbital in neonates and infants of epileptic mothers. *Eur. J. Clin. Pharmacol.* **18,** 31–42.

Nau, H., Rating, D., Häuser, I., and Helge, H. (1981). Valproic acid and its metabolites: Placental transfer, neonatal pharmacokinetics, transfer into mother's milk and clinical status in neonates of epileptic mothers. *J. Pharmacol. Exp. Ther.* **219,** 768–770.

Niebyl, J. R., Blake, D. A., Freeman, J. M., and Luff, R. D. (1979). Carbamazepine levels in pregnancy and lactation. *Obstet. Gynecol.* **53,** 139–140.

Neville, M. C. (2001). Anatomy and physiology or lactation. *Pediatr. Clin. North. Am.* **48,** 13–34.

Ohman, I., Vitols, S., Luef, G., Söderfeldt, B., and Tomson, T. (2002). Topiramate Kinetics during Delivery, Lactation, and in the Neonate: Preliminary Observations. *Epilepsia* **43,** 1157–1160.

Ohman, I., Vitols, S., and Tomson, T. (2000). Lamotrigine in Pregnancy: Pharmacokinetics during Delivery, in the Neonate, and during Lactation. *Epilepsia* **41,** 709–713.

Ohman, I., Vitols, S., and Tomson, T. (2005). Pharmacokinetics of Gabapentin during delivery, in the neonatal period and lactation: Does fetal accumulation occur during pregnancy? *Epilepsia* **46,** 1621–1624.

Page-Sharp, M., Kristensen, J. H., Hackett, L. P., Beran, R. G., Rampono, J., Hale, T. W., Kohan, R., and Ilett, K. F. (2006). Transfer of lamotrigine into breast milk. *Ann. Pharmacother.* **40,** 1470–1471.

Perucca, E. (2006). Clinical pharmacokinetics of new-generation antiepileptic drugs at the extremes of age. *Clin. Pharmacokinet.* **45,** 351–363.

Pynnonen, S., and Sillanpaa, M. (1975). Carbamazepine and mother's milk. *Lancet.* **306,** 563.

Pynnonen, S., Kanto, J., Sillanpää, M., and Erkkola, R. (1977). Carbamazepine: placental transport, tissue concentrations in foetus and newborn, and level in milk. *Acta. Pharmacol. Toxicol. (Copenh)* **41,** 244–253.

Rane, A., Bertilsson, L., and Palmer, L. (1975). Disposition of placentally transferred carbamazepine (Tegretol) in the newborn. *Eur. J. Clin. Pharmacol.* **8,** 337–341.

Rane, A., and Tunell, R. (1981). Ethosuximide in human milk and in plasma of a mother and her nursed infant. *Br. J. Clin. Pharmacol.* **12,** 855–858.

Shimoyama, R., Ohkubo, T., Sugawara, K., Ogasawaea, T., Ozaki, T., Kagiya, A., and Saito, Y. (1998). Monitoring of phenytoin in human breast milk, maternal and cord blood plasma by solid-phase extraction and liquid chromatography. *J. Pharm. Biomed. Anal.* **17,** 863–869.

Shimoyama, R., and Ohkubo, T. (1999). Monitoring of zonisamide in human breast milk and maternal plasma by solid-phase extraction HPLC method. *Biomed. Chromatogr.* **13,** 370–372.

Sills, G. J., and Brodie, M. J. (2007). Pharmacokinetics and drug interactions with zonisamide. **48,** 435–441.

Soderman, P., and Rane, A. (1986). Ethosuximide in human milk and in plasma of a mother and her nursed infant. *Acta. Pharmacol. Toxicol.* **59**(Suppl 5 pt 2), 513.

Stahl, M. M. S., Neiderud, J., and Vinge, E. (1997). Thrombocytopenia purpura and anemia in a breast-fed infant whose mother was treated with valproic acid. *J. Pediatr.* **130,** 1001–1003.

Steen, B., Rane, A., Lönnerholm, G., Falk, O., Elwin, C. E., and Sjöqvist, F. (1982). Phenytoin excretion in human breast milk and plasma levels in nursed infant. *Ther. Drug. Monit.* **4,** 331–334.

Syme, M. R., Paxton, J. W., and Keelan, J. A. (2004). Drug transfer and metabolism by human placenta. *Clin. Pharmacokinet.* **43,** 487–514.

Takeda, A., Okada, H., Tanaka, H., Izumi, M., Ishikawa, S., and Noro, T. (1992). Protein binding of four antiepileptic drugs in maternal and umbilical cord serum. *Epilepsy Res.* **13,** 147–151.

Tallian, K. B., Nahata, M. C., and Lo, W. (2004). Pharmacokinetics of gabapentin in paediatric patients with uncontrolled seizures. *J. Clin. Pharm. Ther.* **29,** 511–515.

Tomson, T., and Villen, T. (1994). Ethosuximide enantiomers in pregnancy and lactation. *Ther. Drug. Monit.* **16,** 621–623.

Tomson, T., Palm, R., Källen, K., Ben-Menachem, E., Söderfeldt, B., Danielsson, B., Johansson, R., Luef, G., and Ohman, I. (2007). Pharmacokinetics of levetiracetam during pregnancy, delivery, in the neonatal period, and lactation. *Epilepsia* **48,** 1111–1116.

U.S. Department of Health and Human Services, FDA (2005). Guidance for Industry [draft]. Clinical lactation studies-Study design, data analysis, and recommendations for labeling February 2005.

Von Unruh, G. E., Froescher, W., Hoffmann, F., and Niesen, M. (1984). Valproic acid in breast milk. How much is really in there? *Ther. Drug. Monit.* **6,** 272–276.

Wisner, K. L., and Perel, J. M. (1998). Serum levels of valproate and carbamazepine in breastfeeding mother-infant pairs. *J. Clin. Psychopharmacol.* **18,** 167–169.

Yerby, M. S., Friel, P. N., McCormick, K., Koerner, M., Van Allen, M., Leavit, A. M., Sells, C. J., and Yerby, J. A. (1990). Pharmacokinetics of anticonvulsants in pregnancy: Alterations in plasma protein binding. *Epilepsy Res.* **5,** 223–228.

SEIZURES IN PREGNANCY: DIAGNOSIS AND MANAGEMENT

Robert L. Beach* and Peter W. Kaplan†

*Department of Neurology, Upstate Medical University, Syracuse, New York 13210, USA
†Department of Neurology, Johns Hopkins University School of Medicine, Johns Hopkins
Bayview Medical Center, Baltimore, Maryland 21224, USA

I. Introduction
   A. Seizures in Pregnancy
   B. Effects of Pregnancy on Seizure Control in WWE
   C. Status Epilepticus
II. AED Pharmacokinetics in Pregnancy
III. Seizures in Nonepileptic Patients During Pregnancy
   A. Intracranial Hemorrhage
   B. Subarachnoid Hemorrhage
   C. Cerebral Venous Thrombosis
   D. Metabolic Causes of Stroke in Pregnancy
IV. Eclampsia
   A. Management of Eclampsia
   B. Prognosis
   C. Eclampsia; Summary
   References

Most seizures during pregnancy occur in women who already have epilepsy. During pregnancy most women will continue their previous level of seizure control, although 15–30% may experience an increase in seizures. Pregnancy-induced changes in antiepileptic drug pharmacokinetics are a major factor affecting changes in seizure control during pregnancy, although compliance is also a significant factor. Status epilepticus occurs in only 1–2% of pregnancies, and if treated appropriately and aggressively carries a fairly low risk of morbidity and mortality. Structural and metabolic changes may precipitate new-onset seizures during pregnancy. The structural causes include intracranial hemorrhage of multiple types, cerebral venous sinus thrombosis, and ischemic stroke. Metabolic causes include hyperemesis gravidarum; acute hepatitis (due to fatty liver of pregnancy or viral hepatitis); metabolic diseases, such as acute intermittent porphyria; infections, such as malaria; and eclampsia.

INTERNATIONAL REVIEW OF
NEUROBIOLOGY, VOL. 83
DOI: 10.1016/S0074-7742(08)00015-9

I. Introduction

A. SEIZURES IN PREGNANCY

The majority of seizures during pregnancy are due to already declared epilepsy (To and Cheung, 1997). *De Novo* seizures in the absence of signs of preeclampsia require exclusion of acute metabolic alterations [e.g., hyponatremia, hypoglycemia, hyperglycemia or acute hepatic failure from fatty liver of pregnancy or viral hepatitis, and structural lesions] (Donaldson *et al.*, 1983; Tank *et al.*, 2002). Gestational epilepsy refers to seizures occurring only during pregnancy. Gestational- onset epileptic patients have their initial seizure during pregnancy and then have recurrent unprovoked seizures. Eclampsia is the most common cause of new-onset seizures during pregnancy.

B. EFFECTS OF PREGNANCY ON SEIZURE CONTROL IN WWE

Two thirds of women with epilepsy (WWE) will continue their prior level of seizure control during pregnancy or will improve (Bardy, 1987; Gjerde *et al.*, 1988; Schmidt *et al.*, 1983). Nearly 60% are likely to remain seizure-free, whereas 15–30% may have an increase in frequency during pregnancy (EURAP Study Group, 2006). Risk for deterioration in seizure control has been associated with focal onset epilepsy, polytherapy, monotherapy with oxcarbazepine or lamotrigine, and poor compliance associated with lack of prepregnancy planning (de Haan *et al.*, 2004; EURAP Study Group, 2006; Lopes-Cendes *et al.*, 1992; Tomson *et al.*, 1994). There is intraindividual variability in patterns of seizure control in successive pregnancies, and interindividual variability among WWE (Kilpatrick and Matthay, 1992; Shehata and Okosun, 2004). Several factors, such as hormonal hepatic microsomal enzyme induction affecting the metabolism of antiepileptic drugs (AEDs); alterations in protein binding and changes in the volume of distribution affecting unbound AED and total AED levels; increased renal clearance; impaired intestinal absorption; and variable compliance, influence seizure control during pregnancy.

It has been recommended to make only essential changes to AEDs once pregnancy is confirmed in WWE.

For valproate or phenobarbital, Meador (2007) make a persuasive argument that with such a significant risk for IQ drops on these agents when measured in the children at 2–3 years, that perhaps we should switch them off these agents, particularly if they are not brittle epileptics. There is some evidence that a moderate dose, frequent low dosing, or long-acting formulations of valproate, which reduce peak levels, may reduce risk. It is important to ensure good compliance with AEDs throughout pregnancy to avoid relapse of seizures, especially because some patients may discontinue AEDs due to a perceived risk, without discussing these issues with their doctors (EURAP Study Group, 2006).

Seizures are most likely to occur in the first trimester and in the peripartum period. Nearly 5% of WWE will have peripartum seizures, representing a threefold increase compared to the rest of pregnancy. This is likely due to factors such as poor compliance, dehydration, decreased oral intake, and intercurrent medications (Bardy, 1987; EURAP Study Group, 2006; Gjerde et al., 1988). During pregnancy, AED dose may require an increase in some patients, if free drug levels fall, or if simple partial seizures or nonconvulsive generalized seizures increase, or if complex partial or generalized seizures occur.

C. STATUS EPILEPTICUS

The risk for status epilepticus during pregnancy is about 1–2%. Status had been reported to have high risk for maternal morbidity and mortality as well as fetal mortality in older studies, but this risk appears to be lower with modern care (EURAP Study Group, 2006). In this study of 1956 pregnancies, there were 36 cases of status epilepticus of which 12 were convulsive. These resulted in no maternal mortality or miscarriage, but a single stillbirth. Standard treatment protocols for SE should be employed quickly; as the duration of convulsive status is the primary risk factor for morbidity and mortality.

Seizures during pregnancy create risk to both mother and fetus, convulsions may cause lactic acidosis and transient increases in uterine pressure and blood flow. It is recommended for the patient to be placed in the left lateral decubitus position to facilitate fetal blood flow and to reduce the possibility of aspiration (Barrett and Richens, 2003).

Oxygen, intravenous fluids, and glucose should be given; lorazepam should be used initially to stop the seizures (Pennell, 2003). Electrolytes, complete blood count (CBC), calcium, magnesium, glucose, and antiepileptic drug levels should be obtained quickly. Intramuscular thiamine should be administered if there is any possibility of deficiency or alcoholism. Although intravenous magnesium is the agent of choice for eclampsia, it is not used for noneclamptic seizures, and conventional AEDs are appropriate. If the patient is already taking a known AED, then additional doses of that medication should be given. Although no drugs are absolutely contraindicated for status treatment during pregnancy, unless valproate or phenobarbital are already part of the patient's regimen, the seizures are related to valproate or phenobarbital withdrawal, or have responded well in the past to valproate or phenobarbital, then these drugs should be avoided. As seizures are more frequent and problematic during labor, potential causes such as dehydration, sleep deprivation, and analgesics which decrease seizure threshold (such as meperidine) should be avoided.

II. AED Pharmacokinetics in Pregnancy

Knowledge of the pharmacokinetics of the different AEDs during pregnancy is necessary to appropriately anticipate and implement necessary medication changes (Perucca, 1987). A major factor is decreased binding to plasma proteins, which causes lower total plasma levels, but generally free (unbound) and active drug concentrations remain stable. Thus total serum levels may be misleading, unfortunately free levels often require more time before getting results.

Battino et al. (1984) found that total and unbound plasma concentrations of phenobarbital decline throughout pregnancy by nearly 50%. Yerby et al. (1992) reported no significant changes in free valproate levels, although total levels declined significantly. They also reported a 42% decrease in total plasma carbamazepine levels along with a 22% decrease in free carbamazepine. However, Tomson et al. (1994) found much less reduction in levels. Both these groups found a 40% decrease in total phenytoin levels and a 20% decrease in free levels.

Levels of lamotrigine are dramatically affected during pregnancy (Öhman et al., 2000). By the 32nd week of gestation, clearance may increase more than threefold (Pennell et al., 2004; Tran et al., 2002). This is a greater decrease in drug levels compared to older AEDs and may cause increased seizure frequency or severity, which can be addressed by escalating doses. If raised during pregnancy, the dose needs to be reduced after delivery to reduce postpartum toxicity (de Haan et al., 2004).

The effects of pregnancy on the pharmokinetics of the other newer AEDs are not clear, although oxcarbazepine's monohydroxy derivative (its active metabolite) may also be reduced by induction of hepatic glucuronidation. If steady-state drug levels prior to pregnancy are available, they can guide timing for diagnostic and therapeutic changes during pregnancy. Monitoring of drug levels is probably most useful for phenytoin, lamotrigine, and oxcarbazepine, although it is probably appropriate for all of the newer drugs where pregnancy-induced metabolic changes have not yet been fully identified. Some authors recommend checking levels each trimester and after delivery, or even more frequently with some AEDs.

III. Seizures in Nonepileptic Patients During Pregnancy

There are both structural and metabolic changes that may precipitate seizures during pregnancy. The structural causes include intracranial hemorrhage of multiple types, cerebral venous sinus thrombosis, ischemic stroke and eclampsia (which is addressed later in this chapter). Metabolic causes include hyperemesis gravidarum, acute hepatitis (due to fatty liver of pregnancy or viral hepatitis; Jaiswal et al., 2001), rare metabolic diseases, such as AIP, or infections, such as malaria.

A. INTRACRANIAL HEMORRHAGE

Munnur *et al.* (2005) reported that intracranial hemorrhage was seen in 1% of ICU pregnancy cases. In other studies, mortality from intracerebral hemorrhage (ICH) ranges from 40% to 70% (Shehata and Okosun, 2004). Typical causes include rupture of aneurysms or arteriovenous malformations (AVMs), or more rarely from bleeding into a tumor. Intraparenchymal hemorrhage may be related to hypertension, or therapeutic, autoimmune, or genetic anticoagulation. Kittner *et al.* (1996) reported the relative risk of ICH during pregnancy was 2.5 and increased to 18.2 in the immediate postpartum period in a large study from Baltimore.

B. SUBARACHNOID HEMORRHAGE

Carhuapoma *et al.* (1999) report a threefold increase in subarachnoid hemorrhage in pregnancy, with 85% of occurring after the first trimester; and into the puerperal period. This is likely related to increases in blood and stroke volume and increased cardiac output; as well as hormonal effects on the vasculature (Gonik *et al.*, 1991). Initial mortality approaches 50%, and overall mortality may be as high as 75%. Diagnosis and treatment are similar to that for nonpregnant patients with appropriate protection to the fetus. Similar problems occur with eclampsia, more often with the HELLP syndrome (see below).

Early surgery is favored as in nonpregnant patients. Awake patients, with grades I to III Hunt and Hess scores, should probably have aneurysm clipping within the first few days (Dias and Sekhar, 1990). In the event of vasospasm, hypervolumic, hypertensive therapy is helpful once the aneurysm has been clipped (Roman *et al.*, 2004). Patients with more severe initial insults have a high operative mortality and are usually treated medically. Appropriate antiepileptic drug treatment should be instituted.

AVMs appear more than 10 times more likely to bleed during pregnancy, and account for nearly half of ICH in pregnancy (Trivedi and Kirkpatrick, 2003). Bleeding risk is highest during the first pregnancy, but after the initial hemorrhage, about 30% of AVMs tend to rebleed in subsequent pregnancies.

Diagnosis can be made by MRA or intravenous contrast angiography. Treatment should include reduction of intracranial pressure and prophylactic antiepileptic drug treatment, using oral or currently available intravenous drugs such as levetiracetam and phenytoin or fosphenytoin. Valproate may be more risky due to its effect on platelet function (Gidal *et al.*, 1994).

Surgical removal, focused radiation, or endovascular embolization have all been used effectively, although the timing of these interventions is dependent on factors such as the size of the hematoma, stage of pregnancy, extent of neurologic deficit, and other risk factors. Small AVMs with minor hemorrhage and associated small deficits can probably have treatment deferred until after delivery (Trivedi and Kirkpatrick, 2003).

Embolization of aneurysms and AVMs with interventional radiology has an expanding role, although careful fetal protection is required (Kizzilkilic *et al.*, 2003). Patients with adequately embolized aneurysms and AVMs may be treated primarily according to obstetric concerns. Obstetrical considerations may also determine the need for Caesarian section, although vaginal birth is safe with adequate pain and blood pressure control and facilitated delivery.

C. Cerebral Venous Thrombosis

Although about three quarters of cerebral venous thromboses (CVT) occur peripartum, there is an increased risk throughout pregnancy (Ferro *et al.*, 2004). The prothrombotic state associated with pregnancy may be due to increases in factors II, VII, and X, in addition to impaired fibrinolysis, and/or to a decrease in anticoagulant factors such as protein S (Toglia and Weg, 1996). The hypercoagulable state in pregnancy is enhanced by dehydration, hyperemesis, infection, and hypertension (Kimber, 2002). Cerebral venous thrombosis and dural sinus thrombosis appear to be more prevalent underdeveloped nations (Munnur *et al.*, 2005).

Cerebral venous thrombose presents with headache in 95% of patients; about 50% will have seizures or focal neurologic deficits. Papilledema or altered mental status is present in about a third of patients (Kimber, 2002). The "empty delta sign," where the clot is a delta-shaped or circular-filling defect near the confluence of the sagittal and transverse sinuses, is the classical finding with contrast computerized tomography (CT). Magnetic resonance venography is more sensitive and specific, generally avoiding contrast angiography. Treatment includes anticoagulation with heparin. Hemorrhagic cerebral infarcts are also common.

D. Metabolic Causes of Stroke in Pregnancy

In addition to acute electrolyte disturbances, hepatic failure, renal insufficiency, and AIP may first present with seizures in pregnancy, often associated with confusion, abdominal pain, and weakness (Jaiswal *et al.*, 2001; Kaupinnen, 2005). Because some of these symptoms also occur in eclampsia, porphyria should be considered in the differential diagnosis of eclampsia.

The various porphyrias are diagnosed by urine porphyrins and porphoblinogens, and by specific assays of their metabolic enzymes. Stress, dehydration, infection, and enzyme-inducing drugs, as well as hormonal changes during pregnancy, may precipitate the syndrome. Because the older AEDs and some of the newer ones (in a dose-dependent manner) may exacerbate or precipitate porphyria, the initial choice of AED should be narrowed to gabapentin, pregabalin, and levetiracetam (Hahn *et al.*, 2006). Treatment also requires high doses glucose and sometimes intravenous infusion of hematin (Kaupinnen, 2005). Refractory status epilepticus may occur.

IV. Eclampsia

Eclampsia is one of the most frequent causes of seizures during pregnancy and remains a significant cause of perinatal morbidity and death. Worldwide, there are about 600,000 maternal deaths with maternal mortality ranging from 1.8% to 5% (Cunningham *et al.*, 1993; WHO/UNICEF, 1990). Even in Western countries, it occurs in about 1 in 2000 pregnancies, with an even higher incidence of 1 per 33–1700 pregnancies in third world nations (Douglas and Redman, 1994). It is still a major cause of death in the United States, United Kingdom, and Scandinavia (Roberts and Redman, 1993). In the United States, 5–10% of Caucasian women are affected, and an even greater percentage of black primigravida women (15–20%) are affected (Sibai *et al.*, 1986). Furthermore, one study indicated that subsequent pregnancies were prone to a 46.8% incidence of eclampsia if the first pregnancy was eclamptic (Sibai *et al.*, 1986).

The hallmark of eclampsia is the presence of hypertension in pregnancy. The typical triad of clinical features in preeclampsia consists of gestational hypertension along with edema and proteinuria (preeclampsia), which is termed eclampsia once seizures or coma appear. Of diagnostic importance is that the full triad is often not present, with one of the three features missing. Even so, most women have one or more heralding features prior to the seizure. A retrospective study of 383 cases of eclampsia in Great Britain noted about 60% (227/383) had visual changes, headache, or epigastric pain. In 38%, seizures occurred before the appearance of either proteinuria or hypertension had been noted (Douglas and Redman, 1994). Eclampsia can thus supervene without the appearance of the apparently heralding features of preclampsia, and there is compelling opinion that the different clinical manifestations and their severity do not represent a continuum that predicts subsequent, signs, symptoms or progression to eclampsia (Katz *et al.*, 2000), HELLP or intracranial hemorrhage. In any case, other causes or explanations for seizures must be excluded to make the diagnosis.

Gestational hypertension (GH) has replaced pregnancy-induced hypertension when referring to an elevated blood pressure without proteinuria after 20 weeks of gestation (NHBPEPWG, 2000). The cut-off is a systolic pressure above 140 mm Hg or a diastolic pressure above 90 mm Hg. About a quarter of women with GH develop proteinuria. Other frequent features are epigastric pain (often from intrahepatic hemorrhage), headache, and visual loss. Visual changes may affect the visual pathways anywhere between the retina (detached) through to pre- and postchiasmatic pathways and the visual cortex (edema, micro-, and macrohemorrhages; Sheehan and Lynch, 1973). There are several CNS problems that may supervene in the pre-, intra-, and postpartum periods including small and large forebrain and brainstem bleeds, edema and raised intracranial pressure, and venous sinus thrombosis.

A clotting disorder and bleeding diathesis that further complicates the brain compromise in the presence of intracranial hypertension is that of the HELLP syndrome (Lain and Roberts, 2002). This condition is characterized by hemolysis, elevated liver enzymes, and low platelets, and may lead to devastating intracranial hemorrhage with a high morbidity and mortality (Redman and Roberts, 1993), even in the absence of hypertension. End-organ damage from hypertension with or without HELLP can lead to cardiac decompensation, renal damage, pulmonary and peripheral edema, hepatic pain and clotting abnormalities, and myriad neurological problems.

Eclampsia has been subdivided according to whether it presents before (antepartum), during (intrapartum), shortly after (early postpartum), or late (>48 h) after birth of the child. About 44% of cases occur postpartum, 12% after the first 2 days (Roberts and Redman, 1993). Some patients present more than 7–25 days after delivery. Postpartum eclampsia often includes severe headache, visual changes, photophobia, scotomata, epigastric pain, and increased uric acid (Lubarsky et al., 1994). Confusing the issue, is that in many cases, GH was the principal or only heralding feature. This is all the more concerning, as postpartum eclampsia carries a worse prognosis with more frequent associated adult respiratory distress syndrome and disseminated intravascular coagulation.

Proteinuria (protein in the urine), is defined as >300 mg/24 h, but with a dipstick, 1+ proteinuria in the absence of a urinary tract infection is concerning (ACOG, 1996). Fifteen to twenty percent of eclamptic women have no proteinuria before the eclamptic seizure.

Severe preeclampsia is defined by BP >160 mm Hg systolic or 110 mm Hg diastolic on two occasions at least 6 h apart; proteinuria >5g/24 h or 3+ dipsticks on two random samples 4 h apart. Other features include abnormal liver function, cyanosis, pulmonary edema, cerebral, or visual problems, epigastric pain, low platelets, impaired fetal growth, or urine output < 0.5 liter/24 h (ACOG, 2002).

HELLP syndrome is defined as the presence of hemolysis (abnormal peripheral blood smear; bilirubin > 1.2 mg/dl or LDH > 600 IU/liter), and a platelet count <100–150,000/μl with elevated liver enzymes (more than twice normal AST; Martin et al., 2002; Sibai et al., 1993, 1995; Sullivan et al., 1994; Weinstein, 1982). This dire condition may affect up to one fifth of women with severe eclampsia and along with a ruptured liver have a much increased morbidity and mortality (Martin et al., 2002; Sibai et al., 1993, 1995; Sullivan et al., 1994).

There are many theories about the causes of preeclampsia and eclampsia with one, suggesting that there is impaired and abnormal cytotrophoblastic invasion of the uterine myometrium. This decreases the release of blood pressure-lowering modulators, thus favoring hypertension. Maternal mitochondrial defects (Widschwendter *et al.*, 1998) with loss of cristae and swelling (Clarke, 1990) have been found to be associated with eclampsia. The eNOS gene has been suggested (Amgrmsson *et al.*, 1997).

Along with the clinical features suggesting an eclamptic diagnosis, MRI can show characteristic serpiginous, multifocal curvi-linear T2 weighted changes along the watershed zones (Crawford *et al.*, 1987; Digre *et al.*, 1993; Raroque *et al.*, 1980), particularly in the occipital lobes. Additionally, changes indicative of edema, of small and large hemorrhages or infarcts, can be identified. Hemorrhage aside, CT head scans are much less sensitive. These typical radiological features are essential in distinguishing eclampsia from other causes of seizures.

A. Management of Eclampsia

The great majority of eclamptic patients are treated by obstetricians with neurologists having a consultative role for neurologic problems. Therapy is largely aimed at controlling hypertension, identifying and treating coagulopathy and other target organ decompensation including pulmonary edema, ARDS, renal failure, and intracranial swelling, infarcts, and bleeds. Antihypertensive agents favored include hydralazine, labetalol, nicardipine, and nifedepine, and are used often when diastolic pressure exceed 100 mm Hg, or a mean arterial blood pressure of 125 mm Hg (Easton *et al.*, 1998; Sibai and Ustav, 1995). Several trials over the last dozen years have suggested the benefit of magnesium sulfate in decreasing progression from GH to eclampsia (Lucas *et al.*, 1995), and the recurrence of seizures in eclampsia (Duley and Johanson, 1994). Empirically magnesium sulfate has been demonstrated to confer a 67% lower risk than phenytoin, and 52% lower risk than diazepam in this study of 1687 randomized patients (Duley and Johanson, 1994). Study drawbacks were the lack of blinding by physicians to the treatment arm, lack of data on phenytoin levels and individual patient blood pressures. The Parkland Study in 2138 women with GH (Lucas *et al.*, 1995) found that 10 of 1089 women on phenytoin, versus none of 1049 on magnesium sulfate progressed from GH to having seizures. This represented only a 1% absolute decrease in seizures. Furthermore, only 20% of women with GH had other signs of preeclampsia. In addition to magnesium sulfate, AEDs have been used successfully to decrease recurrent seizures (Appleton *et al.*, 1991; Coyaji and Otiv, 1990; Crowther, 1990; Slater *et al.*, 1987; Tuffnell *et al.*, 1989). Parenteral anticonvulsants including phenytoin and benzodiazepines have also been used (Tufnell *et al.*, 1984). The role of newer agents such as levetiracetam is unknown. It would seem inadvisable to use valproate (with its platelet-lowering effect) in this condition.

The cornerstone of treatment remains the expeditious delivery of a viable baby which often reverses the course of this progressive and fatal disease. After delivery, maternal hypertension can be more intensively managed without risk to the fetus of placental hypo-perfusion.

Although magnesium sulfate is not a true anticonvulsant, it exhibits an anti-vasospastic effect beyond its transient lowering of blood pressure. There is a consequent increase in cerebral blood flow and middle cerebral artery perfusion (Belfort and Moise, 1992), thus decreasing cerebral ischemia. Furthermore, it increases prostacyclin production which in turn acts as an endothelial vasodilator (Sipes et al., 1994).

B. Prognosis

Ten percent of eclamptic women have repeated seizures if not treated, but a similar percentage will have repeated seizures even when treated with magnesium sulfate. One fifth of maternal deaths are attributable to intracerebral hemorrhage, frequently in patients with a blood pressure of over 170/120 mm Hg (Sibai, 1990).

Hepatic, renal, and pulmonary damage largely reverse with treatment of hypertension and delivery of the baby, in the absence of intraorgan hemorrhage. Similarly, cerebral edema reverses.

C. Eclampsia; Summary

Eclampsia poses a significant worldwide risk for seizures and combined maternal–fetal morbidity and mortality. More intensive treatment, earlier diagnosis and management in intensive care setting by obstetricians with the help of neurologists have lowered the death rate. Expeditious fetal delivery, the correct use of antihypertensive drugs, magnesium sulfate, and antiepileptic medications, and the management of multiorgan failure are key to a good maternal–fetal outcome.

References

American College of Obstetricians and Gynecologists. ACOG Technical Bulletin 219 (1996). Hypertension in pregnancy, Washington, DC.

American College of Obstetricians and Gynecologists. (2002). Practice bulletin. Diagnosis and management of preeclampsia and eclampsia. Number 33, 1/2002.

Amgrmsson, R., Hayward, C., Nadaud, S., Baldursdottir, A., Walker, J. J., Liston, W. A., et al. (1997). Evidence for a familial pregnancy-induced hypertension locus in the eNOS-gene region. Am. J. Hum. Genet. **61,** 354–362.

Appleton, M. P., Kuehle, T. J., Raebel, M. A., Adams, H. R., Knight, A. B., and Gold, W. R. (1991). Magnesium sulfate versus phenytoin for seizure prophylaxis in pregnancy-induced hypertension. Am. J. Obstet. Gynecol. **165,** 907–913.

Bardy, A. H. (1987). Incidence of seizures during pregnancy, labor and puerperium in epileptic women: A prospective study. Acta Neurol. Scand. **75,** 356–360.

Barnett, C., and Richens, A. (2003). Epilepsy and pregnancy: Report of an Epilepsy Research Foundation Workshop. Epilepsy Res. **52,** 147–187.

Battino, D., Binelli, S., Bossi, L., et al. (1984). Changes in Primidone/phenobarbital ratio during pregnancy and the puerperium. Clin. Pharmacokinet. **9,** 252–260.

Belfort, M. A., and Moise, K. J. (1992). Effect of magnesium sulfate on maternal brain blood flow in preeclampsia: A randomized placebo controlled study. Am. J. Obstet. Gynecol. **167,** 661–666.

Carhuapoma, J. R., Tomlinson, M. W., and Levine, S. R. (1999). Neurologic diseases. In "High Risk Pregnancy: Management Options" (D. K. James, P. J. Steer, C. P. Weiner, and B. Gonic, Eds.), 2nd ed., pp. 803–836. WB Saunders, London.

Clarke, A. (1990). Mitochondrial genome: Defects, disease, and evolution. J. Med. Genet. **27,** 451–456.

Coyaji, K. J., and Otiv, S. R. (1990). Single high dose of intravenous phenytoin sodium for the treatment of eclampsia. Acta Obstet. Gynecol. Scand. **69,** 115.

Crawford, S., Varner, M. W., Digre, K. B., et al. (1987). Cranial magnetic resonance imaging in eclampsia. Obstet. Gynecol. **70,** 474–477.

Crowther, C. (1990). Magnesium sulphate versus diazepam in the management of eclampsia: A randomized controlled trial. Br. J. Obstet. Gynaecol. **97,** 110–117.

Cunningham, F. G., MacDonald, P. C., Gant, N. F., Leveno, K. J., and Gilstrap, L. C. (1993). Hypertensive disorders in pregnancy. In "Williams Obstetric" (F. G. Cunningham, P. C. MacDonald, and N. F. Gant, Eds.), 19th ed., pp. 763–817. Appleton & Lange, Norwalk (CT).

de Haan, G. J., Edelbroek, P., Segers, J., et al. (2004). Gestation-induced changes in lamotrigine pharmacokinetics: A monotherapy study. Neurology **63,** 571–573.

Dias, M. S., and Sekhar, L. N. (1990). Intracranial hemorrhage from aneurysms and arteriovenous malformations during pregnancy and puerperium. Neurosurgery **27,** 855–866.

Digre, K. B., Varner, M. W., Osborn, A. G., and Crawford, S. (1993). Cranial magnetic resonance imaging in severe preeclampsia vs. eclampsia. Arch. Neurol. **50,** 399–406.

Donaldson, J. O. (1983). Neurologic emergencies during pregnancy. In "Critical Care of the Obstetric Patient" (R. L. Berkowitz, Ed.), pp. 367–383. Churchill Livingstone, New York.

Douglas, K., and Redman, C. W. (1994). Eclampsia in the United Kingdom. BMJ **309,** 1395–1400.

Duley, L., and Johanson, R. (1994). Magnesium sulphate for preeclampsia and eclampsia: The evidence so far. Br. J. Obstet. Gynaecol. **101,** 565–567.

Easton, J. D., Mas, J. L., Lamy, C., Digre, K. B., Varner, M. W., Redman, C. W. G., et al. (1998). Severe preeclampsia/eclampsia: Hypertensive encephalopathy of pregnancy? Cerebrovasc. Dis. **8,** 53–58.

Ferro, J. M., Canhao, P., Stam, J., et al. (2004). Prognosis of cerebral vein and dural sinus thrombosis: Results of the international study on cerebral vein and dural sinus thrombosis (ISCVT). Stroke **35,** 664–670.

Gidal, B. E., Spencer, N. W., Collins, D. M., et al. (1994). Valproate mediated disturbances of hemostasis: Relationship to concentration and dose. Neurology **44,** 1418–1422.

Gonik, B., Gietzentanner, A., Daily, W. H., et al. (1991). Intracranial hemorrhage in pregnancy. In "Critical Care Obstetrics" 2nd ed. Clark SL.

Gjerde, I. O., Strandjord, R. E., and Ulstein, M. (1988). The course of epilepsy during pregnancy: A study of 78 cases. Acta Neurol. Scand. **78,** 198–205.

Hahn, M., Gildemeister, O. S., Krauss, G. L., Pepe, J. A., Lambrecht, R. W., Donohue, S., and
  Bonkovsky, H. L. (1997). Effects of new anticonvulsant medications on porphyrin synthesis in
  cultured liver cells: Potential implications for patients with acute porphyria. *Neurology* **49**(1), 97–106.
Jaiswal, S. P., Jain, A. K., Naik, G., *et al.* (2001). Viral hepatitis during pregnancy. *Int J Gynaecol Obstet*
  72, 103–108.
Katz, V. L., Farmer, R., and Kuller, J. A. (2000). Preeclampsia into eclampsia: Toward a new
  paradigm. *Am. J. Obstet. Gynecol.* **182,** 1389–1396.
Kaupinen, R. (2005). *Lancet* **365,** 241–252.
Kilpatrick, S. J., and Matthay, M. A. (1992). Obstetric patients requiring critical care: A five year
  review. *Chest* **101,** 1407–1412.
Kimber, J. (2002). Cerebral venous sinus thrombosis. *QJ Med.* **95,** 137–142.
Kittner, S. J., Stern, B. J., Feeser, B. R., *et al.* (1996). Pregnancy and the risk of stroke. *N. Engl. J. Med.*
  335, 768–774.
Kizzilkilic, O., Albayram, S., Adaletli, I., *et al.* (2003). Endovascular treatment of ruptured intracra-
  nial aneurysms during pregnancy: Report of three cases. *Acta Gynecol. Obstet.* **268,** 325–328.
Lain, K. Y., and Roberts, J. M. (2002). Contemporary concepts of the pathogenesis and management
  of preeclampsia. *JAMA* **287,** 3183–3186.
Lopes-Cendes, I. E., Andermann, E., Cendes, L., Dansky, L., and Andermann, F. (1992). Risk factors
  for changes in seizure frequency during pregnancy of epileptic women: A cohort study. *Epilepsia*
  33(Suppl. 3), 57.
Lubarsky, S. L., Barton, J. R., Friedman, S. A., Nasreddine, S., Ramadan, K., and Sibai, B. M. (1994).
  Late postpartum eclampsia revisited. *Obstet. Gynecol.* **83,** 502–505.
Lucas, L., Leveno, K., and Cunningham, G. (1995). A comparison of magnesium sulfate with
  phenytoin for the prevention of eclampsia. *N. Engl. J. Med.* **333,** 201–205.
Martin, J. N., Magann, E. F., and Isler, C. M. (2002). HELLP syndrome: The scope of disease and
  treatment. *In* "Hypertension in Pregnancy" (M. A. Belfort, S. Thornton, and G. R. Saade, Eds.),
  pp. 141–188. Marcel Dekker, New York.
Meador, K. J., Baker, G., Cohen M. J., Gaily E., and Westerveld, M. (2007). Cognitive/behavioral
  teratogenetic effects of antiepileptic drugs. *Epilepsy and Behavior* **11**(3), 292–302.
Munnur, U., Karnad, D. R., Bandi, V. D. P., *et al.* (2005). Critically ill obstetric patients in an
  American and an Indian public hospital: Comparison of case-mix, organ dysfunction, intensive
  care requirements and outcomes. *Intensive Care Med.* **31,** 1087–1094.
Öhman, I., Vitols, S., and Tomson, T. (2000). Lamotrigine in pregnancy: Pharmacokinetics during
  delivery, in the neonate, and during lactation. *Epilepsia* **41,** 709–713.
Pennell, P. B. (2003). Antiepileptic drug pharmacokinetics during pregnancy and lactation. *Neurology*
  61(Suppl. 2), S35–S42.
Pennell, P. B., Newport, D. J., Stowe, Z. N., *et al.* (2004). The impact of pregnancy and childbirth on
  the metabolism of lamotrigine. *Neurology* **62,** 292–295.
Perucca, E. (1987). Drug metabolism in pregnancy, infancy and childhood. *Pharmacol. Ther.* **34,**
  129–143.
Raroque, H. G., Orrison, W. W., and Rosenberg, G. A. (1980). Neurologic involvement in toxemia of
  pregnancy: Reversible MRI lesions. *Neurology* **40,** 167–169.
Redman, C. W., and Roberts, J. M. (1993). Management of preeclampsia. *Lancet* **341,** 1451–1454.
Roberts, J. M., and Redman, C. W. G. (1993). Preeclampsia: More than pregnancy-induced
  hypertension. *Lancet* **341,** 1447–1451.
Roman, H., Descargues, G., Lopes, M., *et al.* (2004). Subarachnoid hemorrhage due to cerebral
  aneurismal rupture during pregnancy. *Acta Obstet. Gynecol. Scand.* **83,** 330–334.
NHBPEPWG (2000). Report of the National High Blood Pressure Education Program Working
  Group on high blood pressure in pregnancy. *Am. J. Obstet. Gynecol.* **183,** S1–S22.
Schmidt, D., Canger, R., Avanzini, G., Battino, D., Cusi, C., Beck-Mannagetta, G., Koch, S.,
  Rating, D., and Janz, D. (1983). Change of seizure frequency in pregnant epileptic women.
  J. Neurol. Neurosurg. Psych. **46**(8), 751–755.

Sheehan, H. L., and Lynch, J. B. (1973). "Pathology of Toxaemia of Pregnancy." Churchill Livingston, Edinburgh.

Shehata, H. A., and Okosun, H. (2004). Neurological disorders in pregnancy. *Curr. Opin. Obstet. Gynecol.* **16,** 117–122.

Sibai, B. M. (1990). Eclampsia: VI. Maternal-perinatal outcome in 254 consecutive cases. *Am. J. Obstet. Gynecol.* **163,** 1049–1055.

Sibai, B. M., el-Nazer, A., and Gonsalez-Ruiz, A. (1986). Severe preeclampsia-eclampsia in young primigravid women: Subsequent pregnancy outcome and remote prognosis. *Am. J. Obstet. Gynecol.* **155,** 1011–1016.

Sibai, B. M., Ramadan, M. K., Usta, I., Salama, M., Mercer, B. M., and Friedman, S. A. (1993). Maternal morbidity and mortality in 442 pregnancies with hemolysis, elevated liver enzymes, and low platelets (HELLP syndrome). *Am. J. Obstet. Gynecol.* **169,** 1000–1006.

Sibai, B. M., Ramadan, M. K., Chari, R. S., and Friedman, S. A. (1995). Pregnancies complicated by HELLP syndrome (hemolysis, elevated liver enzymes, and low platelets): Subsequent pregnancy outcome and long-term prognosis. *Am. J. Obstet. Gynecol.* **172,** 125–129.

Sibai, B. M., and Ustav, I. M. (1995). Emergent management of puerperal eclampsia. *Obstet. Gynecol. Clin. North Am.* 315–335.

Sipes, S. L., Weiner, C. P., Gellhaus, T. M., *et al.* (1994). Effects of magnesium sulfate infusion upon plasma prostaglandins in pre-eclampsia and preterm labor. *Hypertens Pregn.* **13,** 293–302.

Slater, R. M., Wilcox, F. L., Smith, W. D., *et al.* (1987). Phenytoin infusion in severe preeclampsia. *Lancet* **1,** 1417–1421.

Sullivan, C. A., Magann, E. F., Perry, K. G., Jr., Roberts, W. E., Blake, P. G., and Martin, J. N. Jr. (1994). The recurrence risk of the syndrome of hemolysis, elevated liver enzymes, and low platelets (HELLP) in subsequent gestations. *Am. J. Obstet. Gynecol.* **171,** 940–943.

Steer, P. J., Weiner, C. P., and Gonic, B. (1999). WB Saunders, London, pp. 803–836.

Tank, P. D., Nandanwar, Y. S., and Mayadeo, N. M. (2002). Outcome of pregnancy with severe liver disease. *Int. J. Gynecol. Obstet.* **76,** 27–31.

The EURAP Study Group (2006). Seizure control and treatment in pregnancy. Observations from the EURAP Epilepsy Pregnancy Registry. *Neurology* **66,** 354–360.

To, W. K., and Cheung, R. T. F. (1997). Neurological disorders in pregnancy. *Hong Kong Med. J.* **3,** 400–408.

Toglia, M. R., and Weg, J. G. (1996). Venous thromboembolism during pregnancy. *N. Engl. J. Med.* **335,** 108–114.

Tomson, T., Lindbom, U., Ekqvist, B., and Sundqvist, A. (1994). Epilepsy and pregnancy: A prospective study of seizure control in relation to free and total plasma concentrations of carbamazepine and phenytoin. *Epilepsia* **35,** 122–130.

Tran, T. A., Leppik, I. E., Blesi, K., *et al.* (2002). Lamotrigine clearance during pregnancy. *Neurology* **59,** 251–255.

Trivedi, R. A., and Kirkpatrick, P. J. (2003). Arteriovenous malformations of the cerebral circulation that rupture in pregnancy. *J. Obstet. Gynaecol.* **23,** 484–489.

Tuffnell, D., O'Donovan, P., Lilford, R. J., Prys-Davies, A., and Thornton, J. G. (1989). Phenytoin in preeclampsia. *Lancet* **2,** 273–274.

Weinstein, L. (1982). Syndrome of hemolysis, elevated liver enzymes, and low platelet count: A severe consequence of hypertension in pregnancy. *Am. J. Obstet. Gynecol.* **142,** 159–167.

WHO. UNICEF (1996). Revised 1990 estimates of maternal mortality: WHO/FRH/MSM/96.11 WHO, Geneva.

Widschwendter, M., Schrocksnadel, H., and Mortl, M. G. (1998). Opinion: Pre-eclampsia: A disorder of placental mitochondria? *Mol. Med. Today* **4,** 286–291.

Yerby, M. S., Friel, P. N., and McCormick, K. (1992). Antiepileptic drug disposition during pregnancy. *Neurology* **42**(Suppl. 5), 12–16.

MANAGEMENT OF EPILEPSY AND PREGNANCY: AN OBSTETRICAL PERSPECTIVE

Julian N. Robinson* and Jane Cleary-Goldman†

*Brigham and Women's Hospital, Maternal-Fetal Medicine, Boston,
Massachusetts 02115, USA
†Englewood Hospital, Maternal Fetal Medicine, Englewood, NJ 07631, USA

   I. Introduction
  II. Preconception
 III. Assessment of Seizure Control
  IV. Considerations for Antiseizure Medicine Management During Pregnancy
   V. Prenatal Vitamins and Seizure Disorder
  VI. Prenatal Care
 VII. Screening for Fetal Abnormalities
VIII. Obstetrical Risks and Management During Labor
  IX. Conclusion
      References

Women with epilepsy who take antiseizure medicines have successful and unremarkable pregnancies the majority of the time. Achieving seizure freedom is important for successful pregnancies, and it is also highly predictive of seizure freedom during pregnancy. From data derived from the general population, vitamin supplementation is important to prevent birth defects, and women with epilepsy of child-bearing potential should be encouraged to take folic acid supplements daily. Pregnant women with epilepsy should have their pregnancies screened for neural tube defects with a maternal serum alpha-feto-protein level at 15–16 weeks of gestational age and an anatomical survey by ultrasound at 18–22 weeks of gestation. Pregnant women with epilepsy do face a higher risk of both non-proteinuric hypertension and induction of labor than do then general population, as well as an approximately twofold risk of cesarean section. However, the indication for cesarean section is unclear and appears not to be related to fetal distress and may in part be influenced by caution at the time of delivery for such patients. Collaboration between the patient, neurologist, and obstetrician is important for managing this dynamic and complex clinical situation.

INTERNATIONAL REVIEW OF
NEUROBIOLOGY, VOL. 83
DOI: 10.1016/S0074-7742(08)00016-0

273

I. Introduction

The management of a pregnant woman with seizure disorder is optimized if a neurologist and an obstetrician collaborate and if the patient receives preconceptual counseling. Nonetheless, a considerable number of pregnancies are unplanned, and an obstetrician may not become involved until the pregnancy is well into the first trimester or even later. Therefore, it is essential that neurologists looking after women in their reproductive years be well versed in the management of seizure disorders during this life epoch. This chapter focuses on the management of epilepsy in pregnancy.

II. Preconception

Preconception counseling is important for women with epilepsy and is a time to educate and inform these patients about optimal care before, during, and after pregnancy. It should be acknowledged that once women become of reproductive age the pregnancy is possible, whether planned or not, and preconception counseling should be an ongoing conversation over the years of routine neurological visits. It is important that women with a history of seizure disorder and those on antiseizure medications realize that the majority of women taking such drugs (80–96%) have successful and unremarkable pregnancies. Before planning a pregnancy, the patient's seizure history and antiepileptic medications should be reviewed to determine if she is on the optimal regimen for pregnancy, regarding low risk to the developing fetus as well as good seizure control. Other issues that should be addressed include the risk of fetal anomalies, prenatal diagnostic procedures, risk for poor maternal and fetal outcome with recurrent seizures, and the importance of the patient's good self-care, including a healthy diet and adequate sleep.

An important part of pregnancy planning is birth control, and the neurologist should routinely inquire if the patient is sexually active and if she is using birth control. All methods of contraception can be considered for women with epilepsy. If hormonal contraception is being used, the health care provider should be aware that estrogen can be excitatory and decrease seizure threshold and that progesterone can be sedative and increase seizure threshold. However, it should be recognized that these theoretical observations rarely affect the choice of hormonal contraception if that is the desired method. For women with increased seizures at menses (catamenial epilepsy) continuous hormonal methods may be considered.

III. Assessment of Seizure Control

The assessment of a woman's seizure activity is imperative when considering reproductive options. It is recognized that seizure activity increases in pregnancy in about a quarter of women, decreases in about a quarter, and has no change in about half. Investigators evaluating the course of epilepsy during pregnancy have shown an increase in 24% (Schmidt, 1982), 37% (Schmidt *et al.*, 1983), and 15% (Tomson *et al.*, 1994); a decrease in 23% (Schmidt, 1982), 13% (Schmidt *et al.*, 1983), and 24% (Tomson *et al.*, 1994); and no change in 53% (Schmidt, 1982), 50% (Schmidt *et al.*, 1983), and 61% (Tomson *et al.*, 1994). These studies and recent work (Vajda *et al.*, 2008) also bear out the finding that being seizure free prior to pregnancy is associated with seizure freedom during pregnancy. In one recent study (Vajda *et al.*, 2008), 80% of women who were seizure free in the year prior to pregnancy also had no seizures during pregnancy. This study also showed that women with epilepsy who had seizures during the pregnancy were 22 times more likely to have a seizure during labor. Status epilepticus is reported in 0.5% of pregnant women, (Schmidt, 1982), which is not greater than that seen in the general population of persons with epilepsy.

When integrating the ramifications of a woman's seizure disorder into her reproductive choices, an assessment of the severity of her seizure disorder is an obvious place to start. How well are her seizures controlled? How often does she have seizures and how severe are they? When was her last seizure? If the last seizure was over 2 years ago and pregnancy is planned, a trial without medication should be considered. What medications is she on and how well do they work?

The rationale for taking antiepileptic medications during pregnancy include: avoidance of maternal injury, prevention of fetal asphyxia (a fetal death has been reported after seizure in pregnancy (Minkoff *et al.*, 1987), prevention of status epilepticus, and psychosocial reasons. Since good seizure control before pregnancy is associated with a seizure-free pregnancy, patients should be informed of the option to defer pregnancy until seizure control has been optimized. Reasons for failure of antiepileptic drugs in pregnancy include, noncompliance, vomiting, decreased intestinal absorption, maternal CVS changes, decreased protein binding, increased hepatic metabolism, increased plasma volume, and increased renal blood flow with increased drug clearance.

IV. Considerations for Antiseizure Medicine Management During Pregnancy

The basic tenet of pharmacotherapeutics during pregnancy is to simplify drug regimens. In particular, polypharmacy with multiple antiepileptic drugs is to be avoided. The rationale for simplicity is the potential for teratogenicity.

In addition, the changes in physiology associated with pregnancy can affect drug levels and, therefore, make the management of multiple agents complicated. It should be recognized that seizure prevention is the main goal of the therapy, and if this can only be achieved by a combination of drugs then that is the appropriate choice.

In the late 1980s, it was reported that polypharmacy was associated with a higher risk of congenital abnormality (Hanson and Smith, 1975). When reports of teratogenicity of antiepileptic medications started appearing, it was thought that there were particular syndromes related to particular medications. For example, the "hydantoin syndrome" was thought to be associated with phenytoin. This syndrome consisted of craniofacial defects, hypoplasia of nails and distal phalanges, and mental retardation (Jones, 1989). Similarly, carbamazepine was reported to be associated with craniofacial defects and nail hypoplasia (Gaily et al., 1988). However, a blinded review of 121 affected children did not confirm a specific pattern of teratogenic pattern for antiepileptic medications (Jones, 1989). It is now thought there is a nonspecific connotation of congenital abnormalities for antiepileptic drug syndrome.

V. Prenatal Vitamins and Seizure Disorder

Vitamin supplementation is routinely used by women planning pregnancy to ensure an adequate nutritional status. The inclusion of vitamin supplementation is important for the prevention of fetal abnormality. An early landmark large, randomized, controlled trial evaluating vitamin dietary supplementation beginning at least 28 days before conception until at least two menses were missed showed fewer malformations in the vitamin supplemented group (13.3 vs 22.9 per 1000). In addition, it was shown that there were no neural tube defects in the vitamin supplemented group (0 vs 6) (Czeizel and Dudas, 1992). Folic acid supplementation appears to be of particular importance in the prevention of neural tube defects. It has been suggested that the incidence of major congenital malformations may be increased where supplemental folic acid is lacking (Vajda et al., 2003; Betts and Fox, 1999).

Centers for Disease Control and Prevention recommends that all women take 0.4 mg/day of folic acid as a dietary supplementation prior to and during pregnancy, and the available evidence suggests that this is a reasonable recommendation for women with epilepsy who are receiving antiepileptic drugs. Women with a history of a prior neural tube defect take 4 mg/day of folic acid. While it may be suggested that women with a history of seizure disorder be encouraged to take between 2 and 4 mg of folic acid daily prior to conception and during pregnancy; the evidence defining the precise dose of folic acid in women receiving antiepileptic drugs is still lacking.

VI. Prenatal Care

During pregnancy, patients with seizure disorder are for the most part cared for like any other pregnant woman. The main differences are that women with epilepsy are followed for their seizure activity and they may be screened more intensively for fetal anomalies.

VII. Screening for Fetal Abnormalities

All pregnant women should be offered screening for aneuploidy and/or invasive diagnosis for chromosomal abnormalities (first trimester chorionic villous sampling or second trimester genetic amniocentesis). There are several screening tests available for trisomy 13, 18, and 21. The most common of which is trisomy 21 which is also known as Down's syndrome. All of these aneuploidies increase in incidence as women age. The number of screening tests available has recently increased. There is now a range of screening tests that combine first trimester ultrasound (measurement of the fetal nuchal translucency, a sonolucent area at the back of the fetus's neck, and the presence or absence of the fetal nasal bone) with first and second trimester maternal serum analytes. These include first trimester placental associated pregnancy protein A [PAPP-A] and beta human chorionic gonadotropin [hCG] and second trimester alpha fetoprotein [MSAFP], inhibin, beta human chorionic gonadotropin [BhCG], and estriol. The choice of test depends on availability depending on where in the country the patient lives as well as the patient's choice. Besides being associated with an increased risk for trisomy 21, an enlarged nuchal translucency measurement may be associated with an increased risk for congenital heart defects and for other fetal anomalies.

In addition to being used in anueploidy screening, maternal serum alpha fetoprotein MSAFP can be used to screen for fetal anatomical defects. AFPis a protein produced in the fetal liver which ends up in the fetal circulation, the amniotic fluid, and to a lesser extent the maternal circulation. A higher level of MSAFP is present in a number of fetal abnormalities including neural tube disorders (spina bifida), anterior abdominal wall defects (omphalocele and gastroschisis), and renal abnormalities.

In routine obstetrics it may be reasonable to choose a screening test which does not include MSAFP. After all, the anatomical ultrasound also screens for neural tube defects and other structural abnormalities associated with a high MSAFP.

However, the authors feel that in a pregnant women with a seizure disorder, who is taking a medication that may increase the risk of a neural tub defect, it is very likely that using a test that includes MSAFP will increase the sensitivity of screening for open neural tube defects. Therefore, such women should be offered an aneuploidy screening test that includes an assay of MSAFP at 15–16 weeks gestational age. If opting to go for a definitive test for prenatal diagnosis, amniocentesis may offer the advantage of being able to screen for neural tube defect with amniotic fluid AFP and acetylcholinesterase. This may guide a woman toward the choice of amniocentesis. However, if the risk of aneuploidy is very high this advantage may be overridden by the much earlier results that are afforded by chorionic villous sampling.

An anatomical survey should be obtained around 18–22 weeks. The purpose of this screening test is to look for possible anatomical abnormalities. All anatomical structures routinely assessed in routine care should b evaluated. Particular to teratogenic effects associated with antiseizure medications, the head and spinal cord should be evaluated to look for signs and symptoms of a neural tube defect (Fig. 1). Views of face and nose are needed to evaluate for cleft lip or palate (Figs. 2 and 3). Likewise, the heart should be evaluated carefully and a fetal echocardiogram may be considered (Fig. 4). The full anatomical survey should also be completed.

VIII. Obstetrical Risks and Management During Labor

For the most part, patients with seizure disorders do well in pregnancy. For example, Richmond et al. reported on 414 births and 314 women from 1978 to 2000 with seizure disorder (Richmond et al., 2004). While they did find an increased risk for nonproteinuric hypertension ($p < 0.05$) and induction of labor ($p < 0.001$), they found that these patients had fewer instrumental vaginal deliveries. More than one antenatal seizure did not have an effect on antenatal outcome. Likewise, there was no difference in other complications of pregnancy and only a small increase in caesarean delivery rates.

Several other studies have shown a clear increased risk of caesarian section in women with epilepsy (Laskowska et al., 2001; Olafsson et al., 1998; Pilo et al., 2006; Sawhney et al., 1996) and no studies show an absence or an increased risk. The overall risk is around twofold; however, the reason for the increased c-section rate is unclear. It does not appear to be related to an increased occurrence of fetal distress (Sawhney et al., 1996) and may, at least in part, be influenced by caution at the time of delivery for these women.

Nonetheless, besides having their antiepileptic drug serum concentrations monitored serially throughout pregnancy, patients with epilepsy should be followed closely for signs and symptoms of pregnancy complications. For example, serial growth scans are suggested to rule out growth abnormalities such as

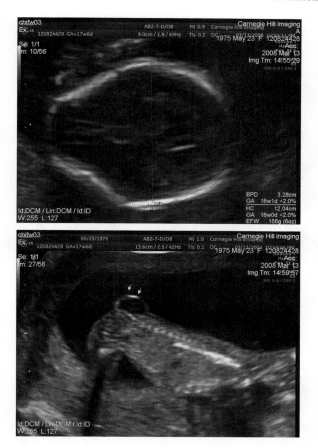

FIG. 1. (A) Lemon sign: Ultrasound finding associated with open neural tube effects. (B) Open neural tube effect.

intrauterine growth restriction. Blood pressure should be monitored for signs and symptoms of preeclampsia. Likewise, they should be watched for signs and symptoms of preterm labor.

The risk of hemorrhage in neonates born to women with epilepsy who were taking enzyme inducing AEDs during pregnancy is also of concern. Prevention of neonate bleeding has only been evaluated in studies where the newborns all received intramuscular vitamin K 1mg at birth. Whether AEDs would be associated with increased rates of hemorrhage in the newborn if this dose of vitamin K were not given remains unclear. Nonetheless, vitamin K supplementation (10–20 mg/day of oral vitamin K during the last 2–4 weeks of pregnancy or 10 mg intravenously during labor) is suggested, but again not proven, to prevent bleeding in newborn.

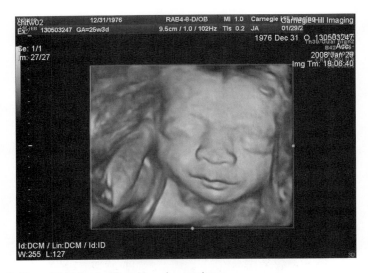

FIG. 2. Normal fetal face in 3D at 25 weeks gestation.

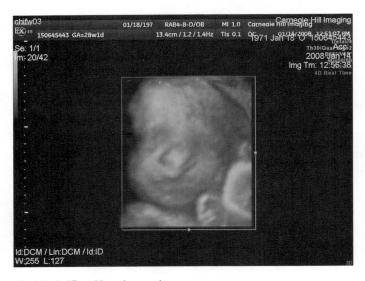

FIG. 3. Cleft lip in 3D at 28 weeks gestation.

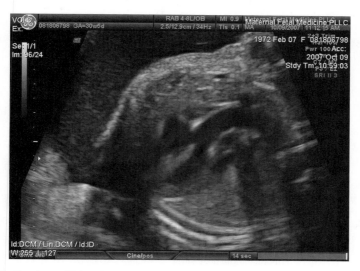

FIG. 4. Tetrology of Fallot: Overring aorta.

Once in labor, they should be continued on their antiepileptic drug regimen. If required, intravenous phenytoin can be used (10–15 mg/kg; max rate 50 mg/min with cardiac monitoring), as can intramuscular phenobarbital (60–90 mg). If preeclampsia is suspected, parenteral magnesium sulfate may be used.

In the postpartum period, medications will likely need readjustment. While breast feeding is not discouraged, the mother should be aware of neonatal absorption of medications and potential sequelae. In addition, contraception should be addressed.

IX. Conclusion

In conclusion, for the most part patients with seizure disorder who become pregnant have good perinatal outcomes. Nonetheless, epilepsy is a significant issue in pregnancy and specialist care is required. Collaboration between neurology and obstetrics is optimal as is careful pregnancy planning. Medications should be prescribed appropriately and monitored throughout pregnancy and the postpartum periods. Monotherapy is preferred. The best medication is the safest one that controls seizures for the particular patient. It is hoped that the new generation of antiepileptic drugs will be associated with fewer fetal risks; this remains to be borne out in emerging research. In addition to routine obstetric care, these patients require careful screening for fetal anatomical abnormalities.

Likewise, women with seizure disorder should be followed for signs and symptoms of pregnancy complications. Antiepileptic drug treatment should be continued during labor and readjusted in the postpartum period.

References

Bells, T., and Fox, C. (1999). Proactive preconception counseling for women with epilepsy-is it effective? *Seizure* **8,** 322–327.

Czeizel, A. E., and Dudas, I. (1992). Prevention of the first occurrence of neural-tube defects by periconceptional vitamin supplementation. *N. Engl. J. Med.* **327,** 1832–1835.

Fox, C., and Betts, T. (1999). How much risk does a woman with active epilepsy pose to her newborn in the puerperium? A pilot study. *Seizure* **8,** 367–369.

Gaily, E., Granstrom, M. L., Hiilesmaa, V., and Bardy, A (1988). Minor anomalies in offspring of epileptic mothers. *J. Pediatr.* **112,** 520–529.

Hanson, J., and Smith, D. (1975). The fetal hydantoin syndrome. *J. Pediatr.* **87,** 285–290.

Jones, K. L. (1989). Pattern of malformations in the children of women treated with carbamazepine during pregnancy. *N. Engl. J. Med.* **320,** 1661–1666.

Laskowska, M., Leszczyriska-Gorzelak, B., and Oleszczuk, J. (2001). Pregnancy in women with epilepsy. *Gynecol. Obstet. Invest.* **51,** 99–102.

Minkoff, H., Nanda, D., Menez, R., and Fikrig, R. (1987). Pregnancies resulting in infants with acquired immunodeficiency syndrome or AIDS-related complex: Follow-up of mothers, children, and subsequently born siblings. *Obstet. Gynecol.* **69,** 288–291.

Olafsson, E., Hallgrimsson, J. T., Hauser, W. A., Ludvigsson, P., and Gudmundsson, G. (1998). Pregnancies of women with epilepsy: A population-based study in Iceland. *Epilepsia* **39**(8), 887–892.

Pilo, C., Wide, K., and Winbladh, B. (2006). Pregnancy, delivery, and neonatal complications after treatment with antiepileptic drugs. *Acta Obstet. Gynecol.* **85,** 643–646.

Richmond, J. R., Krishnamoorthy, P., Andermann, E., and Benjamin, A. (2004). Epilepsy and pregnancy: An obstetric perspective. *Am. J. Obstet. Gynecol.* **190,** 371–379.

Sawhney, H., Vasishta, K., Suri, V., Khunnu, B., Goel, P., and Sawhney, I. M. S. (1996). Pregnancy with epilepsy—a retrospective analysis. *Int. J. Gynecol. Obstet.* **54,** 17–22.

Schmidt, D. (1982). Pregnancy & the Child.. *In* "Epilepsy" (D. Janz *et al.* Eds.). New York.

Schmidt, D., Canger, R., Avanzini, G., Battino, D., Cusi, C., Beck-Mannagetta, G., Koch, S., Rating, D., and Janz, D. (1983). Change of seizure frequency in pregnant epileptic women. *J. Neurol. Neurosurg. Psychiatry* **46,** 751–755.

Tomson, T., Lindbom, U., Ekqvist, B., and Sundqvist, A. (1994). Epilepsy and pregnancy: Prospective study of seizure control in relation to free and total plasma concentrations of carbamazepine and phenytoin. *Epilepsia* **35,** 122–130.

Vajda, F. J., O'Brien, T. J., Hitchcock, A., Graham, J., and Lander, C. (2003). The Australian registry of antiepileptic drugs in pregnancy: Experience after 30 months. *J. Clin Neurosci.* **10,** 543–549.

Vajda, F. J., Hitchcock, A., Graham, J., O'Brien, T., Lander, C., and Eadie, M. (2008). Seizure control in antiepileptic drug-treated pregnancy. *Epilepsia* **49**(1), 172–176.

PREGNANCY REGISTRIES: STRENGTHS, WEAKNESSES, AND BIAS INTERPRETATION OF PREGNANCY REGISTRY DATA

Marianne Cunnington* and John Messenheimer[†]

*GlaxoSmithKline Research and Development, Harlow, United Kingdom
[†]GlaxoSmithKline Research and Development, North Carolina, USA

I. Introduction
II. Background
    A. What Is a Pregnancy Registry?
    B. Pregnancy Registries: When do we Need Them?
III. Design of a Pregnancy Registry
    A. Objectives and Sample Size
    B. Selection of Comparison Group
    C. Eligibility Requirements
    D. Source of Exposure and Outcome Data
    E. Definition of Pregnancy Outcomes
    F. Data Collection
    G. Data Presentation
    H. Use of Independent Data Monitoring Committee
    I. Strategy for Patient Privacy and Human Subject Data Protection
IV. A Brief History of AED Pregnancy Registries
V. Impact of Registry Design on Data Interpretation
    A. Patient Eligibility
    B. Patient Recruitment and Data Collection
    C. Outcome Ascertainment/Classification
    D. Length of Follow-up
    E. Comparators
VI. Interpretation of Signals
    A. What is a Signal?
    B. Using Pregnancy Registry Data to Interpret Signals
    C. Methodologies Beyond Registries
VII. The Future
    A. When to Stop a Registry
    B. Future Roles and Responsibility
    References

The chronic nature of epilepsy treatment, as well as the peak in incidence in children and adolescents, makes it likely that women of childbearing age will be exposed to antiepileptic drugs (AEDs). This has led to the establishment of several pregnancy registries to monitor the safety of anticonvulsants in terms of the risk of major birth defects following *in utero* exposure. Many registries are now

INTERNATIONAL REVIEW OF
NEUROBIOLOGY, VOL. 83
DOI: 10.1016/S0074-7742(08)00017-2

283

approaching their second decade of data collection. With the release of substantial information on a range of AEDs (both older and newer generation drugs), it becomes increasingly important to understand how the methodological variations between cohorts may affect the risks of major birth defects being reported. This chapter explores the key methodological elements of these registries in terms of patient enrolment, the source of exposure and outcome information, outcome definition and ascertainment and comparator groups and how these elements may influence the reported risk estimates.

With multiple registries collecting and releasing substantial data on AED safety in pregnancy, the chapter also reflects on how an increasing number of "signals" around increased risk of specific birth defects is likely. Possible methods for interpreting such signals, that the registries were not originally designed to detect and interpret, are also discussed.

I. Introduction

Since the thalidomide disaster of the mid-1950s, the United States (US) Food and Drug Administration (FDA) has required, that prior to approval, all new medicinal products undergo animal testing to assess the potential teratogenic effects of exposure during pregnancy. However, the results of animal experiments do not always transfer to the clinic (Mitchell, 2003) and given the necessity of excluding pregnant women from clinical trials, robust data on the safety of a new medication in pregnancy are extremely limited both pre- and post-approval.

Until the 1980s, postmarketing assessment of drug safety in pregnancy relied upon a spontaneous reporting system with healthcare professionals and patients reporting adverse events to the pharmaceutical companies who were required to report these events in turn to the regulators. While such reports can generate signals that should be further investigated through pharmacoepidemiological studies, case reports tend to be biased toward the reporting of more severe events and may not be reflective of the pattern of events in the general exposed population. In addition, they cannot differentiate between coincidence and causation and cannot be used to quantify the risk associated with the exposure of interest (US DHHS FDA, 2005). This failure to systematically collect robust data on pregnancy outcomes following *in utero* drug exposure led to the establishment of pregnancy registries from the late 1980s onward. This methodological progress coincided with the development and launch of a new generation of antiepileptic drugs (AEDs), and pregnancy registries have proved a popular tool for monitoring the safety of both the older and newer generations of AEDs (Cunnington and

Tennis, 2005; Holmes *et al.*, 2004; Morrow *et al.*, 2006; Tomson *et al.*, 2004). While the epilepsy field is fortunate to have several independent registries amassing substantial safety data, an understanding of the methodological differences that can exist between pregnancy registries is vital to ensure correct interpretation and comparison of these data.

II. Background

A. What Is a Pregnancy Registry?

A pregnancy registry is a prospective, observational, exposure-registration, and follow-up study. Data collection within the registry is active with women being enrolled prior to knowledge of the pregnancy outcome and as close to the time of exposure as possible (prospective recruitment). The primary endpoint of a pregnancy registry is an estimate of the overall risk of major birth defects (though some are now extending infant follow-up to capture the risk of developmental delay; Keppra Pregnancy Registry, Magnus, 2004). Although a teratogen is unlikely to result in increases in all birth defect types simultaneously, a major teratogen will increase the risk of a spectrum of defects or a specific defect sufficiently for an increase in the overall risk of all defects to be noted. Pregnancy registries are therefore powered to detect a signal of major teratogenicity and can provide margins of risk associated with a drug. Because the background risk of any single defect is low (e.g., for the more common birth defects approximately 1 in 1000 for oral clefts and 4.5 in 1000 for ventricular septal defects, Correa *et al.*, 2007), registries are not designed to detect increases in single defects unless those increases are in the 10- to 100-fold range and thus affect the overall defect rate significantly. The registries may also generate hypotheses around more moderate teratogenic effects on specific defects types or effects by dose and timing of exposure (US DHHS FDA, 2002). Pregnancy registries may collect data on a single drug or many drugs within a class. The registries may be based in a single country or may involve international networks.

B. Pregnancy Registries: When do we Need Them?

Despite the paucity of data on drug safety during pregnancy, it is clear that pregnancy registries are not in existence for the majority of currently marketed drugs. As active surveillance through a pregnancy registry is a large task, both practically and financially, guidelines have been issued by both FDA and the European Medicines Evaluation Agency (EMEA) on when it is appropriate to establish a pregnancy registry (Table I; US DHHS FDA, 2002; CHMP, 2005).

TABLE I

GUIDELINES ON WHEN TO ESTABLISH A PREGNANCY REGISTRY

- When the medication has a high likelihood of being used in women of childbearing age making inadvertent exposure to the drug in pregnancy likely.
- When the medication is for chronic therapy that should not be discontinued in pregnancy.
- The medication represents special circumstances such as potential for maternal fetal infection through administration of live attenuated vaccines.
- Animal reproductive studies have shown the potential for fetal harm.
- Human case reports have shown the potential for fetal harm.
- When the medication belongs to a class of substances, having similar chemical structure or mechanism of action, with suspected or proven teratogenic effects.

AEDs meet many of these criteria. Epilepsy is a chronic, often lifelong neurological condition with incidence peaks in infancy through to adolescence and in the elderly. With onset of epilepsy early in life, it is common for women of childbearing age to need to be exposed to AEDs and failure to continue medication during pregnancy could result in harm to both mother and fetus. The teratogenic effects of some of the older AEDs (e.g. hydantoins) have long been suspected (Hanson 1976). Despite the differences in chemical structure and mechanism of action between the older and newer generations of AEDs, the safety concerns associated with the older generation have increased interest in the safety of the newer AEDs. This interest has led to the establishment of several pregnancy registries monitoring various combinations of AEDs across different countries.

III. Design of a Pregnancy Registry

The past decade has seen an increasing number of US government initiatives and updated European pharmacovigilance legislation to facilitate a discussion of the issues associated with the design and implementation of studies to monitor drug safety in pregnancy. Such initiatives included the development and review of FDA guidance on methodological and logistical points to consider when establishing a pregnancy registry. The critical elements to consider are described below (Table II). The guidelines encompass broad recommendations with a description of a number of methodological options to consider.

A. OBJECTIVES AND SAMPLE SIZE

The desired sample size for a registry will depend on the aim of the registry (magnitude of increase in risk to be detected), the frequency of the outcome of interest in both the exposed and comparator group, and the frequency of

TABLE II

CRITICAL ELEMENTS TO CONSIDER WHEN DESIGNING A PREGNANCY REGISTRY

- Objectives of registry
- Sample size to rule out a difference between exposed and comparator groups or to detect a predetermined level of risk (and how long it may take to reach this sample size)
- Comparison groups
- Eligibility for enrolment
- Source of information on drug exposure and pregnancy outcome
- Definition of congenital defects (inclusion/exclusion criteria) and period of time for defect ascertainment after birth
- Data to be collected on mother, pregnancy, and infant
- Methods to be used in assessing drug associated risk—statistical plan
- Importance of independent data monitoring committee
- Method of obtaining institutional review board review and informed consent
- Criteria for closing a registry

Adapted from US DHHS FDA guidance for industry: Establishing pregnancy exposure registries, 2002.

exposure in the population. Although all AED pregnancy registries aim to detect or refute a signal of major teratogenicity, a failure to quantify this signal and differences in the comparator groups have led to a lack of *a priori* sample size and power calculations. The underlying assumptions can significantly impact the required sample size. For example, a cohort of 280 individuals is needed to detect, with 80% power a twofold increase in risk, assuming a background population birth defect risk of 3%. The cohort size increases to 420 exposed individuals if the underlying population risk is assumed to be 2% and nearly 2000 individuals are needed to detect a 1.5-fold increase with 80% power, given the same 2% baseline (Fleiss *et al.*, 2003; Machin *et al.*, 1997).

B. SELECTION OF COMPARISON GROUP

The comparator group can be either internal or external. Within multidrug pregnancy, registries internal comparator groups can include women with the same underlying indication taking different medications or not taking medication.

External comparator groups use data collected by different investigator groups for different underlying reasons and can include other pregnancy registries, other cohort studies targeted to the same outcomes of interest, or surveillance systems at the hospital, state, or national level. While smaller population-based surveillance programs (e.g., Metropolitan Atlanta Congenital Birth Defects Program; Correa *et al.*, 2007) may allow more active identification of defects to a more defined case definition, the results may not be generalizable to the population at the country level (e.g., different ethnic distribution, smoking patterns). Larger population-based surveillance programs (e.g., March of Dimes, www.marchofdimes.com) reflect data from a wider population base, but data from national defect registries should be viewed with caution as passive reporting may underestimate defect rates (though this varies greatly by country) and are often fail to mirror the strict case definitions and inclusion/exclusion criteria applied by pregnancy registries reducing comparability. As external comparators do not commonly reflect a population with the same underlying condition, descriptive comparisons may be more appropriate.

C. Eligibility Requirements

Prospective enrolment into pregnancy registries is the key eligibility requirement meaning the pregnancy should be registered with exposure to the drug of interest prior to conception and prior to knowledge of the pregnancy outcome, including results of ultrasound studies.

Retrospectively reported pregnancy outcomes may be collected and reviewed by the registries, but should not be included in risk estimates.

D. Source of Exposure and Outcome Data

Active recruitment of exposed pregnancies, and data collection, is recommended either indirectly through healthcare providers (e.g., neurologists, epilepsy specialists, primary care practitioners, obstetricians, midwives) or directly with pregnant women telephoning an advertised toll free number.

The method of data collection will depend on the method of patient recruitment and can include mailed questionnaires, telephone interviews, or medical record reviews.

E. Definition of Pregnancy Outcomes

Pregnancy outcomes include spontaneous losses (before 20 weeks gestation), induced terminations, fetal/stillbirths (loss after 20 weeks gestation), and live births. The presence or absence of birth defects should be assessed within each outcome group.

As birth defect outcomes are not consistently ascertained across induced terminations and fetal/stillbirths, most pregnancy registries exclude those pregnancy outcomes without reported defects as one cannot be certain this is an accurate reflection. Including defect cases from pregnancy losses within the numerator, while excluding pregnancy losses without reported defects from the denominator, reflects a conservative approach biasing the risk estimate upward.

In addition, spontaneous losses are commonly excluded from risk analyses as reported rates of spontaneous loss underestimate this outcome which is very difficult to capture accurately, especially when occurring in the very early stages of pregnancy.

All pregnancy registries are focused on the overall rate of congenital malformations. The precise definition of birth defects differs somewhat between registries and although there is no universally accepted definition scheme, the pregnancy defects to be included in risk estimates should be defined *a priori*. For example, some birth classification schemes include chromosomal defects (e.g., Center for Disease Control and Prevention (CDC), Metropolitan Atlanta Congenital Defects Monitoring Program (MACDP), 1998), while others exclude both chromosomal and Mendelian genetic disorders (e.g., Brigham and Women's Hospital Survillence Program; Nelson and Holmes, 1989). It is also necessary to define a period of ascertainment of defects (e.g., within the first 5 days of life, up to 3 months after birth). Ideally, reports of congenital abnormalities should be reviewed by a specialist in the field, which will prevent misclassification or inappropriate groupings of defects which could hide teratogenic patterns. A consistent method of ascertainment and classification of outcomes is recommended for the comparator group to increase the robustness of comparisons.

F. Data Collection

The critical data to be collected at enrolment include the following:

- Patient identifier;
- Healthcare provider details;
- Date of last menstrual period and expected delivery date;
- Exposure to medication of interest (including date and dose);
- Indication for taking medication of interest;
- Additional exposures of interest (other prescription and over the counter medications, dietary supplements specifically folic acid, vaccines, insertable/implantable medical devices); and
- Other medical conditions of interest.

Patient follow-up will provide the opportunity to review the exposure data, especially any changes in medication exposure during pregnancy, and the relevant information on the infant:

- Gestational age
- Gestational outcome
- Mode of delivery
- Results of neonatal physical examination
- Neonatal illnesses, hospitalization, drug therapy

Additional information on the mother and infant may be available (e.g., maternal race, occupation, obstetric history) but will depend on the source of the data.

G. DATA PRESENTATION

FDA recommends the separate presentation of prospectively and retrospectively collected data; the inclusion of only prospectively collected data in risk estimates of birth defects and the presentation of all risk estimates with 95% confidence intervals. Confidence intervals are commonly calculated with a continuity correction method (e.g., Wilson Score method) to account for the relatively small numerical risks under consideration (Fleiss et al., 2003; Newcombe, 1998). Separate risk estimates are calculated by trimester of exposure and by therapy type (monotherapy vs polytherapy).

H. USE OF INDEPENDENT DATA MONITORING COMMITTEE

To ensure scientific integrity, pregnancy registries are advised to use independent data monitoring committees comprising of experts in epilepsy, obstetrics, teratology, pediatrics, epidemiology, and pharmacology. The committee should be involved in the review of data, classification of birth defects, and dissemination of data.

I. STRATEGY FOR PATIENT PRIVACY AND HUMAN SUBJECT DATA PROTECTION

Although it is recommended for each pregnancy registry to consult with an institutional review board, informed consent is commonly waived for registries recruiting women indirectly through healthcare providers where patient anonymity is maintained. Applying informed consent to such a model would likely result in greatly reduced response rates. However, in those registries enrolling women directly, or requesting a review of the maternal or infant medical records, informed consent must be obtained.

IV. A Brief History of AED Pregnancy Registries

The first pregnancy registry to monitor the safety of an AED was the International Lamotrigine Pregnancy Registry, established by Burroughs Wellcome (now GlaxoSmithKline) in 1992 (Cunnington and Tennis, 2005). This followed the design of the original pregnancy registry, established by Burroughs Wellcome for acyclovir in 1984, with healthcare providers enrolling women exposed to lamotrigine within the month prior to becoming pregnant or at some point during pregnancy on a voluntary basis. Close to the expected date of delivery the reporting healthcare provider is approached to report data on the primary endpoint of interest: major structural birth defects. The International Lamotrigine Registry is coordinated by a contract research organization (Kendle International) and data are reviewed by an independent scientific committee who endorse biannual reports.

Subsequent AED pregnancy registries have been established by independent academic groups or physician networks with the exception of the single drug Keppra Pregnancy Registry established in 2004 by UCB Pharma (Magnus, 2004). The first multidrug AED pregnancy registry was initiated in the UK in 1996 with educational grants from the Epilepsy Research Foundation and various pharma companies. In addition to voluntary reports from healthcare providers, women can directly enroll themselves in the UK Epilepsy and Pregnancy Registry by telephoning a toll free number, though all exposure and follow-up information is sought through the healthcare provider (Russell et al., 2004). The multipharma company-sponsored North American AntiEpileptic Drug (NAAED) registry (also known as the AED Pregnancy Registry), also established in 1996, followed collecting data across the United States and Canada. This was the first registry to rely solely on women directly enrolling themselves with telephone interviews at enrolment, during pregnancy and after delivery. Informed consent is additionally sought for medical record review of outcomes (Holmes et al., 2004).

The European Registry for AntiEpileptic Drugs (EURAP) was the last multi-AED registry to be formed in 2000 and has grown to collect data in more than 40 countries across Europe, Asia, and South America (Tomson et al., 2004). Although an international registry offers many advantages, including increased recruitment and greater generalizability, there are also significant challenges in working across different healthcare settings. EURAP has met these logistic challenges by working to a standardized protocol and ensuring a consistent case definition with all defects reviewed by two physicians at the central coordinating center (Tomson et al., 2004). The single country AED pregnancy registries in the UK and Australia also report into EURAP. A reflection of the methodological variations across these AED pregnancy registries is presented in Table III.

Although not strictly pregnancy exposure registries, additional data on exposure to AEDs in pregnancy can be collected through teratology information services and through national birth registries. Women, or patients of healthcare providers, contacting local teratology information services due to concerns around exposure to drugs in pregnancy can be recruited into cohorts and followed throughout pregnancy. However, the large services such as the Organization for Teratology Information and Specialists (OTIS, www.otispregnancy.org) in the

TABLE III

OVERVIEW OF METHODOLOGY OF EXISTING AED PREGNANCY REGISTRIES

Registry	Eligibility[a]	Recruitment	Latest enrolment	Data collection	Follow-up after birth	Definition of major birth defects	Comparator
LTG International	Prospective	Indirect through healthcare providers	Anytime in pregnancy if outcome not known	Questionnaire to healthcare provider	Mostly at birth. Can be up to 6 years	MACDP	External—MACDP
EURAP International	Prospective	Indirect through healthcare providers	16 weeks gestation	Questionnaire to healthcare provider	14 months	EUROCAT	Internal—other AEDS and women with epilepsy not taking AEDs
UK	Prospective	Indirect through healthcare providers and direct	Anytime in pregnancy if outcome is not known	Questionnaire to healthcare provider	3 months	EUROCAT	Internal—other AEDs and women with epilepsy not taking AEDs
NAAED US and Canada	Prospective	Direct	Anytime in pregnancy if outcome is not known	Telephone interview with women and medical record review	5 days	Structural defect of surgical, medical or cosmetic importance	External—Brigham and Women's Hospital Surveillance program
Keppra North America	Prospective	Indirect through healthcare providers and direct	Anytime in pregnancy if outcome is not known	Questionnaire to healthcare provider	five years after birth	MACDP	External - MACDP

[a]For inclusion in risk estimates.

United States and the European Network of Teratology Information Services (ENTIS, www.entis-org.com) have yet to publish on cohorts of women exposed to AEDs. Data have been published from several large European population-based birth and pharmacy registries, including the Swedish Medical Birth Register. This collects drug exposure data through midwife interviews in the first trimester of pregnancy. Exposure data are then linked to birth outcomes captured through the national birth, hospital, and congenital defects registers using unique individual identifiers (Wide *et al.*, 2004). As reporting to these registers is mandatory, the Swedish medical birth register is estimated to capture over 95% of national births.

V. Impact of Registry Design on Data Interpretation

Current regulatory guidance on establishing pregnancy registries offers many methodological options while maintaining scientific rigor. While there are no strictly right or wrong approaches, an understanding of the potential biases introduced through the different approaches and the impact on the final risk estimates is essential for data interpretation. This is particularly pertinent given the number of "mature" registries in the field of AED surveillance with substantial data being released and compared across registries.

A. PATIENT ELIGIBILITY

The key strength of the pregnancy registry design is enrolment of women exposed to the AED prior to conception and before the pregnancy outcome is known. This increases the accuracy of the exposure reporting and reduces the bias associated with retrospective reporting which can overrepresent more severe and unusual cases. However, the prevalence and timing of antenatal testing has made it increasingly difficult to recruit women into the registries before they have any knowledge of fetal health. Various approaches have been taken to deal with this issue.

The International Lamotrigine Registry includes pregnancies as prospective, if enrolment occurs prior to prenatal screening and as long as a defect was not identified through prenatal screening. If an exposed pregnancy is reported after a defect has been identified through prenatal screening, the pregnancy is classed as retrospective. The differential inclusion of pregnancies without a defect identified through prenatal screening could introduce a selection bias, though 70% of pregnancies are enrolled before 20 weeks gestation (60% before week 16) when targeted ultrasound investigations for birth defects are unlikely to have occurred (http://pregnancyregistry.gsk.com). This potential bias is offset against the recruitment issues that would arise if women were required to have had no prenatal screening prior to enrolment.

The North American Anti-Epileptic Drug (NAAED) has addressed this potential bias by introducing a subdivision of prospective enrolment. "Pure prospective" cases are defined as women enrolled prior to prenatal testing (an amniocentisis or chorionic villus sampling, though a women with a nuchal translucency test before 15 weeks gestation are included). "Traditional prospective" enrolment allows the inclusion of women with prenatal tests or an ultrasound after gestational week 15 as long as the pregnancy was enrolled prior to delivery (Holmes *et al.*, 2004). To date, the two groups have been combined for the calculation of risk estimates to increase the denominator and power to detect a signal, but as the registry grows a comparison of risk estimates between the two prospective enrolment groups may give insight into any bias introduced through the inclusion of women with knowledge of fetal health through prenatal screening.

The effect of this potential bias on risk estimates is difficult to predict. Several issues may arise:

- The exclusion of defects identified by prenatal screening, but inclusion of pregnancies without any evidence of a defect on the same prenatal tests could differentially exclude high-risk pregnancies biasing the estimate downward.
- A failure to report evidence of prenatal screening, despite knowledge of the defect by the women or healthcare provider, could increase the probability of participation in the registry and inclusion of high-risk pregnancies biasing the risk estimate upward.

To overcome these uncertainties, registries can only encourage recruitment as early in pregnancy as possible prior to prenatal screening. This most rigorous approach has been adopted by EURAP, which only includes pregnancies enrolled prior to 16 weeks gestation when the likelihood of detailed ultrasound examinations to identify birth defects is low (Tomson *et al.*, 2004).

B. PATIENT RECRUITMENT AND DATA COLLECTION

The two options for patient recruitment into an AED pregnancy registry are direct enrolment by the patient or indirect enrolment through a healthcare provider. While many pregnancy registries rely on a single reporting physician, most commonly the obstetrician, the chronic and continuous nature of epilepsy management means that AED registries have advertised to a broader range of healthcare workers including neurologists, general practitioners and epilepsy nurses, to report AED exposures during pregnancy.

Each reporting source has advantages and disadvantages. Reporting by healthcare providers may provide more detailed and accurate medical information (e.g., exposure dose, infant outcome). However, the primary reporting healthcare provider may not have direct access to all the necessary medical information which can increase the chance of the case being lost to follow-up. For example, if the neurologist reports the exposure during pregnancy, he or she will rely on the infant's pediatrician to provide accurate outcome information. While a woman directly enrolling herself in a registry may not be expected to provide detailed medical information, inaccuracies, and missing data can be assessed by asking permission for the release of medical records for review. This practice has been adopted by NAAED which is the only registry to rely solely on direct enrolment by the women themselves (Holmes *et al.*, 2004). Conversely, being able to interview the women directly may allow the collection of data on a wider range of covariates that are not always captured in medical records (e.g., socio-demographics, family history).

Whatever the mode of enrolment, participation is on a voluntary basis and it is this that can increase the risk of loss to follow-up. Loss to follow-up tends to be highest in those registries relying on voluntary reporting through healthcare providers where traditionally incentives for complete reporting have not been provided (Table IV). The exception to this rule is the UK register (Morrow *et al.*, 2006), which may be explained by reporting through general practitioners, who in the UK, act as a central coordinating point in the healthcare system for medical data collection and patient follow-up.

Loss to follow-up in EURAP may be amplified by a calculation of the rate of loss after 14-month follow-up, a much longer follow-up than in the other AED registries increasing the opportunities for a case to be lost to follow-up (www.eurapinternational.org/registry/reports). However, this may be offset by the more complete reporting of defects, data on the natural history of outcomes in

TABLE IV

EXPOSED PREGNANCIES LOST TO FOLLOW-UP OR WITHDRAWN FROM SEVERAL LARGE AED PREGNANCY REGISTRIES

Registry	Follow-up after birth	Loss to follow-up
International Lamotrigine[a]	At birth, can be for up to 6 years	24.5%
EURAP[b]	14 months after birth	22.3%
UK[c]	3 months after birth	8.1%
NAAED[d]	5 days after birth	7.2%

[a]Cunnington and Tennis (2005).
[b]www.eurapinternational.org/registry/reportsDecember 2006.
[c]Morrow *et al.* (2006).
[d]Holmes *et al.* (2004).

exposed infants and multiple opportunities to collect a richer dataset with more information on potential confounders including family history.

The loss to follow-up rate in NAAED has to date been low, reflecting the increased motivation of women who enroll themselves in the registry.

It is very important to minimize loss to follow-up as high rates introduce more uncertainty around the risk estimate, making it difficult to assess how generalizable the results are to the general exposed population.

C. Outcome Ascertainment/Classification

While all registries require an expert review of the reported defect cases, the inclusion and exclusion criteria used for major birth defects differs and can therefore influence the final risk estimate.

Antiepileptic drug pregnancy registries concentrate on the risk of major birth defects. The exclusion of minor birth defects or patterns of minor defects (e.g., fetal alcohol or fetal phenytoin syndrome) ensures greater consistency between registries and between reporting centers within a study as minor defects are inconsistently ascertained. There are several classifications of birth defects by independent groups including European network of Congenital Anomoly and Twin registers (EUROCAT, 2002) and CDC (MACDP, 1998). Although these give broadly consistent groupings, there is still scope for individual registries to add different interpretations. For example, most registries exclude chromosomal abnormalities which are very unlikely to be due to drug exposure, but some registries may have more stringent criteria concerning the additional exclusion of monogenic or Mendelian traits (Holmes *et al.*, 2004; eurapinternational.org/registry/reports). However, the length of follow-up of the infant after birth may influence how accurate these exclusion criteria can be (i.e., will the necessary confirmatory tests be possible). It is important to ascertain whether such defects are included or excluded when comparing risk estimates across registries (Table V).

TABLE V

EXCLUSION OF CHROMOSOMAL ABNORMALITIES FROM RISK ESTIMATE IN AED PREGNANCY REGISTRIES

Registry	Chromosomal abnormalities
Lamotrigine International	Excluded
EURAP	Excluded plus monogenic traits
UK Epilepsy and Pregnancy	Excluded
NAAED	Excluded plus Mendelian traits
Keppra	Excluded

Further diagnostic criteria may be applied to the recognition of birth defects. For example, NAAED recognizes major birth defects within the first 5 days of birth as those of externally visible in the delivery room and of major structural importance requiring intervention (Holmes *et al.*, 2004). As some defects may not be externally evident (e.g., ventricular septal defects), this could bias the risk estimate downward compared to registries allowing the inclusion of defects only evident through various imaging examinations before or after birth.

D. LENGTH OF FOLLOW-UP

The length of follow-up in a registry can influence the probability that a birth defect is recognized and the corresponding risk estimate. Therefore, the chance of defects being diagnosed is higher for registries, such as the UK register (Morrow *et al.*, 2006) and EURAP (Tomson *et al.*, 2004), following infants for 3 months and 14 months, respectively, compared to the International Lamotrigine Registry where the majority of defects are reported at birth (Cunnington and Tennis *et al.*, 2005). The impact of length of follow-up on the risk estimate may vary by defect type differentially affecting those defects not visible externally at birth (e.g., ventricular septal defects).

Longer follow-up and an increased number of contact points with patients and infants can allow additional opportunities to confirm exposure and outcome data increasing the robustness of the data. It may also result in the collection of a richer dataset in terms of covariates of interest (e.g., underlying seizure type, family history). Some registries are now extending infant follow-up out for several years to extend the outcomes of interest to developmental delay (EURAP and Keppra) (Tomson, personal communication; Magnus, 2004).

E. COMPARATORS

The choice of comparator groups for AED pregnancy registries has proved challenging. Multi-AED pregnancy registries have the advantage of utilizing different AEDs acting as internal comparators. As lack of therapy is not an option for the majority of women with epilepsy, it is most useful for the patient and physician to be able to directly compare the safety profile of the different treatment options. Another internal comparator used by the multi-AED registries is women with epilepsy not taking medication. In theory, this is the ideal comparator with the same underlying indication making medication exposure the only difference. However, the severity of epilepsy in women not taking or requiring medication is likely to be very different from those on chronic therapy. Therefore, any comparisons should be viewed with caution due to potential confounding by indication. Alternative internal comparators include women exposed to AEDs in the second or third trimester of pregnancies after the period organogenesis. However, this option has not been used within AED pregnancy registries probably reflecting the chronic nature of AED therapy.

Over recent years a complication associated with the use of internal comparators has arisen with the inclusion of women taking an AED for an indication other than epilepsy. For example, lamotrigine is now indicated for bipolar disorder and gabapentin is indicated for neuropathic pain. To date, this may have affected relatively small numbers of women being recruited into the registries, but should be borne in mind when comparisons are being made between drugs in case there are substantial differences in the underlying birth defect risks associated with different indications.

Single drug pregnancy registries do not enjoy these internal comparator options and a range of external comparators are more commonly used. These include data from general population surveillance programs or studies of birth defects in epileptic and general populations. Although it is useful to provide a general population context, only descriptive comparisons are appropriate given potential difference in the underlying risk of birth defects between the general and epileptic populations as well as differences in the selection of the patient populations and reporting of birth defects. One solution is to employ several comparator groups allowing a check of consistency against the risk comparisons generated (US DHHS FDA, 2005). Using data from a pregnancy registry for a drug known not to be a teratogen (e.g., acyclovir) would be one way of solving this last issue around population selection differences, but this option has yet to be explored by the AED pregnancy registries.

The choice of comparator group will greatly influence any relative risk calculations when the risk of birth defects in the exposed treatment group is compared with the risk in the comparator group. Such calculations are only appropriate when data are collected consistently across the exposed and comparator groups and the comparator groups are representative of the same overall population. Additional caution is needed when comparing relative risks for the same AED across different pregnancy registries as these will be highly dependent on the birth defect risk in the comparator group (see Table VI for general population risk range). Therefore,

TABLE VI

RISK OF MAJOR BIRTH DEFECTS ACROSS GENERAL POPULATION SURVEILLANCE PROGRAMS

General population surveillance program	Risk of major birth defects
Brigham and Women's hospital surveillance program[a]	1.6–2.2%
CDC's metropolitan Atlanta congenital birth defects program[b]	2.7%
March of Dimes[c]	3%

[a]Nelson and Holmes (1989).
[b]Correa et al. (2007).
[c]http://www.marchofdimes.com/peristats/.

a high relative risk associated with a treatment group in one registry could be partly due to the low birth defect risk in the comparator group used by that registry. The great variation in comparator groups used by the different registries is one of the main issues in comparing data from the different studies.

VI. Interpretation of Signals

A. WHAT IS A SIGNAL?

Pregnancy registries aim to determine the overall prevalence of all major birth defects, following *in utero* drug exposure and therefore detect or refute a signal of major teratogenicity. In addition, signals may be generated around specific defects as well as for trends with dose and timing of exposure. A signal can be defined as a report or reports of an event with an unknown causal relationship to treatment that is recognized as worthy of further exploration and continued surveillance. A signal is not a confirmed finding, but is generally referred to as a hypothesis-generating situation that must be confirmed or refuted (CIOMS, 2005).

Although FDA guidance indicates that registries may serve as hypothesis generating tools, there is no indication of what may constitute a signal worthy of further assessment. Many pregnancy registries have adopted the "rule of three," originally developed by the Antiretroviral Pregnancy Registry (APR) scientific committee. This rule considers three of the same defect type to constitute a signal as in a cohort ≥ 600 the probability of observing three of the same defect type is $<5\%$ (Covington et al., 2004). Even then, it is difficult to put the signal into a context that will help inform patients and physicians. The confidence intervals around the absolute risk estimate are likely to be very wide and the relative risk estimate can vary widely depending on the comparator group employed by the individual registry. With several AED registries reaching substantial sample sizes, there is an increasing probability of signals, both real and spurious, due to registries achieving adequate power for detection or through chance associated with study multiplicity. There is, therefore, a growing need for a scientific framework to interpret these signals.

B. USING PREGNANCY REGISTRY DATA TO INTERPRET SIGNALS

FDA guidelines state that data from all available sources should be reviewed to assess the strength and validity of any observed association between drug exposure and pregnancy outcome. The existence of multiple AED pregnancy registries with substantial data offers the opportunity to follow this guidance.

The simplest approach is to review the data from each individual registry to ascertain whether there is consistency across registries in the reproduction of the specific signal. However, as registries are not generally powered to detect all but very large increases in the risk of specific defect types, a failure to replicate a signal may represent a power issue.

The combination of data from different registries, most commonly in aggregate form, may appear attractive to increase the power to detect increases in rare events and this can take several approaches: pooling or meta-analysis. Pooling is the simple combination of data where all registries are given an equal weighting. No account is taken of differences in the robustness of data due to variation in registry sample sizes or methodologies. If one calculates a relative risk estimate, one chooses a single comparator group which will not take into account underlying population differences reflected by the various registries.

Some of these issues can be overcome by using a meta-analysis. A meta-analysis is a statistical technique for combining data from independent studies. The individual relative risks (risk of outcome in treated versus untreated group) from each registry are entered in a regression model which weights the different studies according to their size. More complex weights can be developed that account for other methodological strengths and weaknesses across studies. The meta-analysis gives an overall estimate of the treatment effect on outcome (relative risk). The robustness of a given signal can be investigated through a sensitivity analysis including and excluding the registry data providing the signal to give a measure of the heterogeneity the signal generator is introducing (i.e., how much of an outlier it is?).

Although the meta-analysis is also reliant on the comparator group of each registry, the approach is more flexible as each individual registry can utilize the most appropriate comparator to calculate the registry specific relative risks that are inputted into the meta-analysis regression model. However, this does mean that the choice of individual comparators for each registry included in the analysis can inflate or decrease the individual relative risks being considered and therefore the final relative risk estimate. To remove this issue of the impact of heterogeneous comparator groups, individual level data from each registry is needed which to date has not been provided through any collaborations. Without individual level data, the interpretation of summary relative risks from meta-analyses is additionally problematic due to an inability to assess the role of potential confounders for which information is not available.

A further complication of both the pooled and meta-analysis approaches is the assumption that the registries are independent. It is possible for a women exposed to an AED to be enrolled in multiple registries; for example, her healthcare provider may enroll her in the Lamotrigine Pregnancy Registry, and she may then directly enroll herself in NAAED. Indeed, a study of these two registries identified a 7.5% overlap in lamotrigine monotherapy exposed individuals (using the International Lamotrigine Registry as denominator—Wysynski personal communication). Some registries do not collect patient identifiers, as a means of dealing with data privacy issues, and others cannot share identifiers to protect patient confidentiality. It is, therefore, very difficult to identify duplicates between registries, especially where no birth defect was recorded. As such, it is very unlikely that any data combination technique would be able to remove all duplicates invalidating the assumption of data independence.

C. METHODOLOGIES BEYOND REGISTRIES

Case control studies are often considered more efficient for the study of rare outcomes presenting the opportunity to test hypotheses generated by pregnancy registries. Rolling case control studies to monitor birth defects in relation to maternal drug exposure during pregnancy now exist across the United States and in Europe (Slone—Mitchell *et al.*, 1981; CDC National Birth Defects Prevention Study—Yoon *et al.*, 2001; Hungarian case control study—Czeizel, 1997; EUROCAT—www.eurocat.ac.uk). However, these studies tend to rely on maternal interviews after birth to establish data on drug exposure during exposure which can introduce some recall bias (Mitchell *et al.*, 1981; Yoon *et al.*, 2001). There are also variations in the available control group. The Slone rolling case control study includes a group of normal infant controls (Mitchell *et al.*, 1981), whereas the EUROCAT network of congenital malformation registries only collects data on malformed individuals meaning control groups consist of infants with chromosomal abnormalities (where the outcome is considered very unlikely to be related to drug exposure) or infants with malformations other than the defect of interest (www.eurocat.ac.uk). The latter control groups complicate the interpretation of the treatment effect estimate as there is no general population baseline.

Large computerized healthcare databases are increasingly being used to monitor exposure during pregnancy with the development of maternal–infant record linkage algorithms. These databases, based on primary care data in Europe and health maintenance organization, private insurance claims, or medicaid data in the United States, represent large populations giving studies substantial power. Internal control groups are available representing the general population and women with the same underlying condition exposed to no drug or other drugs within the class of interest. Many of the logistical issues associated with registries are avoided due to the data already being in place for purposes other than epidemiological surveillance. Although, the bias associated with self-reported exposure data does not exist with these data sets, exposure data are based on prescription records which assume that the women took the medication close to the time the prescription was written as instructed. Validation of birth defects data is also needed if a medical record review is not possible and data on confounding variables are commonly more limited. In addition, these databases will be of only limited use in the first few years after the drug is launched until sufficient numbers of exposures have been amassed. The initial surveillance for a signal of teratogenicity, therefore, remains with the pregnancy registries.

VII. The Future

A. When to Stop a Registry

Extensive guidance exists on when to establish a registry, but there is little direction on when to close a registry. Monitoring the power of a registry to detect certain levels of increased risk above a baseline can indicate when a signal of major teratogenicity can be refuted (e.g., the registry has the power to detect a 1.2-/1.5-/2.0-fold increase in risk). However, guidance is needed as to the definition of the level of risk that should be refuted, and the feasibility of detecting this increase will depend on the comparator used which varies across registries.

Few registries have been established with predefined closure or data release criteria. The NAAED offers the clearest direction only releasing data on a specific AED when a twofold increase in risk has been proven or refuted against the risk of 1.6% in the general population comparator utilized by the registry (Holmes *et al.*, 2004). However, this low baseline risk means relatively large sample sizes are needed to detect even a twofold increase in risk reflected by data release on only two AEDs (phenobarbital and valproate) over the first 10 years of data collection (Holmes *et al.*, 2004; Wyszynski *et al.*, 2005). Other registries have opted to release data at regular intervals which ensures transparency, but an ever increasing sample size can lead to the generation of increasing numbers of signals that are difficult to interpret.

Many AED pregnancy registries are struggling to meet the balance between ensuring that robust data are available to prescribers and patients in a timely and transparent manner without misinterpretation of data that may still be underpowered. Guidance is lacking in this area and could greatly facilitate the communication of important safety data to prescribers and patients.

B. Future Roles and Responsibility

To date the primary responsibility of monitoring for the potential teratogenic effects of drugs has rested with the pharmaceutical companies through the direct coordination of pregnancy registries or through the sponsorship of registries coordinated by independent research groups. The recognition of the critical nature of postmarketing monitoring of drug safety in pregnancy due to the serious individual and societal consequences of birth defects, as well as the potential harm of withholding important treatments due to lack of knowledge, means that the number of studies monitoring for teratogenicity is set to increase. While regulatory bodies have recognized this expansion and have attempted to give direction through guidelines for establishing pregnancy registries, there is still great variation in the conduct of pregnancy registries making it difficult to directly compare studies and use all available data. Concern around the safety of AEDs in pregnancy has led to the establishment of several large registries. If this trend continues across different therapy areas, greater methodological consistency will become increasingly important to ensure that all data can be used informatively and that resources are not wasted.

Methodological variation can have substantial impact on the robustness of data and on interpretation. Greater consistency may also allow potential collaborations to monitor for drug effects on rarer outcomes (specific defects or by dose). AED pregnancy registries are increasingly facing the challenge of interpreting signals for specific defects, signals that are ever more common due to the existence of multiple pregnancy registries of substantial size. The availability of multiple data sources should offer the answer as to how to interpret such signals, but this can only be the case if registries employ more consistent methodologies and are open to collaboration. These have been few and far between in the epilepsy world and rarely result in publication. In the future, the outstanding questions of importance to patients and physicians are increasingly likely to need the large datasets that only registry collaborations can bring as well as an understanding of methodological subtleties that will determine if and how data should be combined and presented.

References

CIOMS (2005). Report of the CIOMS Working Group VI. Management of safety information from clinical trials. ISBN 92 9036 079 8.

Committee for Medicinal Products for Human Use (CHMP) (2005). Guideline on exposure to medicinal products during pregnancy: Need for post-authorisation data. EMEA/CHMP/313666/2005. http://www.emea.europa.eu/pdfs/human/phvwp/31366605en.pdf.

Correa, A., Cragan, J. D., Kucik, J. E., Alverson, C. J., Gilboa, S. M., Balakrishnan, R., Strickland, M. J., Duke, C. W., O'Leary, L. A., Riehle-Colarusso, T., Siffal, C., Gambrell, D., et al. (2007). MACDP: 40th Anniversary Special Edition Surveillance Report. Birth Defects Res. A Clin. Mol. Teratol. **79**(2), 1–177.

Covington, D., Tilson, H., and Elder, J. (2004). Assessing teratogenicity of antiretroviral drugs: Monitoring and analysis plan of the antiretroviral pregnancy registry. *Pharmacoepidemiol. Drug Saf.* **13,** 537–545.

Cunnington, M., and Tennis, P. (2005). International Lamotrigine Pregnancy Registry Scientific Advisory Committee. Lamotrigine and the risk of malformations in pregnancy. *Neurology* **64,** 955–960.

Czeizel, A. E. (1997). First 25 years of the Hungarian Congenital Abnormalities Register. *Teratology* **55,** 299–305.

Fleiss, J. L., Levin, B., and Paik, M. C. (2003). "Statistical Methods for Rates and Proportions," 3rd ed. John Wiley and Sons, New York.

Hanson, J. W., Myrianthopoulos, N. C., Harvey, M. A., and Smith, D. W. (1976). Risks to the offspring of women treated with hydantoin anticonvulsants with emphasis on fetal hydantoin syndrome. *J. Paediatr.* **89,** 662–668.

Holmes, L. B., Wyszynski, D. F., and Lieberman, E. (2004). The AED (Antiepileptic Drug) pregnancy registry. A 6-year experience. *Arch. Neurol.* **61,** 673–678.

Machin, D., Campbell, M., Fayers, P., and Pinol, A. (1997). "Sample Size Tables for Clinical Studies," 2nd ed. Blackwell Science, Madden, MA.

Magnus, L. (2004). The Keppra (levetiracetam) Pregnancy Registry. Presented 58th Annual Meeting of the American Epilepsy Society.

Metropolitan Atlanta Congenital Defects Program (1998). *In* "Surveillance Procedure Manual and Guide to Computerized Anomaly Record." Centers for Disease Control, Atlanta, GA.

Mitchell, A. (2003). Systematic identification of drugs that cause birth defects – a new opportunity. *N. Eng. J. Med.* **349,** 2556–2559.

Mitchell, A., Rosenberg, L., Shapiro, S., and Slone, D. (1981). Birth defects related to Bendectin use in pregnancy. Oral clefts and cardiac defects. *JAMA* **245,** 2311–2314.

Morrow, J. I., Russell, A., Gutherie, E., *et al.* (2006). Malformation risks of antiepileptic drugs in pregnancy: A prospective study from the UK Epilepsy and Pregnancy Register. *J. Neurol. Neurosurg. Psychiatry* **77,** 193–198.

Nelson, K., and Holmes, L. B. (1989). Malformations due to presumed spontaneous mutations in newborn infants. *N. Eng. J. Med.* **320,** 19–23.

Newcombe, R. (1998). Two-sided confidence intervals for the single proportion: Comparison of seven methods. *Stat. Med.* **17,** 857–872.

Russell, A. J. C., Craig, J. J., Morrison, P., Irwin, B., Waddell, R., Parsons, L., *et al.* (2004). UK epilepsy and pregnancy group. *Epilepsia* **45,** 1467.

Tomson, T., Battino, D., Bonizzoni, E., *et al.* (2004). EURAP: An international registry of antiepileptic drugs and pregnancy. *Epilepsia* **45,** 1463–1464.

US Department of Health and Human Sciences Food and Drug Administration (2002). Guidance for Industry. Establishing Pregnancy Exposure Registries.

US Department of Health and Human Sciences Food and Drug Administration (2005). Reviewer Guidance. Evaluating the risks of drug exposure in human pregnancies.

Wide, K., Winbladh, B., and Kallen, B. (2004). Major malformations in infants exposed to antiepileptic drugs *in utero* with emphasis on carbamazepine and valproic acid: A nation-wide, population based register study. *Acta Paediatr.* **93,** 174–176.

Wyszynski, D. F., Nambisan, M., Surve, T., *et al.* (2005). Increased rate of major malformations in offspring exposed to valproate during pregnancy. *Neurology* **64,** 961–965.

Yoon, P., Ramussen, S. A., and Lynberg, M. (2001). The National Birth Defects Prevention Study. *Public Health Rep.* **116**(S1), 32–40.

BONE HEALTH IN WOMEN WITH EPILEPSY: CLINICAL FEATURES AND POTENTIAL MECHANISMS

Alison M. Pack and Thaddeus S. Walczak*

Columbia University, New York, NY 10032, USA
*MINCEP Epilepsy Care, Minnea Polis, MN 55416, USA

I. Introduction
II. Bone Physiology
III. Assessment of Bone Health
    A. Bone Mineral Density
    B. Calcitropic Hormones and Vitamin D Metabolites
    C. Bone Turnover Markers
IV. Fracture Risk in Persons with Epilepsy
V. AED Effects on Bone
VI. Potential Mechanisms to Explain Changes in Bone Health in Persons with Epilepsy
    A. A Statement of the Prevailing Model
    B. Evidence Supporting the Prevailing Model
    C. Evidence Against the Prevailing Model
    D. Alternative Mechanisms for Poorer Bone Health in Persons with Epilepsy
VII. Treatment
VIII. Conclusion and Recommendations
    References

Bone disease is recognized as an important pathologic process to identify and treat in women. Women are at greater risk than men secondary to multiple factors including estrogen loss in menopause. The most important consequence of bone disease is fracture. Fracture rates are higher in persons with epilepsy treated with antiepileptic drugs (AEDs). Increased bone turnover secondary to AED exposure, higher rates of osteoporosis, adverse effects on bone quality, seizures, and impaired coordination may all contribute. There is a differential effect of AEDs on bone. Although results are mixed for some AEDs, phenytoin use is consistently associated with lower bone mineral density (BMD). As most evidence associates cytochrome P450 enzyme-inducing AEDs with abnormalities in bone, the induction of these enzymes has been proposed as the main mechanism to describe this effect. However, data suggest that this theory does not explain all findings. Many therapies are available for the treatment of bone disease, but there is limited study in persons with epilepsy. All patients should receive at least the recommended daily allowance of calcium and vitamin D and obtain vitamin D status screening. For prolonged AED exposure, BMD screening is available, particularly if the patient has other risk factors.

INTERNATIONAL REVIEW OF
NEUROBIOLOGY, VOL. 83
DOI: 10.1016/S0074-7742(08)00018-4

I. Introduction

Bone disease is increasingly recognized as an important pathologic process to identify and treat, particularly in women. Although men and women may be affected, women are at greater risk secondary to multiple factors including estrogen loss in menopause. The most important consequence or sequelae of bone disease is fracture. It is estimated that 1.5 million Americans suffer fracture secondary to weak bones and by the year 2020, more than 50% of Americans over age 50 will be at risk for a fracture (U.S. Department of Health and Human Services, 2004). In recognition of this growing concern, the United States is currently participating in a WHO-sponsored worldwide initiative, the Decade of the Bone and Joint (2001–2011), to promote education and research about the importance of bone health. In addition, the US Surgeon General issued the first ever report on bone health and osteoporosis in 2004. The report aims to improve individual's literacy about bone health and calls on health care professionals to help Americans maintain healthy bones by evaluating risks for bone disease and fracture (U.S. Department of Health and Human Services, 2004).

Fracture rates are higher in persons with epilepsy treated with antiepileptic drugs (AEDs). Increased bone turnover secondary to AED exposure, higher rates of osteoporosis, adverse effects on bone quality, seizures themselves, and impaired coordination secondary to AEDs may all contribute. As neurologists, it is important and necessary that we recognize persons at risk for bone disease. The costs associated with fractures are tremendous. Caring for bone fractures costs the United States at least $18 billion a year in direct medical costs including visits to doctor's offices and emergency rooms, hospitalizations, and admissions to nursing homes (U.S. Department of Health and Human Services, 2004). The total cost is even higher secondary to loss of daily functioning and jobs and increased caretaker burden.

II. Bone Physiology

Before discussing the pathology in bone associated with epilepsy and AED exposure, the question of why is bone important should be addressed. Bone has multiple functions. Strong bones support us and allow us to move. Bones are a storehouse for vital minerals including calcium and play an integral role in the homeostasis of these minerals. Finally, they protect vital organs including the heart and lungs.

The life span of bone has several distinct phases in women. In childhood, bone elongates and increases in diameter, with the most dramatic changes being in infancy and adolescence. Peak bone mineral density (BMD) is then obtained between the ages 20 and 30. Throughout the remaining years of a woman's life, BMD typically decreases, with the most significant loss occurring in the early menopausal years. The processes of increasing and maintaining BMD is the result of a coupling of bone cells responsible for resorption (osteoclasts) and formation (osteoblasts). An uncoupling of these cells functions results in either high bone turnover or low bone turnover. In childhood, this uncoupling would affect accumulation of peak BMD whereas in adulthood there would be loss in BMD.

Calcium homeostasis is a tightly regulated process and an integral function of bone. Of the three fractions of calcium, the ionized one is most significantly maintained. Vitamin D, the parathyroid gland, and calcitonin are all directly and indirectly involved.

As the concentration of the ionized fraction of calcium changes, the parathyroid gland alters parathyroid hormone (PTH) levels. If the calcium concentration is low, PTH is elevated. PTH acts to restore the ionized calcium concentration level in several ways, including increasing distal renal tubule reabsorption and facilitating bone resorption. PTH enhances renal synthesis of the most active metabolite of vitamin D, 1,25-dihydroxyvitamin D [1,25(OH)2D] and also slows its degradation. As part of a feedback mechanism, 1,25(OH)2D decreases secretion of PTH by inhibiting PTH gene transcription.

Vitamin D plays a critical role in calcium homeostasis and has direct effects on bone such as promoting differentiation of osteoclasts. There are two formulations of vitamin D: vitamin D2 or ergocalciferol and vitamin D3 or cholecalciferol. Vitamin D2 is synthesized by irradiation of ergosterol and is used in many vitamin D supplements. Vitamin D3 is the predominant source of vitamin D as it is synthesized by solar irradiation of 7-dehydrocholesterol in the skin and can be obtained from a few naturally occurring dietary sources or from vitamin supplements. As vitamin D3 has been more extensively studied, its metabolism will be discussed.

Vitamin D3 metabolism occurs through a series of oxidative pathways involving multiple hepatic and renal cytochrome (CYP) 450 isoenzymes (Table I).

TABLE I

HEPATIC AND RENAL CYP450 ISOENZYMES RESPONSIBLE FOR VITAMIN D METABOLISM

CYP450 Isoenzyme	Function
Hepatic CYP27A	• Hydroxylates D3 to 25OHD
Hepatic CYP2R1	• Hydroxylates D3 to 25OHD
Renal CYP27B1	• Hydroxylates 25OHD3 to 1,25(OH)2D
Hepatic CYP24A1	• Catabolizes majority of 25OHD
	• Inactivates majority of 1,25(OH)2D

CYP, cytochrome.

Vitamin D3 is hydroxylated to 25-hydroxyvitamin D3 (25OHD3), the major circulating form of vitamin D, in the liver. Although 25OHD3 is the most commonly used index of vitamin D status, it probably has little direct effect on bone. 25OHD3 is further hydroxylated to several metabolites (Holick and Adams, 1998; Omdahl, 2001) including 24,25-dihydroxyvitamin D3 (24,25(OH)2 D3) and 1,25 (OH)2D3. 24,25(OH)2D3 also has little effect in bone, whereas 1,25(OH)2D3 is responsible for the majority of the biological effects of vitamin D3. 1,25(OH)2D3 binds with a nuclear vitamin D receptor (VDR) which then forms a heterodimeric complex with retinoic acid X receptor (RXR). This complex binds to specific vitamin D response elements to induce gene expression resulting in the various physiologic functions of D3 (DeLuca, 2004; Jones et al., 1998). This same 1,25(OH)2 D3–VDR–RXR complex induces catabolism of 1,25(OH)2D3 by increasing cyp24 gene expression (Pascussi, 2005). 1,25(OH)2D3 maintains calcium concentration by increasing gut absorption of dietary calcium, by facilitating PTH-induced bone resorption, and by increasing distal renal tubule absorption of calcium (DeLuca, 2004; Holick and Adams, 1998). Calcitonin, a hormone secreted from neural crest tissue associated with the thyroid gland, inhibits PTH-induced bone resorption and decreases serum calcium.

Reproductive hormones also directly and indirectly impact bone. Estrogen reduces bone resorption by inhibiting both the genesis and the function of osteoclasts (Waters and Gonadal, 2006). In the menopausal years, estrogen deficiency is thought to result in the reduction seen in bone mass. This is supported by the efficacy of estrogen replacement in treatment of menopausal osteoporosis. Interestingly, estrogen receptors have been identified on both osteoclasts and osteoblasts, suggesting direct effects on these bone cells (Waters and Gonadal, 2006). The role of progesterone is not as well defined. Similar to estrogen, progesterone therapies in the menopausal years improves BMD and osteoblast cells have progesterone receptors (Waters and Gonadal, 2006).

III. Assessment of Bone Health

A. Bone Mineral Density

BMD currently is the most significant predictor of fracture as seen in multiple epidemiological studies. The most sensitive as well as most studied and understood technique to assess BMD is dual-energy X-ray absorptiometry (DXA). Typically, DXA assesses bone mass at central sites, specifically the hip and spine. Devices providing peripheral site measurements such as the heel are available but they are not as accurate. By aiming two X-ray beams at a patient's bones, a DXA device determines BMD by the absorption of each beam by bone after soft tissue absorption is subtracted out. The obtained BMD measurement is in gm/cm^2 and is compared to large databases maintained by the manufacturers of the DXA devices. This comparison yields two standard deviation scores: T-score and Z-score. The T-score compares the obtained BMD measurement to a sex- and race-matched population at peak BMD, whereas the Z-score compares the BMD measurement to an age-matched population. For children and younger persons, it is important to use the Z-score as you may falsely diagnose people with low BMD if they have not yet obtained peak BMD. The WHO defines osteoporosis and osteopenia in postmenopausal women and older men using the T-score (Table II). The International Society of Clinical Densitometry has recently refined its definitions (Table II).

B. Calcitropic Hormones and Vitamin D Metabolites

Calcium, phosphate, and PTH are measured in serum. The obtained calcium concentration reflects total calcium. Vitamin D metabolites are also serologic measurements. 25OHD is the most commonly used index of vitamin D status, but 1,25(OH)2D concentrations can also be ascertained. These measurements are not always reliable as shown in recent studies (Binkley, 2004). They are also sensitive to the time of year when they are drawn; for instance, the concentrations may be lower during the winter months when there are shorter days and less sunlight exposure.

TABLE II

World Health Organization (WHO) and International Society for Clinical Densitometry (ISCD) Criteria for Osteopenia, Osteoporosis, and Low Bone Mineral Density

WHO	Osteopenia
	• In postmenopausal women and older men T-scores between -1.5 and -2.5
	Osteoporosis
	• In postmenopausal women and older men T-scores ≤ -2.5
ISCD	Postmenopausal women and men older than 50
	• Use T-scores
	• Use WHO classification
	Females before menopause and men younger than age 50
	• Use Z-scores
	• Z-score > -2.0 within the expected range for age
	• Z-score < -2.0 below expected range for age

C. Bone Turnover Markers

Bone turnover markers are measurements of bone formation and bone resorption. In the ideal state, bone formation and bone resorption are coupled with no net loss of bone; however, as discussed previously, there may be states of high or low turnover resulting in bone loss. Multiple markers of bone turnover are available (Table III). However, at this time the clinical utility of these markers is limited as they may not be good surrogates for BMD as a predictor of an individual's risk of fracture and standardization among labs has proven to be difficult (Khosla and Kleerekoper, 2006).

Osteoblasts are the cells responsible for bone formation. Individual bone formation markers measure either collagenous or noncollagenous products synthesized by these cells (Table III). The two commonly measured noncollagenous products are osteocalcin and bone-specific alkaline phosphatase. Osteocalcin or bone Gla protein is incorporated into bone and then released into circulation during bone resorption and is therefore really a marker of bone turnover as at any one time it has a component of bone formation and resorption. Total alkaline phosphatase is derived from many tissues. Techniques are available to measure the bone isoenzyme.

As bone is resorbed by osteoclasts, collagen breakdown products are released. These products are further metabolized in the liver and kidney. Assays are available to measure these collagen breakdown products in the urine or serum (Table III).

TABLE III
BONE TURNOVER MARKERS

Bone formation markers	Collageneous
	• Carboxyterminal propeptide of type I collagen (PICP)
	• Aminoterminal propeptide of type I collagen (PINP)
	Non-collageneous
	• Osteocalcin
	• Bone-specific alkaline phosphatase
Bone resorption markers	Urine
	• Free and total pyridinolines (Pyd)
	• Free and total deoxy pyridinolines (Dpd)
	• N-telopeptide of collagen cross-links (NTx)
	• C-telopeptide of collagen cross-links (CTx)
	Serum
	• Cross-linked C-telopeptide of type I collagen (ICTP)
	• Tartrate-resistant acid phosphatase 5b (TRACP5b)
	• N-telopeptide of collagen cross-links (NTx)
	• C-telopeptide of collagen cross-links (CTx)

IV. Fracture Risk in Persons with Epilepsy

Multiple studies have identified epilepsy and AED therapy as being associated with fracture. Many factors likely influence the increased fracture rate, including adverse effects of AEDs on bone, side effects of AEDs resulting in instability or poor coordination, and seizure-related injuries. Figure 1 illustrates potential contributing factors and relationships between them. A meta-analysis of 11 studies highlights that multiple factors may be contributing to the increased fracture risk in persons with epilepsy (Vestergaard, 2005). In this analysis, BMD was significantly decreased and fracture risk was significantly increased with a relative risk of 2.2 (95% CI: 1.9–2.5). However, after analyzing the studies associating BMD with fracture risk, the investigators concluded that the observed deficit in BMD was too small to explain all of the observed increase in fracture risk, and therefore bone disease and seizure-related injury together interact to increase the risk of fractures in patients with epilepsy. In support of the concept of seizures contributing to fracture risk, a large case control study of 3478 patients with epilepsy (Souverein, 2006) found that seizure severity was associated with fracture. Characteristics associated with greater severity of epilepsy, including number of medical visits, prescriptions for rectal benzodiazepines, and polypharmacy, were more commonly found in the patients with fractures than in those without fractures. Interestingly, polypharmacy is a marker for more severe seizures and is associated with greater gait instability, and the use of multiple AEDs may have additive effects on bone and mineral metabolism. These studies support that multiple factors may contribute to the increased risk of fracture in persons with epilepsy.

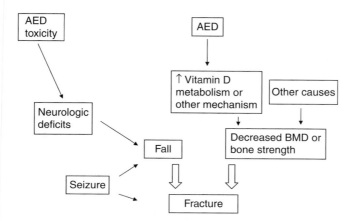

FIG. 1. Factors potentially responsible for fractures in people with epilepsy and their relationships. AED, antiepileptic drug; BMD, bone mineral density.

Different demographic factors are associated with the risk of fracture in persons with epilepsy. Not surprisingly, in patients with epilepsy older age is associated with higher fracture risk (Souverein, 2005). However, children and young adults may also have an increased risk of fractures compared with controls (Sheth, 2004). Some studies suggest that men with epilepsy are at higher risk of fracture than are women, whereas others suggest that the risk is higher in women (Persson, 2002; Souverein, 2005).

Predisposition to fractures is due to an interaction between forces applied to bone and ability of bone to tolerate these forces without fracture. In epilepsy, abnormal forces applied to bone are due to the forces resulting from tonic-clonic seizures or due to increased risks of falls. Falls in turn can be related to the seizures themselves. Multiple studies support that injury secondary to seizures contributes to the increased risk of fracture in persons with epilepsy. Patients with generalized tonic-clonic seizures are at higher risk for fracture than are patients with partial seizures (Persson, 2002). Fracture risk is higher during the first or second year after diagnosis of epilepsy than later (Persson, 2002; Vestergaard, 1999), suggesting that seizure control achieved over time may decrease the risk of fracture. Interestingly, one study in women with epilepsy found a higher relative risk of hip versus forearm fracture (Koppel, 2005). The increased risk for hip fracture compared to that for forearm fracture may be a result of the person being unable to use the hands to break a fall during a seizure.

However, population-based studies (Annegers, 1989; Grisso, 1991) find that trauma related to seizures is not associated with fractures. In persons with epilepsy residing in nursing homes (Lidgren and Walloe, 1977) or presenting to tertiary hospitals (Desai et al., 1996; Nilsson, 1986; Vestergaard, 1999), 0–37% of fractures are potentially related to seizures. Determining the relative contributions of potential causes of fractures in persons with epilepsy requires a multivariate analysis of a large group of subjects and controls. Four studies analyze some of the potential causes outlined in Fig. 1 (Bohannon, 1999; Cummings, 1995; Grisso, 1991; Souverein, 2006), but only one is concerned specifically with persons with epilepsy (Souverein, 2006). Overall, these studies indicate that stroke, generalized weakness, visual impairment, and treatment with AEDs are independent risk factors for fracture. As such, falls may be related to continuously present neurological deficits. These deficits may be due to neurological conditions causing the epilepsy or AED toxicity. Epileptogenic lesions may cause hemiparesis, visual field deficits, or sensory deficits and may increase the risk of fall. There is, surprisingly, little high-quality information regarding incidence of and risk factors for falls in persons with epilepsy. In large hospital-based studies, falls are more common in people with epilepsy (Guse and Porinsky, 2003; Stolze, 2004), but reasons have not been well studied and to our knowledge there are no prospective studies that might inform strategies for prevention in this population.

AED exposure may contribute to fracture risk. For instance, the Study of Osteoporotic Fractures found that postmenopausal Caucasian women treated with AEDs had double the rate of hip fracture compared to a control group of postmenopausal women (Cummings, 1995). Similarly, a meta-analysis of five studies found AED use to be a significant risk factor for fracture, with a relative risk or odds ratio of 2.64 (95% CI: 1.82–3.82) (Espallargues, 2001). A case control study among over 3000 patients with epilepsy found that the risk of fractures increased with duration of AED therapy; treatment longer than 12 years was associated with an adjusted odds ratio of 4.15 (95% CI: 2.7–6.34) for fracture (Souverein, 2006). However, these studies are not able to control for previously discussed factors associated with epilepsy including seizures that result in falls. Interestingly in the Study of Osteoporotic Fractures (Cummings, 1995) after adjustment for previous fractures or calcaneal BMD, AED use was no longer associated with fracture, suggesting that the risk for fractures conferred by AEDs is related to the effect of AEDs on BMD.

There may be a differential effect of individual AEDs on fracture risk. A population-based study in Denmark supports this potential effect (Vestergaard *et al.*, 2004). Over one hundred thousand subjects who had had a fracture from a national hospital discharge register were identified and matched by age and gender to three controls. Drug exposure was assessed through a national pharmacologic database. After adjusting for possible confounders, including a diagnosis of epilepsy, certain AEDs (carbamazepine, clonazepam, phenobarbital, and valproate) were statistically associated with fracture risk (relative risk varied between 1.14 and 1.79). Other AEDs were not statistically associated with fracture risk. However, the estimated relative risks were modest and in the same range for both significant and nonsignificant associations. A dose relationship was found for those AEDs that were significantly associated with fractures. These studies suggest that prolonged AED treatment increases the risk of fracture.

V. AED Effects on Bone

Early studies found that AED exposure resulted in osteomalacia or rickets. Osteomalacia literally means softening of bone and occurs after cessation of growth. Rickets is a pathologic process in children involving the growth plate. Drug-induced osteomalacia and rickets occur secondary to either insufficient availability of calcium, phosphate, and active vitamin D or interference with the deposition of calcium and phosphate in bone. Osteomalacic biopsy specimens exhibit abnormally thick osteoid (unmineralized bone) seams, a prolonged mineralization lag time, and a decrease in the adjusted apposition rate. However, these studies primarily included institutionalized patients treated with phenytoin, primidone, and phenobarbital.

In current reports of ambulatory persons, osteomalacia and rickets are rarely seen. Recent biopsy studies have found normal osteoid seam width and mineralization rates that are consistently normal or increased (Mosekilde and Melsen, 1980; Weinstein, 1984). These results suggest that bone disease in persons with epilepsy treated with AEDs is a disorder of increased remodeling rather than abnormal mineralization, resulting in osteoporosis.

Osteoporosis is a skeletal disorder characterized by decreased bone strength leading to an increased risk of fracture. Osteoporosis, whether manifested by low BMD or fractures, is most common in postmenopausal women in whom the effects of aging and estrogen deficiency cause bone to be lost more rapidly. Secondary osteoporosis may develop because of lifestyle and nutrition factors, underlying medical conditions, or medications (Table IV) (Painter *et al.*, 2006). Studies suggest that AED use can result in secondary osteoporosis (Painter *et al.*, 2006).

TABLE IV
SECONDARY CAUSES OF OSTEOPOROSIS

Lifestyle/Nutrition	Eating disorders
	Vitamin D and/or calcium deficiency
	Alcoholism
	Smoking
Medical diseases	Hyperthyroidism
	Hyperparathyroidism
	Gastrointestinal malabsorption (e.g., celiac disease, postoperative states)
	Cushing's syndrome
	Hypogonadism
	Hypercalciuria
	Renal disease
	Liver disease
	Osteogenesis imperfecta
	Marfan's syndrome
	Homocystinuria
	Rheumatoid arthritis
Medications	Glucocorticosteroids
	Immunosuppressants (cyclosporine)
	Antiepileptic drugs
	GnRH agonists
	Heparin
	Chemotherapeutics
	Depot medroxyprogesterone acetate
	Excess thyroid hormone
	Antiretroviral drugs
	Proton pump inhibitors

GnRH, gonadotropin-releasing hormone.

The advent of DXA allowed noninvasive measurement of bone health in persons with epilepsy. BMD measurements found osteopenia or osteoporosis in 38–60% of persons with epilepsy treated with AEDs in tertiary epilepsy clinics (Andress, 2002; Farhat, 2002; Sato, 2001). Longer AED use was associated with decreased BMD in studies examining this association (Andress, 2002; Farhat, 2002; Sheth, 1995).

Several studies reported effects of individual AEDs on BMD. Phenytoin use was associated with decreased BMD in four of five studies examining the association (Chung and Ahn, 1994; Kubota, 1999; Pack, 2005; Sato, 2001; Valimaki, 1994), phenobarbital in two of two studies (Chung and Ahn, 1994; Kubota, 1999), and valproic acid in three of four studies (Kafali *et al.*, 1999; Pack, 2005; Sato, 2001; Sheth, 1995). Interestingly, carbamazepine use was associated with decreased BMD in only one of five studies examining this association (Kafali *et al.*, 1999; Kim, 2007; Pack, 2005; Sheth, 1995; Valimaki, 1994), though serologic indicators of increased bone turnover have been occasionally reported in persons with epilepsy treated with this medication (Bramswig *et al.*, 2003; Mintzer, 2006; Verrotti, 2000, 2002). BMD following brief treatment with lamotrigine did not differ from BMD following longer treatment with inducing AEDs in a single study (Pack, 2005). There is no other information regarding effects of newer AEDs on BMD.

Most of these studies are difficult to interpret for several reasons. First, the majority have cross-sectional design rendering the findings difficult to interpret as BMD has different rates and directions of change throughout the life cycle. Longitudinal evaluation of serial BMD measures in persons with epilepsy treated with AEDs and age-matched controls permits an assessment as to whether AEDs cause BMD changes different from those expected in a population not using AEDs. Second, many factors have been conclusively associated with decreased BMD (Cummings, 1995; Eastell, 1998). Of these, decreased physical activity, inadequate calcium and protein intake, poorer general health, and depression are likely to be more common among persons with epilepsy and may account for the decreased BMD. For instance, in one study of children treated with valproic acid and lamotrigine, reduced BMD was most significantly associated with reduced exercise in the children with epilepsy (Guo *et al.*, 2001). Third, the above studies are typically based at tertiary epilepsy clinics where severe epilepsy is more prevalent, limiting their generalizability to the general community.

Several longitudinal studies address these limitations (Ensrud, 2004; Kim, 2007). The Study of Osteoporotic Fractures (Ensrud, 2004) is a population-based study that measured serial BMD determinations at both the hip and calcaneus together with many clinical risk factors for low BMD in more than 6000 postmenopausal women. Although depression, poorer general health, and decreased physical activity were more common in postmenopausal women treated with phenytoin, BMD at both the hip and calcaneus declined twice as fast in women treated with phenytoin after adjustment for the above and other factors. Furthermore, decline in BMD statistically attributable to phenytoin was the most significant of the factors found to affect BMD, exceeding the benefit conferred by hormone replacement therapy. Similarly, a prospective study of premenopausal women treated with phenytoin sustained significant bone loss at the femoral neck of the hip (Pack *et al.*, 2008). This bone loss was not seen in the women treated with carbamazepine, valproic acid, or lamotrigine. Significant factors affecting bone loss, including age at menarche, exercise, and diet, did not differ among the groups of women. A 6-month longitudinal study of Korean AED naïve men and women with epilepsy found a significant decrease in BMD and a decrease in vitamin D metabolites in association with carbamazepine but not lamotrigine or valproate treatment (Kim, 2007). Overall, there is strong evidence that phenytoin use is an important factor in decline of BMD in women with epilepsy treated with this drug. However, information regarding other AEDs is not as convincing.

Bone turnover markers may also be obtained as elevated bone turnover markers reflect increased bone remodeling activity, are associated with higher rates of bone loss, and are independent predictors of fracture (Khosla and Kleerekoper, 2006). Elevations in bone formation and resorption markers have been reported during long-term AED therapy (Akin, 1998; Ensrud, 2004; Oner, 2004; Pack, 2005; Sato, 2001; Valimaki, 1994), as well as after initiation of AED therapy (Verrotti, 2000, 2002). For instance, serum alkaline phosphatase including the bone-specific isoenzyme (Okesina *et al.*, 1991; Pack, 2005; Skillen and Pierides, 1976) as well as osteocalcin and C-terminal extension peptide of type I procollagen have been reported as being increased in adults receiving some AEDs (Gough, 1986; Valimaki, 1994; Verrotti, 2000). Not surprisingly, markers of bone resorption such as carboxylterminal telopeptide of human type I collagen and cross-linked N-telopeptides of type I collagen may be elevated as well (Sato, 2001; Valimaki, 1994; Verrotti, 2000, 2002). These findings although not always consistent have been described in association with phenytoin, carbamazepine, valproic acid, and lamotrigine. However, as discussed above, there are limitations to the interpretation of these results. The most interesting findings are in those studies of patients with new-onset epilepsy and no prior exposure to AEDs. Verrotti and colleagues (Verrotti, 2000, 2002) found significant changes in markers of bone turnover when compared to a matched control population after 1 and 2 years of carbamazepine treatment. However, as mentioned previously, the utility of these markers in clinical practice at this time is limited.

VI. Potential Mechanisms to Explain Changes in Bone Health in Persons with Epilepsy

As most evidence associates CYP450 enzyme-inducing AEDs with abnormalities in bone, the induction of these enzymes have been proposed as being the main mechanism to describe this effect. However, there is data to suggest that this theory does not wholly explain previously discussed findings. This section will review the prevailing model as to why persons with epilepsy treated with AEDs are at risk for changes in bone and mineral metabolism. This discussion will include supportive and contradictory data. In addition, other potential mechanisms will be presented.

A. A STATEMENT OF THE PREVAILING MODEL

The prevailing model explaining AED-associated bone disease states that AED-induced disruption of vitamin D metabolism causes osteopenia and osteomalacia (Drezner, 2004; Fitzpatrick, 2004; Hahn, 1972a; Heller and Sakhaee, 2001). According to this model, treatment with liver-inducing AEDs increases the activity of hepatic mixed function oxidases and thus accelerates metabolism of vitamin D and its various metabolites. Furthermore, the majority of the resulting compounds are polar metabolites with no biological activity (Hahn, 1972b). Because the available supply of vitamin D is shunted into these inactive metabolites, less biologically active 1,25(OH)2D is available. This results in decreased intestinal calcium absorption, decreased serum calcium concentration, and a compensatory increased serum PTH concentration (Heller and Sakhaee, 2001). Initially, this secondary hyperparathyroidism increases bone turnover but BMD is maintained. At this point, markers of bone turnover may be increased but BMD measurements are normal. With persistent hyperparathyroidism, BMD decreases at which point standard clinical tests demonstrate osteopenia and osteoporosis and fracture risk is increased. Chronic depletion of vitamin D and calcium eventually results in overt mineralization defect and the clinical picture of osteomalacia (Drezner, 2004; Pack, 2005).

Recent work suggests that an important means of regulating enzymes and transporters responsible for elimination of potentially toxic compounds is involved in disruption of vitamin D metabolism. This may provide a molecular biological explanation for this model. Interestingly, the pregnane X receptor (PXR) and the VDR share a significant homology of amino acid sequence in the DNA-binding domain of the promoter region of CYP24 (Pascussi, 2005; Pascussi et al., 2006). PXR activated by compounds such as phenobarbital could therefore mimic an activated VDR, increase CYP24 expression, shift vitamin D metabolism toward the production of inactive metabolites (Fig. 2), and disrupt

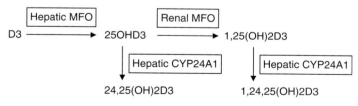

FIG. 2. Important vitamin D metabolites and responsible enzymes (see text). MFO, mixed function oxidase.

bone health. A series of experiments in human hepatocyte preparations strongly supported this mechanism (Pascussi, 2005; Pascussi *et al.*, 2006); however, another group (Xu, 2006; Zhou, 2006) found that this mechanism does not appear to play a large role.

B. EVIDENCE SUPPORTING THE PREVAILING MODEL

Direct measurements of tritiated vitamin D found increased half lives (Hahn, 1972b) and clearance (Matheson, 1976) in a total six patients treated with phenobarbital. Chromatographic evidence suggested increased levels of 25OHD products with high polarity in three of the above subjects (Hahn, 1972b). Most evidence supporting the prevailing model is indirect. Almost all studies demonstrate lower serum calcium concentrations in persons with epilepsy treated with inducing AEDs than in normal controls though overt hypocalcemia is rare (Gough, 1986; Hahn, 1972a; Valimaki, 1994; Weinstein, 1984). Serum 25OHD is lower in many (Gough, 1986; Hahn, 1972a; Mintzer, 2006; Sato, 2001; Stephen, 1999) but not other (Pack, 2005; Verrotti, 2000, 2002; Weinstein, 1984) studies. Furthermore, serum 25OHD is abnormally low in 8–35% of ambulatory persons with epilepsy treated with hepatic enzyme-inducing AEDs (Gough, 1986; Weinstein, 1984) but is normal in ambulatory persons with epilepsy treated with AEDs that do not induce hepatic enymes (Gough, 1986; Sato, 2001; Stephen, 1999). Finally, serum PTH levels in persons with epilepsy treated with AEDs are higher than in control subjects in some (Sato, 2001; Valimaki, 1994; Weinstein, 1984) but not other (Pack, 2005; Verrotti, 2000, 2002) studies.

C. EVIDENCE AGAINST THE PREVAILING MODEL

It is increasingly recognized that vitamin D deficiency is distressingly common. Although the precise definition of vitamin D deficiency continues to be debated, most authorities now believe that 20–50% of healthy individuals suffer from vitamin D deficiency or insufficiency and the rates are even higher in populations with chronic disease similar to persons with epilepsy (Holick, 2006; Holick, 2007; MacFarlane, 2004; Nesby-O'Dell, 2002). Because vitamin D deficiency is so very common in the general population, it will be difficult to demonstrate that AED use specifically plays a role in the vitamin D deficiency. Furthermore, risk factors for vitamin D deficiency (poorer nutrition, less mobility, less sunlight exposure) may be more prevalent among persons with epilepsy and account for the vitamin D deficiency found in this population (Ensrud, 2004). None of the studies reporting decreased vitamin D deficiency in persons with epilepsy measure or adjust for these potential confounders. Therefore, vitamin D deficiency in persons with epilepsy may be due to baseline high rates in the general population or to other accepted etiologies rather than due to AED use.

Other observations also argue against the model. First, the reported effects of specific AEDs on BMD are not consistent with what the model would predict. Carbamazepine, a known inducer of hepatic mixed function oxidases, is not associated with decreased BMD in recent studies (Kafali et al., 1999; Pack, 2005; Sheth, 1995; Valimaki, 1994) while valproic acid, which does not induce liver mixed function oxidases, often is (Kafali et al., 1999; Sato, 2001; Sheth, 1995). Second, 25OHD levels do not differ significantly between persons with epilepsy treated with inducing AEDs and noninducing AEDs when these groups are compared in the same study (Pack, 2005; Stephen, 1999). Third, the amount of vitamin D supplementation needed to maintain normal levels of 25OHD in vitamin D deficient persons with epilepsy is in the range necessary to maintain normal levels in control subjects (Collins, 1991; Heaney, 2003; Mikati, 2006). This argues that the prevailing risk factors for vitamin D deficiency in persons with epilepsy do not differ from those found in the general population. Finally, significant osteopenia and other convincing evidence of increased bone turnover has been found in a series of persons treated with AEDs even though 25OHD3 (Verrotti, 2000, 2002; Weinstein, 1984) and PTH levels (Verrotti, 2000, 2002) were normal. These data indicate that aberrant vitamin D metabolism does not account for all of the changes in bone health observed in persons with epilepsy treated with AEDs.

D. Alternative Mechanisms for Poorer Bone Health in Persons with Epilepsy

Mechanisms other than disruption of vitamin D metabolism may explain poor bone health in many persons with epilepsy treated with AEDs, but their contribution has not been extensively studied. Several possibilities have been suggested. AEDs could have a direct impact on calcium absorption or on bone cells themselves. AEDs could disrupt vitamin K metabolism in a manner similar to that proposed for vitamin D. AEDs could affect calcitonin secretion. Finally, there is the intriguing possibility that epilepsy disrupts central nervous system control of bone metabolism and that AEDs do not play an important role.

AEDs may have direct effect on intestinal calcium absorption that is independent of the effect of vitamin D. For example, phenytoin inhibited calcium absorption from the gut in some (Corradino, 1976) but not other (Bell, 1979) studies. Phenytoin (Feldkamp, 2000; Hahn et al., 1978; Jenkins et al., 1974), phenobarbital (Hahn et al., 1978), carbamazepine (Feldkamp, 2000; Verrotti, 2000, 2002), and valproic acid (Cho, 2005; Schroeder and Westendorf, 2005) have direct effect on cultured bone cells. Different effects are reported in different studies of the same AED (see Nissen-Meyer, 2007, for review), and phenytoin appears to have different effects at low and high levels (Feldkamp, 2000). Levetiracetam in low levels but not high levels decreases bone strength without affecting BMD (Nissen-Meyer, 2007). This is associated with lower osteocalcin levels and increased amounts of cartilage remnants with electron microscopy and mechanism remains unclear (Nissen-Meyer, 2007). Thus, there is strong evidence that AEDs can affect bone directly but no consistent pattern emerges.

AEDs may disrupt vitamin K metabolism in a manner similar to that proposed for vitamin D and may thus impair bone health. Vitamin K is a cofactor required for the carboxylation of Gla-proteins. Three of these are synthesized by osteoblasts of which osteocalcin is the most abundant. Poorly carboxylated osteocalcin is associated with decreased BMD and increased fracture risk (Knapen, 1998; Vergnaud, 1997). High-dose vitamin K2 supplementation modestly increases BMD (Iwamoto et al., 2006; Shiraki, 2000), increases bone strength (Iwamoto et al., 2006; Knapen et al., 2007), and decreases vertebral fracture risk (Shiraki, 2000). Phenytoin administration decreases serum vitamin K2, serum osteocalcin, and BMD in animal models and these effects are reversed with aggressive vitamin K2 supplementation (Onodera, 2002, 2003; Vernillo et al., 1990). This is consistent with the idea that inducing AEDs increase vitamin K2 clearance in a manner similar to that thought to occur with vitamin D. Vitamin K2 deficiency or clearance has not been investigated in persons with epilepsy though high-dose K2 supplementation improved BMD in a small group of persons with epilepsy treated with inducing AEDs. Thus, some data suggest that AED disruption of vitamin K metabolism or function may worsen bone health in persons with epilepsy but many questions remain.

AEDs may disrupt calcitonin secretion. It will be recalled that calcitonin inhibits PTH-induced bone resorption (see the earlier description), and indeed salmon calcitonin modestly increases BMD in humans and is used to treat osteoporosis. Phenytoin treatment decreases calcitonin secretion in animal models (Pento et al., 1973, 1996). Treatment with a variety of AEDs is associated with decreased serum calcitonin in humans (Bogliun, 1986; Kruse, 1980). Calcium-stimulated secretion of calcitonin is decreased in pediatric persons with epilepsy treated with phenytoin or primidone but not in pediatric persons with epilepsy treated with valproic acid or carbamazepine (Kruse, 1987). Although data is sparse, AEDs appear to decrease calcitonin secretion in humans by a mechanism not associated with hepatic induction. The resulting calcitonin deficiency may further aggravate bone resorption due to secondary hyperparathyroidism.

Finally, recent discoveries that the central nervous system plays an important role in regulating bone metabolism (Ducy et al., 2000) raise the possibility that epilepsy rather than AEDs may play a role in decreased bone health in persons with epilepsy. Brain regulation of bone metabolism is thought to be mediated by the hormone leptin. Leptin is secreted by adipocytes, crosses the blood–brain barrier, and binds with specific hypothalamic receptors resulting in activation of the sympathetic nervous system. The consequent activation of adrenergic receptors on the surface of osteoblasts decreases osteoblast numbers and bone formation (Cock and Auwerx, 2003; Ducy et al., 2000; Karsenty, 2006; Takeda, 2002). Interestingly, recurrent seizures in kindled mice increase serum leptin levels (Bhatt, 2006) and could thus potentially decrease bone formation. Persistent seizures could also disrupt brain leptin signaling. While the discovery that the brain has an effect on bone metabolism is an important recent advance, many questions remain regarding its relevance even in the healthy human condition. For example, the fact that both leptin levels and BMD are elevated in obesity in humans appears inconsistent with the notion of leptin as anorexiant and antiosteogenic consistently found in animal studies. This and other questions are being actively addressed (Coen, 2004; Morberg, 2003; Thomas, 2004). Clarifying these issues could inform attempts to untangle the more complex relationships between weight change, leptin signaling, AED treatment, and BMD in persons with epilepsy.

Bone metabolism is complex, and it is likely that multiple pathophysiologic mechanisms are operational in a complex and variable pathologic state such as epilepsy that is treated with different AEDs, each of which can have a variety of effects. The challenge of future research will be to confirm some of the promising mechanisms for which data are presently incomplete and then sort through the relative importance of multiple mechanisms simultaneously in relevant models.

VII. Treatment

Multiple therapies are available for the treatment of bone disease (Table V). Some are recommended in specific clinical situations. For instance, hormone replacement therapy may be useful in a menopausal woman with other significant symptoms including hot flashes. However, if the woman has epilepsy she may be at risk for increased seizure activity (Harden, 2006). Bisphosphonates are known to increase BMD and reduce the risk of fracture but are not routinely recommended in premenopausal women particularly as the teratogenic potential is unknown. Limited study is available on these treatments in persons with epilepsy treated with AEDs. A recent randomized double blind trial over 1 year compared low-dose (400 IU/day for adults and children) and high-dose (4000 IU/day for adults and 2000 IU/day for children) vitamin D supplementation (Mikati, 2006). In the adults, the baseline BMD was reduced at all sites when compared to age- and gender-matched controls. After 1 year, there were significant increases in BMD at all sites in those receiving high-dose vitamin D but not in those receiving

TABLE V

AVAILABLE TREATMENTS FOR OSTEOPOROSIS

- Calcium and vitamin D supplementation
- Bisphosphonates

  Alendronate sodium
  Alendronate sodium plus 2800 IU vitamin D3
  Ibandronate sodium
  Risedronate sodium
  Risedronate sodium plus 500 mg calcium carbonate

- Hormone therapy
- Selective estrogen receptor modulators

  Raloxifene

- Parathyroid hormone

IU, international unit.

low-dose vitamin D. The children had normal BMD when compared to age- and gender-matched controls and had significant and comparable increases in BMD in both treatment groups. This study suggests that persons with epilepsy treated with AEDs should be counseled about adequate vitamin D intake. For those taking enzyme-inducing AEDs, higher doses of vitamin D than currently recommended are suggested. In addition, adequate calcium intake and supplementation if necessary are advised.

VIII. Conclusion and Recommendations

Persons with epilepsy and, in particular, women are at increased for bone diseases, most notably fracture. Fractures rates are higher in persons with epilepsy when compared to the general population. The increased risk is likely secondary to multiple factors including adverse effects of AEDs on bone, side effects of AEDs resulting in instability or poor coordination, and seizure-related injuries. Although results are mixed for some of the AEDs, phenytoin use is consistently associated with lower BMD. It is recommended that all patients receive at least the recommended daily allowance of calcium and vitamin D and that routine screening of vitamin D status be performed to avoid vitamin D insufficiency (current standard for 25OHD: >30 ng/ml). For prolonged AED exposure, BMD screening should be performed particularly if the patient has other risk factors for low BMD (Table IV). If evidence of osteoporosis or low BMD is found, we suggest evaluating the patient for fracture risk including factors discussed above, consider changing AED therapy if the woman is prescribed phenytoin, and refer for possible intervention as many therapies exist for the treatment of osteoporosis.

References

Akin, R, Okutan, V, Sarici, U, Altunbas, A, and Gökçay, E (1998). Evaluation of bone mineral density in children receiving antiepileptic drugs. *Pediatr. Neurol.* **19**(2), 129–131.

Andress, D. L., Ozuna, J., Tirschwell, D., Grande, L., Johnson, M., Jacobson, A. F., and Spain, W. (2002). Antiepileptic drug-induced bone loss in young male patients who have seizures. *Arch. Neurol.* **59**(5), 781–786.

Annegers, J. F., Melton, L. J., 3rd, Sun, C. A., and Hauser, W. A. (1989). Risk of age-related fractures in patients with unprovoked seizures. *Epilepsia* **30**(3), 348–355.

Bell, R. D., Pak, C. Y., Zerwekh, J., Barilla, D. E., and Vasko, M. (1979). Effect of phenytoin on bone and vitamin D metabolism. *Ann. Neurol.* **5**(4), 374–378.

Bhatt, R., Bhatt, S., Hameed, M., Rameshwar, P., and Siegel, A. (2006). Amygdaloid kindled seizures can induce functional and pathological changes in thymus of rat: Role of the sympathetic nervous system. *Neurobiol. Dis.* **21**(1), 127–137.

Binkley, N., Krueger, D., Cowgill, C. S., Plum, L., Lake, E., Hansen, K. E., DeLuca, H. F., and Drezner, M. K. (2004). Assay variation confounds the diagnosis of hypovitaminosis D: A call for standardization. *J. Clin. Endocrinol. Metab.* **89**(7), 3152–3157.

Boglium, G., Beghi, E., Crespi, V., Delodovici, L., and d'Amico, P. (1986). Anticonvulsant drugs and bone metabolism. *Acta Neurol. Scand.* **74**(4), 284–288.

Bohannon, A. D., Hanlon, J. T., Landerman, R., and Gold, D. T. (1999). Association of race and other potential risk factors with nonvertebral fractures in community-dwelling elderly women. *Am. J. Epidemiol.* **149**(11), 1002–1009.

Bramswig, S., Zittermann, A., and Berthold, H. K. (2003). Carbamazepine does not alter biochemical parameters of bone turnover in healthy male adults. *Calcif. Tissue Int.* **73**(4), 356–360.

Cho, H. H., Park, H. T., Kim, Y. J., Bae, Y. C., Suh, K. T., Jung, J. S., Collins, N., Maher, J., Cole, M., and Baker, M. (2005). Induction of osteogenic differentiation of human mesenchymal stem cells by histone deacetylase inhibitors. *J. Cell Biochem.* **96**(3), 533–542.

Chung, S., and Ahn, C. (1994). Effects of antiepileptic drug therapy on bone mineral density in ambulatory epileptic children. *Brain Dev.* **16**(5), 382–385.

Cock, T. A., and Auwerx, J. (2003). Leptin: Cutting the fat off the bone. *Lancet* **362**(9395), 1572–1574.

Coen, G. (2004). Leptin and bone metabolism. *J. Nephrol.* **17**(2), 187–189.

Collins, N., *et al.* (1991). A prospective study to evaluate the dose of vitamin D required to correct low 25-hydroxyvitamin D levels, calcium, and alkaline phosphatase in patients at risk of developing antiepileptic drug-induced osteomalacia. *Q. J. Med.* **78**(286), 113–122.

Corradino, R. A. (1976). Diphenylhydantoin: Direct inhibition of the vitamin D3-mediated calcium absorptive mechanism in organ-cultured duodenum. *Biochem. Pharmacol.* **25**(7), 863–864.

Cummings, S. R., Nevitt, M. C., Browner, W. S., Stone, K., Fox, K. M., Ensrud, K. E., Cauley, J., Black, D., and Vogt, T. M. (1995). Risk factors for hip fracture in white women. Study of Osteoporotic Fractures Research Group. *N. Engl. J. Med.* **332**(12), 767–773.

DeLuca, H. F. (2004). Overview of general physiologic features and functions of vitamin D. *Am. J. Clin. Nutr.* **80**(Suppl. 6), 1689S–1696S.

Desai, K. B., Ribbans, W. J., and Taylor, G. J. (1996). Incidence of five common fracture types in an institutional epileptic population. *Injury* **27**(2), 97–100.

Drezner, M. K. (2004). Treatment of anticonvulsant drug-induced bone disease. *Epilepsy Behav.* **5** (Suppl. 2), S41–S47.

Ducy, P., Schinke, T., and Karsenty, G. (2000). The osteoblast: A sophisticated fibroblast under central surveillance. *Science* **289**(5484), 1501–1504.

Eastell, R. (1998). Treatment of postmenopausal osteoporosis. *N. Engl. J. Med.* **338**(11), 736–746.

Ensrud, K. E., Walczak, T. S., Blackwell, T., Ensrud, E. R., Bowman, P. J., and Stone, K. L. (2004). Antiepileptic drug use increases rates of bone loss in older women: A prospective study. *Neurology* **62**(11), 2051–2057.

Espallargues, M., Sampietro-Colom, L., Estrada, M. D., Solà, M., del Rio, L., Setoain, J., and Granados, A. (2001). Identifying bone-mass-related risk factors for fracture to guide bone densitometry measurements: A systematic review of the literature. *Osteoporos. Int.* **12**(10), 811–822.

Farhat, G., Yamout, B., Mikati, M. A., Demirjian, S., Sawaya, R., and Fuleihan, GE-H (2002). Effect of antiepileptic drugs on bone density in ambulatory patients. *Neurology* **58**(9), 1348–1353.

Feldkamp, J., Becker, A., Witte, O. W., Scharff, D., and Scherbaum, W. A. (2000). Long-term anticonvulsant therapy leads to low bone mineral density—evidence for direct drug effects of phenytoin and carbamazepine on human osteoblast-like cells. *Exp. Clin. Endocrinol. Diabetes* **108**(1), 37–43.

Fitzpatrick, L. A. (2004). Pathophysiology of bone loss in patients receiving anticonvulsant therapy. *Epilepsy Behav.* **5**(Suppl. 2), S3–S15.

Gough, H., Goggin, T., Bissessar, A., Baker, M., Crowley, M., and Callaghan, N. (1986). A comparative study of the relative influence of different anticonvulsant drugs, UV exposure and diet on vitamin D and calcium metabolism in out-patients with epilepsy. *Q. J. Med.* **59**(230), 569–577.

Grisso, J. A., Kelsey, J. L., Strom, B. L., Chiu, G. Y., Maislin, G., O'Brien, L. A., Hoffman, S., and Kaplan, F. (1991). Risk factors for hip fractures in men: A preliminary study. *J. Bone Miner. Res.* **6** (8), 865–868.

Guo, C. Y., Ronen, G. M., and Atkinson, S. A. (2001). Long-term valproate and lamotrigine treatment may be a marker for reduced growth and bone mass in children with epilepsy. *Epilepsia* **42**(9), 1141–1147.

Guse, C. E., and Porinsky, R. (2003). Risk factors associated with hospitalization for unintentional falls: Wisconsin hospital discharge data for patients aged 65 and over. *Wmj* **102**(4), 37–42.

Hahn, T. J., Birge, S. J., Scarp, C. R., and Avioli, L. V. (1972a). Effect of chronic anticonvulsant therapy on serum 25-hydroxycalciferol levels in adults. *N. Engl. J. Med.* **287**(18), 900–904.

Hahn, T. J., Hendin, B. A., Scarp, C. R., and Haddad, J. G. (1972b). Phenobarbital-induced alterations in vitamin D metabolism. *J. Clin. Invest.* **51**(4), 741–748.

Hahn, T. J., Scharp, C. R., Richardson, C. A., Halstead, L. R., Kahn, A. J., and Teitelbaum, S. L. (1978). Interaction of diphenylhydantoin (phenytoin) and phenobarbital with hormonal mediation of fetal rat bone resorption in vitro. *J. Clin. Invest.* **62**, 406–414.

Harden, C. L., Herzog, A. G., Nikolov, B. G., Koppel, B. S., Christos, P. J., Fowler, K., Labar, D. R., and Hauser, W. A. (2006). Hormone replacement therapy in women with epilepsy: A randomized, double-blind, placebo-controlled study. *Epilepsia* **47**(9), 1447–1451.

Heany, R. P., Davies, K. M., Chen, T. C., Holick, M. F., and Barger-Lux, M. J. (2003). Human serum 25-hydroxycholecalciferol response to extended oral dosing with cholecalciferol. *Am. J. Clin. Nutr.* **77**(1), 204–210.

Heller, H. J., and Sakhaee, K. (2001). Anticonvulsant-induced bone disease: A plea for monitoring and treatment. *Arch. Neurol.* **58**(9), 1352–1353.

Holick, M. F. (2006). High prevalence of vitamin D inadequacy and implications for health. *Mayo Clin. Proc.* **81**(3), 353–373.

Holick, M. F. (2007). Vitamin D deficiency. *N. Engl. J. Med.* **357**(3), 266–281.

Holick, M. F., and Adams, A. J. (1998). Vitamin D metabolism and biological function. *In* "Metabolic Bone Disease" (L. V. Avioli and S. M. Krane, Eds.). Academic Press, San Diego.

Iwamoto, J., Takeda, T., and Sato, Y. (2006). Menatetrenone (vitamin K2) and bone quality in the treatment of postmenopausal osteoporosis. *Nutr. Rev.* **64**(12), 509–517.

Jenkins, M. V., Harris, M., and Wills, M. R. (1974). The effect of phenytoin on parathyroid extract and 25-hydroxycholecalciferol-induced bone resorption: Adenosine 3, 5 cyclic monophosphate production. *Calcif. Tissue Res.* **16**(2), 163–167.

Jones, G., Strugnell, S. A., and DeLuca, H. F. (1998). Current understanding of the molecular actions of vitamin D. *Physiol. Rev.* **78**(4), 1193–1231.

Kafali, G., Erselcan, T., and Tanzer, F. (1999). Effect of antiepileptic drugs on bone mineral density in children between ages 6 and 12 years. *Clin. Pediatr. (Phila)* **38**(2), 93–98.

Karsenty, G. (2006). Convergence between bone and energy homeostases: Leptin regulation of bone mass. *Cell Metab.* **4**, 341–348.

Khosla, S., and Kleerekoper, M. (2006). Biochemical markers of bone turnover. *In* "Primer on the Metabolic Bone Diseases and Disorders of Mineral Metabolism" (M. Favus, Ed.), Lippincott Williams & Williams, New York.

Kim, S. H., Lee, J. W., Choi, K. G., Chung, H. W., and Lee, H. W. (2007). A 6-month longitudinal study of bone mineral density with antiepileptic drug monotherapy. *Epilepsy Behav.* **10**(2), 291–295.

Knapen, M. H., Nieuwenhuijzen Kruseman, A. C., Wouters, R. S., and Vermeer, C. (1998). Correlation of serum osteocalcin fractions with bone mineral density in women during the first 10 years after menopause. *Calcif. Tissue Int.* **63**(5), 375–379.

Knapen, M. H., Schurgers, L. J., and Vermeer, C. (2007). Vitamin K2 supplementation improves hip bone geometry and bone strength indices in postmenopausal women. *Osteoporos. Int.* **18**(7), 963–972.

Koppel, B. S., Harden, C. L., Nikolov, B. G., and Labar, D. R. (2005). An analysis of lifetime fractures in women with epilepsy. *Acta Neurol. Scand.* **111**(4), 225–228.

Kruse, K., Bartels, H., Ziegler, R., Dreller, E., and Kracht, U. (1980). Parathyroid function and serum calcitonin in children receiving anticonvulsant drugs. *Eur. J. Pediatr.* **133**(2), 151–156.

Kruse, K., Süss, A., Büsse, M., and Schneider, P. (1987). Monomeric serum calcitonin and bone turnover during anticonvulsant treatment and in congenital hypothyroidism. *J. Pediatr.* **111**(1), 57–63.

Kubota, F., Kifune, A., Shibata, N., Akata, T., Takeuchi, K., Takahashi, S., Ohsawa, M., and Takama, F. (1999). Bone mineral density of epileptic patients on long-term antiepileptic drug therapy: A quantitative digital radiography study. *Epilepsy Res.* **33**(2-3), 93–97.

Lidgren, L., and Walloe, A. (1977). Incidence of fracture in epileptics. *Acta Orthop. Scand.* **48**(4), 356–361.

MacFarlane, G. D., Sackrison, J. L., Body, J. J., Ersfeld, D. L., Fenske, J. S., and Miller, A. B. (2004). Hypovitaminosis D in a normal, apparently healthy urban European population. *J. Steroid. Biochem. Mol. Biol.* **89–90**(1–5), 621–622.

Matheson, R. T., Herbst, J. J., Jubiz, W., Freston, J. W., and Tolman, K. G. (1976). Absorption and biotransfomation of cholecalciferol in drug-induced osteomalacia. *J. Clin. Pharmacol.* **16**(8–9), 426–432.

Mikati, M. A., Dib, L., Yamout, B., Wawan, R., Rahi, A. C., and Fuleihan, Gel-H (2006). Two randomized vitamin D trials in ambulatory patients on anticonvulsants: Impact on bone. *Neurology* **67**(11), 2005–2014.

Mintzer, S., Boppana, P., Toguri, J., and DeSantis, A. (2006). Vitamin D levels and bone turnover in epilepsy patients taking carbamazepine or oxcarbazepine. *Epilepsia* **47**(3), 510–515.

Morberg, C. M., Tetens, I., Black, E., Toubro, S., Soerensen, T. I., Pedersen, O., and Astrup, A. (2003). Leptin and bone mineral density: A cross-sectional study in obese and nonobese men. *J. Clin. Endocrinol. Metab.* **88**(12), 5795–5800.

Mosekilde, L., and Melsen, F. (1980). Dynamic differences in trabecular bone remodeling between patients after jejunoileal bypass for obesity and epileptic patients receiving anticonvulsant therapy. *Metab. Bone Dis. Relat. Res.* **2**, 77–82.

Nesby-O'Dell, S., Scanlon, K. S., Cogswell, M. E., Gillespie, C., Hollis, B. W., Looker, A. C., Allen, C., Dougherty, C., Gunter, E. W., and Bowman, B. A. (2002). Hypovitaminosis D prevalence and determinants among African American and white women of reproductive age: Third National Health and Nutrition Examination Survey, 1988–1994. *Am. J. Clin. Nutr.* **76**(1), 187–192.

Nilsson, O. S., Lindholm, T. S., Elmstedt, E., Lindbäck, A., and Lindholm, T. C. (1986). Fracture incidence and bone disease in epileptics receiving long-term anticonvulsant drug treatment. *Arch. Orthop. Trauma. Surg.* **105**(3), 146–149.

Nissen-Meyer, L. S., Svalheim, S., Taubøll, E., Reppe, S., Lekva, T., Solberg, L. B., Melhus, G., Reinholt, F. P., Gjerstad, L., and Jemtland, R. (2007). Levetiracetam, phenytoin, and valproate act differently on rat bone mass, structure, and metabolism. *Epilepsia* **48**(10), 1850–1860.

Okesina, A. B., Donaldson, D., and Lascelles, P. T. (1991). Isoenzymes of alkaline phosphatase in epileptic patients receiving carbamazepine monotherapy. *J. Clin. Pathol.* **44**(6), 480–482.

Omdahl, J. L., Bobrovnikova, E. A., Choe, S., Dwivedi, P. P., and May, B. K. (2001). Overview of regulatory cytochrome P450 enzymes of the vitamin D pathway. *Steroids* **66**(3–5), 381–389.

Oner, N., Kaya, M., Karasalihoğlu, S., Karaca, H., Celtik, C., and Tütüncüler, F. (2004). Bone mineral metabolism changes in epileptic children receiving valproic acid. *J. Paediatr. Child Health* **40**(8), 470–473.

Onodera, K., Takahashi, A., Sakurada, S., and Okano, Y. (2002). Effects of phenytoin and/or vitamin K2 (menatetrenone) on bone mineral density in the tibiae of growing rats. *Life Sci.* **70**(13), 1533–1542.

Onodera, K., Takahashi, A., Wakabayashi, H., Kamei, J., and Sakurada, S. (2003). Effects of menatetrenone on the bone and serum levels of vitamin K2 (menaquinone derivatives) in osteopenia induced by phenytoin in growing rats. *Nutrition* **19**(5), 446–450.

Pack, A. M., Morrell, M. J., Marcus, R., Holloway, L., Flaster, E., Done, S., Randall, A., and Seale, C. S. (2005). Bone mass and turnover in women with epilepsy on antiepileptic drug monotherapy. *Ann. Neurol.* **57**(2), 252–257.

Pack, A. M., Morrell, M. J., Randall, A., McMahon, D., and Shane, E. S. (2008). Bone health in young women with epilepsy after one year of antiepileptic drug monotherapy. *Neurology* 2008 Apr 29;**70** (18):1586–93.

Painter, S. E., Kleerekoper, M., and Camacho, P. M. (2006). Secondary osteoporosis: A review of the recent evidence. *Endocr. Pract.* **12**(4), 436–445.

Pascussi, J. M., Robert, A., Nguyen, M., Walrant-Debray, O., Garabedian, M., Martin, P., Pineau, T., Saric, J., Navarro, F., Maurel, P., and Vilarem, M. J. (2005). Possible involvement of pregnane X receptor-enhanced CYP24 expression in drug-induced osteomalacia. *J. Clin. Invest.* **115**(1), 177–186.

Pascussi, J. M., Maurel, P., and Vilarem, M. J. (2006). Osteomalacia is a frequent complication resulting from long-term therapy with drugs such as phenytoin, carbamazepine, and phenobarbital. *J. Clin. Invest.* **116**(10), 2564.

Pento, J. T., Glick, S. M., and Kagan, A. (1973). Diphenylhydantoin inhibition of calcitonin secretion in the pig. *Endocrinology* **92**(1), 330–333.

Pento, J. T., Hurt, G. M., and Rajah, T. (1996). Evaluation of calcium-mediated calcitonin secretion from the isolated perfused porcine thyroid using secretory inhibitors. *Horm. Metab. Res.* **27**, 107–109.

Persson, H. B. I., Alberts, K. A., Farahmand, B. Y., and Tomson, T. (2002). Risk of extremity fractures in adult outpatients with epilepsy. *Epilepsia* **43**(7), 768–772.

Quigg, M., Kiely, J. M., Johnson, M. L., Straume, M., Bertram, E. H., and Evans, W. S. (2006). Interictal and postictal circadian and ultradian luteinizing hormone secretion in men with temporal lobe epilepsy. *Epilepsia* **47**(9), 1452–1459.

Sato, Y., Kondo, I., Ishida, S., Motooka, H., Takayama, K., Tomita, Y., Maeda, H., and Satoh, K. (2001). Decreased bone mass and increased bone turnover with valproate therapy in adults with epilepsy. *Neurology* **57**(3), 445–449.

Schroeder, T. M., and Westendorf, J. J. (2005). Histone deacetylase inhibitors promote osteoblast maturation. *J. Bone Miner. Res.* **20**(12), 2254–2263.

Sheth, R. D. (2004). Bone health in pediatric epilepsy. *Epilepsy Behav.* **5**(Suppl. 2), S30–S35.

Sheth, R. D., Wesolowski, C. A., Jacob, J. C., Penney, S., Hobbs, G. R., and Riggs, J. E. (1995). Effect of carbamazepine and valproate on bone mineral density. *J. Pediatr.* **127**(2), 256–262.

Shiraki, M., Shiraki, Y., Aoki, C., and Miura, M. (2000). Vitamin K2 (menatetrenone) effectively prevents fractures and sustains lumbar bone mineral density in osteoporosis. *J. Bone Miner. Res.* **15** (3), 515–521.

Skillen, A. W., and Pierides, A. M. (1976). Serum gamma glutamyl transferase and alkaline phosphatase activities in epileptics receiving anticonvulsant therapy. *Clin. Chim. Acta* **72**(2), 245–251.

Souverein, P. C., Webb, D. J., Petri, H., Weil, J., Van Staa, T. P., and Egberts, T. (2005). Incidence of fractures among epilepsy patients: A population-based retrospective cohort study in the General Practice Research Database. *Epilepsia* **46**(2), 304–310.

Souverein, P. C., Webb, D. J., Weil, J. G., Van Staa, T. P., and Egberts, A. C. G. (2006). Use of antiepileptic drugs and risk of fractures: Case-control study among patients with epilepsy. *Neurology* **66**(9), 1318–1324.

Stephen, L. J., McLellan, A. R., Harrison, J. H., Shapiro, D., Dominiczak, M. H., Sills, G. J., and Brodie, M. J. (1999). Bone density and antiepileptic drugs: A case-controlled study. *Seizure* **8**(6), 339–342.

Stolze, H., Klebe, S., Zechlin, C., Baecker, C., Friege, L., and Deuschl, G. (2004). Falls in frequent neurological diseases—-prevalence, risk factors and aetiology. *J. Neurol.* **251**(1), 79–84.

Takeda, S., Elefteriou, F., Levasseur, R., Liu, X., Zhao, L., Parker, K. L., Armstrong, D., Ducy, P., and Karsenty, G. (2002). Leptin regulates bone formation via the sympathetic nervous system. *Cell* **111** (3), 305–317.

Thomas, T. (2004). The complex effects of leptin on bone metabolism through multiple pathways. *Curr. Opin. Pharmacol.* **4**(3), 295–300.

U.S. Department of Health and Human Services (2004). Bone health and osteoporosis: A report of the Surgeon General, U.D.O.H.a.H. Services, Editor.

Välimäki, M. J., Tiihonen, M., Laitinen, K., Tähtelä, R., Kärkkäinen, M., Lamberg-Allardt, C., Mäkelä, P., and Tunninen, R. (1994). Bone mineral density measured by dual-energy x-ray absorptiometry and novel markers of bone formation and resorption in patients on antiepileptic drugs. *J. Bone Miner. Res.* **9**(5), 631–637.

Vergnaud, P., Garnero, P., Meunier, P. J., Bréart, G., Kamihagi, K., and Delmas, P. D. (1997). Undercarboxylated osteocalcin measured with a specific immunoassay predicts hip fracture in elderly women: The EPIDOS study. *J. Clin. Endocrinol. Metab.* **82**(3), 719–724.

Vernillo, A. T., Rifkin, B. R., and Hauschka, P. V. (1990). Phenytoin affects osteocalcin secretion from osteoblastic rat osteosarcoma 17/2.8 cells in culture. *Bone* **11**(5), 309–312.

Verrotti, A., Greco, R., Morgese, G., and Chiarelli, F. (2000). Increased bone turnover in epileptic patients treated with carbamazepine. *Ann. Neurol.* **47**(3), 385–388.

Verrotti, A., Greco, R., Latini, G., Morgese, G., and Chiarelli, F. (2002). Increased bone turnover in prepubertal, pubertal, and postpubertal patients receiving carbamazepine. *Epilepsia* **43**(12), 1488–1492.

Vestergaard, P. (2005). Epilepsy, osteoporosis and fracture risk—a meta-analysis. *Acta Neurol. Scand.* **112** (5), 277–286.

Vestergaard, P., Tigaran, S., Rejnmark, L., Tigaran, C., Dam, M., and Mosekilde, L. (1999). Fracture risk is increased in epilepsy. *Acta Neurol. Scand.* **99**(5), 269–275.

Vestergaard, P., Rejnmark, L., and Mosekilde, L. (2004). Fracture risk associated with use of antiepileptic drugs. *Epilepsia* **45**(11), 1330–1337.

Waters, K. S., and Gonadal, T. C. (2006). Steroids and Receptors.. *In* "Primer on the Metabolic Bone Diseases and Disorders of Bone and Mineral Metabolism" (M. Favus, Ed.), pp. 104–110. Lippincott Williams and Wilkins, New York.

Weinstein, R. S., Bryce, G. F., Sappington, L. J., King, D. W., and Gallagher, B. B. (1984). Decreased serum ionized calcium and normal vitamin D metabolite levels with anticonvulsant drug treatment. *J. Clin. Endocrinol. Metab.* **58**(6), 1003–1009.

Xu, Y., Hashizume, T., Shuhart, M. C., Davis, C. L., Nelson, W. L., Sakaki, T., Kalhorn, T. F., Watkins, P. B., Shuetz, E. G., and Thummel, K. E. (2006). Intestinal and hepatic CYP3A4 catalyze hydroxylation of 1{alpha},25-dihydroxyvitamin D3: Implications for drug-induced osteomalacia. *Mol. Pharmacol.* **69**(1), 56–65.

Zhou, C., Assem, M., Tay, J. C., Watkins, P. B., Blumberg, B., Schuetz, E. G., and Thummel, K. E. (2006). Steroid and xenobiotic receptor and vitamin D receptor crosstalk mediates CYP24 expression and drug-induced osteomalacia. *J. Clin. Invest.* **116**(6), 1703–1712.

METABOLIC EFFECTS OF AEDs: IMPACT ON BODY WEIGHT, LIPIDS AND GLUCOSE METABOLISM

Raj D. Sheth* and Georgia Montouris[†]

*Department of Neurology, University of Wisconsin, Madison, Wisconsin 53792, USA
[†]Department of Neurology, Boston University Medical Center, Boston, Massachusetts 02118, USA

I. Introduction
II. Body Weight and AEDs
   A. Weight Gain Associated with AEDs
   B. Weight Loss Associated with AEDs
   C. Body Weight and Nonepileptic Events
III. Lipid Metabolism and AEDs
   A. Serum Lipid Concentrations
   B. Glucose, Insulin, and Leptin Levels
IV. Metabolic Acidosis
V. Renal Stones
   References

Epilepsy is a chronic disorder often requiring years of treatment. Accordingly, adverse effects of epilepsy and its treatment can impact general health for many decades. The psychological consequences of epilepsy are well documented, although the metabolic consequences of the treatment of epilepsy have only recently received attention. Antiepileptic drugs (AEDs) are well known to alter weight, causing either weight gain or weight loss. The mechanism by which this occurs remains to be fully understood, although there appears to be an effect on lipid and glucose metabolism. This chapter examines current data available on the adverse effects of individual AEDs on somatic weight, serum lipid profile, and glucose metabolism. These issues are of importance to neurologists caring for patients with epilepsy.

I. Introduction

The relationship between epilepsy and metabolic disorders is multifaceted. Metabolic disorders such as mitochondrial disorders and etiologies associated with the progressive myoclonus epilepsies are an important cause of seizures

INTERNATIONAL REVIEW OF
NEUROBIOLOGY, VOL. 83
DOI: 10.1016/S0074-7742(08)00019-6

329

(Acharya *et al.*, 1995). Furthermore, acute metabolic derangements can cause seizures or alter the frequency of seizures in an otherwise stable epilepsy. On the contrary, seizures, particularly if prolonged, can result in a variety of metabolic derangement (Lothman, 1990). Aspects of the relationship between epilepsy and metabolic disorders have been previously addressed and will not be reviewed in the current chapter (Boggs, 1997; DeLorenzo *et al.*, 1995).

The focus of this chapter will be the metabolic changes, including weight, lipid metabolism, and g changes, that can be associated with antiepileptic drug (AED) treatment. Many patients, however, face lifelong exposure to medication treatment and such changes can be cumulative. Accordingly, minor metabolic derangements that may not be seen over several weeks or months have the potential over many years to become an issue due to concern about the cumulative adverse effects of treatment. Hormonal changes associated with AEDs are an important issue that will be addressed in a different section.

This chapter will address AED-associated changes in body weight, bone disorders, metabolic acidosis, and renal stones. These issues have important implications for the optimal long-term management of epilepsy and will be the major focus of this chapter.

II. Body Weight and AEDs

Obesity has become a national epidemic (Aronne, 2002a). Obesity trends have steadily increased since the 1960s, where ~25–30% of the adult population met criteria for being either overweight (body mass index, BMI >25) or obese (BMI >30). Currently, more than half of the adult US population is categorized as being either overweight or obese (Fig. 1) (Willett *et al.*, 1999). Patients with epilepsy have an increased rate of obesity, some iatrogenically related to the prescribed AED treatment and others linked to the high prevalence of depression in patients with epilepsy (Thearle and Aronne, 2003).

The pathologic consequences of obesity include deleterious effects on insulin resistance, reproductive disorders, cardiovascular disorders, gall bladder disease, bone and joint disease, and cancer (Aronne, 2002b). Insulin resistance is strongly linked to intra-abdominal fat which is the characteristic location of adipose tissue that is seen in the metabolic syndrome (Prabhakaran and Anand, 2004). Furthermore, iatrogenic weight gain often results in medication noncompliance and increased seizures. Often, less well recognized is the psychological effect (Nelson *et al.*, 2004) of increased weight. Increases in body weight often adversely impacts body image and self-confidence. This can be a difficult problem at any age but can be particularly problematic in adolescence, which is a period of heightened awareness of body image and body weight (Sheth, 2002). AEDs are often

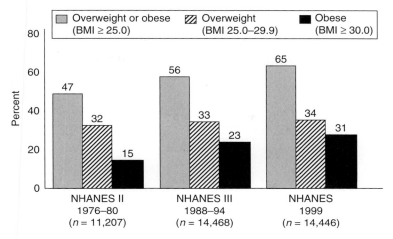

FIG. 1. Prevalence of overweight and obesity among US adults aged 20–74 years old. Note the 100% increase in proportion of the population who are obese over the duration 1976–1999. Age adjusted by the direct method to the year 2000 U.S. Bureau of the Census estimates using age groups 20–34, 35–44, 45–54, and 65–74 years.

associated with a modest increase in weight, although increases in body weight as little as 5–7 kg weight are associated with increased risk of cardiovascular complications (Must *et al.*, 1999).

A. WEIGHT GAIN ASSOCIATED WITH AEDs

AEDs can be associated with either an increase or a reduction in body weight, although most medications are weight neutral (Biton, 2003). However, since most reported retrospective studies are not powered to examine the effects on weight, these should be interpreted cautiously. Pooled data from clinical trials with valproate showed the incidence of weight gain to be as low as 3%, whereas studies specifically assessing weight show up to 71% of patients treated with valproate gaining weight (Biton, 2003).

AEDs that appear to be most consistently associated with weight increase include valproate (+40 to +50%), carbamazepine (+32%), gabapentin (+15 to 20%), and pregabalin (+10 to 15%). Valproate treatment can be associated with weight gain in 40– 50% of patients. Biton *et al.* (2001) examined weight-associated changes in a double-blind controlled study designed to evaluate weight changes with valproate and lamotrigine treatment. They found that patients treated with 10–60 mg/kg/day of valproate had a 5.8 ± 4.2 kg increase in weight compared

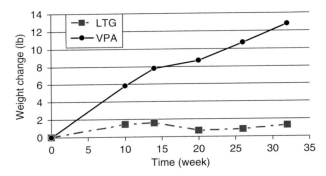

FIG. 2. Mean weight change over time for valproate (VPA) and lamotrigine (LTG) treatment (Biton *et al.*, 2001).

to the lamotrigine-treated group where weight changes of 0.6 ± 5.4 kg were noted. Interestingly, over the 32 weeks of the study there appeared to be steady weight increase (Fig. 2). The absence of a trend toward plateau in weight change is of concern, suggesting that over the course of many years of treatment there could be a cumulative effect on weight.

1. *Valproate*

The predictors of valproate-associated weight gain remain unclear. A mismatch between energy expenditure over caloric consumption was suggested as one mechanism that may underlie this process (Gidal *et al.*, 1996). More recently, valproate-induced hyperinsulinemia is thought to cause the metabolic syndrome with centripetal obesity, lipid abnormalities, and polycystic ovaries/hyperandrogenism in women with epilepsy (Isojarvi *et al.*, 1998). Recently, Luef *et al.* (2004) found that 61% of their patients treated with valproate had hepatic steatosis on ultrasonic examination of the liver compared to 21% for carbamazepine-treated patients. This nonalcoholic intrahepatic accumulation of fat is seen in patients with insulin resistance. Importantly, increased body weight appears to be an important risk factor for the development of nonalcoholic fatty liver disease (Luef *et al.*, 2004). The authors found that patients treated with valproate had higher insulin levels compared to the carbamazepine-treated group. This raises the possibility that valproate-associated weight gain may be an effect of relative insulin resistance.

2. *Carbamazepine*

Carbamazepine treatment can be associated with weight gain in up to one quarter of patients (Corman *et al.*, 1997; Mattson *et al.*, 1992; Richens *et al.*, 1994). Although this figure is lower than that for valproate, carbamazepine is the most commonly used AED after phenytoin, and has the potential to impact a larger number of patients. Interestingly, the widespread awareness of the weight gain potential for valproate may have reduced the expectation for carbamazepine. In an interesting study on 260 children, Easter *et al.* found that by report patients and physicians were more likely to identify valproate-associated weight increase; however, when actual weight measurements were analyzed they found that the incidence of weight gain was similar for both agents. They did find that the degree of weight gain was higher for valproate.

3. *Oxcarbazepinearbazepine*

Oxcarbazepinearbazepine is not reported to be associated with significant change in weight. In randomized control trials, increases in body weight were reported in 2% of patients taking 1200–2400 mg of oxcarbazepinearbazepine per day compared to a 1% rate for the placebo group (Glauser, 2001). However, as with other agents in the absence of trials designed to assess weight changes, the apparent absence of effect should be interpreted cautiously.

4. *Gabapentin and Pregabalin*

Gabapentin was associated with weight gain consistently found in six reported studies. Over half of the 44 patients treated for epilepsy with gabapentin experienced weight gain (DeToledo *et al.*, 1997). The authors found that at least a 10% increase in basal weight occurred in 10 patients and that 15 patients gained 5–10%. Of the 44 patients 16 patients had no change in weight while 3 patients lost 5–10% of their initial weight. Weight increase started between the second and third months of therapy and stabilized after 6–9 months of the study. As with other AEDs, the mechanism of the weight increase remains unknown with gabapentin. Interestingly, pregabalin, a new AED, appears to be also associated with dose-related weight gain (Arroyo *et al.*, 2004). Pregabalin at doses of 600 mg/day was associated with weight gain in 14% compared to 7% on 150 mg/day and 2% for control patients (Arroyo *et al.*, 2004). In a long-term trial, vigabatrin also appeared to be associated with a weight gain of 3.7 ± 0.2 kg over the study period (Guberman and Bruni, 2000).

AED-associated body weight changes are also seen in the pediatric population. Adolescence is a period of heightened awareness of body image and body weight. As in adults with epilepsy, AEDs such as valproate, carbamazepine, and gabapentin are associated with significant weight gain in adolescents. Adolescents who perceive that their AED is causing an increase in weight often become noncompliant with treatment. Ideally, weight-neutral medications such as lamotrigine and leviteracetam are ideally suited for use in adolescents (Devinsky *et al.*, 2000; Gidal *et al.*, 2003).

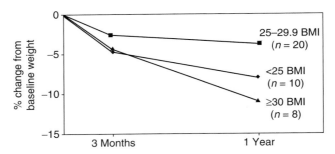

FIG. 3. Percentage change from baseline body weight at 3 months and 1 year of topiramate treatment versus baseline BMI (Ben-Menachem *et al.*, 2003).

B. WEIGHT LOSS ASSOCIATED WITH AEDs

AEDs most consistently associated with weight loss include felbamate (-2% to -75%) and topiramate (-10% to -20%) (Corman *et al.*, 1997; Dinesen *et al.*, 1984; Ketter *et al.*, 1999; Novak *et al.*, 1999). With topiramate, weight loss is dose related and can range from 9% to 11% when used in a dosage of 100–200 mg/ day. Ben-Menachem *et al.* (2003) showed in an uncontrolled prospective topiramate trial for patients 16 years and older that 82% of patients lost weight after 3 months of treatment and 86% lost weight after 12 months of treatment. The average weight loss was 3.0 kg (a 3.9% reduction from baseline body weight). In obese patients ($\text{BMI} > 30 \text{ kg/m}^2$), mean weight loss was 4.2 kg at 3 months and 10.9 kg at 12 months of treatment. They found that patients with a BMI > 30 lost 12% of body weight compared to those with a BMI < 30 who lost 5% of body weight. Importantly, they found that body fat loss represented 60–70% of the weight loss. Interestingly, serum glucose levels and glucose tolerance test and blood lipid profiles also improved and serum leptin levels were reduced (Fig. 3) (Ben-Menachem *et al.*, 2003). These findings offer the possibility in the obese patient of selecting an agent in an appropriate clinical setting such as topiramate to treat seizures as well as to induce weight loss. In clinical practice, discussing adverse effect profiles of AEDs and treatment options many patients appear to favor topiramate.

Felbamate is associated with anorexia and weight loss of 3–5% of body weight in children occurs mostly during the first 3 months of therapy (Bourgeois, 1997). However, in some patients the degree of weight loss can be severe, leading to discontinuation of the medication.

C. BODY WEIGHT AND NONEPILEPTIC EVENTS

It has been long recognized that patients with epilepsy have an increase in psychiatric comorbidity (Gilliam *et al.*, 2003). Psychiatric illness can be associated with weight increase. Marquez *et al.* (2004) examined BMI in patients with video-EEG confirmed nonepileptic events. They found that patients with nonepileptic events had a BMI of 30.5 compared to controls in whom the index was 26.1. Importantly, this effect was present even after controlling for weight-gain properties of antiepileptic drugs.

III. Lipid Metabolism and AEDs

Antiepileptic medications have been shown to affect serum lipid concentration and glucose, insulin, and leptin levels to varying degrees. In some patients the metabolic impact of AEDs may be significant and may be associated with clinical consequences.

A. Serum Lipid Concentrations

Changes in serum lipid concentrations have been associated with AEDs for some time now. Most of the published studies evaluating the effects of antiepileptic medications on lipids have been conducted in children, although a few studies in adults have also been reported.

Total cholesterol, triglycerides, low- and high-density lipoprotein cholesterol (including the high-density lipoprotein-2 and high-density lipoprotein-3 subtractions), and apolipoproteins A1 and B were measured in 120 adult epileptic patients treated with carbamazepine ($n = 42$), sodium valproate ($n = 38$), and phenytoin ($n = 40$) and compared with the values of 48 healthy subjects(Pita-Calandre et al., 1998). They found that carbamazepine-treated subjects showed specifically an increase in the high-density lipoprotein-2 cholesterol, whereas phenytoin-treated subjects showed specifically an increase in triglycerides. These changes with the exception of high-density lipoprotein cholesterol and apolipoprotein all were significantly elevated in women but not in men. There was no correlation with serum concentrations of AEDs and specific lipid changes. Interestingly, valproate-treated patients had no significant differences from controls. These findings suggest that enzyme-inducing antiepileptic medications alter serum lipid concentrations, whereas those not affecting the cytochrome P450 system were not associated with lipid changes. This study suggested that there were gender-specific differences in serum lipid changes (Pita-Calandre et al., 1998).

Serum lipid changes appear to occur across the life cycle. Children appear to experience similar changes in serum lipid concentrations as adults. In 208 children with epilepsy, the influence of AEDs on total cholesterol, high-density lipoprotein cholesterol, and triglyceride levels was compared to that in 175 normal children. As in adults, a significant increase in total cholesterol plasma levels was observed with enzyme-inducing AEDs, including carbamazepine, phenobarbital, and phenytoin. Children treated with valproate had similar lipid profiles as the control population. Hepatic induction by AEDs altering the cytochrome P450 system may underlie these findings. High-density lipoprotein and triglycerides were not altered by any of the AEDs. The authors recommended monitoring of total cholesterol levels in patients receiving carbamazepine, phenobarbital, and phenytoin (Franzoni *et al.*, 1992).

More recently, 64 children between the ages of 1 and 15 years and treated with phenobarbital, carbamazepine, and valproate were studied with regards to the serum lipid profiles and lipoprotein. In a longitudinal study, plasma lipoprotein, total cholesterol, triglycerides, low-density lipoprotein cholesterol, high-density lipoprotein cholesterol, apolipoprotein A and apolipoprotein B levels, and liver enzymes alanine aminotransferase, aspartate aminotransferase, alkaline phosphatase, and γ-glutamyltransferase were examined before the initiation of treatment and at 3, 6, and 12 months of the treatment period. Mean lipoprotein levels were significantly increased in all groups at 3, 6, and 12 months of the treatment period. The increase in alanine aminotransferase, aspartate aminotransferase, alkaline phosphatase, total cholesterol, low-density lipoprotein cholesterol, high-density lipoprotein cholesterol at 3, 6, and 12 months was statistically significant in the phenobarbital-treated group. The higher levels of lipoprotein were observed only in the carbamazepine-treated group at 6 and 12 months. The percentage of children with lipoprotein levels over 30 mg/dl was 44%, 63%, and 33% in the phenobarbital-, carbamazepine-, and valproate-treated children, respectively (Sonmez *et al.*, 2006).

Diet may also alter the impact of enzyme-inducing antiepileptic medications on lipid concentrations. Castro-Gago *et al.* (2006) reported on the evolution of serum lipids and lipoprotein(a) levels in children with epilepsy treated with carbamazepine, valproate, and phenobarbital with diet. In this study, the concentration levels of serum lipids and lipoprotein(a) were measured in 20 children receiving carbamazepine, 25 receiving valproate, and 5 children receiving phenobarbital while consuming a normal diet and subsequently following the initiation of a low-fat diet (children treated with carbamazepine and phenobarbital with high levels of total cholesterol, high-density lipoprotein cholesterol, and low-density lipoprotein cholesterol) and 3 months after the end of treatment with antiepileptic drugs. They found that patients consuming a regular diet had significant changes in lipids, but those receiving a low-fat diet had normalized all lipid parameters. These findings suggest that changes associated with AED treatment could be reversed by diets with lowered fat content.

In another study of 30 children treated with carbamazepine monotherapy, ages 30 months to 14 years, with idiopathic or cryptogenic partial or generalized tonic clonic seizures, serum lipids were evaluated at the onset and at the third month of therapy. Again, mean total cholesterol, low-density lipoprotein, very low-density lipoprotein, and triglyceride levels were found to be significantly increased during treatment, but mean high-density lipoprotein levels were not found to be significantly changed during the study. This study adds further support to previous findings that carbamazepine treatment alters the serum lipid profile in children and could predispose these children to the possibility of developing atherosclerosis later in life (Mahmoudian et al., 2005).

Further studies evaluating alterations in lipid concentration in patients treated with carbamazepine and valproate following 2 years of treatment confirm the findings seen in earlier studies. In a comparison of treatment of children with carbamazepine versus valproate monotherapy, serum total cholesterol, triglycerides, high- and low-density lipoprotein cholesterol, apolipoproteins AI and B concentrations, and serum concentration of biochemical markers of liver and renal function were measured before and at 6, 12, and 24 months of treatment. Serum concentration of lipoprotein(a) was found to be increased at 6, 12, and 24 months of carbamazepine and valproate monotherapy. These authors also suggested measuring serum lipoprotein (a) concentration routine in epileptic children taking these AEDs (Voudris et al., 2006).

The clinical relevance of the alterations in lipid concentrations and the long-term effects were addressed by Isojarvi et al. (1993). As previously shown, serum lipid levels change during treatment with carbamazepine. The increase in serum concentrations of total cholesterol and high-density lipoprotein cholesterol appear to persist, but the increase in serum low-density lipoprotein cholesterol and triglyceride levels were transient. Change in lipid metabolism may be associated with induction of the liver enzymes during carbamazepine medication. The increase in serum cholesterol and high-density lipoprotein cholesterol levels may have clinical relevance with regard to the incidence of atherosclerosis and coronary heart disease in patients with epilepsy receiving carbamazepine medication (Isojarvi et al., 1993). Eiris et al. (1995) also confirm that the risk of atherosclerosis-related disease may be related to the effects of long-term treatment with drugs such as phenobarbital and carbamazepine in children with epilepsy.

The onset of changes in lipid concentration have been shown to occur early in treatment. In a study comparing phenobarbital, carbamazepine, and valproate-treated children, ($n = 53$), serum total cholesterol levels increased after 3 months of treatment with carbamazepine and with phenobarbital and remained high for 1 year. Serum lipid concentration did not change during valproate treatment (total cholesterol, high- and low-density lipoprotein, triglycerides) (Yilmaz et al., 2001).

In a study comparing enzyme-inducing antiepileptic medications and none-nzyme inducers, Nikolaos et al. (2004) reported the long-term effects of carbamazepine, phenobarbital, valproate, and phenytoin treatment on cholesterol and lipoprotein serum levels . The findings related to carbamazepine and phenobarbital demonstrated the same results as described in previous studies. Patients on phenytoin showed significantly higher low-density lipoprotein-C values and non-significant differences in the rest of the parameters, while those on valproate showed significantly lower total cholesterol, low-density lipoprotein-C, and tri-glyceride values and nonsignificant differences in high-density lipoprotein-C values. As noted elsewhere, dietary changes may be of benefit. A low-cholesterol diet was suggested in those patients treated with carbamazepine and phenytoin (Nikolaos *et al.*, 2004).

B. GLUCOSE, INSULIN, AND LEPTIN LEVELS

Glucose, insulin, and leptin levels are also impacted by antiepileptic medications. Both first-generation and second-generation antiepileptic medications have been reported to alter insulin and glucose levels. Data available for phenytoin, gabapentin, valproate, and topiramate will be reviewed.

1. *Phenytoin*

Phenytoin is known to induce hyperglycemia. The mechanism has generally been considered primarily an inhibition of insulin release. In a case report, al-Rubeaan and Ryan reported a case of a patient who became hyperglycemic on phenytoin and whose markedly increased insulin requirements suggested an insulin-resistant state. Reduction of the phenytoin dose resulted in amelioration of the hyperglycemia. *In vitro* studies of phenytoin in a primary culture system of adipocytes that allowed assessment of both insulin receptor-binding and post-binding function showed a 57% reduction in maximum [14C]3-0-methylcglucose transport in the presence of phenytoin while having no effect on maximum insulin binding. These results suggest that phenytoin administration can result in insulin insensitivity by inducing a post-binding defect in insulin action (al-Rubeaan and Ryan, 1991).

Carter *et al.* (1981) reported a case of phenytoin-induced hyperglycemia prescribed following a right-sided focal seizure during a hospitalization for non-ketotic hyperosmolar coma. In this case, phenytoin was discontinued as the seizure disorder was considered to be secondary to the previous episode of hyperosmolar coma. The authors suggest that if "hyperglycemia occurs in a patient taking phenytoin, especially after starting phenytoin therapy of increasing the dose, drug-induced hyperglycemia should be considered in the differential diagnosis. Phenytoin inhibits glucose-induced insulin release from pancreatic islets by a mechanism that is unknown. In a study published in 2006 (Nabe *et al.*, 2006) phenytoin was shown to suppress glucose-induced insulin release concentration dependently. This study noted that phenytoin increased cytoplasmic pH in the presence of high glucose, but was abolished under Na^+-deprived conditions and HCO_3^--deprived conditions, suggesting that the Na^+ and HCO_3^- transport across the plasma membrane are involved in the increase in cytoplasmic pH by phenytoin. Phenytoin was also shown to suppress mitochondrial ATP production by reducing the H^+ gradient across mitochondrial membrane. Phenytoin inhibits glucose-induced insulin secretion not only by inhibiting mitochondrial ATP production but also by reducing Ca^{2+} efficacy in the exocytotic system through its alkalizing effect on cytoplasm.

2. Gabapentin

Gabapentin-induced hypoglycemia is reported in a single case of long-term peritoneal dialysis. This patient was treated with gabapentin and was noted to have high insulin and C-peptide levels during the hypoglycemic episode which returned to normal after gabapentin was discontinued. Since the discontinuation of gabapentin, no further hypoglycemic episodes were reported (Penumalee et al., 2003).

3. Topiramate

Topiramate reduces body weight and ameliorates glycemic control in obese patients with diabetes. In rodent models of obesity and diabetes, topiramate treatment counteracts hyperglyemcia and increases insulin levels on glucose tolerance test. These observations suggest that topiramate might exert direct action on insulin-secreting cells, in particular regarding obesity-associated beta-cell dysfunction. In this study, topiramate counteracted oleate-induced lipid load and restored glucose-stimulated insulin secretion, in this case, by maintaining low insulin release at basal glucose (Frigerio et al., 2006).

4. Valproate

Valproate treatment has been reported to be associated with obesity and high fasting serum insulin concentrations, although the mechanism remains to be defined. Pylvanen et al. (2006) examined fasting plasma glucose, serum insulin, proinsulin, and C-peptide concentrations, taken after overnight fast in 51 patients receiving valproate monotherapy, and compared them to those in 45 control subjects. Valproate-treated patients demonstrated a fasting hyperinsulinemia, although the fasting serum proinsulin and C-peptide concentrations were not significantly higher in the patients than in the controls. Proinsulin/insulin and C-peptide concentrations were lower in the valproate-treated group. They also had lower fasting plasma glucose concentrations. The findings in this study suggest that valproate does not induce insulin secretion but might interfere with the insulin metabolism in the liver, resulting in higher insulin concentrations in the peripheral circulation. These findings were seen irrespective of concomitant weight gain, suggesting that increased insulin concentrations induce weight gain and not vice versa.

Age-related insulin resistance is reported by Tan et al. (2005). In this study, prepubertal girls with epilepsy were evaluated analyzing fasting serum insulin and glucose levels as well as hormonal levels. The findings demonstrated that valproate may lead to hyperinsulinemia which may not require a mature adult endocrine system. As previously described, weight gain has been associated with valproate among other antiepileptic medications (carbamazepine, gabapentin, pregabalin). Studies evaluating valproate have shown that the decreased blood glucose level, impairment of beta-oxidation of fatty acids, and increased insulin levels are some of the possible mechanisms (Aydin *et al.*, 2005). In the study reported by Aydin *et al.* (2005), BMI and fasting insulin glucose ratio were calculated and serum glucose, insulin, cortisol, leptin, and neuropeptide Y levels were measured. At the end of 3 months, the mean BMI values and the mean serum insulin, fasting insulin glucose ratio, and neuropeptide Y levels increased, whereas the serum glucose levels decreased. After 6 months of treatment, the mean serum cortisol and leptin levels were high, in addition to the BMI, neuropeptide Y level, and fasting insulin glucose ratio, suggesting that weight gain may be related to low glucose and high insulin, cortisol, leptin, and neuropeptide Y levels.

Weight gain appears to influence insulin and leptin levels. Greco *et al.* (2005) also noted in 40 patients treated with valproate, 15 (37.2%) having gained weight, that circulating leptin and insulin levels were higher and adiponectin levels were lower in those who did not gain weight.

Similar findings were reported by Verrottti *et al.* (2005) who found during valproate monotherapy, a significant increase in serum leptin levels in epilepsy patients who became obese, whereas valproate-treated patients who remained lean did not show any significant changes in leptin levels. Moreover, insulin resistance was seen only in those who became obese during valproate therapy and not in those who remained lean (Verrotti *et al.*, 2005). The mechanism of insulin level alteration may be related to valproate's mechanism of action. Valproate is a fatty acid derivative, competes with free fatty acids for albumin binding, and acts as a γ-aminobutyric acid (GABA)-ergic agonist, mechanisms which are known to be involved in pancreatic beta-cell regulation and insulin secretion (Luef *et al.*, 2002).

The impact of antiepileptic medications on lipid concentration and glucose, insulin, and leptin levels suggests that monitoring be considered to possibly prevent long-term consequences on general health. The onset of metabolic derangement following initiation of antiepileptic medication should be evaluated carefully as to etiology. In addition, concurrent conditions should be considered when choice in antiepileptic medication is undertaken.

IV. Metabolic Acidosis

Metabolic acidosis results either when the kidney is unable to excrete dietary H^+ load or from an excessive loss of HCO_3^- secondary to reduced renal tubular reabsorption. This latter condition is referred to as renal tubular acidosis and consists of three types. The mildest and self-limiting form is renal tubular acidosis

Type 2 where the primary defect is in the proximal renal tubule. Typically, plasma HCO_3^- concentrations are mildly reduced in the 14–20 mEq/l range. Renal tubular acidosis Type 2 associated with decreased serum bicarbonate is referred to as hyperchloremic, nonanion gap metabolic acidosis.

Three AEDs are typically associated with metabolic acidosis, acetazolamide, zonisamide, and topiramate. This effect appears to be a function of their property to inhibit the enzyme carbonic anhydrase. Acetalzolamide, zonisamide, and topiramate are all associated with varying degrees of renal tubular acidosis (Ballaban-Gil et al., 1998; Bell and Key, 1994; Elinav et al., 2002; Ikeda et al., 2002; Inoue et al., 2000; Izzedine et al., 2004; Ozawa et al., 2001).

Topiramate is associated with a mild hyperchloremic, nonanion gap metabolic acidosis manifested by a persistent low bicarbonate in 23–67% of patients compared to 1–10% of patients receiving placebo. However, the incidence of markedly low serum bicarbonate in clinical trials ranges from 3% to 11% for topiramate and 0–<1% for placebo. Bicarbonate decrements are usually mild-moderate, with an average decrease of 4 mEq/l at daily doses of 400 mg in adults and ~6 mg/kg/day in pediatric patients, although rarely values below 10 mEq/l can be found. The timing of the metabolic acidosis is typically soon after initiation of therapy.

Conditions or therapies that predispose to acidosis (such as renal disease, severe respiratory disorders, status epilepticus, diarrhea, surgery, ketogenic diet, or drugs) may be additive to the bicarbonate-lowering effects of topiramate.

Some manifestations of acute or chronic metabolic acidosis may include hyperventilation, nonspecific symptoms such as fatigue and anorexia, or more severe sequelae including cardiac arrhythmias or stupor. Chronic, untreated metabolic acidosis may increase the risk for nephrolithiasis or nephrocalcinosis, and may also result in osteomalacia (referred to as rickets in pediatric patients) and/or osteoporosis with an increased risk for fractures. Chronic metabolic acidosis in pediatric patients may also reduce growth rates. A reduction in growth rate may eventually decrease the maximal height achieved. The effect of topiramate on growth and bone-related sequelae has not been systematically investigated.

For adults on topiramate, persistent treatment-emergent decrease in serum bicarbonate (defined as <20 mEq/l) occurring on two consecutive visits or at the final visit was 32% for 400 mg/day, compared to 1% for placebo. This effect can be observed on doses of 50 mg/day. In patients younger than 16 years of age with refractory epilepsy treated with topiramate 6 mg/kg/day, the incidence of treatment-emergent decreases in serum bicarbonate was 67% compared to 10% for placebo. Marked reductions in serum bicarbonate occurred in 11% of patients and did not occur in the placebo group. This effect has been observed in infants at doses of 5 mg/kg/day or higher (Philippi et al., 2002).

Measurement of baseline and periodic serum bicarbonate during topiramate treatment is recommended. If metabolic acidosis develops and persists, consideration should be given to reducing the dose or discontinuing topiramate (using dose tapering). If the decision is made to continue patients on topiramate in the face of persistent acidosis, alkali treatment should be considered.

V. Renal Stones

Zonisamide and topiramate are two agents that are associated with a mild increase in the incidence of renal stones. Zonisamide is associated with a 4% rate of renal stones. Of these, 12 were symptomatic, and 28 were described as possible kidney stones based on sonographic detection. In nine patients, the diagnosis was confirmed by a passage of a stone or by a definitive sonographic finding. The rate of occurrence of kidney stones was 28.7 per 1000 patient-years of exposure in the first 6 months, 62.6 per 1000 patient-years of exposure between 6 and 12 months, and 24.3 per 1000 patient-years of exposure after 12 months of use. There are no normative sonographic data available for either the general population or patients with epilepsy. The clinical significance of the sonographic finding is unknown. The analyzed stones were composed of calcium or urate salts. In general, increasing fluid intake and urine output can help reduce the risk of stone formation, particularly in those with predisposing risk factors. It is unknown, however, whether these measures will reduce the formation of renal stones.

Approximately 1.5% of patients treated with topiramate develop kidney stones compared to the 0.5% incidence of renal stones in the general population. Men are more at risk of developing kidney stones and the association has not been reported for children treated with topiramate. This effect may also result from the weak carbonic anhydrase property of the agent. Acetazolamide promotes stone formation by reducing urinary citrate excretion and by increasing urinary pH. Accordingly, it is not advisable to use concomitant treatment with these agents or the ketogenic diet. Factors that generally appear to reduce the risk of renal stones include increased fluid intake and lowering the concentration of substances involved in stone formation.

Ketogenic diet may be associated with renal stones (Ballaban-Gil *et al.*, 1998; Kossoff *et al.*, 2002; Maydell *et al.*, 2001). This association has given concern for the potential theoretical additive effects of carbonic anhydrase inhibitors with the ketogenic diet. Kossoff *et al.* (2002) examined this issue in 301 children treated with the ketogenic diet. They found that the incidence of renal stones was 6.7% for patients on the ketogenic diet but not receiving a carbonic anhydrase inhibitor compared to 6.5% for the combined use of carbonic anhydrase inhibitor and the ketogenic diet. They recommend increased hydration in patients treated with combination therapy and that urine alkalinization be considered for children having a family history of renal stones or prior history of renal abnormalities.

Clinicians need to become familiar with the metabolic issues that accompany AEDs. Many of the metabolic issues are insidious in presentation and do not manifest for years. Further study is required to better define the differential adverse effect profile of the currently available AEDs.

References

Acharya, J. N., Satishchandra, P., and Shankar, S. K. (1995). Familial progressive myoclonus epilepsy: Clinical and electrophysiologic observations. *Epilepsia* **36,** 429–434.

al-Rubeaan, K., and Ryan, E. A. (1991). Phenytoin-induced insulin insensitivity. *Diabet. Med.* **8,** 968–970.

Aronne, L. J. (2002a). Classification of obesity and assessment of obesity-related health risks. *Obes. Res.* **10**(Suppl. 2), 105S–115S.

Aronne, L. J. (2002b). Obesity as a disease: Etiology, treatment, and management considerations for the obese patient. *Obes. Res.* **10**(Suppl. 2), 95S–96S.

Arroyo, S., Anhut, H., Kugler, A. R., Lee, C. M., Knapp, L. E., Garofalo, E. A., and Messmer, S. (2004). Pregabalin add-on treatment: A randomized, double-blind, placebo-controlled, dose-response study in adults with partial seizures. *Epilepsia* **45,** 20–27.

Aydin, K., Serdaroglu, A., Okuyaz, C., Bideci, A., and Gucuyener, K. (2005). Serum insulin, leptin, and neuropeptide y levels in epileptic children treated with valproate. *J. Child Neurol.* **20,** 848–851.

Ballaban-Gil, K., Callahan, C., O'dell, C., Pappo, M., Moshe, S., and Shinnar, S. (1998). Complications of the ketogenic diet. *Epilepsia* **39,** 744–748.

Bell, N. H., and Key, L. L., Jr. (1994). Acquired osteomalacia. *Curr. Ther. Endocrinol. Metab.* **5,** 495–499.

Ben-Menachem, E., Axelsen, M., Johanson, E. H., Stagge, A., and Smith, U. (2003). Predictors of weight loss in adults with topiramate-treated epilepsy. *Obes. Res.* **11,** 556–562.

Biton, V. (2003). Effect of antiepileptic drugs on bodyweight: Overview and clinical implications for the treatment of epilepsy. *CNS Drugs* **17,** 781–791.

Biton, V., Mirza, W., Montouris, G., Vuong, A., Hammer, A. E., and Barrett, P. S. (2001). Weight change associated with valproate and lamotrigine monotherapy in patients with epilepsy. *Neurology* **56,** 172–177.

Boggs, J. G. (1997). Seizures in medically complex patients. *Epilepsia* **38**(Suppl. 4), S55–S59.

Bourgeois, B. F. (1997). Felbamate. *Semin. Pediatr. Neurol.* **4,** 3–8.

Carter, B. L., Small, R. E., Mandel, M. D., and Starkman, M. T. (1981). Phenytoin-induced hyperglycemia. *Am. J. Hosp. Pharm.* **38,** 1508–1512.

Castro-Gago, M., Novo-Rodriguez, M. I., Blanco-Barca, M. O., Urisarri-Ruiz De Cortazar, A., Rodriguez-Garcia, J., Rodriguez-Segade, S., and Eiris-Punal, J. (2006). Evolution of serum lipids and lipoprotein (a) levels in epileptic children treated with carbamazepine, valproic acid, and phenobarbital. *J. Child Neurol.* **21,** 48–53.

Corman, C. L., Leung, N. M., and Guberman, A. H. (1997). Weight gain in epileptic patients during treatment with valproic acid: A retrospective study. *Can. J. Neurol. Sci.* **24,** 240–244.

DeLorenzo, R. J., Pellock, J. M., Towne, A. R., and Boggs, J. G. (1995). Epidemiology of status epilepticus. *J. Clin. Neurophysiol.* **12,** 316–325.

DeToledo, J. C., Toledo, C., Decerce, J., and Ramsay, R. E. (1997). Changes in body weight with chronic, high-dose gabapentin therapy. *Ther. Drug Monit.* **19,** 394–396.

Devinsky, O., Vuong, A., Hammer, A., and Barrett, P. S. (2000). Stable weight during lamotrigine therapy: A review of 32 studies. *Neurology* **54,** 973–975.

Dinesen, H., Gram, L., Andersen, T., and Dam, M. (1984). Weight gain during treatment with valproate. *Acta Neurol. Scand.* **70,** 65–69.

Eiris, J. M., Lojo, S., Del Rio, M. C., Novo, I., Bravo, M., Pavon, P., and Castro-Gago, M. (1995). Effects of long-term treatment with antiepileptic drugs on serum lipid levels in children with epilepsy. *Neurology* **45,** 1155–1157.

Elinav, E., Ackerman, Z., Gottehrer, N. P., and Heyman, S. N. (2002). Recurrent life-threatening acidosis induced by acetazolamide in a patient with diabetic type IV renal tubular acidosis. *Ann. Emerg. Med.* **40,** 259–260.

Franzoni, E., Govoni, M., D'addato, S., Gualandi, S., Sangiorgi, Z., Descovich, G. C., and Salvioli, G. P. (1992). Total cholesterol, high-density lipoprotein cholesterol, and triglycerides in children receiving antiepileptic drugs. *Epilepsia* **33,** 932–935.

Frigerio, F., Chaffard, G., Berwaer, M., and Maechler, P. (2006). The antiepileptic drug topiramate preserves metabolism-secretion coupling in insulin secreting cells chronically exposed to the fatty acid oleate. *Biochem. Pharmacol.* **72,** 965–973.

Gidal, B. E., Anderson, G. W., Spencer, N. W., Maly, M. M., Murty, J., and Collins, D. M. (1996). Valproate-associated weight gain: Potential relation to energy expenditure and metabolism in patients with epilepsy. *J. Epilepsy* **9,** 234–241.

Gidal, B. E., Sheth, R. D., Magnus, L., and Herbeuval, A. F. (2003). Levetiracetam does not alter body weight: Analysis of randomized, controlled clinical trials. *Epilepsy Res.* **56,** 121–126.

Gilliam, F., Hecimovic, H., and Sheline, Y. (2003). Psychiatric comorbidity, health, and function in epilepsy. *Epilepsy Behav.* **4**(Suppl. 4), S26–S30.

Glauser, T. A. (2001). Oxcarbazepine in the treatment of epilepsy. *Pharmacotherapy* **21,** 904–919.

Greco, R., Latini, G., Chiarelli, F., Iannetti, P., and Verrotti, A. (2005). Leptin, ghrelin, and adiponectin in epileptic patients treated with valproic acid. *Neurology* **65,** 1808–1809.

Guberman, A., and Bruni, J. (2000). Long-term open multicentre, add-on trial of vigabatrin in adult resistant partial epilepsy. The Canadian Vigabatrin Study Group. *Seizure* **9,** 112–118.

Ikeda, K., Iwasaki, Y., Kinoshita, M., Yabuki, D., Igarashi, O., Ichikawa, Y., and Satoyoshi, E. (2002). Acetazolamide-induced muscle weakness in hypokalemic periodic paralysis. *Intern. Med.* **41,** 743–745.

Inoue, T., Kira, R., Kaku, Y., Ikeda, K., Gondo, K., and Hara, T. (2000). Renal tubular acidosis associated with zonisamide therapy. *Epilepsia* **41,** 1642–1644.

Isojarvi, J. I., Pakarinen, A. J., and Myllyla, V. V. (1993). Serum lipid levels during carbamazepine medication. A prospective study. *Arch. Neurol.* **50,** 590–593.

Isojarvi, J. I., Rattya, J., Myllyla, V. V., Knip, M., Koivunen, R., Pakarinen, A. J., Tekay, A., and Tapanainen, J. S. (1998). Valproate, lamotrigine, and insulin-mediated risks in women with epilepsy. *Ann. Neurol.* **43,** 446–451.

Izzedine, H., Launay-Vacher, V., and Deray, G. (2004). Topiramate-induced renal tubular acidosis. *Am. J. Med.* **116,** 281–282.

Ketter, T. A., Post, R. M., and Theodore, W. H. (1999). Positive and negative psychiatric effects of antiepileptic drugs in patients with seizure disorders. *Neurology* **53,** S53–S67.

Kossoff, E. H., Pyzik, P. L., Furth, S. L., Hladky, H. D., Freeman, J. M., and Vining, E. P. (2002). Kidney stones, carbonic anhydrase inhibitors, and the ketogenic diet. *Epilepsia* **43,** 1168–1171.

Lothman, E. (1990). The biochemical basis and pathophysiology of status epilepticus. *Neurology* **40** (Suppl. 2), 13–23.

Luef, G., Abraham, I., Hoppichler, F., Trinka, E., Unterberger, I., Bauer, G., and Lechleitner, M. (2002). Increase in postprandial serum insulin levels in epileptic patients with valproic acid therapy. *Metabolism* **51,** 1274–1278.

Luef, G. J., Waldmann, M., Sturm, W., Naser, A., Trinka, E., Unterberger, I., Bauer, G., and Lechleitner, M. (2004). Valproate therapy and nonalcoholic fatty liver disease. *Ann. Neurol.* **55,** 729–732.

Mahmoudian, T., Iranpour, R., and Messri, N. (2005). Serum lipid levels during carbamazepine therapy in epileptic children. *Epilepsy Behav.* **6,** 257–259.

Marquez, A. V., Farias, S. T., Apperson, M., Koopmans, S., Jorgensen, J., Shatzel, A., and Alsaadi, T. M. (2004). Psychogenic nonepileptic seizures are associated with an increased risk of obesity. *Epilepsy Behav.* **5,** 88–93.

Mattson, R. H., Cramer, J. A., and Collins, J. F. (1992). A comparison of valproate with carbamazepine for the treatment of complex partial seizures and secondarily generalized tonic-clonic seizures in adults. The Department of Veterans Affairs Epilepsy Cooperative Study No. 264 Group. *N. Engl. J. Med.* **327,** 765–771.

Maydell, B. V., Wyllie, E., Akhtar, N., Kotagal, P., Powaski, K., Cook, K., Weinstock, A., and Rothner, A. D. (2001). Efficacy of the ketogenic diet in focal versus generalized seizures. *Pediatr. Neurol.* **25,** 208–212.

Must, A., Spadano, J., Coakley, E. H., Field, A. E., Colditz, G., and Dietz, W. H. (1999). The disease burden associated with overweight and obesity. *JAMA* **282,** 1523–1529.

Nabe, K., Fujimoto, S., Shimodahira, M., Kominato, R., Nishi, Y., Funakoshi, S., Mukai, E., Yamada, Y., Seino, Y., and Inagaki, N. (2006). Diphenylhydantoin suppresses glucose-induced insulin release by decreasing cytoplasmic H+ concentration in pancreatic islets. *Endocrinology* **147,** 2717–2727.

Nelson, T. L., Palmer, R. F., and Pedersen, N. L. (2004). The metabolic syndrome mediates the relationship between cynical hostility and cardiovascular disease. *Exp. Aging Res.* **30,** 163–177.

Nikolaos, T., Stylianos, G., Chryssoula, N., Irini, P., Christos, M., Dimitrios, T., Konstantinos, P., and Antonis, T. (2004). The effect of long-term antiepileptic treatment on serum cholesterol (TC, HDL, LDL) and triglyceride levels in adult epileptic patients on monotherapy. *Med. Sci. Monit.* **10,** MT50–MT52.

Novak, G. P., Maytal, J., Alshansky, A., Eviatar, L., Sy-Kho, R., and Siddique, Q. (1999). Risk of excessive weight gain in epileptic children treated with valproate. *J. Child Neurol.* **14,** 490–495.

Ozawa, H., Azuma, E., Shindo, K., Higashigawa, M., Mukouhara, R., and Komada, Y. (2001). Transient renal tubular acidosis in a neonate following transplacental acetazolamide. *Eur. J. Pediatr.* **160,** 321–322.

Penumalee, S., Kissner, P. Z., and Migdal, S. D. (2003). Gabapentin-induced hypoglycemia in a long-term peritoneal dialysis patient. *Am. J. Kidney Dis.* **42,** E3–E5.

Philippi, H., Boor, R., and Reitter, B. (2002). Topiramate and metabolic acidosis in infants and toddlers. *Epilepsia* **43,** 744–747.

Pita-Calandre, E., Rodriguez-Lopez, C. M., Cano, M. D., and Pena-Bernal, M. (1998). [Serum lipids. lipoproteins, and apolipoproteins in adult epileptics treated with carbamazepine, valproic acid, or phenytoin]. *Rev. Neurol.* **27,** 785–789.

Prabhakaran, D., and Anand, S. S. (2004). The metabolic syndrome: An emerging risk state for cardiovascular disease. *Vasc. Med.* **9,** 55–68.

Pylvanen, V., Pakarinen, A., Knip, M., and Isojarvi, J. (2006). Insulin-related metabolic changes during treatment with valproate in patients with epilepsy. *Epilepsy Behav.* **8,** 643–648.

Richens, A., Davidson, D. L., Cartlidge, N. E., and Easter, D. J. (1994). A multicentre comparative trial of sodium valproate and carbamazepine in adult onset epilepsy. Adult EPITEG Collaborative Group. *J. Neurol. Neurosurg. Psychiatry* **57,** 682–687.

Sheth, R. D. (2002). Adolescent issues in epilepsy. *J. Child Neurol.* **17**(Suppl. 2), 2S23–2S27.

Sonmez, F. M., Demir, E., Orem, A., Yildirmis, S., Orhan, F., Aslan, A., and Topbas, M. (2006). Effect of antiepileptic drugs on plasma lipids, lipoprotein (a), and liver enzymes. *J. Child Neurol.* **21,** 70–74.

Tan, H., Orbak, Z., Kantarci, M., Kocak, N., and Karaca, L. (2005). Valproate-induced insulin resistance in prepubertal girls with epilepsy. *J. Pediatr. Endocrinol. Metab.* **18,** 985–989.

Thearle, M., and Aronne, L. J. (2003). Obesity and pharmacologic therapy. *Endocrinol. Metab. Clin. North Am.* **32,** 1005–1024.

Verrotti, A., Greco, R., Latini, G., and Chiarelli, F. (2005). Endocrine and metabolic changes in epileptic patients receiving valproic acid. *J. Pediatr. Endocrinol. Metab.* **18,** 423–430.

Voudris, K. A., Attilakos, A., Katsarou, E., Drakatos, A., Dimou, S., Mastroyianni, S., Skardoutsou, A., Prassouli, A., and Garoufi, A. (2006). Early and persistent increase in serum lipoprotein (a) concentrations in epileptic children treated with carbamazepine and sodium valproate monotherapy. *Epilepsy Res.* **70,** 211–217.

Willett, W. C., Dietz, W. H., and Colditz, G. A. (1999). Guidelines for healthy weight. *N. Engl. J. Med.* **341,** 427–434.

Yilmaz, E., Dosan, Y., Gurgoze, M. K., and Gungor, S. (2001). Serum lipid changes during anticonvulsive treatment serum lipids in epileptic children. *Acta Neurol. Belg.* **101,** 217–220.

PSYCHIATRIC COMORBIDITIES IN EPILEPSY

W. Curt LaFrance, Jr.,* Andres M. Kanner,[†] and Bruce Hermann[‡]

*Brown Medical School, Rhode Island Hospital, Departments of Psychiatry and Neurology,
Providence, Rhode Island 02903, USA
[†]Rush Epilepsy Center, Chicago, Illinois 60612, USA
[‡]University of Wisconsin, Madison, Wisconsin 53972, USA

I. Comorbid Disorders in Epilepsy
  A. Some General Principles
II. Depression in Epilepsy
  A. Suicidality in Patients with Epilepsy
  B. Depression as a Paraictal Phenomenon
  C. Depression as a CoMorbid Disorder: Interictal Depressive Disorders
  D. Depression as an Iatrogenic Process
  E. Depression Following Epilepsy Surgery
III. Treatment of Depression in Epilepsy
  A. Pharmacokinetic Interactions Between ADs and AEDs
  B. Choice of AD
  C. Other Types of Psychiatric Treatments
IV. Anxiety Disorders in Epilepsy
  A. Anxiety Episodes as Paraictal Processes
  B. Treatment of Anxiety Disorders in Epilepsy
V. Psychosis of Epilepsy
  A. Postictal Psychotic Symptoms and Psychotic Episodes
  B. Alternative Psychosis or "Forced Normalization"
  C. Iatrogenic Psychotic Disorders
  D. Drug Treatment of Psychosis in Patients with Epilepsy
VI. Attention Deficit Disorders and Behavior Disturbances
  A. Preictal Symptoms and Episodes
  B. Postictal Symptoms of ADD and Behavioral Disturbances
  C. ADD and Behavior Disturbances as an Expression of Paraictal Processes
  D. ADD and Behavioral Disturbances as an Interictal Comorbid Disorder
  E. Iatrogenic Behavioral Changes
  F. Treatment of ADHD in PWE
VII. Psychosocial Consequences for Women with Epilepsy
  A. Impact of Depression on Quality of life in Epilepsy Patients
  B. Stigma
VIII. Nonepileptic Seizures
  A. Introduction
  B. Epidemiology and Costs
  C. Pathology
  D. Diagnosis of NES

INTERNATIONAL REVIEW OF
NEUROBIOLOGY, VOL. 83
DOI: 10.1016/S0074-7742(08)00020-2

IX. Treatment of NES
     A. Treatment Literature
     B. Treatment
 X. Conclusions
     References

Psychiatric disorders can be identified in 25–50% of patients with epilepsy, with higher prevalence among patients with poorly controlled seizures. These disturbances include depression, anxiety, psychotic disorders, cognitive, and personality changes occurring in the interictal or ictal/postictal states. In this chapter, we describe four areas of focus in women with epilepsy: comorbid primary psychiatric processes, integrated symptoms secondary to epilepsy, stigma and psychosocial consequences of epilepsy, and nonepileptic seizures.

I. Comorbid Disorders in Epilepsy

Patients with epilepsy (PWE) have been found to be at higher risk of suffering from mood, anxiety, psychotic, and attention deficit disorders (ADDs) (Blum *et al.*, 2002; Bredkjaer *et al.*, 1998; Brown *et al.*, 2001; Currie *et al.*, 1971; Edeh and Toone, 1987; Jacoby *et al.*, 1996; Kessler *et al.*, 1994; Kogeorgos *et al.*, 1982; McDermott *et al.*, 1995; Mendez *et al.*, 1986; O'Donoghue *et al.*, 1999; Onuma *et al.*, 1995; Pariente *et al.*, 1991; Perini *et al.*, 1996; Regier *et al.*, 1993; Roy-Byrne *et al.*, 1999; Rutter *et al.*, 1970; Schmitz and Wolf, 1995; Semrud-Clikeman and Wical, 1999) (see Table I). By the same token, there is evidence of a bidirectional relationship between some psychiatric disorders and epilepsy. Patients with a history of major depressive disorders or suicidality (independent of a major depressive disorder) have a 4 to 7 times greater risk of developing epilepsy (Forsgren and Nystrom, 1990; Hesdorffer *et al.*, 2000, 2006). Further support of the bidirectional relationship comes from a recent study of patients with chronic temporal lobe epilepsy (TLE), revealing progression of psychiatric comorbidity even after controlling for premorbid psychiatric history (Jones *et al.*, 2007a). Children with a history of ADD of the inattentive type have a 3.7-fold higher risk of developing epilepsy (Hesdorffer *et al.*, 2004). Jones *et al.* (2007b) found that 45% of adolescents with new-onset epilepsy met criteria for an axis I diagnosis according to the *Diagnostic and Statistical Manual of Mental Disorders* (*DSM-IV-TR*) classification, while McAfee *et al.* recently reported that children with a psychiatric comorbidity were almost 3 times more likely to develop epilepsy than those without (McAfee *et al.*, 2007). Clearly, the relationship between psychiatric disorders and epilepsy is complex, and the symptoms are not only the consequence of the epilepsy.

TABLE I

PREVALENCE RATES OF PSYCHIATRIC DISORDERS IN EPILEPSY AND THE GENERAL POPULATION

Psychiatric disorder	Prevalence rates (%)	
	Patients with epilepsy	General population
Depression	11–80	3.3: Dysthymia
		4.9–17: Major depression
Psychosis	2–9.1	1: Schizophrenia
		0.2: Schizophreniform disorder
Generalized anxiety disorders	15–25	5.1–7.2
Panic disorder	4.9–21	0.5–3
ADHD	12–37	4–12

ADHD, attention deficit hyperactivity disorder

The wide prevalence ranges reflect the different patient populations surveyed and the different assessment techniques.

A. SOME GENERAL PRINCIPLES

The evaluation of any type of psychopathology in PWE must be approached with the following questions in mind.

(1) Is this psychiatric disturbance temporally related to the occurrence of seizures?
(2) Is the onset of psychiatric symptoms associated with the remission of seizures?

We consider the peri-ictal psychiatric symptoms (preictal and postictal) as well as interictal symptoms associated with the onset or remission of seizures as an expression of a paraictal process.

(3) Are the psychiatric symptoms the result of the introduction of an antiepileptic drug (AED) with potential negative psychotropic properties, or did they appear after discontinuation of an AED with positive psychotropic properties (mood stabilizing, antidepressant, and anxiolytic properties)?
(4) Do the symptoms meet diagnostic criteria of the *DSM-IV,* or the International Classification of Diseases (ICD) or do these symptoms present as an atypical disorder?
(5) What is the impact of the psychiatric disorder at hand on the quality of life of patients?
(6) What is the treatment for the psychiatric disorder? If pharmacotherapy is required, how do psychotropic drugs interact with AEDs and what is the impact of psychotropic drugs on the seizure threshold?

The question of focal epilepsy and its relation to a higher prevalence of psychiatric disorders is raised in temporal and frontal epilepsies. Some researchers have hypothesized that patients with TLE with involvement of temporomesial limbic structures show more psychiatric symptoms compared with extra-TLE patients. While some researchers showed higher depression scores in localization-related epilepsies (Quiske *et al.*, 2000), other researchers did not find symptomatic differences between patients with TLE and extra-TLE patients (Swinkels *et al.*, 2006). Given the frontal lobe dysfunction found in juvenile myoclonic epilepsy (JME), psychiatric disorders have been investigated in this population also. In a comparison of 100 patients with JME with 100 healthy controls, psychiatric diagnoses were found in 49 patients with JME. Anxiety and mood disorders, present in 23 and 19 patients, respectively, were the most frequently observed and 20 had personality disorders (de Araujo Filho *et al.*, 2007).

II. Depression in Epilepsy

Depression is the most frequent psychiatric disorder in PWE. It is more common in patients with partial seizure disorders of temporal or frontal lobe origin and among patients with poorly controlled seizures (Edeh and Toone, 1987; Jacoby *et al.*, 1996; Mendez *et al.*, 1986; O'Donoghue *et al.*, 1999). In three community-based studies, prevalence rates of depression ranged between 21% and 33% among patients with persistent seizures and 4–6% among seizure-free patients (Edeh and Toone, 1987; Jacoby *et al.*, 1996; O'Donoghue *et al.*, 1999). Similar results were found in a recent Canadian population-based study of psychiatric disorders in PWE (Tellez-Zenteno *et al.*, 2007). Ettinger *et al.* reported the results of a population-based survey that investigated a lifetime prevalence of depression, epilepsy, diabetes, and asthma in 185,000 households (Ettinger *et al.*, 2004). Among the 2900 PWE, 32% reported having experienced at least one episode of depression. This contrasted with 8.6% prevalence among healthy respondents, 13% among patients with diabetes, and 16% among people with asthma. Using the same population, these investigators found that 13% of PWE had experienced symptoms of manic depressive illness compared to 2% of healthy controls (Ettinger *et al.*, 2005).

A. SUICIDALITY IN PATIENTS WITH EPILEPSY

The suicide rate in depressed PWE is 9–25 times higher in patients with partial seizures of temporal lobe origin than expected in the overall population (Nilsson *et al.*, 1997; Rafnsson *et al.*, 2001; Robertson, 1997). In a review of the literature, Gilliam and Kanner concluded that suicide has one of the highest standardized mortality rates (SMR) of all causes of death in PWE (Gilliam and Kanner, 2002). Robertson reviewed 17 studies pertaining to mortality in epilepsy and found that suicide was 10 times more frequent than in the general population (Robertson, 1997). Rafnsson *et al.* reported the results of a population-based incidence cohort study in PWE from Iceland in which suicide had the highest SMR (5.8) of all causes of death (Rafnsson *et al.*, 2001). A Swedish study of cause specific mortality among 9000 previously hospitalized PWE found an SMR of 3.5 (Nilsson *et al.*, 1997). In a UK population-based study, the highest risk of suicide in PWE occurred within 6 months after a new diagnosis of epilepsy was made (Christensen *et al.*, 2007).

B. DEPRESSION AS A PARAICTAL PHENOMENON

Preictal symptoms of depression and depressive episodes typically present as a dysphoric mood in which the prodromal symptoms may extend for hours or even 1 to 3 days before the onset of a seizure. In children, this dysphoric mood often takes the form of irritability, poor frustration tolerance, and aggressive behavior. Blanchet and Frommer (1986) assessed mood changes for 56 days in 27 PWE who rated their mood on a daily basis. Mood ratings pointed to a dysphoric state 3 days before a seizure in 22 (81%) patients. This change in mood was greatest during the 24 h preceding the seizure. Patients or parents of children with epilepsy often report that dysphoric symptoms completely resolve the day after the ictus.

Postictal symptoms of depression and depressive episodes have been recognized for decades but have been investigated in a systematic manner in only one study (Kanner *et al.*, 2004). The presence of postictal symptoms of depression was identified in 43 of 100 consecutive patients with refractory partial seizure disorders. These symptoms occurred after more than 50% of seizures and their duration ranged from 0.5 to 108 h, with a median duration of 24 h. Other studies have shown that symptoms of depression can outlast the ictus for up to 2 weeks, and, at times, have led patients to suicide (Anatassopoulos and Kokkini, 1969; Hancock and Bevilacqua, 1971).

Ictal symptoms of depression or a depressive episode are the clinical expression of a simple partial seizure in which the depressive symptoms are the sole (or predominant) semiology. Ictal symptoms of depression ranked second after symptoms of anxiety/fear as the most common type of ictal affect in one study (Williams, 1956). This presentation occurred in 21% of 100 PWE who reported auras consisting of psychiatric symptoms (Daly, 1958; Weil, 1955). Yet, the actual prevalence of ictal symptoms of depression is yet to be established in larger studies. The most frequent symptoms include feelings of anhedonia, guilt, and suicidal ideation. Such mood changes are typically brief, stereotypical, occur out of context, and are associated with other ictal phenomena. More typically, however, ictal symptoms of depression are followed by an alteration of consciousness as the ictus evolves from a simple to a complex partial seizure.

C. DEPRESSION AS A COMORBID DISORDER: INTERICTAL DEPRESSIVE DISORDERS

Interictal forms of depression in epilepsy can be identical to depressive disorders described in patients without epilepsy (i.e., major depression, bipolar disorder, cyclothymia, dysthymia, and minor depression). Nevertheless, a review of the literature has clearly shown an atypical clinical presentation of interictal depressive episodes that fail to meet any of the *DSM* categories. Blumer coined the term, Interictal Dysphoric Disorder, to describe this atypical presentation, found in about one third of patients with mood disorders in epilepsy (Blumer and Altshuler, 1998). It is characterized by a chronic "dysthymic-like" state, where symptoms tend to occur intermittently, intermixed with brief euphoric moods, explosive irritability, anxiety, paranoid feelings, and somatoform symptoms (anergia, atypical pain, and insomnia). This type of depression is often unrecognized in epilepsy.

D. DEPRESSION AS AN IATROGENIC PROCESS

AEDs can cause psychiatric symptoms (McConnell and Duncan, 1998). AEDs with GABAergic properties, primarily phenobarbital, primidone, the benzodiazepines, tiagabine, and vigabatrin (Barabas and Matthews, 1988; Brent *et al.*, 1987; Ferrari *et al.*, 1983; Ring and Reynolds, 1990; Smith *et al.*, 1987), are more likely to cause depression. Other AEDs that have been linked to depression include felbamate, topiramate, levetiracetam, and zonisamide (Kanner *et al.*, 2003; McConnell *et al.*, 1994; Mula and Trimble, 2003). The addition of AEDs with mood-stabilizing properties, such as carbamazepine, valproic acid, and lamotrigine, can occasionally cause depressive episodes, albeit with a significantly lower frequency than other AEDs. More often than not, these AEDs are associated with the occurrence of depression *upon their discontinuation* in patients with a prior history of depression or panic disorder, which had been kept in remission by these AEDs (Ketter *et al.*, 1994).

E. DEPRESSION FOLLOWING EPILEPSY SURGERY

There have been an increasing number of reports of depressive disorders following an antero-temporal lobectomy (Savard *et al.*, 1998). It is not unusual to see "mood lability" within the initial 6 weeks to 3 months after surgery. Often these symptoms subside, but in up to 30% of patients, overt symptoms of depression become apparent within the first 6 months. Characteristically, symptoms of depression vary in severity from mild to very severe, including suicide attempts. In most instances, these depressive disorders respond readily to pharmacologic treatment with antidepressant drugs (ADs) (see below). Patients with a prior history of depression are at greater risk. A German study found that patients with personality disorders are at higher risk of suffering from postoperative psychiatric complications as compared with patients with other preoperative psychiatric conditions (such as depression) or with patients with no preoperative psychiatric diagnosis whatsoever (Koch-Stoecker, 2002). While some studies have not found a relation between depression with the postsurgical control of seizures, others have (Balabanov and Kanner, in press; Pintor et al., 2007). All patients undergoing epilepsy surgery, therefore, should be advised of this potential complication, *prior to surgery*.

III. Treatment of Depression in Epilepsy

Before starting a patient on an AD, it is important to determine if the seizures maybe related to starting or stopping an AED.

In all cases inquiry into suicidality is mandatory.

Do ADs worsen seizures? A review of the literature has found an increased incidence of seizures with the use of four specific ADs : maprotiline, amoxepine, clomipramine, and bupropion (McConnell and Duncan, 1998; Swinkels and Jonghe, 1995). Increased seizures have been identified in patients without epilepsy taking tricyclic antidepressants (TCAs), but these seizures have been associated with the following variables: (1) high plasma serum concentrations; (2) rapid dose increments; (3) the presence of other drugs with proconvulsant properties; and (4) the presence of central nervous system (CNS) pathology, abnormal electroencephalographic (EEG) recording, and personal and family history of epilepsy (Curran and de Pauw, 1998; Preskorn and Fast, 1992; Rosenstein et al., 1993; Swinkels and Jonghe, 1995). Based on the evidence suggesting a bidirectional relation between depression and epilepsy that suggests a higher incidence of seizures in patients with depression, it is important to reconsider the question of whether ADs increase the risk of seizures or whether we are identifying the seizure occurrence associated with such increased risk. A recent study appears to support this view.

Alper et al. (2007) compared the incidence of seizures between depressed patients randomized to selective serotonin reuptake inhibitors (SSRIs), serotonin-norepinephrine reuptake inhibitors (SNRIs), or mirtazapine and placebo in the course of multicenter placebo-controlled studies of these drugs submitted to the Food and Drug Administration for approval. Compared to the expected incidence of seizures in the general population, all depressed patients had a higher incidence. Nonetheless, patients randomized to placebo had a significantly higher incidence of seizures than did those treated with the actual ADs.

In general, the SRI class is safe in PWE. In one study, sertraline was found to *definitely* worsen seizures in *only* 1 out of 100 patients with refractory epilepsy

(Kanner *et al.*, 2000). Blumer has also reported using TCAs alone and in combination with SSRIs in PWE without seizure exacerbation (Blumer and Zielinksi, 1988). Monoamine oxidase-A-inhibitors (MAO-I) are not known to cause seizures in patients without epilepsy. Patients treated with TCAs should be started at low doses with small increments until the desired clinical response is reached. This will minimize the risk of causing or exacerbating seizures.

A. PHARMACOKINETIC INTERACTIONS BETWEEN ADs AND AEDs

Most ADs are metabolized in the liver, and their metabolism is accelerated in the presence of AEDs with enzyme-inducing properties, which include phenytoin, carbamazepine, phenobarbital, primidone at regular doses, and oxcarbazepine and topiramate at higher doses. This pharmacokinetic effect is not observed with the new AEDs gabapentin, lamotrigine, tiagabine, levetiracetam, and zonisamide. Conversely, some of the SSRIs are inhibitors of one or more isoenzymes of the cytochrome P450 (CYP 450) system. These include fluoxetine, paroxetine, fluvoxamine, and, to a lesser degree, sertraline (Fritze *et al.*, 1991; Grimsley *et al.*, 1991; Pearson, 1990). Citalopram on the contrary does not have pharmacokinetic interactions with AEDs (McConnell and Duncan, 1998). Sertraline has been shown rarely to increase phenytoin levels, and this is thought to be associated with displacement by tight protein binding, or by inhibition of the CYP 450 system (Haselberger *et al.*, 1997; PDR, 2002).

B. CHOICE OF AD

The SSRI class should be considered as the first-line treatment in depressed PWE. They are safe with respect to seizure propensity, are less likely to result in fatalities after an overdose, and generally have a favorable adverse effects profile. Furthermore, their efficacy in dysthymic disorders and in symptoms of irritability and poor frustration tolerance makes this class of ADs more attractive among PWE that have atypical forms of depression. SSRIs with no or minimal effects on CYP 450 isoenzymes, such as citalopram and sertraline, should be considered in patients taking hepatically metabolized AEDs to avoid pharmacokinetic interactions.

In open, uncontrolled trials, TCAs have also been reported to yield a good clinical response, but the cardiotoxic effects and severe complications seen in overdose make these drugs a second-line AD choice. Blumer has anecdotal reports of the utility of low-dose TCAs in PWE and interictal dysphoric disorder (Blumer and Zielinksi, 1988).

A cautionary note is in order. Before starting an AD, clinicians must rule out a history of a manic or hypomanic episode that maybe suggestive of a bipolar disorder, as ADs can potentially trigger a manic or hypomanic episode in the short term, while it may worsen the course of the bipolar disorder in the long term, particularly in the case of rapid cycling bipolar disease. In such cases, an AED with mood stabilizing and antidepressant properties, such as lamotrigine, must be considered. Carbamazepine and valproate maybe added in case of persistent symptoms. Lithium should be considered if these AEDs cannot yield a euthymic state. If an antidepressant is required, it should not be started in the absence of a mood stabilizing drug in the patient with mania.

C. OTHER TYPES OF PSYCHIATRIC TREATMENTS

Lithium was the first "mood stabilizing drug" used for the treatment of patients with bipolar disorder. Its use in epileptic patients with affective disorders, however, has been fraught with several problems, including changes in EEG recordings and proconvulsant effects at therapeutic serum concentrations in patients without epilepsy (Bell *et al.*, 1993). Lithium's neurotoxicity and related seizure risk increase with the concurrent use of neuroleptic drugs, in the presence of EEG abnormalities and with a history of CNS disorder.

Electroconvulsive therapy (ECT) is not contraindicated in depressed PWE (Fink *et al.*, 1999; Regenold *et al.*, 1998; Sackeim *et al.*, 1983). It is a well-tolerated treatment and is worth considering in PWE with very severe depression that fails to respond to ADs. Furthermore, there is no evidence that ECT increases the risk of epilepsy (Blackwood *et al.*, 1980).

In addition to pharmacological intervention, the value of psychotherapy for the treatment of depression in PWE should not be overlooked. Surveys reveal that fear of the next seizure is rated as the greatest concern in PWE (Fisher *et al.*, 2000). Counseling and psychotherapy can be very useful in helping the patient deal with the stressors and limitations of living with epilepsy. Studies reveal that psychotherapy may also reduce epileptic seizures (Reiter and Andrews, 2000).

IV. Anxiety Disorders in Epilepsy

Anxiety is the second most common psychiatric comorbidity in PWE, with an estimated prevalence between 15% and 25% (Edeh and Toone, 1987; Jacoby *et al.*, 1996; Jones *et al.*, 2003; O'Donoghue *et al.*, 1999; Vazquez and Devinsky, 2003). In 174 consecutive PWE from five epilepsy centers, a current *DSM-IV* diagnosis of anxiety disorder was found in 30% of patients (Jones *et al.*, 2003).

The various forms of anxiety disorders (generalized anxiety disorder, panic disorder, phobias, obsessive compulsive disorder, and post-traumatic stress disorder) can present *interictally* with the same clinical manifestations as anxiety disorders in the general population. The peri-ictal presentations of anxiety symptoms often differ from their interictal manifestations, however.

A. ANXIETY EPISODES AS PARAICTAL PROCESSES

Ictal fear or panic is the most frequent ictal psychiatric symptom. It is the sole or predominant clinical expression of a simple partial seizure (aura) or the initial symptom of a complex partial seizure and usually has a mesial temporal lobe origin. Seizures of mesial frontal origin involving the cyngulate gyrus can also be associated with a panic feeling as an expression of the aura. Relying on electrographic interictal and ictal data to document a diagnosis may often yield false negative results. Indeed, simple partial seizures originating from mesial frontal regions are often undetected in scalp EEG recordings as the location of the epileptogenic zone (in cyngulate gyrus) relative to the angle subtended by scalp electrodes positioned at the midline and over suprasylvian regions may not permit the detection of the epileptiform discharges or ictal patterns. Likewise, scalp recordings are unlikely to detect any epileptiform activity from simple partial seizures of mesial temporal lobe origin, particularly those in which the epileptogenic area is in the amygdala, as this structure generates epileptiform discharges with a very narrow electric field. By the same token, interictal recordings may fail to recode any interictal discharges, even with the use of basal and antero-temporal electrodes. In these instances, the use of sphenoidal electrodes placed under fluoroscopic guidance will be necessary. It should be emphasized that the placement of sphenoidal electrodes without fluoroscopic guidance does not yield any advantage over antero-temporal and basal temporal electrodes (Kanner and Jones, 1997).

A careful history can help distinguish interictal panic from ictal panic. Ictal panic is typically less than 30 s in duration, is stereotypical, occurs out of context to concurrent events, and is associated with other ictal phenomena such as periods of confusion of variable duration and subtle or overt automatisms. The intensity of the sensation of fear is mild to moderate and rarely reaches the intensity of a panic attack. On the contrary, interictal panic attacks consist of episodes of 5–20 minutes duration, which at times may persist for several hours. The feeling of fear or panic is very intense ("feeling of impending doom") and is associated with a variety of autonomic symptoms, including tachycardia, diffuse diaphoresis, and dyspnea. Patients may become so completely absorbed by the panic that they may not be able to report what is going on around them; however, there is no confusion or loss of consciousness, as seen in complex partial seizures. It is not infrequent for patients to develop agoraphobia due to the fear of experiencing a panic attack. As stated above, EEG recordings with sphenoidal electrodes placed under fluoroscopic guidance may be necessary to demonstrate the mesial temporal lobe epileptiform activity that generates ictal panic (Kanner and Jones, 1997; Kanner *et al.*, 1995).

Patients with ictal panic may also suffer from interictal panic attacks, which have been identified in up to 25% of PWE (Vazquez and Devinsky, 2003).

Postictal symptoms of anxiety can be relatively frequent among patients with refractory partial epilepsy. In a recently published study of 100 consecutive patients with pharmacoresistant partial epilepsy, we identified a mean of 2 ± 1 postictal symptoms of anxiety (range: 1–5; median = 2) in 45 patients (Kanner *et al.*, 2004). These symptoms occurred after more than 50% of their seizures and had a median duration of 24 h (range: 0.5–148 h). Thirty-two patients reported symptoms of generalized anxiety and/or panic; an additional 10 patients also reported symptoms of compulsions and 29 patients experienced postictal symptoms of agoraphobia. In 44 of these 45 patients, postictal symptoms of depression were also reported, which included anhedonia, feelings of helplessness, crying bouts, suicidal ideation, and feelings of guilt.

B. Treatment of Anxiety Disorders in Epilepsy

Antidepressants belonging to the SSRI class can prevent the occurrence of interictal panic attacks as well as treat generalized anxiety disorders. On the contrary, there is as of yet no evidence that these drugs have any impact on postictal psychiatric symptoms. ADs of the SNRI family have also been used with success, but no controlled studies exist in PWE. Benzodiazepines have been used for years in the management of anxiety disorders. We do not recommend their chronic use because of the development of tolerance and sedating adverse events. However, short trials with clonazepam can be quite effective.

V. Psychosis of Epilepsy

Psychotic disorders are more frequent in PWE than in the general population, with some studies suggesting prevalence rates of up to 10%. Psychotic disorders can present as a schizophreniform disorder, indistinguishable from those of patients without epilepsy. However, the term psychosis of epilepsy (POE) implies the presence of certain characteristics that distinguish these disorders from those of patients without epilepsy.

A. Postictal Psychotic Symptoms and Psychotic Episodes

Postictal psychotic phenomena can present in the form of isolated symptoms or as psychotic episodes defined as a cluster of symptoms of at least 24-h duration. The prevalence of postictal psychotic disorders in PWE is yet to be established, but has been estimated to range between 6% and 10% (Dongier, 1959; Kanner *et al.*, 1996). Recurrent postictal psychotic symptoms have been found in 7% of 100 consecutive patients with refractory partial epilepsy (Kanner *et al.*, 2004). Common findings include the following: (1) A delay between the onset of psychiatric symptoms and the time of the last seizure. (2) A relatively short duration (from hours up to a few weeks long). (3) An affect-laden symptomatology. (4) The clustering of symptoms into delusional and affective-like psychosis. (5) An increase in the frequency of secondarily generalized tonic-clonic seizures preceding the onset of postictal psychosis (PIP). (6) The onset of PIP after having seizures for a mean period of more than 10 years. (7) A prompt response to low-dose neuroleptic medication or benzodiazepines (Devinsky *et al.*, 1995; Kanner *et al.*, 1996; Lancman *et al.*, 1994; Logsdail and Toone, 1988; Umbricht *et al.*, 1995). In a study with eight years of follow-up on patients with PIP, three developed chronic psychosis and four of 14 patients died (Logsdail and Toone, 1988).

In most cases, insomnia is the initial presenting symptom. In patients with recurrent postictal psychotic episodes, families need to learn to recognize these symptoms so that a timely administration of 1–2 mg of risperidone may avert the episode. It should be given for 2 to 5 days and then discontinued.

The occurrence of postictal psychotic episodes also has important localizing implications. PIP suggests the presence of bilateral independent *ictal foci* (Devinsky *et al.*, 1995; Logsdail and Toone, 1988; Umbricht *et al.*, 1995). In a recent study, Kanner and Ostrovskaya have demonstrated that the presence of postictal psychotic episodes suggest the presence of bilateral ictal foci in close to 90% of patients with refractory partial epilepsy (Kanner and Ostrovskaya, 2008). Accordingly, patients undergoing surgical evaluation may require longer video EEG (vEEG) monitoring studies and possibly the use of intracranial electrodes. If recordings with depth or subdural electrodes are used, prophylactic treatment with low-dose risperidone or haloperidol can avert the occurrence of such episodes during the invasive vEEG monitoring studies (Kanner *et al.*, 1996).

Ictal psychotic symptoms or episodes should always be considered in the differential diagnosis of PIP and POE, as a whole. It is typically due to nonconvulsive status epilepticus. The presence of unresponsiveness and automatisms should increase the suspicion. Yet, confirmation with EEG recordings is of the essence as certain psychotic processes, such as catatonic states, can be associated with unresponsiveness and mannerisms that mimic automatisms.

B. ALTERNATIVE PSYCHOSIS OR "FORCED NORMALIZATION"

The concept of alternative psychosis, developed from observations by Land-oldt in 1953 (Blanchet and Frommer, 1986; Landoldt, 1953), implies an inverse relation between seizure control and psychotic symptom occurrence. He de-scribed a "normalization" of EEG recordings with the appearance of psychiatric symptoms and coined the term "forced normalization." Forced normalization has been reported in patients with TLE and generalized epilepsies. Dongier reported the disappearance of a focal discharge during a psychotic episode in 15% of 318 patients with peri-ictal psychoses (Dongier, 1959). Prevalence rates of alternative psychosis are reported to be 11–25% (Trimble and Schmitz, 2002). As with other forms of POE, the psychotic manifestations were identified after a 15.2-year history of epilepsy in 23 patients reported by Wolf (Wolf and Trimble, 1985). The dopamine (DA) system has been implicated in forced normalization. DA antagonists provoke seizures, and DA agonists have anticonvulsant properties but may precipitate psychosis. Both Landoldt and Wolf reported a pleomorphic clinical presentation with a paranoid psychosis without clouding of consciousness being the most frequent manifestation. A premonitory phase involving insomnia, anxiety, a feeling of oppression, and social withdrawal may occur in a prodromal phase. Forced normalization may then manifest as psychosis, conversion symp-toms, hypochondriasis, depression, or mania.

Interictal psychotic disorders can present with delusions, hallucinations, ref-erential thinking, and thought disorders, as in patients without epilepsy. Slater coined the term interictal POE to describe certain clinical characteristics, particu-larly, psychotic episodes seen interictally in patients with chronic epilepsy (Slater et al., 1963). The description of these cases is remarkable for *the absence* of negative symptoms, better premorbid history, and less common deterioration of the patients' personality. The psychosis is less severe and more responsive to therapy.

C. IATROGENIC PSYCHOTIC DISORDERS

1. AED-Related Psychosis

Psychotic disorder as an expression of a drug toxicity has been reported with several AEDs, most prominently ethosuximide, phenobarbital, and primidone as well as the newer AEDs topiramate and levetiracetam (McConnell and Duncan, 1998). Psychotic disorders can occasionally follow the discontinuation of AEDs, particularly those with mood-stabilizing properties. Ketter et al. reported the development of some cases who experienced psychosis among 32 inpatients who were withdrawn from carbamazepine, phenytoin, and valproic acid (Ketter *et al.*, 1994). Acute withdrawal from benzodiazepines is well known to result in an acute psychotic episode (Sironi *et al.*, 1979).

2. *Psychosis Following Temporal Lobectomy*

Temporal lobectomy has been associated with postoperative psychosis. In a series of 100 of Falconer's patients, Taylor reported seven with *de novo* postoperative psychosis (Taylor, 1972). Jensen and Vaernet reported *de novo* psychotic disorders in nine of 74 patients (Jensen and Vaernet, 1977). Trimble calculated postoperative *de novo* psychoses to range between 3.8% and 35.7% (mean, 7.6%) of patients and suggested that in at least some cases a causal relation by way of forced normalization was possible (Trimble, 1992).

Many epilepsy centers currently do not consider patients with a preoperative history of psychosis candidates for epilepsy surgery. Thus, more recent reports of postsurgical psychosis in patients are primarily *de novo* psychoses, which would be expected to be of lower incidence than postoperative exacerbations of preexisting psychosis.

Yet, a history of psychosis should not be considered an absolute contraindication to epilepsy surgery, provided that the patient can cooperate during the presurgical evaluation, has a clear understanding of the nature of the surgical procedure, and can provide a fully informed consent.

D. DRUG TREATMENT OF PSYCHOSIS IN PATIENTS WITH EPILEPSY

Antipsychotic drugs (APDs) are necessary in the management of psychotic disorders in patients with epilepsy despite their proconvulsant properties. While it is essential that the risk of seizure occurrence be always carefully considered when starting APDs in these patients, it should never be a reason not to treat a patient in need of antipsychotic medication. APDs can be separated into two classes: the "conventional" APDs (CAPDs) and "atypical" APDs (AAPDs). The former include 18 drugs developed between the 1950s and the 1970s. Their mechanism of action resides in their ability to block DA-2 receptors, both at the level of meso-cortical, nigrostriatal and tubero-infundibular DA pathways (Stahl, 2000). Blockade of the DA receptors at the former pathways is responsible for their antipsychotic effect, but results as well in "emotional blunting" and cognitive symptoms that often lead to confusion with the "negative" symptoms of schizophrenia. Blockade at the nigrostriatal pathways results in acute and chronic movement disorders, presenting as Parkinsonian symptoms, as well as dystonic and dyskinetic movements, while blockade at the tubero-infundibular pathways results in increased secretion of prolactin. In addition to their DA blockade properties, most of these CAPDs have muscarinic cholinergic, alpha-1-, and histaminic-blocking properties, responsible for anticholinergic adverse effects, weight gain, sedation, dizziness, and orthostatic hypotension.

AAPDs are dopamine-serotonin antagonists that target DA-2 and 5HT-2A receptors (Stahl, 2000). Their main difference with CAPDs is the absence or mild occurrence of extrapyramidal adverse events and of hyperprolactinemia. In addition, this class of drugs has a lesser blunting of affect and several of these AAPDs have mood-stabilizing properties. Hence, AAPDs have in large part replaced conventional APDs. Today, seven AAPDs have been introduced in the USA: clozapine (Clozaril), risperidone (Risperidal), olanzapine (Zyprexa), ziprasidone (Geodon), quetiapine (Seroquel), aripiprazole (Abilify), and paliperidone (Invega).

The seizure rate associated with the use of APDs has ranged between 0.5% and 1.2% among nonepileptic patients (Whitworth and Fleischhacker, 1995). The risk is higher with certain drugs, and in the presence of the following factors: (1) a history of epilepsy; (2) abnormal EEG recordings; (3) history of CNS disorder; (4) rapid titration of the APD dose; (5) high doses of APD; and (6) the presence of other drugs that lower the seizure threshold (McConnell and Duncan, 1998). For example, when chlorpromazine is used at doses above 1000 mg/day, the incidence of seizures was reported to increase to 9%, in contrast to a 0.5% incidence when lower doses are taken (Logothetis, 1967). Clozapine has been reported to cause seizures in 4.4% when used at doses above 600 mg/day, while at a doses lower than 300 mg, the incidence of seizures is less than 1% (Toth and Frankenburg, 1994). While these two drugs have been associated with the higher frequencies of seizures, most APDs have been associated with seizure occurrence in the presence of the risk factors cited above.

With the exception of clozapine, AAPD-related seizure incidence has not been higher than expected in the general population (Toth and Frankenburg, 1994). This finding was confirmed by Alper et al. in a study comparing the incidence of seizures of psychotic patients without epilepsy randomized to either placebo or one of the AAPDs (risperidone, olanzapine, quetiapine, and aripiprazole) in regulatory studies submitted to the FDA. Thus, during premarketing studies of patients without epilepsy taking AAPDs, seizures were reported in 0.3% of patients given risperidone, 0.9% given olanzapine, 0.8% given quietapine (vs 0.5% on placebo), and 0.4% of patients treated with ziprasidone [data in PDR] (PDR, 2002).

The risk of seizure occurrence or worsening of seizures with AAPDs in PWE has not been well studied. Pacia and Devinsky reviewed the incidence of seizures among 5629 patients treated with clozapine (Pacia and Devinsky, 1994). Sixteen of these patients had epilepsy before the start of this APD and all patients experienced worsening of seizures while on the drug: eight patients at doses lower than 300 mg/day, three patients at doses between 300 and 600 mg/day, and five at doses higher than 600 mg/day. Higher doses of clozapine were associated with greater risk of seizures than lower dose therapy (Pacia and

Devinsky, 1994). It goes without saying that clozapine should be avoided or used in exceptional circumstances with extreme caution in PWE.

Most APDs can cause EEG changes consisting of slowing of the background activity particularly when used at high doses. In addition some of these drugs, particularly clozapine, can cause paroxysmal electrographic changes in the form of interictal sharp waves and spikes. This type of epileptiform activity, however, is not predictive of seizure occurrence. Data from studies by Tiihonen *et al.* suggest that a severe disorganization of the EEG recordings is a better predictor of seizure occurrence (Tiihonen *et al.*, 1991).

Clozapine followed by chlorpromazine and loxapine are the three APDs with the highest risk of seizure occurrence. Those with a lower seizure risk include haloperidol, molindone, fluphenazine, perphenazine, trifluoperazine, and the atypical, risperidone. The PDR data available on the atypicals report seizures during clinical trials occurring with olanzapine (0.9%), quetiapine (0.8%), risperidone (0.3%), and ziprasidone (0.4%) (PDR, 2002) Whether the presence of AEDs at adequate levels protects PWE from breakthrough seizures upon the introduction of APDs with proconvulsant properties is yet to be established. AEDs are sometimes started when clozapine is used at greater than 600 mg/day.

In addition to the proconvulsant properties of APDs, clinicians must also consider the pharmacokinetic and pharmacodynamic interactions between APDs and AEDs. Induction of hepatic enzymes upon the introduction of enzyme-inducing AEDs may result in an increase in the clearance of most APDs. By the same token, discontinuation of an AED with enzyme-inducing properties may result in a decrease in the clearance of APD, which in turn can lead to extrapyramidal side effects caused by an increase of their serum concentrations. Finally, certain AEDs, like valproic acid, can inhibit the glucuronidation metabolism of APDs like clozapine.

VI. Attention Deficit Disorders and Behavior Disturbances

While the adult epilepsy literature has characterized the full spectrum of *DSM-* and ICD-defined psychiatric disorders (Swinkels *et al.*, 2005), similar efforts in the pediatric epilepsy literature have essentially just begun (Caplan *et al.*, 2005; Jones *et al.*, 2007b; McLellan *et al.*, 2005; Ott *et al.*, 2001), again with a focus on children with chronic epilepsy. Of the potential psychiatric comorbidities of childhood epilepsy, attention deficit hyperactivity disorder (ADHD) has been of long-standing interest. Ounsted (1955) was among the first to call attention to the syndrome of hyperkinetic disorder and its complications in children with epilepsy. A growing literature has characterized disorders of attention in youth with epilepsy using a diversity of methods including proxy (parent, teacher) rating scales, behavioral checklists, or formal cognitive tests (Dunn and Kronenberger, 2005). However, only three investigations determined the rate of ADHD and its subtypes in pediatric epilepsy using contemporary diagnostic criteria that now recognize specific subtypes of the disorder (*DSM-IV*) (TaskForceonDSM-IV, 1994). One of these studies was population based (Hesdorffer *et al.*, 2004), while the others were derived from tertiary care clinical settings (Dunn *et al.*, 2003; Sherman *et al.*, 2007). All studies reported a significantly elevated rate of ADHD in childhood epilepsy with an overrepresentation of the inattentive subtype; a distribution that appears different compared to clinically derived samples of ADHD children seen in tertiary care centers where the combined subtype predominates. None of the studies of ADHD in epilepsy examined the neurobehavioral or neuroradiological complications compared to children with epilepsy without ADHD or healthy controls.

In a population-based study carried out in the Isle of White in Great Britain, Rutter and collaborators found behavioral disorders in 28.6% of children with uncomplicated seizures, and 58.3% of children with both seizures and additional CNS pathology (Rutter *et al.*, 1970). In a separate population-based study of children with seizures, cardiac disorders, and controls, McDermott and collaborators found that children with epilepsy had more behavioral problems than either the children with cardiac disease or the controls. The children with epilepsy presented with higher rates of hyperactive behavior (28.1% vs 12.6% in cardiac children and 4.9% in controls), headstrong or oppositional behavior (28.1% vs 18.3% of cardiac children and 8.6% of controls), and antisocial behavior (18.2% vs 11.6% of cardiac children and 8.8% of controls) (McDermott *et al.*, 1995).

A. PREICTAL SYMPTOMS AND EPISODES

Preictal irritability, impulsive behavior, and poor frustration tolerance have been frequently reported by parents of children with epilepsy without ADHD. Their actual prevalence rates are yet to be established, however. Blanchet and Frommer identified preictal irritability as a prominent symptom, associated with symptoms of depression (Blanchet and Frommer, 1986). These changes were more accentuated during the 24 h preceding the seizure.

B. POSTICTAL SYMPTOMS OF ADD AND BEHAVIORAL DISTURBANCES

In the study on clinical characteristics and prevalence of postictal psychiatric symptoms cited above (Kanner *et al.*, 2004), we found postictal irritability in 30 patients and poor frustration tolerance in 36, with a median duration of 24 h for each symptom (range: 0.5 –108 h).

C. ADD AND BEHAVIOR DISTURBANCES AS AN EXPRESSION OF PARAICTAL PROCESSES

Behavior disturbances and ADD are frequent expressions of paraictal processes, remitting or improving significantly upon reaching seizure control. Examples include "epileptic encephalopathies" such as the acquired epileptic aphasia of childhood (also known as Landau-Kleffner Syndrome) (Morrell *et al.*, 1995).

Aggressive behavior and ADD can be seen in children with gelastic seizures associated with hypothalamic hamartomas. These psychiatric symptoms remit with cessation of epilepsy (Fohlen *et al.*, 2003).

D. ADD AND BEHAVIORAL DISTURBANCES AS AN INTERICTAL COMORBID DISORDER

The prevalence of ADHD in PWE is reported to range between 10% and 40% (McDermott *et al.*, 1995; Rutter *et al.*, 1970; Semrud-Clikeman and Wical, 1999). These data reflect statistics from pediatric populations with epilepsy. In fact there are no data on the incidence or prevalence of ADD in adults with epilepsy. Theoretically, if ADD were to follow the same natural course in PWE than primary ADD, 50–75% of children with epilepsy and ADD would be expected to display symptoms of ADD when entering adulthood. This question will need to be answered in future studies. Furthermore, the clinical manifestations of ADD in adults with epilepsy are yet to be described in a systematic manner.

E. IATROGENIC BEHAVIORAL CHANGES

Many of the AEDs can cause symptoms of behavioral disturbances. The most frequent offenders include GABAergic drugs such as the barbiturates, benzodiazepines, and vigabatrin. Among the newer AEDs, topiramate and levetiracetam have been implicated. Valproic acid can cause behavioral disturbances at higher doses and encephalopathy even with therapeutic doses.

F. TREATMENT OF ADHD IN PWE

The pharmacologic treatment of ADHD in PWE is the same as that of patients without seizures. In general, there is no pharmacokinetic interaction between CNS stimulants and AEDs, though there have been two reports that methylphenidate can increase blood levels of phenytoin and phenobarbital (McConnell and Duncan, 1998).

VII. Psychosocial Consequences for Women with Epilepsy

A. Impact of Depression on Quality of Life in Epilepsy Patients

Psychiatric symptoms in general are found to have a greater impact on quality of life in patients with TLE than in healthy controls (Hermann *et al.*, 2000). Depression, specifically, has a significant negative impact on the quality of life of PWE. Lehrner *et al.* (1999) found that depression was the single strongest predictor for each domain of health-related quality of life which persisted after controlling for seizure frequency, seizure severity, and other psychosocial variables. Perrine *et al.* (1995) found that mood had the highest correlations with scales of the Quality of Life in Epilepsy Inventory-89 (QOLIE-89) and was the strongest predictor of poor quality of life in regression analyses. In a study of patients with pharmacoresistant TLE, Gilliam *et al.* found that high ratings of depression and neurotoxicity from AEDs were the only independent variables significantly associated with poor quality of life scores on the QOLIE-89 summary score. The authors *did not* find any correlation between the type and/or the frequency of seizures. Gilliam *et al.* also found that mood status was the strongest predictor of the patients' assessment of their own health status in a group of 125 patients more than 1 year after temporal lobe surgery (Gilliam, 2002; Gilliam *et al.*, 1997).

B. Stigma

The statement that treating the seizure is not the sum of treating the patient with epilepsy is most apparent in the psychosocial consequences and familial impact of epilepsy. While the practice of "sterilization of the epileptic" seems archaic, laws were in place in four US states in the early 20th century that ratified this policy (Friedlander, 2001). Sadly, in the 21st century, research in developing countries reveals that the stigma of epilepsy still affects women. Santosh *et al.* point out that "The psychosocial consequences of the stigma potentials of epilepsy are nowhere more evident than in the case of women with epilepsy of the marriageable age in a developing country." They examined the prevalence of concealment/disclosure of the history of epilepsy and its consequences on the married life of women with epilepsy in southern India (Santosh *et al.*, 2007). The authors found that 55% of 82 women with epilepsy concealed their history of epilepsy before marriage, and 38% of those who concealed were separated or divorced. Concealment was described as a coping strategy for anticipated negative consequences of disclosure of the stigmatized disease. Unfortunately, this attitude is not solely a reflection of a developing country's practice. Researchers in Japan who studied marital statistics in a population of 278 PWE found that in one quarter of PWE who divorced, the reason for divorce was epilepsy (Wada *et al.*, 2004). Kleinman *et al.* found that family, marriage, financial, and moral consequences of the social experience of epilepsy as a chronic disease demonstrated the importance of the social impact of epilepsy (Kleinman *et al.*, 1995).

Along with the stigma of epilepsy itself, the comorbidities of epilepsy, including depression, anxiety, and nonepileptic seizures (NES), bear a psychosocial burden unto themselves. Because of stigmatizing attitudes, patients may avoid or delay medical care and treatment for their mental health problems (Andrews *et al.*, 2001). In a survey of 1400 respondents with depression and anxiety, one quarter of individuals did not present their symptoms to a physician, with reasons including fear of stigma (Meltzer *et al.*, 2003). The importance of early detection of mental illness in patients with chronic somatic disorders is paramount to initiate psychiatric treatment in order to prevent chronification (Gatchel *et al.*, 1995). Freidl *et al.* investigated the impact of perceptions of stigma in PWE, with NES, and with somatoform pain disorders in 101 in- and outpatients (Freidl *et al.*, 2007). The authors found a high stigmatization concerning psychiatry even in PWE and somatoform/dissociative symptoms with psychiatric comorbidity, concluding that perceived stigma is a barrier to recovery. In the next section, we discuss another comorbidity in epilepsy, NES.

VIII. Nonepileptic Seizures

A. Introduction

Nonepileptic events are either physiologic or psychological in origin. Psychological NES resemble epileptic seizures (ES) presenting as a sudden, involuntary, time-limited alteration in behavior, motor activity, autonomic function, consciousness, or sensation. However, unlike epilepsy, NES do not result from epileptogenic pathology and are not accompanied by an epileptiform electrographic ictal pattern. Patients with NES are often disabled and difficult to treat.

B. Epidemiology and Costs

Of the 1% of the US population with epilepsy, 5–20% have NES (Gates *et al.*, 1991). They are usually women (∼80%) and are aged between 15 and 35 (∼80%) (Shen *et al.*, 1990), though young children and the elderly can also develop NES. The patients, their family, and society bear an enormous cost if psychiatric care is not provided or if inappropriate neurological therapy is instituted (LaFrance and Benbadis, 2006). Patients with NES take double the number of medications than do PWE (Hantke *et al.*, 2007), and while NES are not directly treated by AEDs, most patients with NES receive unnecessary AEDs (de Timary *et al.*, 2002). Extensive observational data suggest that AEDs are ineffective or may worsen NES (Krumholz *et al.*, 1980). In some cases, potentially dangerous invasive diagnostic studies, toxic parenteral medications, or emergent intubation are administered. Diagnostic and therapeutic challenges are complicated by the 10–30% rate of comorbid NES and ES. Misdiagnosis and mistreatment of NES as ES costs an estimated $110–920 million annually on diagnostic evaluations, inappropriate administration of AEDs, and emergency department utilization (Martin *et al.*, 1998).

C. Pathology

While we do not have a specific "lesion" that explains NES, we do have an understanding of the comorbid psychopathology in patients with NES. The phenomenology of NES, also referred to as pseudoseizures, is well defined, with systematic assessments of diagnostic comorbidities and psychological testing (Gates and Rowan, 2000; Gram *et al.*, 1993). Studies have informed us of risk factors for NES (e. g., sexual or physical abuse, head injury) (Alper *et al.*, 1993; Westbrook *et al.*, 1998), and good prognostic features for NES resolution (e.g., female, independent lifestyle, short duration of NES) (Barry, 2001; Bowman, 1999; Chabolla *et al.*, 1996; Ettinger *et al.*, 1999). Negative prognostic factors include longer duration of NES, comorbid neurologic, and/or psychiatric disease and pending litigation, among others. Interestingly, CNS pathology and abnormal EEG recordings did not predict outcome in two studies (Kanner *et al.*, 1999; Lelliott and Fenwick, 1991).

No single psychopathogenic process causes NES. NES are clinically classified under different *DSM-IV* diagnoses, including conversion, somatization, and dissociation disorders, and a much smaller percentage as factitious disorder and malingering. A psychosocial stressor (e.g., sexual or physical abuse, loss of a relationship, work stress, parental divorce) (Wyllie *et al.*, 1999) is often identified but may take time to uncover. Many patients with NES also suffer from mood (12–100%), anxiety (11–80%), personality (33–66%), nonseizure conversion/somatoform (20–100%), and nonseizure dissociative disorders (up to 90%) co-occurring with their primary NES diagnosis of conversion, somatoform, or dissociative disorder (Bowman, 1999).

1. *Gender Differences in NES*

Oto *et al.* evaluated the differences between women and men with NES and found many similarities between the genders, but a few significant differences were noted (Oto *et al.*, 2005a). Event semiology was similar, but women were more likely to weep after events ($p = 0.017$). Males were more likely to be unemployed ($p = 0.028$) than were women with NES. Females were 6 times more likely to self-harm than were men ($P = 0.050$), though the numbers were small in these categories. O'Sullivan *et al.* found that men with NES had higher seizure frequencies than did women with NES (O'Sullivan *et al.*, 2007). The study also found that males were found to have taken larger numbers of AEDs per patient before the diagnosis of NES than were women.

Perception of causation of NES was different, as men were more likely to attribute their NES to a predisposing factor for epilepsy ($P = 0.001$) (Oto *et al.*, 2005a). Women were over eight times more likely to report sexual abuse ($P = 0.001$); however, this may have been underestimated, as seen in the clinic, men sometimes do not disclose abuse in the initial evaluation. The caretakers and family of men with NES were three times less likely to accept the diagnosis of NES ($P = 0.017$). The scores on the majority of Oto's variables were similar across gender; however, the above noted differences could have implications on treatment outcomes.

D. DIAGNOSIS OF NES

Obtaining an accurate diagnosis of NES is the essential first step for instituting proper therapy and avoiding unnecessary and potentially dangerous therapies. Clinical features of epileptic and NES overlap, however, and there is no one clinical feature that reliably distinguishes ES from NES. Subjective visceral, sensory, or psychic phenomena, alterations in responsiveness, and convulsive motor activity can be present in both disorders. Ictal presentations range from uncoordinated disorganized motor activity to unresponsiveness without motor signs in NES. Clinical differentiation between NES and epilepsy has also been based on other identifiers such as the presence of preictal pseudosleep (where the patient reports being asleep but EEG shows them to be awake), geotropic eye movements (forced downward deviation of the eyes toward the floor with head turning), eye closure and postictal whispering with NES, and the presence of postictal headache and postictal nose rubbing with epilepsy (LaFrance, 2008). The use of suggestion to both provoke and to stop NES is documented. With the issue of disclosure and informed consent, activation procedures have drawn fire recently as a potentially unethical intervention (Smith *et al.*, 1997). However, when properly employed, seizure induction can act as a "stepping stone" to treatment if the patient develops insight into the events (Devinsky and Fisher, 1996). The distinction between physiologic nonepileptic events and psychological NES is based on the combination of thorough history, physical exam in the peri-ictal period, and neurophysiologic monitoring.

Video-electroencephalographic monitoring (vEEG) led to an explosion of NES knowledge beginning in the 1980s (Boon and Williamson, 1993; Desai *et al.*, 1979; Jedrzejczak *et al.*, 1999; Penin, 1968). An article reviewing the diagnostic tests, including EEG, neuroimaging, prolactin levels, and personality testing, provides the sensitivities and specificities for each of these tests (Cragar *et al.*, 2002). It was once thought that absence of physical injury sustained during a seizure was a diagnostic indicator differentiating NES from ES; however, more than half of all patients with NES actually do have physical injury associated with their NES (Kanner, 2003). Other injuries occur as a result of iatrogenic issues which are also prevalent in NES, and death has resulted in medically aggressive treatment of NES (Reuber *et al.*, 2004). Up to half of NES patients have had "pseudo-status epilepticus" and 27.8% of patients with NES are admitted to intensive care units inappropriately for treatment (Reuber *et al.*, 2003).

NES are not associated with epileptiform discharges on vEEG recordings, the gold standard for NES diagnosis (Ghougassian *et al.*, 2004). Humility in diagnosing NES without vEEG—and sometimes with vEEG—is critical. In one study, prediction of the nature of unusual seizures by the admitting neurologist was accurate in only 67% of cases. When observing these events without accompanying EEG, determination from observations of unit personnel and neurologists was correct in less than 80% of episodes (King *et al.*, 1982). Lancman *et al.* strongly assert "no matter how suggestive the clinical manifestation of a paroxysmal event maybe of pseudoseizures, such diagnosis should never be made without electrographic confirmation" (Lancman *et al.*, 2001). The co-occurrence of ES and NES in a patient further complicates diagnosis and therapy. The diagnosis comes through careful history and thorough review of medical records that can identify different episode types and assess the supportive data.

EEG abnormalities in patients with NES do not necessarily confirm the diagnosis of ES. For example, EEGs showing "sharpish waves" or paroxysmal slowing provide little support of ES. A positive neurologic history was present in a quarter of patients with NES and a positive family history of epilepsy was present in 37.6% of NES patients (Lancman *et al.*, 1993). While neurologic signs, symptoms and history are important to note in seizure patients, they are in no way pathognomic in distinguishing NES from ES. A recent paper described three criteria in NES patients admitted for vEEG, yielding a positive predictive value of 85% (Davis, 2004). The criteria were (1) at least 2 NES per week, (2) refractory to at least 2 AEDs, and (3) at least 2 EEGs without epileptiform activity. Using "the rule of 2's" documenting seizure frequency, EEG abnormalities, and drug treatment response before vEEG may help establish the diagnosis of NES.

IX. Treatment of NES

A. TREATMENT LITERATURE

Despite diagnostic advances, there is no standardized, effective treatment for NES. Even as our knowledge of NES phenomenology continues to grow, there are no published randomized placebo-controlled trials (RCTs) for treatment of

NES. The literature provides divergent views on natural history and outcome, as well as the value of psychotherapy, psychotropic medication, and other interventions for NES (Aboukasm *et al.*, 1998; Barry, 2001; Ramani, 2000; Walczak *et al.*, 1995). More than a century after this disorder was clearly identified, we still need controlled studies on treatment of this costly and disabling disorder.

The NES treatment literature has been systematically reviewed and published in the literature (LaFrance and Devinsky, 2004; LaFrance and Barry, 2005). Four references to a prospective series in the NES treatment literature are published. Ataoglu *et al.* (2003) randomized 30 patients with NES, half to paradoxical intention (PI) inpatient psychotherapy, and the other half to oral benzodiazepine therapy. PI consists of the therapist suggesting that the patient engage in the undesired activity intentionally. The authors found greater improvements in anxiety scores and mildly better seizure control in the PI group than in the diazepam group. An uncontrolled individualized psychological therapeutic program for 16 patients with NES for an average of 12 weeks resulted in complete cessation of NES in half of the patients (McDade and Brown, 1992). More recently, two prospective, open trials of cognitive behavioral therapy and group psychotherapy showed reduction in NES frequency and post-traumatic symptoms, respectively (Goldstein *et al.*, 2004; Zaroff *et al.*, 2004).

In a follow-up cohort study, 11 of 14 (79%) inpatients with NES experienced cessation or significant improvement after receiving a combination of hypnosis, group therapy, family therapy, and individual therapy (Kim *et al.*, 1998). A follow-up study at a comprehensive epilepsy center (CEP) (Aboukasm *et al.*, 1998) suggested that CEP psychotherapists and CEP neurologists have a similar favorable treatment outcome, underscoring the beneficial impact of continuity of care and explanation of the nature of the seizures. The study also showed that the absence of communication with a NES patient about the diagnosis yields no improvement or worsening in their seizures. Rusch *et al.* (2001) found that matching specific psychotherapies to the patient's comorbid diagnoses produced greater seizure-free rates, with 21 of 33 patients (63%) reaching event-free status at the end of treatment.

B. TREATMENT

Despite our preliminary understanding of risk factors, treatment for patients with NES is poorly understood. One of the main reasons for this is the lack of systematic intervention studies. The void of generalizable, effective treatments for NES leaves only consensus recommendations (Ramani, 2000). Although psychotherapy is the mainstay of treatment recommendations (Aboukasm *et al.*, 1998; Ramani, 2000), its efficacy remains unproven. Further, no medications have been proven effective in the treatment of NES. Clinicians do, however, use psychotropic medications to treat comorbid mood, anxiety, and elements of personality disorders, which often occur in patients with NES.

1. Treatment Theories

Etiological approaches for NES include *biomedical, psychodynamic, cognitive behavioral*, and *family theory* models (Krawetz *et al.*, 2001; Swingle, 1998; Ziegler and Imboden, 1962). The diagnosis of NES is often seen as a unitary disorder or syndrome. Just as the behavioral manifestations of NES vary tremendously, the underlying etiologies are also varied. Precursors to psychogenic NES include childhood sexual abuse, physical abuse, comorbid psychiatric conditions, minor head trauma, disability claims, and reinforced behavioral patterns, among others. In identifying signs, symptoms, and situations that are associated with NES in a patient, we can then provide interventions to promote the mental, physical, and social health of the patient (LaFrance and Devinsky, 2002).

Biomedical approaches highlight the absence of epileptiform activity during NES, demonstrating a functional-neuroanatomic dissociation model for NES (Blumer, 2000; Brown and Trimble, 2000). AEDs do not treat NES and in some patients can worsen NES (Niedermeyer *et al.*, 1970). Conversely, withdrawal of AEDs has been shown to be safe in patients with lone NES (Oto *et al.*, 2005b). Antidepressant, antianxiety, and antipsychotic therapies (e.g., medication, relaxation techniques, etc.) can treat symptomatic comorbid disorders and are currently being studied to evaluate if medications may indirectly improve NES frequency or severity (LaFrance *et al.*, 2007).

NES are currently treated as a neuropsychiatric illness with psychological underpinnings. Both psychotherapeutic and psychopharmacologic interventions are used to treat psychological conflicts and to treat the psychiatric comorbid diagnoses. These approaches fall under the headings of Psychodynamic Psychotherapy, Cognitive Behavioral Therapies, Family Systems Therapies, Behavioral Modification (mainly for mentally handicapped individuals), and Biological Psychiatric Treatments.

2. Conceptualization for Treatment Recommendations

Bowman recommends the "4 E's" for interventions by neurologists: Explanation, Exploration, Exportation (for treatment), and do not Exile. The circumspect neurologist will exercise caution when deciding whether or not to "explore" a patient's trauma history. The "exile" issue is of greatest importance because it must be realized that once the vEEG diagnosis of NES is confirmed by the neurologist, the difficult work of collaboratively treating the patient with psychiatry is just begun.

Treatment and outcome vary considerably with the underlying psychopathology. Patients with NES generally have poor to fair treatment outcomes, but children and adolescents tend to do better than adults. In one study, outcome was significantly better for the younger patients at 1, 2, and 3 years after diagnosis (seizure-free percentages: children 73%, 75%, 81%, and adults 25%, 25%, 40%, respectively). The authors proposed that different psychological mechanisms at different ages of onset and greater effectiveness with earlier intervention may be factors leading to better outcome for children and adolescents (Wyllie *et al.*, 1991).

The higher success rates are noted in the treatment articles and chapters describing longer inpatient admissions where patients were managed by a multi-disciplinary team familiar with NES (Ramani and Gumnit, 1982). More recent reviews, however, reveal that roughly one third of the patients have NES cessation, and another third have reduction in their NES (Reuber and Elger, 2003). In one NES outcome study, 71% of patients reported persistence of their seizures, in spite of 41% of the patients having had inpatient psychiatric treatment (Reuber *et al.*, 2003). Of the patients with lone NES, 40% continued to receive AEDs inappropriately, impacting quality of life. Patients with NES rate their quality of life more poorly than those with epilepsy (Testa *et al.*, 2007). Quigg *et al.* found that quality-of-life measures improve, however, when patients reach NES freedom, and not when their NES are merely reduced (Quigg *et al.*, 2002). Even with NES improvement, up to half of the patients remain on government or family support and are unemployed (Krawetz *et al.*, 2001), and patients with NES generally do not expect to return to work (Pestana *et al.*, 2003). One study found that patients with NES scored higher on hypochondriasis and somatic-complaint scales of the Minnesota Multiphasic Personality Inventory when compared with PWE, reflective of a focus on bodily function and neurologic complaints (Owczarek, 2003). Poor quality of life in patients with NES may partly result from their somatic focus. A factor analysis of predictors of health-related quality of life revealed that patients with NES had more bodily concern than those with epilepsy (Testa *et al.*, 2003), and that somatic focus may influence health-related quality of life.

Noting the good prognosis if NES has a recent onset, Gates suggested that psychiatric treatment be based on NES chronicity: short-term psychotherapy for those with NES less than 6 months, and more intensive inpatient therapy for long-standing NES (Gates, 1998). Although patients who receive feedback about their diagnosis and psychotherapy have better outcomes than those who do not (Aboukasm *et al.*, 1998), the difference may reflect baseline characteristics of the groups, rather than the effects of intervention.

On the basis of clinical and research reports to date, we suggest the following assessment and treatment approach by a multispecialty neuropsychiatric team:

(1) Proper diagnosis—vEEG for each patient with suspected NES, refractory or pharmacoresistant seizures.
(2) Presentation—explain the NES diagnosis in a clear, positive, non-pejorative manner. The patient may make the diagnosis presentation to the family members if cognitively and emotionally capable. This process

helps reveal the level of understanding and initial acceptance of the diagnosis by the patient. Clarifications can be made by the physician who is present. Communicate the diagnosis unambiguously to the referring physician and explain the need to eliminate unnecessary medications.

(3) Psychiatric treatment—conduct a thorough psychiatric assessment to identify predisposing factors (including comorbid psychiatric disorders), seizure precipitants, and perpetuating factors. As diagnosis informs treatment, a dual-armed approach ensues with pharmacotherapy and/or psychotherapy, as indicated by the individual needs of the patient with NES.

Psychopharmacology begins with tapering and discontinuing ineffective AEDs for patients with lone NES, unless a specific AED has a documented beneficial psychopharmacologic effect in the patient. In patients with mixed ES/NES, reduce high-dose or multiple AED therapy if possible. Use psychopharmacologic agents to treat mood, anxiety, or psychotic disorders (LaFrance and Devinsky, 2002).

Psychological NES are likely the result of a complex interaction between psychiatric disorders, psychosocial stressors, dysfunctional coping styles, and CNS vulnerability (Mokleby *et al.*, 2002). Identifying the underlying stressors and providing supportive psychotherapy can help some patients but is often insufficient or ineffective. Studies consistently identify three main comorbid diagnoses in patients with NES: major depressive disorder, post-traumatic stress disorder, and cluster B personality traits characterized by impulsivity/hostility (Bowman and Markand, 1996; Rechlin *et al.*, 1997). Three additional critical areas of dysfunction in the NES population are emotion regulation, family dynamics, and unemployment/disability (Griffith *et al.*, 1998; Holmes *et al.*, 2001; Walczak *et al.*, 1995). Poorer outcomes to treatment maybe associated with the high number of comorbid psychiatric disorders and psychosocial stressors (Carson *et al.*, 2000). Therefore, therapy for patients with NES may require combined psychological education, psychotherapy, and pharmacotherapy, while simultaneously eliminating ineffective AEDs. An NINDS/NIMH/AES workshop emphasized that there is a great need for these interventions to be studied in randomized, controlled trials (LaFrance *et al.*, 2006).

Prior-published treatment reports reveal that coordination between neurologists and psychiatrists/psychologists with accurate diagnosis and prompt initiation of psychotherapy and communication between care providers, patients, and family yields higher treatment success.

X. Conclusions

In conclusion, a significant number of PWE have psychiatric disorders that accompany their seizures, and/or integrated mood/anxiety/psychotic and personality integrated symptoms secondary to their epilepsy. Quality of life and stigma associated with epilepsy has a significant impact on the lives of PWE. Management of epilepsy is also complicated by the presence of NES. Further research in these four areas is needed to inform diagnosis, pathophysiology, and treatment of these neuropsychiatric aspects of epilepsy.

References

Aboukasm, A., Mahr, G., Gahry, B. R., Thomas, A., and Barkley, G. L. (1998). Retrospective analysis of the effects of psychotherapeutic interventions on outcomes of psychogenic nonepileptic seizures. *Epilepsia* **39,** 470–473.

Alper, K., Devinsky, O., Perrine, K., Vazquez, B., and Luciano, D. (1993). Nonepileptic seizures and childhood sexual and physical abuse. *Neurology* **43,** 1950–1953.

Alper, K., Schwartz, K. A., Kolts, R. L., and Khan, A. (2007). Seizure incidence in psychopharmacological clinical trials: An analysis of food and drug administration (FDA) summary basis of approval reports. *Biol. Psychiatry* **62,** 345–354.

Anatassopoulos, G., and Kokkini, D. (1969). Suicidal attempts in psychomotor epilepsy. *Behav. Neuropsychiatry* **1,** 11–16.

Andrews, G., Henderson, S., and Hall, W. (2001). Prevalence, comorbidity, disability and service utilisation. Overview of the Australian National Mental Health Survey. *Br. J. Psychiatry* **178,** 145–153.

Ataoglu, A., Ozcetin, A., Icmeli, C., and Ozbulut, O. (2003). Paradoxical therapy in conversion reaction. *J. Korean Med. Sci.* **18,** 581–584.

Balabanov, A., and Kanner, A. M. (in press). Psychiatric outcome of epilepsy surgery. *In* "Textbook of Epilepsy Surgery" (H. O. Lüders, W. Bongaman, and I. M. Najim, Eds.). Lippincott, Williams and Wilkins.

Barabas, G., and Matthews, W. S. (1988). Barbiturate anticonvulsants as a cause of severe depression. *Pediatrics* **82,** 284–285.

Barry, J. J. (2001). Nonepileptic seizures: An overview. *CNS Spectr.* **6,** 956–962.

Bell, A. J., Cole, A., Eccleston, D., and Ferrier, I. N. (1993). Lithium neurotoxicity at normal therapeutic levels. *Br. J. Psychiatry* **162,** 689–692.

Blackwood, D. H., Cull, R. E., Freeman, C. P., Evans, J. I., and Mawdsley, C. (1980). A study of the incidence of epilepsy following ECT. *J. Neurol. Neurosurg. Psychiatry* **43,** 1098–1102.

Blanchet, P., and Frommer, G. P. (1986). Mood change preceding epileptic seizures. *J. Nerv. Ment. Dis.* **174,** 471–476.

Blum, D., Reed, M., and Metz, A. (2002). Prevalence of major affective disorders and manic/hypomanic symptoms in persons with epilepsy: A community survey. *Neurology* Suppl. 3, A–175.

Blumer, D. (2000). Chapter 24. On the Psychobiology of Non-Epileptic Seizures. *In* "Non-Epileptic Seizures" (J. R. Gates and A. J. Rowan, Eds.), pp. 305–310. Butterworth-Heinemann, Boston.

Blumer, D., and Altshuler, L. L. (1998). Affective disorders. *In* "Epilepsy: A Comprehensive Textbook" (J. Engel and T. A. Pedley, Eds.), pp. 2083–2099. Lippincott-Raven, Philadelphia.

Blumer, D., and Zielinksi, J. (1988). Pharmacologic treatment of psychiatric disorders associated with epilepsy. *J. Epilepsy* **1,** 135–150.

Boon, P. A., and Williamson, P. D. (1993). The diagnosis of pseudoseizures. *Clin. Neurol. Neurosurg.* **95,** 1–8.

Bowman, E. S. (1999). Nonepileptic seizures: Psychiatric framework, treatment, and outcome. *Neurology* **53,** S84–S88.

Bowman, E. S., and Markand, O. N. (1996). Psychodynamics and psychiatric diagnoses of pseudo-seizure subjects. *Am. J. Psychiatry* **153,** 57–63.

Bredkjaer, S. R., Mortensen, P. B., and Parnas, J. (1998). Epilepsy and non-organic non-affective psychosis. National epidemiologic study. *Br. J. Psychiatry* **172,** 235–238.

Brent, D. A., Crumrine, P. K., Varma, R. R., Allan, M., and Allman, C. (1987). Phenobarbital treatment and major depressive disorder in children with epilepsy. *Pediatrics* **80,** 909–917.

Brown, R. J., and Trimble, M. R. (2000). Editorial: Dissociative psychopathology, non-epileptic seizures, and neurology. *J. Neurol. Neurosurg. Psychiatry* **69,** 285–288.

Brown, R. T., Freeman, W. S., Perrin, J. M., Stein, M. T., Amler, R. W., Feldman, H. M., Pierce, K., and Wolraich, M. L. (2001). Prevalence and assessment of attention-deficit/hyperactivity disorder in primary care settings. *Pediatrics* **107,** E43.

Caplan, R., Siddarth, P., Gurbani, S., Hanson, R., Sankar, R., and Shields, W. D. (2005). Depression and anxiety disorders in pediatric epilepsy. *Epilepsia* **46,** 720–730.

Carson, A. J., Ringbauer, B., MacKenzie, L., Warlow, C., and Sharpe, M. (2000). Neurological disease, emotional disorder, and disability: They are related: A study of 300 consecutive new referrals to a neurology outpatient department. *J. Neurol. Neurosurg. Psychiatry* **68,** 202–206.

Chabolla, D. R., Krahn, L. E., So, E. L., and Rummans, T. A. (1996). Psychogenic nonepileptic seizures. *Mayo Clin. Proc.* **71,** 493–500.

Christensen, J., Vestergaard, M., Mortensen, P. B., Sidenius, P., and Agerbo, E. (2007). Epilepsy and risk of suicide: A population-based case-control study. *Lancet Neurol.* **6,** 693–698.

Cragar, D. E., Berry, D. T., Fakhoury, T. A., Cibula, J. E., and Schmitt, F. A. (2002). A review of diagnostic techniques in the differential diagnosis of epileptic and nonepileptic seizures. *Neuropsychol. Rev.* **12,** 31–64.

Curran, S., and de Pauw, K. (1998). Selecting an antidepressant for use in a patient with epilepsy. Safety considerations. *Drug Saf.* **18,** 125–133.

Currie, S., Heathfield, K. W., Henson, R. A., and Scott, D. F. (1971). Clinical course and prognosis of temporal lobe epilepsy. A survey of 666 patients. *Brain* **94,** 173–190.

Daly, D. (1958). Ictal affect. *Am. J. Psychiatry* **115,** 97–108.

Davis, B. J. (2004). Predicting nonepileptic seizures utilizing seizure frequency, EEG, and response to medication. *Eur. Neurol.* **51,** 153–156.

de Araujo Filho, G. M., Pascalicchio, T. F., Sousa Pda, S., Lin, K., Ferreira Guilhoto, L. M., and Yacubian, E. M. (2007). Psychiatric disorders in juvenile myoclonic epilepsy: A controlled study of 100 patients. *Epilepsy Behav.* **10,** 437–441.

de Timary, P., Fouchet, P., Sylin, M., Indriets, J. P., De Barsy, T., Lefebvre, A., and Van Rijckevorsel, K. (2002). Non-epileptic seizures: Delayed diagnosis in patients presenting with electroencephalographic (EEG) or clinical signs of epileptic seizures. *Seizure* **11,** 193–197.

Desai, B. T., Porter, R. J., and Penry, J. K. (1979). Abstract GS 43: The psychogenic seizure by videotape analysis: A study of 42 attacks in 6 patients. *Neurol. (Minneap.)* **29,** 602.

Devinsky, O., and Fisher, R. (1996). Ethical use of placebos and provocative testing in diagnosing nonepileptic seizures. *Neurology* **47,** 866–870.

Devinsky, O., Abramson, H., Alper, K., FitzGerald, L. S., Perrine, K., Calderon, J., and Luciano, D. (1995). Postictal psychosis: A case control series of 20 patients and 150 controls. *Epilepsy Res.* **20,** 247–253.

Dongier, S. (1959). Statistical study of clinical and electroencephalographic manifestations of 536 psychotic episodes occurring in 516 epileptics between clinical seizures. *Epilepsia* **1,** 117–142.

Dunn, D. W., and Kronenberger, W. G. (2005). Childhood epilepsy, attention problems, and ADHD: Review and practical considerations. *Semin. Pediatr. Neurol.* **12,** 222–228.

Dunn, D. W., Austin, J. K., Harezlak, J., and Ambrosius, W. T. (2003). ADHD and epilepsy in childhood. *Dev. Med. Child. Neurol.* **45,** 50–54.

Edeh, J., and Toone, B. (1987). Relationship between interictal psychopathology and the type of epilepsy. Results of a survey in general practice. *Br. J. Psychiatry* **151,** 95–101.

Ettinger, A. B., Dhoon, A., Weisbrot, D. M., and Devinsky, O. (1999). Predictive factors for outcome of nonepileptic seizures after diagnosis. *J. Neuropsych. Clin. Neurosci.* **11,** 458–463.

Ettinger, A., Reed, M., and Cramer, J. (2004). Depression and comorbidity in community-based patients with epilepsy or asthma. *Neurology* **63,** 1008–1014.

Ettinger, A. B., Reed, M. L., Goldberg, J. F., and Hirschfeld, R. M. (2005). Prevalence of bipolar symptoms in epilepsy vs other chronic health disorders. *Neurology* **65,** 535–540.

Ferrari, M., Barabas, G., and Matthews, W. S. (1983). Psychologic and behavioral disturbance among epileptic children treated with barbiturate anticonvulsants. *Am. J. Psychiatry* **140,** 112–113.

Fink, M., Kellner, C. H., and Sackeim, H. A. (1999). Intractable seizures, status epilepticus, and ECT. *J. Ect.* **15,** 282–284.

Fisher, R. S., Vickrey, B. G., Gibson, P., Hermann, B., Penovich, P., Scherer, A., and Walker, S. (2000). The impact of epilepsy from the patient's perspective I. Descriptions and subjective perceptions. *Epilepsy Res.* **41,** 39–51.

Fohlen, M., Lellouch, A., and Delalande, O. (2003). Hypothalamic hamartoma with refractory epilepsy: Surgical procedures and results in 18 patients. *Epileptic Disord.* **5,** 267–273.

Forsgren, L., and Nystrom, L. (1990). An incident case-referent study of epileptic seizures in adults. *Epilepsy Res.* **6,** 66–81.

Freidl, M., Spitzl, S. P., Prause, W., Zimprich, F., Lehner-Baumgartner, E., Baumgartner, C., and Aigner, M. (2007). The stigma of mental illness: Anticipation and attitudes among patients with epileptic, dissociative or somatoform pain disorder. *Int. Rev. Psychiatry* **19,** 123–129.

Friedlander, W. J. (2001). Chapter 9. Societal Aspects. *In* "The History of Modern Epilepsy: The Beginning, 1865–1914" Vol. 45, pp. 239–275. Greenwood Press, Westport, CT.

Fritze, J., Unsorg, B., and Lanczik, M. (1991). Interaction between carbamazepine and fluvoxamine. *Acta Psychiatr. Scand.* **84,** 583–584.

Gatchel, R. J., Polatin, P. B., and Kinney, R. K. (1995). Predicting outcome of chronic back pain using clinical predictors of psychopathology: A prospective analysis. *Health Psychol.* **14,** 415–420.

Gates, J. R. (1998). Diagnosis and treatment of nonepileptic seizures. *In* "Psychiatric Comorbidity in Epilepsy. Basic Mechanisms, Diagnosis, and Treatment" (H. W. McConnell and P. J. Snyder, Eds.), pp. 187–204. American Psychiatric Press, Inc., Washington, DC.

Gates, J. R., and Rowan, A. J. (2000). "Non-Epileptic Seizures," pp. 1–323. Butterworth-Heinemann, Boston MA.

Gates, J. R., Luciano, D., and Devinsky, O. (1991). Chapter 18. The Classification and Treatment of Nonepileptic Events. *In* "Epilepsy and Behavior" (O. Devinsky and W. H. Theodore, Eds.), Vol. 12, pp. 251–263. Wiley-Liss, New York.

Ghougassian, D. F., d'Souza, W., Cook, M. J., and O'Brien, T. J. (2004). Evaluating the utility of inpatient video-EEG monitoring. *Epilepsia* **45,** 928–932.

Gilliam, F. (2002). Optimizing health outcomes in active epilepsy. *Neurology* **58,** S9–S20.

Gilliam, F., and Kanner, A. M. (2002). Treatment of depressive disorders in epilepsy patients. *Epilepsy Behav.* **3,** S2–S9.

Gilliam, F., Kuzniecky, R., Faught, E., Black, L., Carpenter, G., and Schrodt, R. (1997). Patient-validated content of epilepsy-specific quality-of-life measurement. *Epilepsia* **38,** 233–236.

Goldstein, L. H., Deale, A. C., Mitchell-O'Malley, S. J., Toone, B. K., and Mellers, J. D. C. (2004). An evaluation of cognitive behavioral therapy as a treatment for dissociative seizures: A pilot study. *Cogn. Behav. Neurol.* **17,** 41–49.

Gram, L., Johannessen, S. I., Oterman, P. O., and Sillanpää, M. (1993). "Pseudo-Epileptic Seizures," pp. 1–165. Wrightson Biomedical Publishing, LTD, Petersfield, UK.

Griffith, J. L., Polles, A., and Griffith, M. E. (1998). Pseudoseizures, families, and unspeakable dilemmas. *Psychosomatics* **39,** 144–153.

Grimsley, S. R., Jann, M. W., Carter, J. G., D'Mello, A. P., and D'Souza, M. J. (1991). Increased carbamazepine plasma concentrations after fluoxetine coadministration. *Clin. Pharmacol. Ther.* **50,** 10–15.

Hancock, J. C., and Bevilacqua, A. R. (1971). Temporal lobe dysrhythmia and impulsive or suicidal behavior: Preliminary report. *South. Med. J.* **64,** 1189–1193.

Hantke, N. C., Doherty, M. J., and Haltiner, A. M. (2007). Medication use profiles in patients with psychogenic nonepileptic seizures. *Epilepsy Behav.* **10,** 333–335.

Haselberger, M. B., Freedman, L. S., and Tolbert, S. (1997). Elevated serum phenytoin concentrations associated with coadministration of sertraline. *J. Clin. Psychopharmacol.* **17,** 107–109.

Hermann, B. P., Seidenberg, M., Bell, B., Woodard, A., Rutecki, P., and Sheth, R. (2000). Comorbid psychiatric symptoms in temporal lobe epilepsy: Association with chronicity of epilepsy and impact on quality of life. *Epilepsy Behav.* **1,** 184–190.

Hesdorffer, D. C., Hauser, W. A., Annegers, J. F., and Cascino, G. (2000). Major depression is a risk factor for seizures in older adults. *Ann. Neurol.* **47,** 246–249.

Hesdorffer, D. C., Hauser, W. A., Olafsson, E., Ludvigsson, P., and Kjartansson, O. (2006). Depression and suicide attempt as risk factors for incident unprovoked seizures. *Ann. Neurol.* **59,** 35–41.

Hesdorffer, D. C., Ludvigsson, P., Olafsson, E., Gudmundsson, G., Kjartansson, O., and Hauser, W. A. (2004). ADHD as a risk factor for incident unprovoked seizures and epilepsy in children. *Arch. Gen. Psychiatry* **61,** 731–736.

Holmes, M. D., Dodrill, C. B., Bachtler, S., Wilensky, A. J., Ojemann, L. M., and Miller, J. W. (2001). Evidence that emotional maladjustment is worse in men than in women with psychogenic nonepileptic seizures. *Epilepsy Behav.* **2,** 568–573.

Jacoby, A., Baker, G. A., Steen, N., Potts, P., and Chadwick, D. W. (1996). The clinical course of epilepsy and its psychosocial correlates: Findings from a U.K. Community study. *Epilepsia* **37,** 148–161.

Jedrzejczak, J., Owczarek, K., and Majkowski, J. (1999). Psychogenic pseudoepileptic seizures: Clinical and electroencephalogram (EEG) video-tape recordings. *Eur. J. Neurol.* **6,** 473–479.

Jensen, I., and Vaernet, K. (1977). Temporal lobe epilepsy. Follow-up investigation of 74 temporal lobe resected patients. *Acta Neurochir. (Wien)* **37,** 173–200.

Jones, J. E., Hermann, B. P., Barry, J. J., Gilliam, F. G., Kanner, A. M., and Meador, K. J. (2003). Rates and risk factors for suicide, suicidal ideation, and suicide attempts in chronic epilepsy. *Epilepsy Behav.* **4,** 31–38.

Jones, J. E., Bell, B., Fine, J., Rutecki, P., Seidenberg, M., and Hermann, B. (2007a). A controlled prospective investigation of psychiatric comorbidity in temporal lobe epilepsy. *Epilepsia* **48,** 2357–2360.

Jones, J. E., Watson, R., Sheth, R., Caplan, R., Koehn, M., Seidenberg, M., and Hermann, B. (2007b). Psychiatric comorbidity in children with new onset epilepsy. *Dev. Med. Child. Neurol.* **49,** 493–497.

Kanner, A. M. (2003). Psychogenic nonepileptic seizures are bad for your health. *Epilepsy Curr.* **3,** 181–182.

Kanner, A. M., and Jones, J. C. (1997). When do sphenoidal electrodes yield additional data to that obtained with antero-temporal electrodes? *Electroencephalogr. Clin. Neurophysiol.* **102,** 12–19.

Kanner, A. M., Ramirez, L., and Jones, J. C. (1995). The utility of placing sphenoidal electrodes under the foramen ovale with fluoroscopic guidance. *J. Clin. Neurophysiol.* **12,** 72–81.

Kanner, A. M., Stagno, S., Kotagal, P., and Morris, H. H. (1996). Postictal psychiatric events during prolonged video-electroencephalographic monitoring studies. *Arch. Neurol.* **53,** 258–263.

Kanner, A. M., Parra, J., Frey, M., Stebbins, G., Pierre-Louis, S., and Iriarte, J. (1999). Psychiatric and neurologic predictors of psychogenic pseudoseizure outcome. *Neurology* **53,** 933–938.

Kanner, A. M., Kozak, A. M., and Frey, M. (2000). The use of sertraline in patients with epilepsy: Is it safe? *Epilepsy Behav.* **1,** 100–105.

Kanner, A. M., and Ostrovskaya, A. (2008). Long-term significance of postictal psychotic episodes I. Are they predictive of bilateral ictal foci? *Epilepsy Behav.* **12,** 150–153.

Kanner, A. M., Wuu, J., Faught, E., Tatum, W. O., IV, Fix, A., and French, J. A. (2003). A past psychiatric history may be a risk factor for topiramate-related psychiatric and cognitive adverse events. *Epilepsy Behav.* **4,** 548–552.

Kanner, A. M., Soto, A., and Gross-Kanner, H. (2004). Prevalence and clinical characteristics of postictal psychiatric symptoms in partial epilepsy. *Neurology* **62,** 708–713.

Kessler, R. C., McGonagle, K. A., Zhao, S., Nelson, C. B., Hughes, M., Eshleman, S., Wittchen, H. U., and Kendler, K. S. (1994). Lifetime and 12-month prevalence of DSM-III-R psychiatric disorders in the United States. Results from the National Comorbidity Survey. *Arch. Gen. Psychiatry* **51,** 8–19.

Ketter, T. A., Malow, B. A., Flamini, R., White, S. R., Post, R. M., and Theodore, W. H. (1994). Anticonvulsant withdrawal-emergent psychopathology. *Neurology* **44,** 55–61.

Kim, C. M., Barry, J. J., and Zeifert, P. A. (1998). Abstract 7.078. The use of inpatient medical psychiatric treatment for nonepileptic events. *Epilepsia* **39,** 242–243.

King, D. W., Gallagher, B. B., Murvin, A. J., Smith, D. B., Marcus, D. J., Hartlage, L. C., and Ward, L. C., 3rd (1982). Pseudoseizures: Diagnostic evaluation. *Neurology* **32,** 18–23.

Kleinman, A., Wang, W. Z., Li, S. C., Cheng, X. M., Dai, X. Y., Li, K. T., and Kleinman, J. (1995). The social course of epilepsy: Chronic illness as social experience in interior China. *Soc. Sci. Med.* **40,** 1319–1330.

Koch-Stoecker, S. (2002). Personality disorders as predictors of severe postsurgical psychiatric complications in epilepsy patients undergoing temporal lobe resections. *Epilepsy Behav.* **3,** 526–531.

Kogeorgos, J., Fonagy, P., and Scott, D. F. (1982). Psychiatric symptom patterns of chronic epileptics attending a neurological clinic: A controlled investigation. *Br. J. Psychiatry* **140,** 236–243.

Krawetz, P., Fleisher, W., Pillay, N., Staley, D., Arnett, J., and Maher, J. (2001). Family functioning in subjects with pseudoseizures and epilepsy. *J. Nerv. Ment. Dis.* **189,** 38–43.

Krumholz, A., Niedermeyer, E., Alkaitis, D., and Morel, R. (1980). Abstract: Psychogenic seizures: A 5-year follow-up study. *Neurology* **30,** 392.

LaFrance, W. C., Jr. (2008). Psychogenic nonepileptic seizures. *Curr. Opin. Neurology* **21,** 195–201.

LaFrance, W. C., Jr., and Barry, J. J. (2005). Update on treatments of psychological nonepileptic seizures. *Epilepsy Behav.* **7,** 364–374.

LaFrance, W. C., Jr., and Benbadis, S. R. (2006). Avoiding the costs of unrecognized psychological nonepileptic seizures. *Neurology* **66,** 1620–1621.

LaFrance, W. C., Jr., and Devinsky, O. (2002). Treatment of nonepileptic seizures. *Epilepsy Behav.* **3,** S19–S23.

LaFrance, W. C., Jr., and Devinsky, O. (2004). The treatment of nonepileptic seizures: Historical perspectives and future directions. *Epilepsia* **45,** 15–21.

LaFrance, W. C., Jr., Alper, K., Babcock, D., Barry, J. J., Benbadis, S., Caplan, R., Gates, J., Jacobs, M., Kanner, A., Martin, R., Rundhaugen, L., Stewart, R., *et al.* (2006). Nonepileptic seizures treatment workshop summary. *Epilepsy Behav.* **8,** 451–461.

LaFrance, W. C., Jr., Blum, A. S., Miller, I. W., Ryan, C. E., and Keitner, G. I. (2007). Methodological issues in conducting treatment trials for psychological nonepileptic seizures. *J. Neuropsych. Clin. Neurosci.* **19,** 391–398.

Lancman, M. E., Brotherton, T. A., Asconape, J. J., and Penry, J. K. (1993). Psychogenic seizures in adults: A longitudinal analysis. *Seizure* **2,** 281–286.

Lancman, M. E., Craven, W. J., Asconape, J. J., and Penry, J. K. (1994). Clinical management of recurrent postictal psychosis. *J. Epilepsy* **7,** 47–51.

Lancman, M. E., Lambrakis, C. C., and Steinhardt, M. I. (2001). Psychogenic pseudoseizures: A general overview. *In* "Psychiatry Issues in Epilepsy: A Practical Guide to Diagnosis and Treatment" (A. B. Ettinger and A. M. Kanner, Eds.), pp. 341–354. Lippincott, Williams & Wilkins, Philadelphia, PA.

Landoldt, H. (1953). Some clinical electroencephalographical correlations in epileptic psychosis (twilight states). *Electroencephalogr. Clin. Neurophysiol.* **5,** 121 (abstract).

Lehrner, J., Kalchmayr, R., Serles, W., Olbrich, A., Pataraia, E., Aull, S., Bacher, J., Leutmezer, F., Groppel, G., Deecke, L., and Baumgartner, C. (1999). Health-related quality of life (HRQOL), activity of daily living (ADL) and depressive mood disorder in temporal lobe epilepsy patients. *Seizure* **8,** 88–92.

Lelliott, P. T., and Fenwick, P. (1991). Cerebral pathology in pseudoseizures. *Acta Neurol. Scand.* **83,** 129–132.

Logothetis, J. (1967). Spontaneous epileptic seizures and electroencephalographic changes in the course of phenothiazine therapy. *Neurology* **17,** 869–877.

Logsdail, S. J., and Toone, B. K. (1988). Post-ictal psychoses. A clinical and phenomenological description. *Br. J. Psychiatry* **152,** 246–252.

Martin, R. C., Gilliam, F. G., Kilgore, M., Faught, E., and Kuzniecky, R. (1998). Improved health care resource utilization following video-EEG-confirmed diagnosis of nonepileptic psychogenic seizures. *Seizure* **7,** 385–390.

McAfee, A. T., Chilcott, K. E., Johannes, C. B., Hornbuckle, K., Hauser, W. A., and Walker, A. M. (2007). The incidence of first provoked and unprovoked seizure in pediatric patients with and without psychiatric diagnoses. *Epilepsia* **48,** 1075–1082.

McConnell, H., and Duncan, D. (1998). Treatment of psychiatric comorbidity in epilepsy. *In* "Psychiatric Comorbidity in Epilepsy" (H. McConnell, and P. Snyder, Eds.), pp. 245–361. American Psychiatric Press, Washington.

McConnell, H., Duffy, J., and Cress, K. (1994). Behavioral effects of felbamate. *J. Neuropsych. Clin. Neurosci.* **6,** 323.

McDade, G., and Brown, S. W. (1992). Non-epileptic seizures: Management and predictive factors of outcome. *Seizure* **1,** 7–10.

McDermott, S., Mani, S., and Krishnaswami, S. (1995). A population-based analysis of specific behavior problems associated with childhood seizures. *J. Epilepsy* **8,** 100–110.

McLellan, A., Davies, S., Heyman, I., Harding, B., Harkness, W., Taylor, D., Neville, B. G., and Cross, J. H. (2005). Psychopathology in children with epilepsy before and after temporal lobe resection. *Dev. Med. Child. Neurol.* **47,** 666–672.

Meltzer, H., Bebbington, P., Brugha, T., Farrell, M., Jenkins, R., and Lewis, G. (2003). The reluctance to seek treatment for neurotic disorders. *Int. Rev. Psychiatry* **15,** 123–128.

Mendez, M. F., Cummings, J. L., and Benson, D. F. (1986). Depression in epilepsy. Significance and phenomenology. *Arch. Neurol.* **43,** 766–770.

Mokleby, K., Blomhoff, S., Malt, U. F., Dahlstrom, A., Tauboll, E., and Gjerstad, L. (2002). Psychiatric comorbidity and hostility in patients with psychogenic nonepileptic seizures compared with somatoform disorders and healthy controls. *Epilepsia* **43,** 193–198.

Morrell, F., Whisler, W. W., Smith, M. C., Hoeppner, T. J., de Toledo-Morrell, L., Pierre-Louis, S. J., Kanner, A. M., Buelow, J. M., Ristanovic, R., Bergen, D., *et al.* (1995). Landau-Kleffner syndrome. Treatment with subpial intracortical transection. *Brain* **118**(Pt 6), 1529–1546.

Mula, M., and Trimble, M. R. (2003). The importance of being seizure free: Topiramate and psychopathology in epilepsy. *Epilepsy Behav.* **4,** 430–434.

Niedermeyer, E., Blumer, D., Holscher, E., and Walker, B. A. (1970). Classical hysterical seizures facilitated by anticonvulsant toxicity. *Psychiatr. Clin. (Basel.)* **3,** 71–84.

Nilsson, L., Tomson, T., Farahmand, B. Y., Diwan, V., and Persson, P. G. (1997). Cause-specific mortality in epilepsy: A cohort study of more than 9,000 patients once hospitalized for epilepsy. *Epilepsia* **38,** 1062–1068.

O'Donoghue, M. F., Goodridge, D. M., Redhead, K., Sander, J. W., and Duncan, J. S. (1999). Assessing the psychosocial consequences of epilepsy: A community-based study. *Br. J. Gen. Pract.* **49,** 211–214.

Onuma, T., Adachi, N., Ishida, S., Katou, M., and Uesugi, S. (1995). Prevalence and annual incidence of psychosis in patients with epilepsy. *Psychiatry. Clin. Neurosci.* **49,** S267–S268.

O'Sullivan, S. S., Spillane, J. E., McMahon, E. M., Sweeney, B. J., Galvin, R. J., McNamara, B., and Cassidy, E. M. (2007). Clinical characteristics and outcome of patients diagnosed with psychogenic nonepileptic seizures: A 5-year review. *Epilepsy Behav.* **11,** 77–84.

Ott, D., Caplan, R., Guthrie, D., Siddarth, P., Komo, S., Shields, W. D., Sankar, R., Kornblum, H., and Chayasirisobhon, S. (2001). Measures of psychopathology in children with complex partial seizures and primary generalized epilepsy with absence. *J. Am. Acad. Child. Adolesc. Psychiatry* **40,** 907–914.

Oto, M., Conway, P., McGonigal, A., Russell, A. J., and Duncan, R. (2005a). Gender differences in psychogenic non-epileptic seizures. *Seizure* **14,** 33–39.

Oto, M., Espie, C., Pelosi, A., Selkirk, M., and Duncan, R. (2005b). The safety of antiepileptic drug withdrawal in patients with non-epileptic seizures. *J. Neurol. Neurosurg. Psychiatry* **76,** 1682–1685.

Ounsted, C. (1955). The hyperkinetic syndrome in epileptic children. *Lancet* **269,** 303–311.

Owczarek, K. (2003). Somatisation indexes as differential factors in psychogenic pseudoepileptic and epileptic seizures. *Seizure* **12,** 178–181.

Pacia, S. V., and Devinsky, O. (1994). Clozapine-related seizures: Experience with 5,629 patients. *Neurology* **44,** 2247–2249.

Pariente, P. D., Lepine, J. P., and Lellouch, J. (1991). Lifetime history of panic attacks and epilepsy: An association from a general population survey. *J. Clin. Psychiatry* **52,** 88–89.

PDR (2002). "Physicians' Desk Reference." Medical Economics Co., Montvale, NJ.

Pearson, H. J. (1990). Interaction of fluoxetine with carbamazepine. *J. Clin. Psychiatry* **51,** 126.

Penin, H. (1968). Elektonische Patientenuberwachung in der Nervenklinik Bonn [Electronic patient monitoring in the neurologic hospital of Bonn]. *Umsschau in Wissenschaft und Technik* **7,** 211–212.

Perini, G. I., Tosin, C., Carraro, C., Bernasconi, G., Canevini, M. P., Canger, R., Pellegrini, A., and Testa, G. (1996). Interictal mood and personality disorders in temporal lobe epilepsy and juvenile myoclonic epilepsy. *J. Neurol. Neurosurg. Psychiatry* **61,** 601–605.

Perrine, K., Hermann, B. P., Meador, K. J., Vickrey, B. G., Cramer, J. A., Hays, R. D., and Devinsky, O. (1995). The relationship of neuropsychological functioning to quality of life in epilepsy. *Arch. Neurol.* **52,** 997–1003.

Pestana, E. M., Foldvary-Shaefer, N., Marsillio, D., and Morris, H. H., III. (2003). Abstract [P05.023] quality of life in patients with psychogenic seizures. *Neurology* **60,** A355.

Pintor, L., Bailles, E., Fernandez-Egea, E., Sanchez-Gistau, V., Torres, X., Carreno, M., Rumia, J., Matrai, S., Boget, T., Raspall, T., Donaire, A., Bargallo, N., *et al.* (2007). Psychiatric disorders in temporal lobe epilepsy patients over the first year after surgical treatment. *Seizure* **16,** 218–225.

Preskorn, S. H., and Fast, G. A. (1992). Tricyclic antidepressant-induced seizures and plasma drug concentration. *J. Clin. Psychiatry* **53,** 160–162.

Quigg, M., Armstrong, R. F., Farace, E., and Fountain, N. B. (2002). Quality of life outcome is associated with cessation rather than reduction of psychogenic nonepileptic seizures. *Epilepsy Behav.* **3,** 455–459.

Quiske, A., Helmstaedter, C., Lux, S., and Elger, C. E. (2000). Depression in patients with temporal lobe epilepsy is related to mesial temporal sclerosis. *Epilepsy Res.* **39,** 121–125.

Rafnsson, V., Olafsson, E., Hauser, W. A., and Gudmundsson, G. (2001). Cause-specific mortality in adults with unprovoked seizures. A population-based incidence cohort study. *Neuroepidemiology* **20,** 232–236.

Ramani, V. (2000). Chapter 25. Treatment of the Adult Patient with Non-Epileptic Seizures. *In* "Non-Epileptic Seizures" (J. R. Gates and A. J. Rowan, Eds.), pp. 300–316. Butterworth-Heinemann, Boston, MA.

Ramani, V., and Gumnit, R. J. (1982). Management of hysterical seizures in epileptic patients. *Arch. Neurol.* **39,** 78–81.

Rechlin, T., Loew, T. H., and Joraschky, P. (1997). Pseudoseizure "status". *J. Psychosom. Res.* **42,** 495–498.

Regenold, W. T., Weintraub, D., and Taller, A. (1998). Electroconvulsive therapy for epilepsy and major depression. *Am. J. Geriatr. Psychiatry* **6,** 180–183.

Regier, D. A., Farmer, M. E., Rae, D. S., Myers, J. K., Kramer, M., Robins, L. N., George, L. K., Karno, M., and Locke, B. Z. (1993). One-month prevalence of mental disorders in the United States and sociodemographic characteristics: The Epidemiologic Catchment Area study. *Acta Psychiatr. Scand.* **88,** 35–47.

Reiter, J. M., and Andrews, D. J. (2000). A neurobehavioral approach for treatment of complex partial epilepsy: Efficacy. *Seizure* **9,** 198–203.

Reuber, M., and Elger, C. E. (2003). Psychogenic nonepileptic seizures: Review and update. *Epilepsy Behav.* **4,** 205–216.

Reuber, M., Pukrop, R., Bauer, J., Helmstaedter, C., Tessendorf, N., and Elger, C. E. (2003). Outcome in psychogenic nonepileptic seizures: 1 to 10-year follow-up in 164 patients. *Ann. Neurol.* **53,** 305–311.

Reuber, M., Baker, G. A., Gill, R., Smith, D. F., and Chadwick, D. W. (2004). Failure to recognize psychogenic nonepileptic seizures may cause death. *Neurology* **62,** 834–835.

Ring, H. A., and Reynolds, E. H. (1990). Vigabatrin and behaviour disturbance. *Lancet* **335,** 970.

Robertson, M. M. (1997). Suicide, parasuicide, and epilepsy. *In* "Epilepsy: A Comprehensive Textbook" (T. Pedley and J. Engel, Eds.) Lippincott-Raver, Philadelphia.

Rosenstein, D. L., Nelson, J. C., and Jacobs, S. C. (1993). Seizures associated with antidepressants: A review. *J. Clin. Psychiatry* **54,** 289–299.

Roy-Byrne, P. P., Stein, M. B., Russo, J., Mercier, E., Thomas, R., McQuaid, J., Katon, W. J., Craske, M. G., Bystritsky, A., and Sherbourne, C. D. (1999). Panic disorder in the primary care setting: Comorbidity, disability, service utilization, and treatment. *J. Clin. Psychiatry* **60,** 492–499; quiz 500.

Rusch, M. D., Morris, G. L., Allen, L., and Lathrop, L. (2001). Psychological treatment of nonepileptic events. *Epilepsy Behav.* **2,** 277–283.

Rutter, M., Graham, P., and Yule, W. (1970). "A Neuropsychiatric Study in Childhood." JB Lippincott, Philadelphia.

Sackeim, H. A., Decina, P., Prohovnik, I., Malitz, S., and Resor, S. R. (1983). Anticonvulsant and antidepressant properties of electroconvulsive therapy: A proposed mechanism of action. *Biol. Psychiatry* **18,** 1301–1310.

Santosh, D., Kumar, T. S., Sarma, P. S., and Radhakrishnan, K. (2007). Women with onset of epilepsy prior to marriage: Disclose or conceal? *Epilepsia* **48,** 1007–1010.

Savard, G., Andermann, L. F., Reutens, D., and Andermann, F. (1998). Epilepsy, surgical treatment and postoperative psychiatric complications: A re-evaluation of the evidence. *In* "Forced Normalization and Alternative Psychosis of Epilepsy" (M. Trimble and B. Schmitz, Eds.), pp. 179–192. Writson Biomedical Publishing Ltd., Petersfield.

Schmitz, B., and Wolf, P. (1995). Psychosis in epilepsy: Frequency and risk factors. *J. Epilepsy* **8,** 295–305.

Semrud-Clikeman, M., and Wical, B. (1999). Components of attention in children with complex partial seizures with and without ADHD. *Epilepsia* **40,** 211–215.

Shen, W., Bowman, E. S., and Markand, O. N. (1990). Presenting the diagnosis of pseudoseizure. *Neurology* **40,** 756–759.

Sherman, E. M., Slick, D. J., Connolly, M. B., and Eyrl, K. L. (2007). ADHD, neurological correlates and health-related quality of life in severe pediatric epilepsy. *Epilepsia* **48,** 1083–1091.

Sironi, V. A., Franzini, A., Ravagnati, L., and Marossero, F. (1979). Interictal acute psychoses in temporal lobe epilepsy during withdrawal of anticonvulsant therapy. *J. Neurol. Neurosurg. Psychiatry* **42,** 724–730.

Slater, E., Beard, A. W., and Glithero, E. (1963). The schizophrenialike psychoses of epilepsy. *Br. J. Psychiatry* **109**, 95–150.

Smith, D. B., Mattson, R. H., Cramer, J. A., Collins, J. F., Novelly, R. A., and Craft, B. (1987). Results of a nationwide Veterans Administration Cooperative Study comparing the efficacy and toxicity of carbamazepine, phenobarbital, phenytoin, and primidone. *Epilepsia* **28**(Suppl. 3), S50–S58.

Smith, M. L., Stagno, S. J., Dolske, M., Kosalko, J., McConnell, C., Kaspar, L., and Lederman, R. (1997). Induction procedures for psychogenic seizures: Ethical and clinical considerations. *J. Clin. Ethics* **8**, 217–229.

Stahl, S. M. (2000). "Essential Psychopharmacology: Neuroscientific Basis and Practical Applications" Cambridge University Press, Cambridge, UK; New York, NY.

Swingle, P. G. (1998). Neurofeedback treatment of pseudoseizure disorder. *Biol. Psychiatry* **44**, 1196–1199.

Swinkels, J., and Jonghe, F. (1995). Safety of antidepressants. *Int. Clin. Psychopharmacol.* **9**, 19–25.

Swinkels, W. A., Kuyk, J., van Dyck, R., and Spinhoven, P. (2005). Psychiatric comorbidity in epilepsy. *Epilepsy Behav.* **7**, 37–50.

Swinkels, W. A., van Emde Boas, W., Kuyk, J., van Dyck, R., and Spinhoven, P. (2006). Interictal depression, anxiety, personality traits, and psychological dissociation in patients with temporal lobe epilepsy (TLE) and extra-TLE. *Epilepsia* **47**, 2092–2103.

Task Force on DSM-IV (1994). "Diagnostic and Statistical Manual of Mental Disorders: DSM-IV." American Psychiatric Association, Washington, DC.

Taylor, D. C. (1972). Mental state and temporal lobe epilepsy. A correlative account of 100 patients treated surgically. *Epilepsia* **13**, 727–765.

Tellez-Zenteno, J. F., Patten, S. B., Jette, N., Williams, J., and Wiebe, S. (2007). Psychiatric comorbidity in epilepsy: A population-based analysis. *Epilepsia* **48**, 2336–2344.

Testa, S. M., Szaflarski, J. P., Fargo, J. D., Dulay, M. F., and Schefft, B. K. (2003). Abstract [P05.097] Psychological correlates of health-related quality of life (HRQOL) in epileptic and nonepileptic seizures. *Neurology* **60**, A383.

Testa, S. M., Schefft, B. K., Szaflarski, J. P., Yeh, H. S., and Privitera, M. D. (2007). Mood, personality, and health-related quality of life in epileptic and psychogenic seizure disorders. *Epilepsia* **48**, 973–982.

Tiihonen, J., Nousiainen, U., Hakola, P., Leinonen, E., Tuunainen, A., Mervaala, E., and Paanila, J. (1991). EEG abnormalities associated with clozapine treatment. *Am. J. Psychiatry.* **148**, 1406.

Toth, P., and Frankenburg, F. R. (1994). Clozapine and seizures: A review. *Can. J. Psychiatry* **39**, 236–238.

Trimble, M. R. (1992). Behaviour changes following temporal lobectomy, with special reference to psychosis. *J. Neurol. Neurosurg. Psychiatry* **55**, 89–91.

Trimble, M. R., and Schmitz, B. (2002). "The Neuropsychiatry of Epilepsy," p. x, 350 p.: ill.: 26 cm. Cambridge University Press, Cambridge, UK; New York.

Umbricht, D., Degreef, G., Barr, W. B., Lieberman, J. A., Pollack, S., and Schaul, N. (1995). Postictal and chronic psychoses in patients with temporal lobe epilepsy. *Am. J. Psychiatry* **152**, 224–231.

Vazquez, B., and Devinsky, O. (2003). Epilepsy and anxiety. *Epilepsy Behav.* **4**, S20–S25.

Wada, K., Iwasa, H., Okada, M., Kawata, Y., Murakami, T., Kamata, A., Zhu, G., Osanai, T., Kato, T., and Kaneko, S. (2004). Marital status of patients with epilepsy with special reference to the influence of epileptic seizures on the patient's married life. *Epilepsia* **45**(Suppl. 8), 33–36.

Walczak, T. S., Papacostas, S., Williams, D. T., Scheuer, M. L., Lebowitz, N., and Notarfrancesco, A. (1995). Outcome after diagnosis of psychogenic nonepileptic seizures. *Epilepsia* **36**, 1131–1137.

Weil, A. A. (1955). Depressive reactions associated with temporal lobe-uncinate seizure. *J. Nerv. Ment. Dis.* **121**, 505–510.

Westbrook, L. E., Devinsky, O., and Geocadin, R. (1998). Nonepileptic seizures after head injury. *Epilepsia* **39**, 978–982.

Whitworth, A. B., and Fleischhacker, W. W. (1995). Adverse effects of antipsychotic drugs. *Int. Clin. Psychopharmacol.* **9**(Suppl. 5), 21–27.

Williams, D. (1956). The structure of emotions reflected in epileptic experiences. *Brain* **79**, 29–67.

Wolf, P., and Trimble, M. R. (1985). Biological antagonism and epileptic psychosis. *Br. J. Psychiatry* **146**, 272–276.

Wyllie, E., Friedman, D., Luders, H., Morris, H., Rothner, D., and Turnbull, J. (1991). Outcome of psychogenic seizures in children and adolescents compared with adults. *Neurology* **41**, 742–744.

Wyllie, E., Glazer, J. P., Benbadis, S., Kotagal, P., and Wolgamuth, B. (1999). Psychiatric features of children and adolescents with pseudoseizures. *Arch. Pediatr. Adolesc. Med.* **153**, 244–248.

Zaroff, C. M., Myers, L. B., Barr, W., Luciano, D., and Devinsky, O. (2004). Group psychoeducation as treatment for psychological nonepileptic seizures. *Epilepsy Behav.* **5**, 587–592.

Ziegler, F. J., and Imboden, J. B. (1962). Contemporary conversion reactions. II. A conceptual model. *Arch. Gen. Psychiatry* **6**, 279–287.

ISSUES FOR MATURE WOMEN WITH EPILEPSY

Cynthia L. Harden

Department of Neurology, Leonard M. Miller School of Medicine,
University of Miami, Miami, Florida, USA

I. Introduction
II. Premature Ovarian Failure: Early Onset Perimenopause and Menopause
III. Changes in Seizures Related to Perimenopause and Menopause
IV. Hormone Replacement Therapy in Women with Epilepsy
V. Menopause and HRT in Animal Seizure Models
VI. AED Treatment in the Elderly
VII. Conclusion
References

Specific concerns regarding mature women with epilepsy (WWE), specifically epilepsy-associated issues during perimenopause, menopause, and postmenopause, have been emerging in the epilepsy community. This chapter presents evidence that for WWE, seizure frequency may increase during perimenopause and decrease at postmenopause, especially if a catamenial epilepsy pattern was present during the reproductive years. This finding implies that, as in other age groups, a subset of mature WWE are particularly susceptible to endogenous reproductive hormonal changes. An adverse effect on seizure frequency with the use of hormone replacement therapy (HRT) during postmenopause for WWE was reported in surveys, and a dose-related association between standard HRT and increased seizures was later borne out in a double-blind, placebo-controlled, randomized clinical trial. Management of symptomatic postmenopausal WWE using estrogenic and progestogenic compounds that are less likely to promote seizures is discussed.

WWE are at risk for premature ovarian failure and for menopause at a younger age than the general population. This appears to be related to epilepsy severity in terms of seizure frequency and is likely a consequence of adverse effects of seizures and interictal activity on the hypothalamo–pituitary–gonadal axis.

The decline in antiepileptic drug (AED) clearance, as well as alterations in gastric functioning and decreasing albumin levels, with maturity can affect AED use in the aging population; therefore, mature individuals with epilepsy need to be monitored carefully for toxicity and for increasing AED levels that could eventually cause toxicity. Information about gender differences for AED use in the mature population is scant.

INTERNATIONAL REVIEW OF
NEUROBIOLOGY, VOL. 83
DOI: 10.1016/S0074-7742(08)00021-4

385

I. Introduction

Women with epilepsy (WWE) in perimenopause, menopause, and perimenopause often have many questions regarding the effect of these life changes on their epilepsy. In this chapter, associations between these life changes in WWE, seizure frequency, and the use of hormone replacement therapy (HRT) will be presented. Alterations in the expected age at menopause found in several studies will be explored as well as the mechanisms by which this could occur. General antiepileptic drug (AED) biopharmaceutical concerns in the mature population will be presented, although there is little gender-specific information in this area. Suggestions for management of mature WWE, both for the use of HRT and AEDs, will be discussed.

II. Premature Ovarian Failure: Early Onset Perimenopause and Menopause

WWE have a risk of experiencing an early onset of perimenopausal symptoms, often in the late fourth decade or early fifth decade of life (Klein *et al.*, 2001). Klein *et al.* described that 7 of 50 WWE had symptoms or hormonal findings of premature ovarian failure before the age of 42 years, compared to 3 of 82 healthy control women, determining a risk of early perimenopause 4 times greater in WWE than in controls. Furthermore, the severity of epilepsy (i.e., the seizure frequency) is related to a risk for earlier menopause (Harden *et al.*, 2003). Within a group of WWE, those who had only rare seizures (e.g., fewer than 20 in a lifetime) had less risk for earlier menopause and had a normal age at menopause of 50–51 years. However, WWE who had frequent seizures, occurring at least monthly, experienced earlier menopause, at age 46–47 years on average (see Table I). In this study, there was no relationship between early menopause and specific AED

TABLE I
MENOPAUSAL AGE CORRELATED WITH SEIZURE FREQUENCY

Seizure frequency	Number of patients	Mean age	Mean age at last menses[a]
<20 seizures in lifetime	15	55	49.9
>20 seizures in lifetime; <1 seizure per month	25	54	47.7
>1 seizure per month	28	52	46.7

Adapted from Harden *et al.* (2003)
[a]Significantly different between groups ($p = 0.04$).

treatments. Therefore, it is postulated that early menopause is another consequence of reproductive dysfunction caused by epilepsy itself (Harden *et al.*, 2003).

III. Changes in Seizures Related to Perimenopause and Menopause

Although no prospective information is available on the course of epilepsy as WWE progress through perimenopause, menopause, and postmenopause, a questionnaire study was performed in order to obtain information about the effect of menopause and perimenopause on the course of epilepsy. Further, the questionnaire assessed whether a history of a catamenial seizure pattern would influence this course (Harden *et al.*, 1999). These questionnaires were sent to WWE using a mailing list from the local epilepsy consumer advocacy organizations; responses were used from women currently in menopause or perimenopause; respondents who did not have AED changes during these life epochs provided information regarding the course of their epilepsy and treatment, seizure type, relationship of seizures to menses during their reproductive years, specifically the occurrence of seizures in the week before menses and at the onset of menses [catamenial seizure pattern type 1 (Herzog *et al.*, 1997)], and any use of HRT.

Thirty-nine perimenopausal WWE (ages 38–55 years) as defined by a recent change in menstrual pattern and the occurrence of "hot flushes" responded. Nine subjects reported no change in seizures at perimenopause, 5 reported a decrease in seizure frequency, and the majority of women, 25, reported an increase. Twenty-eight (72%) reported having a catamenial seizure pattern before menopause, and eight (15%) subjects took synthetic HRT. HRT had no significant effect on seizures; however, a history of catamenial seizure pattern was significantly associated with an increase in seizures at perimenopause ($p = 0.02$) (see Fig. 1). Considering that estrogen is generally proconvulsant and progesterone is anticonvulsant in animal seizure models (Scharfman and MacLusky, 2006), it can be postulated that reproductive hormonal changes in perimenopause could contribute to increased seizures. Further explanation of this influence is as follows: during perimenopause, estrogen levels remain unchanged or may rise with age until the onset of menopause, presumably in response to the elevated follicle-stimulating hormone (FSH) levels. However, the cyclic progesterone elevation during the luteal phase of the menstrual cycle gradually becomes less frequent throughout perimenopause, resulting in increasing rates of anovulatory cycles (Burger *et al.*, 2002). The elevation of the estrogen-to-progesterone ratio may contribute to the increase in seizure frequency at perimenopause for some WWE.

Forty-two postmenopausal WWE (ages 41–86 years), defined as 1 year without menses, responded. There was no overall directional change in seizure frequency within this group: 12 subjects reported no change in seizures at menopause, 17 reported a decrease in seizure frequency, and 13 reported an increase. Sixteen (38%) took synthetic HRT. Sixteen (38%) additional subjects (having some overlap with the HRT group) reported having a catamenial seizure pattern before menopause. HRT was significantly associated with an increase in seizures during perimenopause ($p = 0.001$). A history of catamenial seizure pattern was significantly associated with a decrease in seizures at menopause ($p = 0.013$) (see Fig. 2) (Harden *et al.*, 1999).

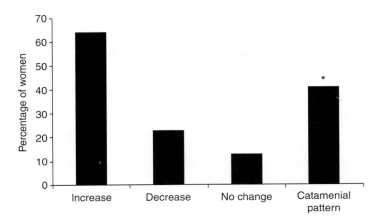

FIG. 1. Perimenopausal women-epilepsy pattern. *Significantly associated with an increase in seizures ($p = 0.02$) Harden (1999).

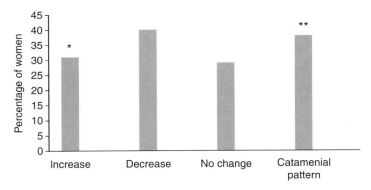

FIG. 2. Postmenopausal women—epilepsy pattern. **Significantly associated with a decrease in seizures ($p = 0.013$). *Hormone replacement therapy (HRT) was associated with seizure exacerbation ($p = 0.001$) Harden (1999).

These cross-sectional data suggest that WWE may be likely to have an increase in seizures at perimenopause and, therefore, may need more careful monitoring at this time for AED adjustment or AED change. Further, these findings indicate that catamenial seizure pattern may be associated with seizure increase during perimenopause but seizure decrease after menopause. This findings are also consistent with the idea that a subset of WWE are especially sensitive to endogenous hormonal changes, associated with increased seizures in response to hormonal fluctuations, but decreased seizures when reproductive hormones stabilize. Further, the results suggest that synthetic HRT may be associated with an increase in seizure frequency in menopausal WWE. The implications of this finding prompted further study whether such an effect of endogenous hormones on WWE was present.

IV. Hormone Replacement Therapy in Women with Epilepsy

The evaluation of HRT in WWE was designed to determine whether adding HRT to the medication regimen of postmenopausal WWE was associated with an increase in seizure frequency (Harden *et al.*, 2006). The study design was a double-blind, randomized, placebo-controlled trial of the effect of HRT on seizure frequency in postmenopausal WWE. Women took stable doses of AEDs, and were within 10 years of their last menses. After a 3-month prospective baseline, subjects were randomized to placebo, Prempro (0.625 mg of conjugated equine estrogens plus 2.5 mg of medroxyprogesterone acetate or CEE/MPA) daily, or double-dose CEE/MPA daily for a 3-month treatment period. This form of HRT was chosen for the trial because it was widely used at the time. Further, it was the same treatment used in the large, long-term, placebo-controlled The Women's Health Initiative (WHI) study which looked at multiple medical outcomes. Therefore, the use of this complex equine-derived estrogen and this synthetic progestin in the WWE study would be appropriate in the WWE trial because the results could be extrapolated to the general population of WWE. Further, this was the most commonly used form of HRT reported in the questionnaire study. The results were analyzed by chi-square for trend, comparing the number of subjects whose seizure frequency increased on treatment compared to baseline versus the number of subjects whose seizures did not increase across treatment arms.

Unfortunately, the first report of the WHI results in 2002 was that HRT in the form of CEE/MPA was associated with an increased risk for breast cancer and stroke (Rossouw *et al.*, 2002). These results were surprising in the light of the long use of this compound, but lead to early termination of the WHI trial as well as the HRT in WWE study due to safety concerns.

Therefore, only 21 subjects were randomized after completing baseline. The subjects' ages ranged from 45 to 62 years (mean, 53 years; SD, ±5), and the number of AEDs used ranged from 0 to 3 (median,1). There were no differences in baseline characteristics including age, age at menopause, number of AEDs, and complex partial and generalized seizure frequency between the three treatment arms.

On HRT treatment compared to placebo, there was a significant trend toward increased seizures in a dose-related manner using several seizure frequency analyses. Five (71%) of seven subjects taking double-dose CEE/MPA had a worsening seizure frequency of at least one seizure type, compared with four (50%) of eight taking single-dose CEE/MPA, and one (17%) of six taking placebo ($p = 0.05$). An increase in seizure frequency of the subject's most severe seizure type was associated with increasing CEE/MPA dose ($p = 0.008$). An increase in complex partial seizure frequency also was associated with increasing CEE/MPA dose ($p = 0.05$) (see Table II). Total seizure number approached significance with increasing CEE/MPA ($p = 0.10$) as well.

Two subjects taking lamotrigine had a decrease of 25–30% in lamotrigine levels while taking CEE/MPA. This is likely due to induction of uridine diphosphate–glucuronosyltransferase (UGT) 1A4 by ethinyl estradiol, which is the predominant metabolic enzyme for lamotrigine, as occurs with hormonal contraceptives (Harden and Leppik, 2006). Therefore, although the small numbers of subjects in this study may limit its generalizability, the results indicate that CEE/MPA is associated with a dose-related increase in seizure frequency in

TABLE II

NUMBER OF SUBJECTS WITH INCREASE IN SEIZURE FREQUENCY BY TREATMENT ARM ($N = 21$)

Treatment group	Simple partial[a]		Complex partial[b]		Secondarily generalized		Total # Sz[c]		Any Sz type[d]		Most severe Sz type[e]	
	n	%	n	%	n	%	n	%	n	%	n	%
Placebo ($n = 6$)	1	16.7	0	0.0	0	0.0	0	0.0	1	16.7	0	0.0
Single CEE/ MPA ($n = 8$)	3	37.5	1	12.5	0	0.0	3	37.5	4	50.0	3	37.5
Double CEE/ MPA ($n = 7$)	1	14.3	3	42.9	1	14.3	3	42.9	5	71.4	5	71.4

Harden et al. (2006).

CEE, conjugated equine estrogens; MPA, medroxyprogesterone acetate.

[a] $p = 0.88$ by chi-square test for trend.
[b] $p = 0.05$ by chi-square test for trend.
[c] $p = 0.10$ by chi-square test for trend.
[d] $p = 0.05$ by chi-square test for trend.
[e] $p = 0.008$ by chi-square test for trend.

postmenopausal WWE. Further, the lamotrigine clearance may be increased with HRT as well.

V. Menopause and HRT in Animal Seizure Models

Although these two clinical reports have consistent outcomes of adverse effects of HRT on seizures, there are no supportive laboratory counterparts of these findings. As an analogous state to menopause, ovariectomy in adult female rat is associated with increased seizure activity in using standard seizure-producing techniques. Using the pilocarpine model, ovariectomized rats showed a significantly more rapid progression to status epilepticus compared with intact animals (Scharfman *et al.*, 2005). With an NMDA seizure-induction model, ovariectomized rats had a significantly increased total seizure number and more severe hippocampal damage compared with age-matched intact female animals (Kalkbrenner and Standley, 2003).

As an analogous state to HRT during menopause, what laboratory evidence is available for how hormone replacement affects seizure activity in a rodent postmenopausal model? Again, contrary to the findings of the recent human studies, several experiments have shown an overall neuroprotective effect of estrogen and progesterone, but little effect on seizure frequency. In a kainate-induced model, estrogen pretreatment had no effect on seizure severity but significantly decreased "spread," neuronal loss, and mortality in ovariectomized rats compared with ovariectomized rats without pretreatment. Progesterone pre-treatment in this model had a slightly different effects; it decreased seizure severity and hippocampal damage (Hoffman *et al.*, 2003). In the NMDA-induced model, estrogen pretreatment decreased total seizure number in ovariectomized rats compared with ovariectomized rats without pretreatment; and in fact, estrogen replacement restored seizure number to that of the intact state (Kalkbrenner and Standley, 2003). In the lithium–pilocarpine model of status epilepticus, estrogen pretreatment is neuroprotective in ovariectomized rats compared with sham-treated ovariectomized controls (Galanopoulou *et al.*, 2003).

Several factors may explain why these laboratory results cannot be extrapolated to the effects of HRT on menopausal WWE. First, ovariectomized rats likely do not have an analogous hormonal brain milieu to naturally menopausal women. The rats were not in surgical postmenopause for a matter of days prior to the experiments, in contrast to postmenopausal women who had years to develop changes to neurons and glia following hormone withdrawal. Second, the doses of HRT used by menopausal women are actually relatively higher than the doses used in these laboratory experiments. Finally, it is possible that the synthetic progestin, MPA, used in human studies could account for the adverse effects on seizures. It is widely accepted that estrogen generally promotes seizure activity, while progesterone (through the action of its reduced metabolite, allopregnanolone) has anticonvulsant properties (Scharfman and MacLusky, 2006). However, MPA clearly has a different profile of activity in the brain, in that it is not metabolized to allopregnanolone and is not neuroprotective in rodents (Ciriza et al., 2006). In one study of ovariectomized rats with and without estrogen replacement, the effect of progesterone versus MPA pretreatment on kainate-induced seizures produced quite differing results for the two compounds. Both progesterone and MPA blocked the neuroprotective effects of estrogen in these experiments (a result differing from previous experiments for progesterone as well), and seizure severity was worse but not significantly so in the MPA-treated group (Rosario et al., 2006). Therefore, several factors, including the possibility of an adverse effect of MPA on seizures, may account for the divergence of the laboratory and clinical experiments.

Since progesterone in its natural form in the FDA-approved form of Prometrium is readily available, it may be a reasonable option as the progestin component when HRT is needed for WWE, especially since there is evidence that it has active anticonvulsant properties (Herzog, 1999). For the estrogen component, a simplified estrogen compound, such as 17-β-estradiol, could be considered. Clinicians must consider these options since HRT will be needed for some WWE; sleep deprivation related to "hot flushes" can have an adverse effect on seizure frequency and, in such cases, HRT may be beneficial by permitting adequate sleep (Peebles et al., 2000).

VI. AED Treatment in the Elderly

One consistent alteration with maturity in the pharmacokinetics of both standard and newer AEDs is a decline in overall clearance of 20–40%. This change is variable and difficult to predict within an individual, and is influenced by medical comorbidities and drug–drug interactions. However, the decline in clearance can be at least partly attributed to a decrease in renal excretion rate and to reduced drug metabolism, both of which decline with age. Another factor important for toxicity related to highly protein-bound AEDs is the decrease in serum albumin that occurs with aging (Perucca, 2007).

Carbamazepine and phenytoin plasma concentrations are more variable in the elderly compared to the adult population, due to alterations in absorption rather than a relatively minor effect on half-life (Cloyd et al., 2007). Variable drug absorption in the elderly is due to slower gastric emptying time and to slower fluctuations in gastric pH in this age group. This could have implications in particular for the absorption of phenytoin, which is itself a weakly acidic drug that absorbs more completely in a gastric environment with higher pH and less well in a lower pH environment (Gidal, 2007).

In addition to the biopharmaceutical considerations in the mature age group, there is some information available on efficacy and tolerability. One randomized, double-blind clinical trial of the treatment of new-onset epilepsy in the elderly showed equal efficacy for the gabapentin, carbamazepine, and lamotrigine treatment arms in 593 randomized subjects. However, lamotrigine was associated with significantly fewer terminations for adverse events than carmbamazepine or gabapentin (Rowan *et al.*, 2005). There is little information regarding gender differences in AED treatment for the mature population. One report of phenytoin use in elderly nursing home residents found that women took higher doses than did men in order to achieve similar serum concentrations, although no other obvious factors, such as complications that would affect phenytoin metabolism or albumin levels, differed between genders.

VII. Conclusion

WWE are at risk for premature ovarian failure and menopause at a younger age than expected. This appears to be related to epilepsy severity in terms of seizure frequency and is likely a consequence of adverse effects of seizures and interictal activity on the hypothalamo–pituitary–gonadal axis.

Overall, WWE seem to be at risk for increased seizure frequency at perimenopause. The presence of a catamenial seizure pattern is especially associated with increased seizures at perimenopause, but decreased seizures after menopause. This finding provides further support for the presence of a subset of WWE, who are particularly sensitive to the neuroactivity of the endogenous hormonal milieu.

A risk of increased seizures with HRT consisting of CEE and MPA appears to be present in postmenopausal WWE, found in a cross-sectional questionnaire and a randomized, double-blinded, placebo-controlled clinical trial. Yet WWE will need to take HRT at times, for symptomatic relief and to allow adequate sleep when "hot flushes" are disruptive. The author suggests that a combination of a single estrogenic compound such as 17-β-estradiol along with natural progesterone be considered in this clinical scenario.

The decline in AED clearance, as well as alterations in gastric functioning and decreasing albumin levels, with maturity can affect AED use in the aging population. These changes could impact all AEDs, but phenytoin is most at risk for having an altered biopharmaceutical profile in the elderly since all of these mechanisms are involved in phenytoin use. Mature individuals with epilepsy need to be monitored carefully for toxicity and for increasing AED levels that could eventually cause toxicity. There is little information about gender differences for AED use in the mature population.

References

Burger, H. G., Dudley, E. C., Robertson, D. M., and Dennerstein, L. (2002). Hormonal changes in the menopause transition. *Recent Prog. Horm. Res.* **57,** 257–275.

Ciriza, I., Carrero, P., Frye, C. A., and Garcia-Segura, L. M. (2006). Reduced metabolites mediate neuroprotective effects of progesterone in the adult rat hippocampus. The synthetic progestin medroxyprogesterone acetate (Provera) is not neuroprotective. *J. Neurobiol.* **66,** 916–928.

Cloyd, J. C., Marino, S., and Birnbaum, A. K. (2007). Factors affecting antiepileptic drug pharmacokinetics in community-dwelling elderly. *Int. Rev. Neurobiol.* **81,** 201–210.

Galanopoulou, A. S., Alm, E. M., and Velísková, J. (2003). Estradiol reduces seizure-induced hippocampal injury in ovariectomized female but not in male rats. *Neurosci. Lett.* **342**(3), 201–205.

Gidal, B. E. (2007). Antiepileptic drug formulation and treatment in the elderly: Biopharmaceutical considerations. *Int. Rev. Neurobiol.* **81,** 299–311.

Harden, C. L., and Leppik, I. (2006). Optimizing therapy of seizures in women who use oral contraceptives. *Neurology* **67**(12 Suppl 4), S56–S58.

Harden, C. L., Pulver, M. C., and Jacobs, A. R. (1999). The effect of menopause and perimenopause on the course of epilepsy. *Epilepsia* **40,** 1402–1407.

Harden, C. L., Koppel, B. S., Herzog, A. G., Nikolov, B. G., and Hauser, W. A. (2003). Seizure frequency is associated with age of menopause in women with epilepsy. *Neurology* **61,** 451–455.

Harden, C. L., Herzog, A. G., Nikolov, B. G., Koppel, B. S., Christos, P. J., Fowler, K., Labar, D. R., and Hauser, W. A. (2006). Hormone replacement therapy in women with epilepsy: A randomized, double-blind, placebo-controlled study. *Epilepsia* **47**(9), 1447–1451.

Herzog, A. G. (1999). Progesterone therapy in women with epilepsy: A 3-year follow-up. *Neurology* **52,** 1917–1918.

Herzog, A. G., Klein, P., and Ransil, B. J. (1997). Three patterns of catamenial epilepsy. *Epilepsia* **38** (10), 1082–1088.

Hoffman, G. E., Moore, N., Fiskum, G., and Murphy, A. Z. (2003). Ovarian steroid modulation of seizure severity and hippocampal cell death after kainic acid treatment. *Exp. Neurol.* **182**(1), 124–134.

Kalkbrenner, K. A., and Standley, C. A. (2003). Estrogen modulation of NMDA-induced seizures in ovariectomized and non-ovariectomized rats. *Brain Res.* **964**(2), 244–249.

Klein, P., Serje, A., and Pezzullo, J. C. (2001). Premature ovarian failure in women with epilepsy. *Epilepsia* **42,** 1584–1589.

Peebles, C. T., McAuley, J. W., Moore, J. L., Malone, H. J., and Reeves, A. L. (2000). Hormone replacement therapy in a postmenopausal woman with epilepsy. *Ann. Pharmacother.* **34**(9), 1028–1031.

Perucca, E. (2007). Age-related changes in pharmacokinetics: Predictability and assessment methods. *Int. Rev. Neurobiol.* **81,** 183–199.

Rosario, E. R., Ramsden, M., and Pike, C. J. (2006). Progestins inhibit the neuroprotective effects of estrogen in rat hippocampus. *Brain Res.* **1099**(1), 206–210.

Rossouw, J. E., Anderson, G. L., Prentice, R. L., *et al.* The Writing Group for the Women's Health Initiative Investigators (2002). Risks and benefits of estrogen plus progestin in healthy post-postmenopausal women: Principal results of the women's health initiative randomized, controlled trial. *JAMA* **288,** 321–333.

Rowan, A. J., Ramsay, R. E., Collins, J. F., Pryor, F., Boardman, K. D., Uthman, B. M., Spitz, M., Frederick, T., Towne, A., Carter, G. S., Marks, W., Felicetta, J., *et al.* VA Cooperative Study 428 Group (2005). New onset geriatric epilepsy: A randomized study of gabapentin, lamotrigine, and carbamazepine. *Neurology* **64**(11), 1868–1873.

Scharfman, H. E., and MacLusky, N. J. (2006). The influence of gonadal hormones on neuronal excitability, seizures, and epilepsy in the female. *Epilepsia* **47**(9), 1423–1440.

Scharfman, H. E., Goodman, J. H., Rigoulot, M. A., Berger, R. E., Walling, S. G., Mercurio, T. C., Stormes, K., and Maclusky, N. J. (2005). Seizure susceptibility in intact and ovariectomized female rats treated with the convulsant pilocarpine. *Exp. Neurol.* **196**(1), 73–86.

PHARMACODYNAMIC AND PHARMACOKINETIC INTERACTIONS OF PSYCHOTROPIC DRUGS WITH ANTIEPILEPTIC DRUGS

Andres M. Kanner* and Barry E. Gidal[†]

*Rush University Medical Center, Chicago, Illinois, USA
[†]School of Pharmacy and Department of Neurology,
University of Wisconsin, Madison, Wisconsin, USA

I. Introduction
II. The Use of Antidepressant Drugs in Epilepsy
  A. Impact on Seizure Threshold
  B. Pharmacokinetic Interactions with AEDs
  C. Pharmacodynamic Interactions with AEDs
III. Anxiolytic Drugs
  A. Pharmacokinetic Interactions with AEDs
  B. Pharmacodynamic Interactions with AEDs
IV. Lithium
  A. Pharmacokinetic Interactions with AEDs
  B. Pharmacodynamic Interactions with AEDs
V. CNS Stimulants
  A. Impact on Seizure Threshold
VI. Other Treatment for ADHD: Atomoxetine
  A. Impact on Seizure Threshold
  B. Pharmacokinetic Interactions of CNSS with AEDs
  C. Pharmacodynamic Interactions of CNSS with AEDs
VII. Antipsychotic Drugs
  A. Impact on Seizure Threshold
  B. Pharmacokinetic Interactions with AEDs
  C. Pharmacodynamic Interactions with AEDs
VIII. Concluding Remarks
  References

Co-morbid psychiatric disorders are relatively frequent in patients with epilepsy. The prevalence rates of mood and anxiety disorders, psychotic disorders and attention deficit/hyperactivity disorder have been found to be significantly higher in patients with epilepsy than in the general population. While co-morbid psychiatric disorders have frequently been considered as complications of the seizure disorder, there is an increasing body of literature that points to a complex relationship between psychiatric and seizure disorders. Because of this, it is crucial that clinicians consider the presence of co-morbid psychiatric disorders when planning the treatment of patients with epilepsy. Having a clear understanding

INTERNATIONAL REVIEW OF
NEUROBIOLOGY, VOL. 83
DOI: 10.1016/S0074-7742(08)00022-6

397

of the pharmacodynamic and pharmacokinetic interactions between antiepileptic drugs and psychotropic drugs is of the essence to avert unnecessary adverse events and loss of efficacy of psychotropic drugs. This chapter provides a practical review on the use of psychotropic drugs for the treatment of these psychiatric co-morbidities in patients with epilepsy.

I. Introduction

Co-morbid psychiatric disorders are relatively frequent in patients with epilepsy (Tellez-Zenteno et al., 2007). The prevalence rates of mood and anxiety disorders, psychotic disorders and attention deficit/ hyperactivity disorder (ADHD) have been found to be significantly higher in patients with epilepsy than in the general population (Dunn and Austin, 1999; Edeh and Toone, 1987; Jacoby et al., 1996; Matsuura, et al., 2005). While co-morbid psychiatric disorders have "typically" been considered as complications of the seizure disorder, or the underlying neurologic condition that caused the epilepsy, there is an increasing body of literature that points to a complex relationship between psychiatric and seizure disorders. In the case of mood disorders and ADHD, there is evidence of a bidirectional relationship between these disorders and epilepsy (Forsgren and Nystrom, 1999; Hesdorffer et al., 2000, 2004, 2006). For example, Hesdorffer et al. found that compared to the expected occurrence rate in the general population, ADHD of the inattentive type occurred 3.7 times more often (95% CI, 1.1–12.8) *before* unprovoked seizures in a population-based case-control study of all newly diagnosed unprovoked seizures among Icelandic children younger than 16 years (aged 3–16 years) (Hesdorffer et al., 2004). The association was restricted to ADHD predominantly of the inattentive type. Data suggestive of a bidirectional relationship between depression and epilepsy were suggested in three population-based case-control studies of patients with newly diagnosed adult-onset epilepsy (Forsgren and Nystrom, 1999; Hesdorffer et al., 2000, 2006). These studies suggested that patients with new-onset epilepsy had a four- to sevenfold higher likelihood of having experienced a depressive episode or suicidal ideation preceding the onset of epilepsy compared to matched controls.

Psychotic disorders are also more frequent in patients with epilepsy than in the general population. While population-based data are not as frequent as that of the other psychiatric disorders, it is estimated that the prevalence rate of psychotic disorders ranges between 6% and 10% in patients with epilepsy compared to 1% in the general population (Matsuura et al., 2005).

Furthermore, other studies have demonstrated the presence of psychiatric disorders in patients with new-onset idiopathic epilepsy by the time of the first seizure. For example, in a population-based study, Austin *et al.* identified higher rates of behaviour disturbances in children with new-onset epilepsy than in their siblings, in the 6 months *preceding* the first recognized seizure (Austin *et al.*, 2001). The psychopathology included symptoms of mood and anxiety disorders, attention disturbances, and thought and somatic complaints. In a study of 50 children and adolescents with new-onset epilepsy and 53 age-matched controls, Jones *et al.* found a significantly higher prevalence of mood and anxiety disorders and ADHD in patients with idiopathic or cryptogenic epilepsy than in controls (Jones, *et al.*, 2007). Among the children with co-morbid psychopathology, 45% already presented a psychiatric disorder (according to *DSMIV-TR* diagnostic criteria) at the time of the diagnosis of epilepsy.

Clearly, these data document the need to factor-in the presence of co-morbid psychiatric disorders when planning the treatment of patients with epilepsy. Having a clear understanding of the pharmacodynamic and pharmacokinetic interactions between antiepileptic drugs (AEDs) and psychotropic drugs is of the essence to avert unnecessary adverse events and loss of efficacy of psychotropic drugs. This chapter provides a practical review on the use of psychotropic drugs for the treatment of these psychiatric co-morbidities in patients with epilepsy.

II. The Use of Antidepressant Drugs in Epilepsy

Antidepressant drugs are the most frequently prescribed psychotropic drugs in patients with epilepsy; they are used for the management of mood and anxiety disorders, including panic, generalized anxiety and obsessive-compulsive disorders as well as social phobia.

A. IMPACT ON SEIZURE THRESHOLD

There is a widespread concern among clinicians to prescribe this type of drug in patients with epilepsy, given a reported "proconvulsant" effect in patients without epilepsy. Yet, a review of the literature reveals the following fact: Seizures have been reported in patients who took overdoses or in whom high serum concentrations were identified, because they were "slow metabolizers"; most of these data were derived from trials with tricyclic antidepressants (TCAs). Furthermore, in assessing the seizure occurrence in patients treated with antidepressant drugs, it is necessary to factor-in the bidirectional relationship between depression and epilepsy alluded to above, which implies an increased risk of depressed patients to experience an epileptic seizure compared to non-depressed people (Forsgren and Nystrom, 1999; Hesdorffer *et al.*, 2000, 2006). Thus, is it possible that a seizure experienced by a depressed patient be the expression of that inherent risk and not related to the use of an antidepressant? Recent studies seem to support this hypothesis. Alper *et al.* compared published rates of unprovoked seizures in the general population and the seizure incidence in patients randomized to placebo and one of the selective serotonin reuptake inhibitors (SSRIs) or mirtazapine in phase II and III regulatory clinical trials submitted to the Food and Drug Administration between 1985 and 2004 (Alper *et al.*, 2007). The incidence of seizures was *significantly lower* among patients *randomized to antidepressants* compared to those given placebo (standardized incidence ratio = 0.48; 95% CI, 0.36–0.61). The seizure incidence was 19 times higher than the published incidence of unprovoked seizures in community non-patient samples in patients randomized to placebo. These data support the findings of population-based studies cited above demonstrating a higher risk of seizures and epilepsy in depressed patients and also indicate that SSRIs can be used safely in patients with epilepsy.

Furthermore, uncontrolled studies in humans with refractory epilepsy have suggested an improvement in seizure frequency in patients with refractory epilepsy treated with fluoxetine and citalopram. For example, Favale *et al.* treated 17 patients with refractory epilepsy with 20 mg of fluoxetine per day in an open trial; six patients became seizure free (Favale *et al.*, 1995). No patient was reported to have an increase in seizure frequency. Of note, since fluoxetine can inhibit the metabolism of several AEDs, the investigators monitored their serum concentrations on a monthly basis. They ruled out an increase in AEDs' serum concentrations as a possible explanation for the improvement in seizure frequency. The same group of investigators treated 11 patients with refractory epilepsy without depression with citalopram at a dosage of 20 mg/day in an open trial (Favale *et al.*, 2003). Nine patients experienced a reduction of at least 50% in seizure frequency, and no patient was reported to have had an increase in seizure frequency. By the same token, Speccio *et al.* reported a 37% overall reduction in seizure frequency in an open trial of citalopram for the treatment of depression in 39 patients with epilepsy (Specchio *et al.*, 2004).

Anticonvulsant effects have been reported with the use of TCAs, specifically imipramine. For example, Fromm *et al.* treated 16 patients with absence and myoclonic seizures in an open trial of imipramine and reported initial reductions in seizure frequency in 10 patients (Fromm *et al.*, 1972). Following this open trial, these investigators carried out a double-blind crossover study with imipramine which yielded initial reductions in seizure frequency in 5 patients, which persisted at 1 year in 2 patients (Fromm *et al.*, 1978). Of note, serum imipramine levels in the patients who showed a long-term response ranged between 40 and 120 ng/ml, which corresponds to one half of the concentrations associated with the therapeutic effectiveness of imipramine for the treatment of depression. Hurst reported his experience with imipramine in an open trial of 15 patients with various types of seizure disorders that were refractory to AED therapy (Hurst, 1986); initial reductions of 80% in seizure frequency were found in 8 patients, particularly in patients with drop attacks, but not in those with partial seizures. Seizure improvement persisted at 1 year in 5 patients, 4 of whom remained completely seizure free.

1. Tricyclic Antidepressants

This was the first class of antidepressant drugs used in the pharmacologic treatment of depression and include eight agents. TCAs were reported to cause seizures in patients without epilepsy, primarily in the setting of *overdoses* or in patients who have *high serum concentrations* attributed to a genetically determined slow metabolic rate. Such proconvulsant effect is not mediated by serotonergic or noradrenergic mechanisms but rather, by their antihistaminergic effect (Ago *et al.*, 2006).

Among the family of TCAs, however, clomipramine was identified as an agent associated with a significantly higher incidence of seizures (1%), and thus it is not recommended that it be used in people with epilepsy (McConnell and Duncan, 1998). Two other antidepressant drugs in the TCA family, amoxepine and maprotiline, were also found to be associated with higher incidences of seizures and are also not recommended in this patient population. With the use of TCAs, it is recommended that the patient be started out at a low dose and that the titration upwards be done at a slow pace. Furthermore, serum concentrations of most antidepressants of this class are available, and it is recommended that they be measured once the desired dose is reached to identify those patients who may be "slow metabolizers". Nonetheless, given the relatively higher frequency of adverse events, which include cardio-toxic effects, their use should be restricted when safer antidepressant drugs such as SSRIs and serotonin-norepinephrine reuptake inhibitors (SNRIs) are not effective (see below).

2. Mono-Amino-Oxidase Inhibitors

This class of antidepressant drugs includes four drugs (McConnell and Duncan, 1998) and in general has been found to be safe in people with epilepsy. Their use, however, has been limited because of the potential adverse events associated with the ingestion of certain tyramine-containing foods that can result in hypertensive crisis. Mono-amino-oxidase inhibitors (MAOIs) today have been restricted to the management of certain patients with atypical depressions, severe anxiety disorders and borderline personality disorders. Since the advent of the SSRIs, MAOIs have been displaced to third-line treatment drugs; thus, psychiatrists should be the only ones prescribing this type of antidepressant drug.

3. Selective Serotonin Reuptake Inhibitors

This is the third family of antidepressants to become available for the treatment of mood and anxiety disorders. In fact, they have become the first-line treatment for these psychiatric entities. They include six drugs (fluoxetine, fluvoxamine, sertraline, paroxetine, citalopram and escitalopram), which have been found to be very safe in patients with epilepsy with respect to the risk of causing seizures. Some of these SSRIs have been used for the management of migraines and other pain disorders.

Occasional reports of seizures have been associated with overdoses or very high serum concentrations. In a study of 100 consecutive patients with pharmaco-resistant epilepsy who were treated with sertraline for a mood and/or anxiety disorder, Kanner et al. found a worsening of seizure frequency that could be attributed to sertraline in only one patient (Kanner et al., 2000).

4. Serotonin-Norepinephrine Reuptake Inhibitors

Serotonin-norepinephrine reuptake inhibitors: The experience with the newer antidepressant drugs in the family of SNRIs, venlafaxine and duloxetine, is very limited, but the incidence of seizures in the regulatory studies compared to placebo-exposed patients does not appear to be increased.

5. Dopamine-Norepinephrine Reuptake Inhibitors

Another class of antidepressant drugs is norepinephrine and dopamine reuptake Inhibitors. Bupropion has relatively weak reuptake properties of dopamine and norepinephrine, but its active hydroxylated metabolite has strong reuptake properties of these neurotransmitters and seems to be responsible for the efficacy of this agent. This drug is used for a certain type of depressive order (i.e. retarded depression), as well as for the management of ADHD. In one study, bupropion appeared to be relatively safe at dosages of up to 450 mg/day, with a seizure frequency ranging from 0.36% to 0.48% (Davidson, 1989). However, bulimic patients were found to be at increased risk of developing generalized tonic–clonic seizures (Horne et al., 1988; Pope et al., 1989). Lower seizure rates, however, were identified with extended- release formulations at dosages of 300 mg/day or less in a study of 3100 patients yielding a seizure frequency of 0.15% (Jefferson et al., 2005). This lower frequency of seizures suggests that avoidance of a peak of dose effect may have an important role in minimizing the proconvulsant properties of this antidepressant medication. Alper et al. found that depressed patients randomized to bupropion had a 1.6 times relative risk of developing seizures compared to those given placebo (Alper et al., 2007). If this medication is to be used today in patients with epilepsy, it should be started at a low dose and dosage should not exceed 300 mg/day. In general, it is recommended that the drug be avoided.

In summary, to date, antidepressant medications can be safely used in patients with epilepsy with drugs of the SSRI type being among the safest ones; TCAs can be safely used but should be started at low doses that can be increased slowly, and serum concentrations should be monitored to identify the patients who may be slow metabolizers. Clomipramine, maprotiline and amoxapine and bupropion as an immediate-release formulation, however, should be avoided in patients with epilepsy. MAOIs can be safely used in patients with epilepsy but should be prescribed only by psychiatrists.

B. PHARMACOKINETIC INTERACTIONS WITH AEDs

The majority of commonly employed psychotropic medications, including antidepressant as well as antipsychotic medications, are substrates for one or more of the cytochrome p450 (CYP) isozymes (Patsalos and Perucca, 2003). Therefore, co-medication with an enzyme-inducing AED would be expected to increase the systemic clearance of these medications, with the result being lower serum concentrations of the psychotropic agent. Given the likelihood of concomitant treatment with these medications, knowledge of potential drug interactions is important.

Older, traditional AEDs such as phenytoin, carbamazepine and phenobarbital are potent inducers of the CYP enzyme system, as well as the UDP-glucuronyl transferase (UGT) enzyme system In contrast, sodium valproate is not an inducer, but rather an inhibitor of certain CYP isozymes (CYP 2C19, 2C9) as well as UGT.

Among the newer generation AEDs, oxcarbazepine and topiramate are also inducers, but appear to be much less potent inducers of CYP 3A4. Other newer agents including gabapentin, pregabalin, levetiracetam, tiagabine, zonisamide and lamotrigine do not appear to interfere with CYP activity.

Clinically, the impact of enzyme induction on certain psychotropic drugs can be substantial. For example, serum concentrations of TCAs such as amitriptyline, nortriptyline, imipramine, desipramine, clomipramine, protriptyline and doxepin, as well as non-TCA agents such as sertraline, paroxetine, mianserin, citalopram and nefazodone, would be expected to be reduced in patients receiving enzyme-inducing AEDs (Trimble and Mula, 2005) Co-medication with enzyme-inducing AEDs such as phenytoin or carbamazepine may significantly reduce sertraline concentrations, and may require marked increases in dosage in order to maintain a therapeutic antidepressant response (Patsalos and Perucca, 2003). In contrast, co-medication with sodium valproate may result in significant increases (50–60%) in serum concentrations of antidepressants such as amitriptyline or nortriptyline (Trimble and Mula, 2005).

It is also important to recognize that AED–antidepressant drug interactions may be bidirectional. For example, anecdotal reports have suggested that SSRIs such as fluoxetine and sertraline have resulted in increased phenytoin and carbamazepine serum concentrations, likely due to fluoxetine inhibition of CYP 3A4 (Spina and Perucca, 2002). Fluoxetine inhibition of CYP 2C19 may also result in increases in serum phenytoin concentration. The active metabolite of fluoxetine, norfluoxetine, has also been shown to inhibit CYP 2D6. Inhibition of CYP 3A4, CYP 2C9 and CYP 2C19 is of the most relevance when considering potential effects on the currently available AEDs (Nelson *et al.*, 2001). *In vitro* experiments examining phenytoin parahydroxylation have found that between fluoxetine, norfluoxetine, sertraline and paroxetine, fluoxetine was the most potent inhibitor, followed by norfluoxetine, sertraline and to a lesser extent, paroxetine (Nelson *et al.*, 2001). While the *in vitro* data certainly suggest a potential pharmacokinetic interaction, they would also suggest that the likelihood of an interaction occurring is relatively low, particularly with paroxetine and sertraline when used at typical doses. Indeed, clinical studies did not find an interaction between either sertraline or paroxetine and carbamazepine or phenytoin (Andersen *et al.*, 1991).

The antidepressant fluvoxamine is an inhibitor of CYP 1A2, 3A4, 2C9 and 2C19. Inhibition of CYP 2C19 and 2C9 is likely to result in marked increases in phenytoin serum concentrations (Mamiya and Kojima, 2001).

In settings where higher SSRI doses are used, or perhaps in elderly patients who may have reduced clearance of both phenytoin and the SSRI, the potential for a clinically meaningful interaction may be increased (Nelson *et al.*, 2001). Nefazodone, a CYP 3A4 inhibitor, has been shown to increase carbamazepine serum concentrations (Laroudie and Salazar, 2000). SSRIs with the least potential for causing inhibitory interactions are citalopram and escitalopram. Venlafaxine and duloxetine also appear unlikely to cause significant interactions with currently available AEDs (Nelson *et al.*, 2001).

While there is less clinical data available regarding pharmacokinetic interactions between antidepressants and the newer generation AEDs, based upon our understanding of the metabolic disposition of these drugs, it would seem likely that there will be fewer pharmacokinetic interactions. Case reports have, however, suggested a possible inhibitory effect of sertraline on lamotrigine, a drug metabolized primarily by *N*-glucuronidation (Kaufman and Gerner, 1998).

C. Pharmacodynamic Interactions with AEDs

One of the concerns that clinicians have to always keep in mind is the potential worsening of adverse events resulting from the combination of antidepressant drugs and AEDs that have common adverse events. From a theoretical standpoint, the following potential synergistic adverse events have to be looked for carefully: (1) Potentiation of weight gain that can be caused by AEDs such as gabapentin, valproic acid, carbamazepine and pregabalin and antidepressant drugs such as sertraline and paroxetine. (2) Potentiation of sexual adverse events. Sexual adverse events, such as decreased libido, anorgasmia and sexual impotence, can be relatively common with AEDs such as the barbiturates (phenobarbital and primidone), but can also be seen with other enzyme-inducing

AEDs. This adverse event has been explained by synthesis of the sex hormone-binding globulin, which binds the free fraction of sex hormones, and hence makes them less accessible to the central nervous system (CNS). Antidepressant drugs of the SSRI, MAOI and TCA type, as well as the SNRI type, are known to cause sexual adverse events. Whether the combination of this type of AEDs and antidepressants has a "synergistic adverse effect" on sexual functions has yet to be established. An additional caveat is the direct impact of the seizure disorder on sexual functions which could, in fact, be the variable responsible for the decreased sexual drive independently of the exposure to the AED (or in combination with).

Single case reports of various pharmacodynamic interactions have been published in the literature. For example, Dursun *et al.* reported one case of serotonin syndrome resulting from a combination of fluoxetine and carbamaze-pine (Dursun *et al.*, 1993). Likewise, Rosenhagen *et al.* recently reported two patients comedicated with escitalopram, the S-enantiomer of citralopram, and lamotrigine who developed myoclonus, a potential symptom of serotonin syn-drome (Rosenhagen *et al.*, 2006). These authors speculate that lamotrigine may amplify the risk of developing myoclonus in patients receiving SSRIs. Finally, Gernat *et al.* have reported on the development of extrapyramidal syndrome when using fluoxetine in combination with AEDs, but again these were isolated reports (Gernaat *et al.*, 1991).

III. Anxiolytic Drugs

A. Pharmacokinetic Interactions with AEDs

1. *Pharmacokinetic Interactions*

Enzyme-inducing AEDs can accelerate the metabolism of various benzodia-zepines. Thus, carbamazepine has been found to accelerate the metabolism of diazepam, clobazam, clonazepam and alprazolam (Anderson and Miller, 2002). Nonetheless, given the wide therapeutic index of these benzodiazepines, the clinical impact is limited. On the one hand, enzyme-inducing AEDs can have a significantly clinical effect on the metabolism of midazolam, by enhancing its metabolic rate. On the other hand, sodium valproate inhibits the metabolism of lorazepam which is also metabolized by UGT (Anderson and Miller, 2002).

By the same token, clobazam and clonazepam have been reported to cause an increase in phenytoin serum concentrations, while clobazam was found to increase the serum concentrations of valproate, carbamazepine and its 1011-epoxide metabolite (Anderson and Miller, 2002).

B. PHARMACODYNAMIC INTERACTIONS WITH AEDS

Benzodiazepines are drugs with sedative adverse events which can be potentiated by AEDs with similar properties such as barbiturates. By the same token, these two classes of drugs can cause a variety of psychiatric adverse events such as aggression, motor hyperactivity, impulsivity, poor frustration tolerance and depression. Whether these adverse events may be potentiated by the combination is yet to be established but, nonetheless, remains a distinct possibility which clinicians should be on the lookout.

Some authors have cautioned against the combination of benzodiazepines such as clonazepam and valproic acid. Jeavons, for example, reported an increase in sedation in 9 of 12 children with absence seizures treated with valproic acid and in whom clonazepam was added (Jeavons *et al.*, 1977). This finding has not been replicated by other investigators, however.

IV. Lithium

A. PHARMACOKINETIC INTERACTIONS WITH AEDS

There does not appear to be substantial risk for pharmacokinetic interactions between lithium and AEDs. Among the newer agents, neither gabapentin nor lamotrigine was found to interact with lithium (Patsalos and Perucca, 2003; Trimble and Mula, 2005; Spina and Perucca, 2002).

B. PHARMACODYNAMIC INTERACTIONS WITH AEDS

Before the discovery of the mood-stabilizing properties of AEDs, lithium was the mood-stabilizing agent par excellence. While today, many AEDs, such as valproic acid, carbamazepine, oxcarbazepine and lamotrigine, have replaced the use of lithium in the management of bipolar patients, lithium continues to play an important role, above all, in patients with more refractory bipolar disease. It is not infrequent that patients with refractory bipolar illness may be placed on a combination of lithium and valproic acid or lithium and carbamazepine, lamotrigine or oxcarbazepine.

The combination of lithium and carbamazepine has been documented for a long time to cause a synergistic toxicity caused by each individual drug when given alone. Shukla *et al.* suggested that carbamazepine enhanced the development of lithium neurotoxicity syndrome characterized by symptoms of confusion, drowsiness, lethargy, tremor and cerebellar signs, including ataxia (Shukla *et al.*, 1984). These symptoms occur in the setting of therapeutic serum levels of lithium and carbamazepine. In addition, synergistic interaction between lithium and carbamazepine was identified by Kramlinger and Post as a reported significant increase in haematologic parameters primarily involving increase in white blood cell counts, as well as decrease in thyroid function test values with lowering of the total and free T4 serum concentrations (Kramlinger and Post, 1990). Finally, when carbamazepine and lithium are given together, lithium counteracts the hyponatremic effect of carbamazepine.

The combination of lithium and valproate could, in theory, result in an exacerbation of weight gain, as well as tremor, although this pharmacodynamic interaction has not been documented in systematic studies. Similarly, one might speculate that co-medication with gabapentin or pregabalin might also contribute to increased weight gain. Finally, increasing tremor can also be expected when lithium is added to lamotrigine, as both drugs have this potential adverse event, but little data have been published with respect to this potential pharmacodynamic interaction.

V. CNS Stimulants

A. IMPACT ON SEIZURE THRESHOLD

Central nervous system stimulants (CNSS) are another class of psychotropic drugs that needs to be prescribed with a relatively high frequency for the treatment of ADHD, given the high prevalence rates of this condition, ranging between 15% and 30% among different studies. They are the first choice of therapy for ADHD, both combined type and predominantly inattentive type (Dunn and Kronenberger, 2005). Methylphenidate and dextroamphetamine are the most frequently prescribed CNSS and have been reported to yield comparable efficacy, though dextroamphetamine has been reported to be associated with more side effects. By the same token, there have been more studies with methylphenidate. Yet, the *Physicians' Desk Reference* (*PDR*) lists seizures as a possible adverse event during treatment with this type of drug and recommends their discontinuation if seizures occur. Such warnings have resulted in a great reluctance by clinicians to use this type of medication in children with epilepsy and ADHD. Yet, patients with ADHD of the inattentive type are at a significant risk of experiencing epileptic seizures. Thus, the same question asked in the case of mood disorders is warranted in these patients, mainly, is a seizure the expression of the inherent risk of the psychiatric disorder or an adverse event of the CNSS? For example, in a study of 234 children with ADHD but without epilepsy for whom electroencephalogram (EEGs) were recorded before starting methylphenidate, Hemmer *et al.* found epileptiform activity on the EEG of 36 children (15.4%) (Hemmer and Pasternak, 2001). Of these 234 patients, 205 were started on methylphenidate and 4 (2%) experienced seizures, 3 of whom had EEG recordings with epileptiform discharges at baseline. Most of the epileptiform discharges consisted of centrotemporal (rolandic) spikes and those were the ones most likely to experience seizures (16.7%). Thus, exposure to methylphenidate may have played no role in the development of seizures, which occurred as an expression of an underlying seizure disorder.

In a review of the literature, Dunn and other others concluded that CNSS are generally safe for their use in patients with epilepsy (Dunn and Kronenberger, 2005). For example, Feldman *et al.* treated children with epilepsy and ADHD with methylphenidate at a dosage of 0.3 mg/kg given twice daily (Feldman *et al.*, 1989); they found an improvement in psychiatric symptoms without an increase in seizure frequency. In a different study, Gross-Tsur *et al.* treated 30 children with epilepsy and ADHD with methylphenidate, 0.3 mg/kg given in a single dose (Gross-Tsur *et al.*, 1997). Twenty-five of the 30 children had been seizure-free for the 2 months before the start of the CNSS and remained without seizures during the trial; 2 who had seizures in the prior 2 months had no change or fewer seizures, and 3 with prior seizures had more seizures, but difference in seizure frequency was not statistically significant. There was no change in AED levels or EEG findings. A significant improvement in symptoms of ADHD was identified in 70% of the children.

In one retrospective study, the efficacy and safety of dextroamphetamine ($n = 17$) and methylphenidate ($n = 19$) were compared in 36 children with epilepsy and ADHD (Gonzalez-Heydrich *et al.*, 2007). An improvement in ADHD symptoms was found in 63% of the children treated with methylphenidate, but only in 24% of those on amphetamine. There was an increase in seizure frequency in 3 of the children with active seizures that improved after discontinuation of stimulant or change in AED dose. This study had too many methodologic problems, and hence these findings were of questionable validity.

Modafinil is another CNSS that has been found to be effective in the treatment of ADHD in children without epilepsy in five double-blind trials involving more than 800 children with dosages as high as 425 mg/day. No seizures were reported in any of these trials. (Biederman *et al.*, 2005, 2006; Greenhill *et al.*, 2006; Rugino and Samsock, 2003; Swanson *et al.*, 2006). This CNSS is rarely used for ADHD, however, because of its association with relatively high incidence of severe dermatologic adverse events, including the risk of developing Stevens-Johnsons syndrome. Neurologists use this drug frequently for the treatment of excessive daytime somnolence in patients with narcolepsy and obstructive sleep apnea.

VI. Other Treatment for ADHD: Atomoxetine

Atomoxetine is a norepinephrine reuptake inhibitor that has been shown to be effective in the treatment of ADHD in adults and children (Hernández and Barragán, 2005; Wernicke *et al.*, 2007). Atomoxetine also increases dopamine levels in the cortex but not in the basal ganglia or nucleus accumbens and its therapeutic actions may partly be due to its effect on dopamine levels in specific areas of the brain.

A. IMPACT ON SEIZURE THRESHOLD

As with TCAs and SSRIs, atomoxetine has been found to have anticonvulsant effects at low doses and proconvulsant effects at high doses in animal models of epilepsy. For example, in mouse models of seizures with electroshock at 50 mg/kg/day, there was evidence of a protective effect against seizures, though seizures were induced at 400 mg/kg/day (Data on File, Eli Lilly and Co., 2002). In animal models with dogs, dosages of 12–25 mg/kg/day protected against seizures. In humans with ADHD, but not epilepsy, Wernicke *et al.* investigated the incidence of seizures in patients exposed to atomoxetine by conducting a systematic review of two Eli Lilly and Company databases (atomoxetine clinical trials database and atomoxetine postmarketing spontaneous adverse event database) (Wernicke *et al.*, 2007). In the clinical trials database, a crude incidence of 0.06–0.2% for seizures was identified among the treated pediatric patients. One of the 1614 children (0.06%) taking atomoxetine in a controlled trial experienced a seizure, and 12 children among 5083 patients (0.2%) in any type of trial experienced a seizure. Five hundred and twenty-three children treated with methylphenidate and 849 with placebo provided a comparison to the atomoxetine-treated group. The crude incidence rates of seizure adverse events did not significantly differ between atomoxetine, placebo and methylphenidate for children or adults.

The data of atomoxetine use in patients with epilepsy are sparse. In a retrospective chart review of atomoxetine treatment for ADHD in 27 children with epilepsy, 90% of whom had failed previous trials with CNSS (Schaller and Behar, 1999), no patients experienced an exacerbation of seizures or serious adverse events.

B. PHARMACOKINETIC INTERACTIONS OF CNSS WITH AEDs

CNSS such as methylphenidate may participate in pharmacokinetic interactions with AEDs. Carbamazepine has been noted to reduce methylphenidate serum concentrations, possibly leading to loss of efficacy (Schaller and Behar, 1999). Methylphenidate may also have modest inhibitory actions on the CYP isozyme system (Markowitz *et al.*, 1999) and has been reported to modestly increase phenytoin serum concentrations. Atomoxetine is primarily metabolized via CYP 2D6, and no pharmacokinetic interactions with AEDs have been noted.

C. PHARMACODYNAMIC INTERACTIONS OF CNSS WITH AEDs

No documentation has been provided of any pharmacodynamic interaction between these classes of drugs. However, from a theoretical standpoint, clinicians should be aware of the potentiation of movement disorders associated with the use of lamotrigine and CNSS, two types of drugs that can cause tics and Tourette's syndrome.

VII. Antipsychotic Drugs

Antipsychotic drugs (APDs) can be separated into two classes: "conventional" APDs (CAPDs) and "atypical" APDs (AAPDs). The former includes 18 drugs developed between the 1950s and the 1970s. Their mechanism of action resides in their ability to block dopamine (DA-2) receptors, at the level of meso-cortical, nigrostriatal and tuberoinfundibular DA pathways (Stahl, 2000). Blockade of the DA receptors at the meso-cortical pathways is responsible for their antipsychotic effect, but results as well in "emotional blunting" and cognitive symptoms that often lead to confusion with the "negative" symptoms of schizophrenia. Blockade at the nigrostriatal pathways results in acute and chronic movement disorders, presenting as parkinsonian symptoms, as well as dystonic and dyskinetic movements, while blockade at the tuberoinfundibular DA pathways results in increased secretion of prolactin. In addition to their DA-blockade properties, most of these CAPDs have muscarinic cholinergic, alpha-1 and histaminic blocking properties, responsible for anticholinergic adverse effects, weight gain, sedation, dizziness and orthostatic hypotension.

AAPDs are dopamine-serotonin antagonists that target DA-2 and 5HT-2A receptors (Stahl, 2000). Their main difference with CAPDs is the absence or mild occurrence of extrapyramidal adverse events and of hyperprolactinemia. In addition, this class of drugs has a lesser blunting of affect and several of these AAPDs have mood-stabilizing properties. Hence, AAPDs have in large part replaced the CAPDs. Today, six AAPDs have been introduced in the USA: clozapine, risperidone, olanzapine, ziprasidone, quietapine and aripiprazole.

A. IMPACT ON SEIZURE THRESHOLD

The proconvulsant properties of CAPD have been recognized for a long time with seizure incidence-rates ranging between 0.5% and 1.2% among patients without epilepsy (Logothetis, 1967; Stahl, 2000; Whitworth and Fleischhacker, 1995). The risk is higher with certain drugs and in the presence of the following factors: (1) a history of epilepsy; (2) abnormal EEG recordings; (3) history of CNS disorder; (4) rapid titration of the CAPD dose; (5) high doses of APDs; (6) the presence of other drugs that lower the seizure threshold. For example, when chlorpromazine is used at dosages above 1000 mg/day, the incidence of seizures was reported to increase to 9%, in contrast to a 0.5% incidence when lower doses are taken (Logothetis, 1967). Haloperidol, molindone, fluphenazine, perfenazine and trifluoperazine are among the CAPDs with a lower seizure risk (Whitworth and Fleischhacker, 1995).

In the study by Alper et al. cited above (Alper et al., 2007), the incidence of seizures identified during regulatory studies of AAPDs carried out between 1985 and 2004 was compared between (non-epileptic) patients randomized to placebo and AAPDs. The incidence of seizures was higher among those randomized to clozapine and olanzapine, but not among those randomized to other AAPDs. Clozapine has been reported to cause seizures in 4.4% of patients without epilepsy when used at dosages above 600 mg/day, while at a dosage lower than 300 mg/day, the incidence of seizures was less than 1% in patients without epilepsy.

With the exception of clozapine, the impact of AAPDs on seizure occurrence has not been properly studied in patients with epilepsy. Pacia and Devinsky reviewed the incidence of seizures among 5629 patients treated with clozapine (Pacia and Devinsky, 1994). Sixteen of these patients had epilepsy before the start of this AAPD and all patients experienced worsening of seizures while on the drug; eight patients at dosages lower than 300 mg/day; three patients at dosages between 300 and 600 mg/day and five at dosages higher than 600 mg/day. It goes without saying that this AAPD should be avoided or used in exceptional circumstances with extreme caution in patients with epilepsy.

Clozapine followed by the two CAPDs chlorpromazine and loxepine is the APD with the highest risk of seizure occurrence. Those with a lower seizure risk include haloperidol, molindone, fluphenazine, perfenazine and trifluoperazine, among the CAPDs, and risperidone, among the AAPDs. Whether the presence of AEDs at adequate levels protects patients with epilepsy from breakthrough seizures upon the introduction of APDs with proconvulsant properties is yet to be established.

Most APDs can cause EEG changes consisting of slowing of the background activity above all when used at high doses. In addition, some of these drugs, and particularly clozapine, can cause paroxysmal electrographic changes in the form of interictal sharp waves and spikes. This type of epileptiform activity, however, is not predictive of seizure occurrence (Tiihonen et al., 1991). There are data suggesting that a severe disorganization of the EEG recordings is a more likely predictor of seizure occurrence. As a rule, any APD should be started at low doses and should undergo slow dose increments to minimize the risk of seizures in patients with epilepsy.

B. Pharmacokinetic Interactions with AEDs

Induction of hepatic enzymes upon the introduction of older enzyme-inducing AEDs such as phenytoin or carbamazepine may result in an increase inthe clearance of most APDs. This is, in fact, the most frequent and clinically relevant pharmacokinetic interaction encountered in clinical practice. Reductions in antipsychotic concentration may be quite marked. For example, co-medication with carbamazepine has been shown to decrease haloperidol concentrations by 50–60% (Jann et al., 1985). It may potentially result in recurrence of psychotic symptoms previously controlled at higher serum concentrations of APDs. By the same token, discontinuation of an AED with enzyme-inducing properties may result in a decrease in the clearance of APDs, which in turn can lead to extrapyramidal adverse events caused by an increase in the serum concentrations of CAPDs. In contrast to the enzyme-inducing AEDs, valproate appears to have minimal pharmacokinetic interactions with these drugs. Several studies have suggested that valproate has only minimal effects on serum concentrations of either haloperidol or risperidone (Hesslinger et al., 1999; Spina et al., 2000). Valproate has been reported to have modest, variable effects on clozapine concentrations.

Among the newer agents, modest increases were seen in haloperidol concentrations in patients comedicated with topiramate (Doose et al., 1999). AEDs that neither substantially induce nor inhibit the CYP isozyme system (e.g. gabapentin, pregabalin, lamotrigine, levetiracetam, zonisamide) are unlikely to result in significant pharmacokinetic interactions with APDs.

APDs are less likely to cause pharmacokinetic interactions with AEDs. Among the typical APDs, both chlorpromazine and thioridazine have been reported to result in increases in phenytoin serum concentrations. With regard to atypical antipsychotics, risperidone has been noted to result in modest decreases in carbamazepine concentrations (Mula and Monaco, 2002). Finally, no significant interaction was noted between olanzapine and lamotrigine (Jann and Hon, 2006).

C. Pharmacodynamic Interactions with AEDs

A potential negative interaction between clozapine and carbamazepine should be kept in mind, as both can cause leucopenia and if combined, a potential synergism of this adverse event. In addition, the combination of these two drugs has been also reported to cause an increased risk of neuroleptic malignant syndrome.

From a theoretical standpoint, the potential for worsening of adverse events caused by both types of drugs, such as increased weight gain and sexual dysfunction, are to be considered, with increased weight gain being a common and significant adverse event for patients taking AAPDs such as quietapine, risperidone, olanzapine and ziprasidone when given in combination with AEDs that are known to cause weight gain as well such as gabapentin, pregabalin, carbamazepine and valproate. Also, it should be remembered that all AAPDs can cause type-II diabetes mellitus. Thus, glycaemic and lipid profiles need to be monitored in all patients on a regular basis. Conversely, co-medication with AEDs associated with weight loss, such as topiramate, may result in weight loss in patients receiving AAPDs. Exacerbation of sexual dysfunction can also be a common adverse event of the older APDs, such as those in the family of the phenothyzines can be in theory accentuated by the use of enzyme-inducing AEDs, due possibly to reductions in serum testosterone concentrations, as well as increases in sex hormone-binding globulin.

VIII. Concluding Remarks

Psychotropic drugs are relatively commonly used in patients with epilepsy. Antidepressants, CNSS and most of the AAPDs are safe in these patients. Their pharmacokinetic interaction with the first-generation AEDs that have enzyme-inducing properties may lower the serum concentrations of most antidepressants and APDs and thus limit their efficacy, while valproic acid may inhibit the clearance of some of the drugs metabolized by glucuronidation. The lack of pharmacokinetic effects of most of the new AEDs (with the exception of felbamate, topiramate and oxcarbazepine) is an advantage in patients who are taking concomitant psychotropic drugs.

On the contrary, some of the SSRIs can inhibit the metabolism of certain AEDs. Recognition of the pharmacokinetic interactions is of the essence to avert loss of efficacy of psychotropic drugs or toxicity of AEDs and psychotropic agents. Finally, AEDs and psychotropic agents can have pharmacodynamic interactions that may result in a variety of adverse events, often requiring the discontinuation of the AED or psychotropic agents.

References

Ago, J., Ishikawa, T., Matsumoto, N., Ashequr Rahman, M., and Kamei, C. (2006). Mechanism of imipramine-induced seizures in amygdala-kindled rats. *Epilepsy Res.* **72,** 1–9.
Alper, K., Schwartz, K. A., Kolts, R. L., and Khan, A. (2007). Seizure incidence in psychopharmacological clinical trials: An analysis of Food and Drug Administration (FDA) summary basis of approval reports. *Biol. Psychiatry* **62**(4), 345–354.

Andersen, B. B., Mikkelsen, M., and Vesterager, A., et al. (1991). No influence of the antidepressant paroxetine on carbamazepine, valproate, and phenytoin. Epilepsy Res. **10**, 201–204.

Anderson, G., and Miller, J. W. (2002). Benzodiazepines: Chemistry, biotransformation and pharmacokinetics. In "Antiepileptic Drugs" (R. H. Levy, R. H. Mattson, B. S. Meldrum, and E. Perucca, Eds.), 5th ed., pp. 187–205. Lippincott Williams and Wilkins, Baltimore.

Austin, J. K., Harezlak, J., Dunn, D. W., et al. (2001). Behavior problems in children before first recognized seizure. Pediatrics **107**, 115–122.

Biederman, J., Swanson, J. M., Wigal, S. B., et al. (2005). Efficacy and safety of modafinil film-coated tablets in children and adolescents with attention-deficit/hyperactivity disorder: Results of a randomized, double-blind, placebo-controlled, flexible-dose study. Pediatrics **116**, e777–e784.

Biederman, J., Swanson, J. M., Wigal, S. B., et al. (2006). A comparison of once-daily and divided doses of modafinil in children with attention-deficit/hyperactivity disorder: A randomized, double-blind, and placebo-controlled study. J. Clin. Psychiatry **67**, 727–735.

Davidson, J. (1989). Seizures and bupropion: A review. J. Clin. Psychiatry **50**, 256–261.

Doose, D. R., Kohl, K. A., and Desai-Krieger, D. (1999). No clinically significant effect of topiramate on haloperidol plasma concentration. Eur. Neuropsychopharmacol. **9**, S357.

Dunn, D. W., and Austin, J. K. (1999). Behavioral issues in pediatric epilepsy. Neurology **53**(Suppl. 2), S96–S100.

Dunn, D. W., and Kronenberger, W. G. (2005). Childhood epilepsy, attention problems, and ADHD: Review and practical considerations. Semin. Pediatr. Neurol. **12**(4), 222–228.

Dursun, S. M., Mathew, V. M., and Reveley, M. A. (1993). Toxic serotonin syndrome after fluoxetine plus carbamazepine. Lancet **342**, 442–443.

Edeh, J., and Toone, B. (1987). Relationship between interictal psychopathology and the type of epilepsy. Br. J. Psychiatry **151**, 95–101.

Favale, E., Rubino, V., Mainardi, P., Lunardi, G., and Albano, C. (1995). The anticonvulsant effect of fluoxetine in humans. Neurology **45**, 1926.

Favale, E., Audenino, D., Cocito, L., and Albano, C. (2003). The anticonvulsant effect of citalopram as an indirect evidence of serotonergic impairment in human epileptogenesis. Seizure **12**, 316–318.

Feldman, H., Crumine, P., Handen, B. L., Alvin, R., and Teodori, J. (1989). Methylphenidate in children with seizures and attention-deficit disorder. Am. J. Dis. Child **143**, 1081–1086.

Forsgren, L., and Nystrom, L. (1999). An incident case referent study of epileptic seizures in adults. Epilepsy Res. **6**, 66–81.

Fromm, G. H., Wessel, H. B., Glass, J. D., Alvin, J. D., and Van Horn, G. (1978). Imipramine in absence and myoclonic-astatic seizures. Neurology **28**, 953–957.

Fromm, G. H., Amores, C. Y., and Thies, W. (1972). Imipramine in epilepsy. Arch. Neurol. **27**, 198–204.

Gernaat, H. B., Van de Woude, J., and Touw, D. J. (1991). Fluoxetine and parkinsonism in patients taking carba-mazepine. Am. J. Psychiatry **148**, 1604–1605.

Gonzalez-Heydrich, J., Dodds, A., Whitney, J., et al. (2007). Psychiatric disorders and behavioral characteristics of pediatric patients with both epilepsy and attention-deficit hyperactivity disorder. Epilepsy Behav. **10**, 384–388.

Greenhill, L. L., Biederman, J., Boellner, S. W., et al. (2006). A randomized, double-blind, placebo-controlled study of modafinil film-coated tablets in children and adolescents with attention-deficit/hyperactivity disorder. J. Am. Acad. Child Adolesc. Psychiatry **45**, 503–511.

Gross-Tsur, V., Manor, O., van der Meere, J., Joseph, A., and Shalev, R. S. (1997). Epilepsy and attention deficit hyperactivity disorder: Is methylphenidate safe and effective? J. Pediatr. **130**, 670–674.

Hemmer, S. A., Pasternak, J. F., et al. (2001). Stimulant therapy and seizure risk in children with ADHD. Pediatr. Neurol. **24**(2), 99–102.

Hernández, A. J. C., and Barragán, P. E. J. (2005). Efficacy of atomoxetine treatment in children with ADHD and epilepsy. Epilepsia **46**(Suppl. 6), 241.

Hesdorffer, D. C., Hauser, W. A., Annegers, J. F., *et al.* (2000). Major depression is a risk factor for seizures in older adults. *Ann. Neurol.* **47,** 246–249.

Hesdorffer, D. C., Ludvigsson, P., Olafsson, E., Gudmundsson, G., Kjartansson, O., and Hauser, W. A. (2004). ADHD as a risk factor for incident unprovoked seizures and epilepsy in children. *Arch. Gen. Psychiatry* **61**(7), 731–736.

Hesdorffer, D. C., Hauser, W. A., Olafsson, E., Ludvigsson, P., and Kjartansson, O. (2006). Depression and suicidal attempt as risk factor for incidental unprovoked seizures. *Ann. Neurol.* **59**(1), 35–41.

Hesslinger, B., Normann, C., Langgosch, J. M., *et al.* (1999). Effects of carbamazepine and valproate on haloperidol levels and on psychopathologic outcome in schizophrenic patients. *J. Clin. Psychopharmacol.* **19,** 310–315.

Horne, R. L., Ferguson, J. M., Pope, H. G., Jr, Hudson, J. I., Lineberry, C. G., Ascher, J., and Cato, A. (1988). Treatment of bulimia with bupropion: A multicenter controlled trial. *J. Clin. Psychiatry* **49,** 262–266.

Hurst, D. L. (1986). The use of imipramine in minor motor seizures. *Pediatr. Neurol.* **2,** 13–17.

Jacoby, A., Baker, G. A., Steen, N., *et al.* (1996). The clinical course of epilepsy and its psychosocial correlates: Findings from a UK community study. *Epilepsia* **37,** 148–161.

Jann, M., Hon, Y., *et al.* (2006). Lack of pharmacokinetic interaction between lamotrigine and olanzapine in healthy volunteers. *Pharmacotherapy* **26,** 627–633.

Jann, M. W., Ereshefsky, L., Saklad, S. R., *et al.* (1985). Effects of carbamazepine on plasma haloperidol levels. *J. Clin. Psychopharmacol.* **5,** 106–109.

Jeavons, P. M., Clark, J. E., and Mahashwari, M. C. (1977). Treatment of generalized epilepsies of childhood and adolescence with sodium valproate. *Dev. Med. Child Neurol.* **19,** 9.

Jefferson, J. W., Pradko, J. F., and Muir, K. T. (2005). Bupropion for major depressive disorder: Pharmacokinetic and formulation considerations. *Clin. Ther.* **27,** 1685–1695.

Jones, J. E., Waston, R., Sheth, R., Caplan, R., Koehn, M., Seidenberg, M., and Hermann, B. (2007). Psychiatric comorbidity in children with new onset epilepsy. *Dev. Med. Child Neurol.* **49**(7), 493–497.

Kanner, A. M., Kozak, A. M., and Frey, M. (2000). The use of sertraline in patients with epilepsy: Is it safe? *Epilepsy Behav.* **1**(2), 100–105.

Kaufman, K. R., and Gerner, R. (1998). Lamotrigine toxicity secondary to sertraline. *Seizure* **7,** 163–165.

Kramlinger, K. G., and Post, R. M. (1990). Addition of lithium carbonate to carbamazepine: Haematological and thyroid effects. *Am. J. Psychiatry* **147,** 615–620.

Laroudie, C., Salazar, D. E., *et al.* (2000). Carbamazepine-nefazodone interaction in healthy subjects. *J. Clin. Psychopharmacol.* **20,** 46–53.

Logothetis, J. (1967). Spontaneous epileptic seizures and EEG changes in the course of phenothiazine therapy. *Neurology* **17,** 869–877.

Mamiya, K., Kojima, K., *et al.* (2001). Phenytoin intoxication induced by fluvoxamine. *Ther. Drug Monit.* **23,** 75–77.

Markowitz, J. S., Morrison, S. D., and DeVane, C. L. (1999). Drug interactions with psychstimulants. *Int. Clin. Psychopharmacol.* **14,** 1–18.

Matsuura, M., Adachi, N., Muramatsu, R., Kato, M., Onuma, T., Okubo, Y., Oana, Y., and Hara, T. (2005). Intellectual disability and psychotic disorders of adult epilepsy. *Epilepsia* **46**(Suppl. 1), 11–14.

McConnell, H., and Duncan, D. (1998). Treatment of psychiatric comorbidity in epilepsy. *In* "Psychiatric Comorbidity in Epilepsy" (H. McConnell and P. Snyder, Eds.), pp. 245–362. Am. Psych. Press, Washington.

Mula, M., and Monaco, F. (2002). Carbamazepine-risperidone interactions in patients with epilepsy. *Clin. Neuropharmacol.* **25,** 97–100.

Nelson, M. H., Birnbaum, A. K., and Remmel, R. P. (2001). Inhibition of phenytoin hydroxylation in human liver microsomes by several selective serotonin re-uptake inhibitors. *Epilepsy Res.* **44,** 71–82.

Pacia, S. V., and Devinsky, O. (1994). Clozapine-related seizures: Experience with 5,629 patients. *Neurology* **44**(12), 2247–2249.

Patsalos, P., and Perucca, E. (2003). Clinically important drug interactions in epilepsy: Interactions between antiepileptic drugs and other drugs. *Lancet Neurol.* **2,** 473–481.

Pope, H. G., Jr, McElroy, S. L., Keck, P. E., Hudson, J. I., Ferguson, J. M., and Horne, R. L. (1989). Electrophysiological abnormalities in bulimia and their implications for pharmacotherapy: A reassessment. *Int. J. Eat. Disord.* **8,** 191–201.

Rosenhagen, M., Schmidt, U., Weber, F., and Steiger, A. (2006). Combination therapy of lamotrigine and escitalopram may cause myoclonus. *J. Clin. Psychopharmacol.* **26,** 346–347.

Rugino, T. A., and Samsock, T. C. (2003). Modafinil in children with attention-deficit/hyperactivity disorder. *Pediatr. Neurol.* **29,** 136–142.

Schaller, J. L., and Behar, D. (1999). Carbamazepine and methylphenidate in ADHD (letter). *J. Am. Acad. Child Adolesc. Psychiatry* **38,** 112–113.

Shukla, S., Godwin, C. D., Long, L. E. B., *et al.* (1984). Lithium-carbamazepine neurotoxicity and risk factors. *Am. J. Psychiatry* **141,** 1604–1606.

Specchio, L. M., Iudice, A., Specchio, N., La Neve, A., Spinelli, A., Galli, R., Rocchi, R., Ulivelli, M., de Tommaso, M., Pizzanelli, C., and Murri, L. (2004). Citalopram as treatment of depression in patients with epilepsy. *Clin. Neuropharmacol.* **27**(3), 133–136.

Spina, E., and Perucca, E. (2002). Clinical significance of pharmacokinetic interactions between antiepileptic and psychtropic drugs. *Epilepsia* **43**(Suppl. 2), 37–44.

Spina, E., Avenoso, A., Facciola, G., *et al.* (2000). Plasma concentrations of risperidone and 9-hydroxyrespiridone; effect of comedication with carbamazepine or valproate. *Ther. Drug Monit.* **22,** 481–485.

Stahl, S. M. (2000). Antipsychotic agents. *In* "Essential Pharmacology: Neuroscientific Basis and Practical Applications" (S. M. Stahl, Ed.), 2nd ed., pp. 401–458. Cambridge University Press, NY, NY.

Swanson, J. M., Greenhill, L. L., Lopez, L. A., *et al.* (2006). Modafinil film-coated tablets in children and adolescents with attention-deficit/hyperactivity disorder: Results of a randomized, double-blind, placebo-controlled, fixed-dose study followed by abrupt discontinuation. *J. Clin. Psychiatry* **67,** 137–147.

Tellez-Zenteno, J. F., Patten, S. B., Jetté, N., Williams, J., and Wiebe, S. (2007). Psychiatric comorbidity in epilepsy: A population-based analysis. *Epilepsia* (Online Early Articles). doi:10.1111/j.1528–1167.2007.

Tiihonen, J., Nousiainen, U., Hakola, P., *et al.* (1991). EEG abnormalities associated with clozapine treatment. (letter). *Am. J. Psychiatry* **148,** 1406.

Trimble, M. R., and Mula, M. (2005). Antiepileptic drug interactions in patients requiring psychiatric drug treatment. *In* "Antiepileptic Drugs. Combination Therapy and Interactions" (J. Majkowski, B. Bourgeois, P. Patsalos, and R. Mattson, Eds.), pp. 350–368. Cambridge University Press, New York.

Wernicke, J. F., Holdridge, K. C., Jin, L., *et al.* (2007). Seizure risk in patients with attention-deficit-hyperactivity disorder treated with atomoxetine. *Dev. Med. Child. Neurol.* **49,** 498–502.

Whitworth, A. B., and Fleischhacker, W. W. (1995). Adverse effects of antipsychotic drugs. *Int. Clin. Psychopharmacol.* **9**(Suppl. 5), 21–27.

HEALTH DISPARITIES IN EPILEPSY: HOW PATIENT-ORIENTED OUTCOMES IN WOMEN DIFFER FROM MEN

Frank Gilliam

Department of Neurology, Columbia University Medical Center,
Comprehensive Epilepsy Center, New York 10032, USA

Epilepsy is a chronic disorder with multiple effects on biological, social, and psychological health. Many of these effects differ between men and women, but only sparse research has specifically addressed the relevance and importance of the differences. Available evidence suggests that men and women with epilepsy have differing rates of employment and driving, and women with epilepsy have increased risk for specific mood disorders such as post-partum depression. National surveys of physicians indicate that many physicians providing care for women with epilepsy have limited knowledge of fundamental concerns such as interactions between antiepileptic drugs and oral contraceptives, and their potential teratogenic effects. Further research and clinical implementation of improved gender-specific care is needed to optimize outcomes for women with epilepsy.

Epilepsy is a complex disorder with multiple clinical syndromes, etiologies, and potential long-term health effects (Fisher et al., 2005). Extensive research in recent decades has enriched our understanding of the intricate hormonal, neuro-chemical, and environmental effects on epileptic neurons and associated cerebral networks (Chang and Lowenstein, 2003). The development of reliable and valid instruments for the evaluation of patient-oriented outcomes has further informed our modern perspective of the effects of epilepsy on psychological, vocational, and social functioning (Baker et al., 1997; Devinsky et al., 1995; Vickrey et al., 1994). Considering the observed gender differences in aspects physiological and behavior functions, it seems very appropriate to study the associations of these differences with specific clinical and biological aspects of epilepsy (Cramer et al., 2007; Scharfman and MacLusky, 2006). The study of relevant aspects of epilepsy in women offers the potential to develop optimal treatment strategies, and may also yield important advances to further our understanding of the complexity of epilepsy intervention and comprehensive outcomes that could benefit both women and men (Zahn et al., 1998).

INTERNATIONAL REVIEW OF
NEUROBIOLOGY, VOL. 83
DOI: 10.1016/S0074-7742(08)00023-8

417

Depression is an important example of the multidimensional health effects of epilepsy in women. Although depression is significantly more prevalent in women than men in the general population, it appears to occur at similar rates in women and men with epilepsy (Mensah *et al.*, 2006). A possible explanation of this lack of difference in persons with epilepsy could be due to interictal brain changes that predispose both sexes with epilepsy to depression (Gilliam *et al.*, 2004). However, certain health states unique to women may increase the risk of depression. For example, a recent study found that postpartum depression was more than twice as frequent in women with epilepsy compared to controls (29% versus 11%; $p < 0.05$). Specific aspects of comorbidities unique to gender must be fully understood in order to develop successful research initiatives and develop optimal diagnostic and research strategies.

Independence appears to be another important aspect of epilepsy that may be underemphasized by clinicians, although it was ranked as the second most common problem spontaneously cited by patients in a subspecialty epilepsy clinic sample (Gilliam *et al.*, 1997). Interestingly, factors critical to independence, such as driving privileges and employment, may be different between men and women in certain situations. For example, men with a childhood history of epilepsy were nearly three times (relative risk 2.7 95% CI 1.1–6.3) more likely to have a driver's license in Finland compared to women with a similar history (Sillanpaa and Shinnar, 2005). Although single women and men were equally likely to be employed in another large cohort in the United Kingdom (78% employed), married women were much less likely to have a job than married men (55% versus 81%) (Jacoby, 1995). Observations such as differences in driving privileges and employment suggest that advances are still needed in our understanding of the role of gender in epilepsy-related social and vocational disabilities.

Aspects of care specific to women with epilepsy have traditionally been neglected, an outlook that is now reversing. A glaring example of the deficiency in delivery of health care to women with epilepsy is the limited knowledge of clinicians regarding the interaction between common antiepileptic drugs and oral contraceptives (Krauss *et al.*, 1996). In a national survey 91% of responding neurologists and 75% of obstetricians reported that they provided care of women of childbearing age with epilepsy, but only 4% of neurologists and none of the obstetricians knew the effects of the six most common antiepileptic drugs on oral contraceptives. Similarly, potential effects of antiepileptic drugs on endogenous hormones may also impact other aspects of quality of life such as sexuality. Unfortunately, relatively little attention has been given to this issue in women with epilepsy as compared to men.

The potential impact of seizures as well as commonly used medications during pregnancy is also of notable concern. Although available evidence at the time indicated that the risk of antiepileptic drug exposure during pregnancy increased birth defect rates from 4% to 6%, the risk was estimated by 44% of neurologist to be 0–3%, and some respondents thought the risk was as high as 50%. Several pregnancy registries are defining more accurately the risk of birth malformations for specific drugs, but very little clinical research has investigated the impact of this information on improved patient education and care.

The past has taught us, therefore, that there are biological, psychosocial, and academic differences regarding gender issues in epilepsy. This volume attests to the growing body of knowledge gender-specific health care, and is intended to present up-to-date information on epilepsy care for women across age groups ranging from adolescents to late maturity.

References

Baker, G. A., Jacoby, A., Buck, D., Stalgis, C., and Monnet, D. (1997). Quality of life of people with epilepsy: A European study. *Epilepsia* **38,** 353–362.

Chang, B. S., and Lowenstein, D. H. (2003). Epilepsy. *N. Engl. J. Med.* **349,** 1257–1266.

Cramer, J. A., Gordon, J., Schachter, S., and Devinsky, O. (2007). Women with epilepsy: Hormonal issues from menarche through menopause. *Epilepsy Behav.* **11,** 160–178.

Devinsky, O., Vickrey, B. G., Cramer, J., *et al.* (1995). Development of the quality of life in epilepsy inventory. *Epilepsia* **36,** 1089–1104.

Fisher, R. S., Boas, W. V. E., Blume, W., *et al.* (2005). Epileptic seizures and epilepsy: Definitions proposed by the International League Against Epilepsy (ILAE) and the International Bureau for Epilepsy (IBE). *Epilepsia* **46,** 470–472.

Gilliam, F., Kuzniecky, R., Faught, E., Black, L., Carpenter, G., and Schrodt, R. (1997). Patient-validated content of epilepsy-specific quality-of-life measurement. *Epilepsia* **38,** 233–236.

Gilliam, F. G., Santos, J., Vahle, V., Carter, J., Brown, K., and Hecimovic, H. (2004). Depression in epilepsy: Ignoring clinical expression of neuronal network Dysfunction? *Epilepsia* **45,** 28–33.

Jacoby, A. (1995). Impact of epilepsy on employment status: Findings from a UK study of people with well-controlled epilepsy. *Epilepsy Res.* **21,** 125–132.

Krauss, G. L., Brandt, J., Campbell, M., Plate, C., and Summerfield, M. (1996). Antiepileptic medication and oral contraceptive interactions: A national survey of neurologists and obstetricians. *Neurology* **46,** 1534–1539.

Mensah, S. A., Beavis, J. M., Thapar, A. K., and Kerr, M. (2006). The presence and clinical implications of depression in a community population of adults with epilepsy. *Epilepsy Behav.* **8,** 213–219.

Scharfman, H. E., and MacLusky, N. J. (2006). The influence of gonadal hormones on neuronal excitability, seizures, and epilepsy in the female. *Epilepsia (Series 4)* **47,** 1423–1440.

Sillanpaa, M., and Shinnar, S. (2005). Obtaining a driver's license and seizure relapse in patients with childhood-onset epilepsy. *Neurology* **64,** 680–686.

Vickrey, B. G., Hays, R. D., Rausch, R., Sutherling, W. W., Engel, J., Jr., and Brook, R. H. (1994). Quality of life of epilepsy surgery patients as compared with outpatients with hypertension, diabetes, heart disease, and/or depressive symptoms. *Epilepsia* **35,** 597–607.

Zahn, C. A., Morrell, M. J., Collins, S. D., Labiner, D. M., and Yerby, M. S. (1998). Management issues for women with epilepsy: A review of the literature. *Neurology* **51,** 949–956.

INDEX

A

AAPDs. *See* Atypical APDs
Acetazolamide therapy
  for catamenial epilepsy, 85
  and renal stones, associations of, 342
  renal tubular acidosis and, 341
N-Acetyltransferase (NAT), 4
Active epilepsy, 13, 23. *See also* Epilepsy
  syndrome
Acyclovir, 291, 298
ADHD. *See* Attention deficit hyperactivity
  disorder
Adolescence, 92
  and AED-associated body weight
    changes, 333
  bone phases in, 306
  depressive disorders, 101
  and epilepsy (*see* Epilepsy, in young women)
  epilepsy and migraine, as neurologic
    disorders in, 102
  quality of life (QOL) in, 98
  seizure-related cause of death in, 21
Adrenal ectomized (ADX), 51
Adrenocorticotropic hormone (ACTH), 50, 53
AED pregnancy registries, 290–293. *See also*
  Pregnancy registry
  choice of comparator groups for, 297
  from Epilepsy Research Foundation and, 291
  by EURAP, 291
  methodology of, 292
  OTITS and ENTIS for, 291, 293
AEDs. *See* Antiepileptic drugs
Alpha 1-acid glycoprotein (α-AGP), 230
Amantadine drug, 161
γ-Aminobutyric acid (GABA), 27, 30, 47–48,
  54, 340
Amitriptyline, 402–403
Amoxapine, 402
Amphetamine, 408
Androgen-dependent hippocampal and
  hypothalamic functions, seizures on, 33

Androgen receptors (ARs), 31
3α-Androstan-17β-diol (3α-diol), role of, 32–33
Anorgasmia drug, 159
Anovulation, in women, 140, 145–146, 148
Anovulatory cycles, 94
Anticonvulsant distribution in neonate,
  factors for
  neonatal pharmacokinetics, 244–245
  placental factors, 243–244
  properties of, 242–243
Antidepressant drugs, 399
  impact on seizure threshold, 399–401
    dopamine-norepinephrine reuptake
      inhibitors, 402–403
    mono-amino-oxidase inhibitors, 401
    selective serotonin reuptake
      inhibitors, 401–402
    serotonin-norepinephrine reuptake
      inhibitors, 402
    tricyclic antidepressants, 401
  pharmacodynamic interactions with
    AEDs, 404–405
  pharmacokinetic interactions with
    AEDs, 403–404
  in sexual dysfunction, 158–162
Antidepressant-induced anorgasmia,
  frequency of, 160
Antiepileptic drugs, 20, 83, 135, 137, 157, 284.
  See also CYP450 enzyme-inducing AEDs;
  Epilepsy syndrome
  birth defect due to, 171–172
    orofacial clefting, 185–186
  body weight and, 330–335
  effect on
    bone, 313–316
    contraception, 96
    quality of life, 418
  in elderly WWE treatment, 392–393
  exposure, resulted in osteomalacia or
    rickets, 313
  exposure risk, during pregnancy, 418

Antiepileptic drugs (*cont.*)
  and hormones, interaction between, 93–94
  lipid metabolism and, 335–340
  MCMs (*see* Major congenital malformations)
  menstrual irregularities, 94
  metabolic acidosis, 340–342
  metabolism mechanisms of
    hydroxylation (oxidative) and
      glucuronidation, 216–217
  pharmacodynamic interactions with
    antidepressant, 404–405
    serotonin syndrome and myoclonus
      development, 405
    synergistic adverse events, 404
  pharmacokinetic characteristics of, 118
  pharmacokinetic interactions with
    antidepressant, 403–404
    co-medication with sodium valproate, 403
    fluvoxamine and phenytoin serum
      concentrations, 404
    impact of enzyme induction, on
      psychotropic drugs, 403
    inhibition, of CYP 2C19, CYP 3A4 and
      CYP 2D6, 403–404
    inhibitory effect of sertraline on
      lamotrigine, 404
    nefazodone and carbamazepine serum
      concentrations, 404
  in placenta and breast milk, 247–254
    factors affecting, 242–245
    identifying exposures of, 245–246
  in pregnancy, 229–237
  pregnancy registries, 296
  and psychotropic drugs, on sexual
    dysfunction, 157–163
  renal stones, 342
  seizure frequency and, 228–229
  and steroid hormones, 56–57
  teratogenicity due to (*see* Teratogenicity,
    AED-related)
  and weight gain in women, 150–151
Antipsychotic drugs, 360, 410
  impact on seizure threshold, 410–411
  pharmacodynamic interactions with
    AEDs, 412–413
  pharmacokinetic interactions with
    AEDs, 412
  on sexual dysfunction, 162–163
Antipsychotics and sexual functioning
  questionnaire, 162

Anxiolytic drugs
  pharmacodynamic interactions, with
    AEDS, 406
  pharmacokinetic interactions, with
    AEDs, 405
APDs. *See* Antipsychotic drugs
Area under curve (AUC), 3, 246
Arene oxides, 186–187
Arousal disorders, 164
Arteriovenous malformations
  (AVMs), 263–264
ASFQ. *See* Antipsychotics and Sexual
  Functioning Questionnaire
Atomoxetine, 408–409
ATPbinding cassette (ABC), 5
Attention deficit hyperactivity
  disorder, 362–364, 398–399, 402,
  407–409
Atypical APDs, 360–361, 410–411, 413

B

Benzodiazepines, 47–48, 86, 311, 352, 357–358,
  360, 364, 405–406
Beta human chorionic gonadotropin
  (BhCG), 277
Birth defects, 171. *See also* Teratogenicity,
  AED-related
  across general population surveillance
    programs, 298
  antiepileptic drug pregnancy registries
    and, 296
  dissemination of data and classification,
    review, 290
  due to AED treatment, 172
    congenital heart disease, 182
    IMEs, 183
    orofacial clefts, 185–186
  effect of folate and AEDs related, 190
  genetic defect in arene oxide detoxification
    and, 187
  maternal factors associated with
    alcohol and tobacco, 174
    endocrine conditions, 173
    folic acid deficiency, 173–174
  Rolling case control studies to monitor, 301
  ultrasound investigations for, 293
BMD. *See* Bone mineral density
Body mass index (BMI), 140, 146, 330,
  334, 340

Bone disease, AED-associated
  multiple therapies for treatment of, 321
  in women, 305
Bone health assessment
  BMD as significant predictor, 308–309
  bone turnover markers, 310
  mechanisms explaining changes, in epilepsy
      patient, 316–321
    AEDs, disrupting vitamin K and calcitonin
        secretion, 320
    AEDs, effecting intestinal calcium
        absorption, 319
    AEDs, inducing, disruption of vitamin D
        metabolism, 317
    CNS, role in, 320–321
    CYP450 enzyme-inducing AEDs, 316
    evidence supporting, prevailing model, 318
    observations, against model, 319
  vitamin D metabolites and calcitropic
      hormones, 309
Bone loss
  in premenopausal women treated with
      phenytoin, 316
  and turnover markers, 310
Bone mineral density, 97, 305, 308, 310–311,
    313, 315–317, 319–322
Bone physiology, 306–308
Bone-specific alkaline phosphatase, 98
Bone turnover markers, 310, 316
Breakthrough bleeding, 86, 116, 122, 129
Bupropion, 159, 161–162, 164, 353, 402

C

Calcium homeostasis, 307
CAPDs. See Conventional APDs
Carbamazepine, 4, 31, 97, 103, 117, 121, 141,
    148, 158, 229, 315, 404, 409
  to accelerate metabolism of diazepam
      and, 405
  associated weight gain, 332–333
  haloperidol concentrations, in co-medication
      with, 412
  metabolism of, 216, 218
  monotherapy on hormones, in women with
      epilepsy, 150
  and phenobarbital, 337
  and phenytoin plasma concentrations in
      elders, 392
  in placenta and breast milk, 247

  in pregnancy, 232, 234
  SB apperta due to, 194–195
  serum lipid concentrations, 335–338
  and valproate, 337, 355
Catamenial epilepsy, 29, 36, 39, 55, 79–80
  define, 79
  epidemiology and patterns of, 81–83
  mechanisms of, 83–85
  patterns of, 82
  treatments for, 85–87
Catamenial seizures, 39, 85, 92–94. See also
    Catamenial epilepsy
CBZ. See Carbamazepine
Centers for Disease Control (CDC), 9
  babies with congenital malformations, reports
      on, 171
  birth classification schemes and chromosomal
      defects, 289
  classifications of birth defects by, 296
  folate supplementation recommendation,
      190, 192
  monitoring birth defects in relation to drug
      exposure, 301
Centers for Disease Control and
    Prevention, 171, 276
Central nervous system (CNS)
  $3\alpha,5\alpha$-THP synthesized de novo in, 45
  active drugs, 216
  $GABA_A$ receptor subunits, 54
  P4's antiseizure effects and, 39
  steroid hormones in, 29–30, 42–43
  stimulants, 407–408
  vulnerability, 373
Central nervous system stimulants (CNSS)
  impact on seizure threshold, 407–408
  pharmacodynamic interactions with
      AEDS, 410
  pharmacokinetic interactions with
      AEDs, 409
Cerebral venous thromboses (CVT), in
    pregnancy, 264
Childhood absence epilepsy (CAE), 18–19
Chlorpromazine, 7, 162, 361–362, 411–412
Citalopram, 160, 354, 400, 402–405
Clobazam, 86, 405
Clomiphene, 36, 86, 136
Clomipramine, 353, 401–403
Clonazepam, 250, 313, 357, 405–406
Clozapine, 361–362, 410–412
COC. See Combined oral contraceptive

Cognitive teratogenesis, maternal intelligence
    quotient (IQ) role in, 207
Combined oral contraceptive
    and AEDs, pharmacokinetics of, 117
        contraceptive patch, 123–124
        cytochrome 3A4 isoenzyme inducers, 118
        cytochrome 3A4 isoenzyme
            noninducers, 119
        emergency contraception, 125
        lamotrigine, 119–120
        NuvaRing®, 124
        oxcarbazepine, 120
        Plan B®, 125
        topiramate and felbamate, 121
    failure risk, 114
    pharmacology of, 116–117
Co-morbid psychiatric disorders, 397–399.
    See also Patients with epilepsy
Complete blood count (CBC), 261
Computerized tomography (CT), 264, 267
Congenital malformations. See also Birth defects
    babies born with, 171
    in children of mothers with epilepsy, 185
    definitions of, 172
    and folic acid supplementation, 276
    Lamictal Pregnancy Registry reevaluating rate
        of, 221
    maternal seizures during pregnancy and, 183
    phenobarbital monotherapy and, 196
    and pregnancy registries, 289
Conjugated equine estrogen (CEE), 46, 389
Conjugated equine estrogens plus
        medroxyprogesterone acetate (CEE/
        MPA), 389–390
Contraceptive counseling, 114
    women requiring AED prescription
        factors affecting contraceptive choice, 128
        hormonal contraception, 129–130
Contraceptive implants, 124
Contraceptive methods
    with AED interaction (see also Combined oral
        contraceptive)
    without AED interaction
        barriers methods, 126–127
        female sterilization, 127
        IUDs, 125–126
        lactational amenorrhea method, 128
Contraceptive patch, 123–124
Contraceptive vaginal ring, 124
Conventional APDs, 360–361, 410–412

Cryptogenic epilepsy, 13, 399
CYP450 enzyme-inducing AEDs, 94
    oral contraception failure risk, 96
    osteoporosis risk, 97–98
CYP isozyme system, 403, 412
Cyproheptadine, 161
Cytochrome 3A4 isoenzyme
    inducers, 118
    noninducers, 119
Cytochrome P-450 (cyt P-450), family of
        enzymes, 1, 4, 43, 117, 216, 230, 232, 245
    in CBZ metabolism, 218
    enzyme-inducing AEDs, 97, 103, 316
    formation of electrophilic reactive
        intermediate by, 217
    genes, role of polymorphisms in, 221–222
    hepatic and renal isoenzymes, 307
    in LTG metabolism, 219
    in PHT metabolism, 218
    relevant to antiepileptic medications, 244
    VPA metabolism, 220–221

D

DA. See Dopamine
Depo-provera, 97
Depot Medroxyprogesterone Acetate or
        Depo-Provera® (DMPA), 122–123, 128
Depressive disorders, 101, 348, 352
Desipramine, 403
Dihydrodiol (DHD), 186–187, 236
5α-Dihydroprogesterone (DHP), 40, 43,
        46–47, 49
Dihydrotestosterone (DHT), 31–32, 51–52
Dopamine, 162, 359, 361, 402, 408, 410
Dopamine-norepinephrine reuptake
        inhibitors, 402–403
Dopamine-serotonin antagonists, 361, 410
Down's syndrome, 277
Doxepin, 403
Drug-induced osteomalacia and rickets, 313
Drug reactions, in females, 7–8
Duloxetine, 160, 402, 404

E

Electroencephalography (EEG), 12, 39, 355,
        357–358, 368, 408, 411
Emergency contraception, 125
Endocrine disorders and epilepsy, 136–137

Enzyme-inducing AEDs, 148
EPIGEN study, 15–16
Epilepsy in women, 136
  evaluation for reproductive endocrine
      disorders, 141–144
  fertility of, 139–141
  menopause, 139
  puberty and menopause in, 138–139
  sexual dysfunction
    antiepileptic and psychotropic drugs effect
        on, 157–163
    treatment for, 163–164
Epilepsy, in young women. *See also* Pregnant
    women with epilepsy
  AEDs and oral contraceptive hormones,
      interaction between
    pregnancy risk, 115–116
  comorbidities associated with
    depression and suicide, 101–102
    migraine, 102
  influence of hormones on, 93
  management of (*see* Patient management)
  psychosocial issues
    driving, 99–100
    educational underachievement, 99
    quality of life, 98–99
    stigma, 100–101
  reproductive health and endocrinal
      disturbances (*see* Reproductive health
      and endocrinal disturbances)
  treatment with valproate
    anovulatory cycles, rate of, 94
Epilepsy-related social disabilities, role of
    gender in, 418
Epilepsy syndrome, 11–12. *See also* Seizure
    disorders
  catamenial epilepsy, 80
    epidemiology and patterns of, 81–83
    mechanisms of, 83–85
    treatments for, 85–87
  classification of, 12–14
  epidemiologic studies, methodology of, 14
  gender differences in epidemiology of
    incidence of, 14–18
    mortality in, 21–22
    prevalence of, 18
    prognosis in, 20
    in specific epilepsy syndromes, 18–20
    status epilepticus, 22–23
  and pregnancy, management of

antiseizure medicine
    management, 275–276
  fetal anatomical defect screening, 277–278
  labor, obstetrical risks and
      management, 278–281
  preconception counseling, 274
  prenatal care, 277
  vitamin supplementation, 276–277
  woman's seizure activity assessment, 275
  in remission, 13, 23
EPIMART study, 15–16
Epoxide hydrolase activity, 186–187
Escitalopram, 160, 402, 404–405
Estrogen (E)
  antagonist, 86
  effects, on seizure disorders, 37–38
  estrogen:progesterone ratio, 93
  exogenous administration of, 116
  levels with concurrent AED use, 122
  oral administration, 117
  as potent pro-convulsant, 84
  reducing bone resorption by, 308
  replacement therapy, 163 (*see also* Hormone
      replacement therapy)
Ethinyl estradiol (EE)
  dose in oral contraceptives, 116
  hydroxylation and conjugation, 117
Ethosuximide (ESX), 4, 119, 247, 250, 359
  in placenta and breast milk, 250
  during pregnancy, 234
Etonogestrel implant, 124
EUROCAT network, of congenital
    malformation registries, 301
European Medicines Evaluation Agency
    (EMEA), 285
European network of Congenital Anomoly and
    Twin registers (EUROCAT), 296
European Registry for AntiEpileptic Drugs
    (EURAP), 291
Excitatory post synaptic potentials (EPSPs), 84

F

Felbamate, 121, 247, 334, 352, 413
Female orgasmic disorder (FOD), 163–164
Female sexual arousal disorder (FSAD), 163–164
Female sexual dysfunction, treatment
    for, 163–164
Females, pharmacological response in, 1–2
Fertility of women with epilepsy, 139–141

Fetal anatomical defects, screening for, 277–278
Fetal valproate syndrome, 194
Fluoxetine, 354, 400, 402–403, 405
Fluphenazine, 162, 362, 411
Fluvoxamine, 354, 402, 404
Focal epilepsies, 20
Folic acid deficiency, 173–174
Follicle stimulating hormone, 35, 80, 116, 139, 144, 146–147, 387
Food and Drug Administration (FDA), 3, 8, 115, 126, 246, 286, 361, 392
Fracture rates, AED-treated patients, 306
FSH. *See* Follicle stimulating hormone

G

GABA$_A$/benzodiazepine receptor complex (GBRs), 47
Gabapentin, 298, 404, 412
  associated weight gain, 333
  insulin and glucose levels, 339
  in placenta and breast milk, 251–252
Gender differences
  in epidemiology of epilepsy, 11–12
    incidence of, 14–18
    mortality in, 21–22
    prevalence of, 18
    prognosis in, 20
    in specific epilepsy syndromes, 18–20
    status epilepticus, 22–23
  in pharmacological response, 2
  in seizure disorders, 27–30
    acute stress-induced steroid biosynthesis and, 50–52
    androgens in, 30–33
    factors affecting, 54–55
    GABA transmitter system, 47–50
    HPG role in, 33–36
    reproductive events and, 36–47
    stress-induced changes in, 52–54
Genetic polymorphisms, in CYP enzymes expression, 5
Gestational epilepsy, 260
Gestational hypertension (GH), 265
Ginkgo biloba, 161
Glucocorticoid receptor, 186
  phenytoin teratogenicity and, 189
  RU5020 binding to, 51
Glucuronidation, 4, 119–120, 217, 220, 230, 260, 362, 404, 413

Glutathione, 186, 188, 193, 217, 220, 222
Gonadotropin releasing hormone (GnRH), 35–36, 80, 145–146

H

HA. *See* Hypothalamic amenorrhea
Haloperidol, 162, 411–412
HELLP syndrome, 266
Hepatic enzymes, function of, 4–5
Histone deacytelase (HDAC), 222
Homeobox (HOX) genes, 189
Hormonal contraception. *See* Oral contraceptives
Hormone replacement therapy, 316, 321, 386, 389–392
HPRL. *See* Hyperprolactinemia
HRT. *See* Hormone replacement therapy
Human chorionic gonadotropin (hCG), 277
Hydantoin syndrome, 276
3α-Hydroxy-5α-pregnan-20-one (3α,5α-THP), 40
  biosynthesis/metabolism of, 42–45
  GBR activity and, 47–48
  variations in, 45–46
3α-Hydroxysteroid dehydrogenase (3α-HSD), 32
Hyperinsulinemia, 145–146, 332, 339
Hyperprolactinemia, 135–136, 361, 410
Hypoactive sexual desire disorder (HSDD), 163–164
Hypogonadotropic hypogonadism, 144
Hypoplasia, 189, 211, 276
Hypothalamic amenorrhea, 135–136, 144, 149
Hypothalamic–pituitary–adrenal (HPA), 50
Hypothalamic–pituitary–gonadal axis (HPG), 33

I

Idiopathic epilepsy, 13–14, 137, 398
Idiopathic generalized epilepsies (IGEs), 11, 18–19, 93, 105
Imipramine, 159, 400, 403
Independence, aspect of epilepsy, 418
Indomethacin therapy, 47
International Lamotrigine Pregnancy Registry, 290
International League Against Epilepsy (ILAE), 11–14

Intracerebral hemorrhage (ICH)
  maternal deaths attributable to, 268
  in pregnancy, 263
Intrauterine devices (IUDs), 114

J

Juvenile absence epilepsy (JAE), 19, 93
Juvenile myoclonic epilepsy (JME), 19, 93, 103, 350

K

Kainate-induced model, 391
Keppra pregnancy registry, 291
Ketogenic diet and renal stones, 342

L

Lamictal Pregnancy Registry, 221
Lamotrigine, 96, 119–120, 216, 219, 229, 298, 316, 404, 406, 412
  metabolism of, 216
  in placenta and breast milk, 252–253
  during pregnancy, 235–236
Leucopenia, 412
Levetiracetam (LEV), 412
  in placenta and breast milk, 252
  during pregnancy, 236–237
Levonorgestrel capsules, 124
Libido and antipsychotic drugs, 162
Lithium
  pharmacodynamic interactions with AEDs, 406–407
  pharmacokinetic interactions with AEDs, 406
Lithium–pilocarpine model. See Status epilepticus
Localization-related epilepsy (LRE), 158
Long QT syndrome, in females, 7
Loxepine, 411
LTG. See Lamotrigine
Luteinizing hormone (LH), 35, 144
Lymphocyte cytotoxicity, 187

M

Major congenital malformations
  AED exposure and, 205
    relationship of dose to, 209
    risk for cleft palate, 209–210

MAOIs. See Monoamine oxidase inhibitors
Maprotiline, 353, 401–402
Maternal epilepsy, and congenital malformation risk, 183–184
Maternal obesity
  and congenital anomalies, 173
  folic acid deficiency risk, 174
Maternal serum alpha fetoprotein (MSAFP), 277
MCMs. See Major congenital malformations
Menstrual cycle, 7, 28, 33, 55, 80, 83, 86–87, 93, 95, 139, 141, 387
Mesial temporal sclerosis, 12, 20
Metabolic acidosis and antiepileptic drugs, association, 340–342
Methylphenidate, 364, 407–409
Mianserin, 403
Migraine and epilepsy, 102
Minor malformations, 211
Mirtazapine, 159, 161, 400
Modafinil, 408
Molindone, 411
Mono-amino-oxidase inhibitors, 159, 401
Monohydroxy derivative (MHD), 230
Multidrug resistance protein (MRP), 244
Myoclonic seizures, 400

N

National General Practice Study of Epilepsy (NGPSE), 20
National Institutes of Health (NIH), 8
Nefazodone, 159, 161, 403–404
Neonatal anticonvulsant exposure, causes of, 242
Neonate bleeding, prevention of, 279
Neural tube defects
  association of valproate with
    dysmorphism, 193–194
    spina bifida (SB), 194
  epidemiology and pathogenesis, 192–193
  and folate supplementation, 190–191
Neuroactive steroids, 42–43
  effects on GBR, 48
  factors affecting, 54–55
  treatment for catamenial epilepsy, 87
Neuroendocrine cycle, in females, 80–81
Neuroleptic malignant syndrome, 412
NMDA seizure-induction model, 391
N-Methyl-d-aspartate (NMDA), 32, 38, 54, 391
Nonepileptic patients, seizure disorder in, 262–265

Nonepileptic seizures. *See also* Patients with
   epilepsy
   gender differences in, 367–368
   misdiagnosis and mistreatment of, 367
   negative prognostic factors, 367
   treatment of, 369–370
      assessment and treatment
         approach, 372–373
      4 E interventions, 371
      etiological and biomedical approaches, 371
      psychopharmacologic effect, 373
      video-electroencephalographic monitoring
         (vEEG), 368–369
Non-TCA agents, 403
North American Anti-Epileptic Drug
   (NAAED), 294–297
Nortriptyline, 403
NTDs. *See* Neural tube defects
NuvaRing®, 124

O

Obesity and AEDs, 330–335
OCP. *See* Oral contraceptives
Olanzapine, 162, 361, 410–413
Oral contraceptives, 117
   and AEDs, pharmacokinetics of, 117
      breakthrough bleeding, 122
      COC failure, 96–97, 114–116
      cytochrome 3A4 isoenzyme inducers, 118
      cytochrome 3A4 isoenzyme
         noninducers, 119
      DMPA, 122–123
      lamotrigine, 119–120
      oxcarbazepine, 120
      POPs, 122
      seizure susceptibility, 121
      topiramate and felbamate, 121
Organization for Teratology Information and
   Specialists (OTIS), 291
Osteocalcin, 310, 316, 320
Osteomalacia, 313–314, 317
Osteoporosis
   with CYP450 enzyme-inducing AEDs, 97–98
   secondary causes of, 314
   treatments for, 322
Osteoporotic fractures, 315–316
Oxcarbazepine (OXC), 5, 103, 120, 158, 230,
   403, 406
   associated weight gain, 333

   in placenta and breast milk, 253
   during pregnancy, 236

P

Parathyroid hormone, 98, 307–308, 317,
   319–320
Parkinsonian symptoms, 360
Paroxetine, 161, 402–404
Patient management, 102
   good nutrition, 103
   medication and contraception choice, 103
   sleep deprivation, 104–105
   specialized teenage clinics for, 105–106
   treatment compliance, 104
Patients with epilepsy (PWE), with comorbid
   disorders, 348
   anxiety disorder, 355–356
      ictal fear or panic, 356–357
      postictal symptoms, 357
      treatment of, 357
   attention deficit hyperactivity disorder
      (ADHD), 362–364
      treatment of, 364
   depression, 350, 418
      following epilepsy surgery, 352–353
      as iatrogenic process, 352
      interictal forms of depression, 352
      preictal and ictal symptoms, 351
      suicidality in patients, 350–351
      treatment of, 353–355
   evaluation of psychopathology, principles
      for, 349–350
   prevalence rates of, 349
   psychosis of epilepsy (POE), 357
      AED-related psychosis, 359–360
      alternative psychosis, 359
      drug treatment of, 360–362
      interictal psychotic disorders, 359
      postictal psychosis (PIP) and ictal psychotic
         symptoms, 358
      temporal lobectomy associated with, 360
PCO in women, prevalence of, 145
PCOS. *See* Polycystic ovarian syndrome
Pelvic ultrasonography, role of, 141
Pentylenetetrazol (PTZ), 28, 52, 84
Perfenazine, 411
Peroxisome proliferator-activated receptor delta
   (PPAR-δ), 222
Persons with epilepsy, fracture risk in, 311–313

demographic factors associated with, 312
drug exposure, assessment, 313
hip *vs.* forearm fracture, 312
osteoporotic fractures, 313
P-glycoprotein (Pgp), 5–6
Pharmacokinetics in females, factors affecting, 1
absorption and bioavailability of drugs, 3–4
body weight, 2–3
distribution and metabolism in, 4–5
pharmacodynamic changes, 7–8
renal clearance of drugs, 6
transporters, 5–6
Phenelzine, 159
Phenobarbital (PB), 229
in placenta and breast milk, 250
during pregnancy, 234
serum lipid concentrations and, 335–338
teratogenicity, 196
in utero exposure to, 210–211
Phenytoin, 158, 229, 315, 404
in elderly WWE treatment, 392–393
and hyperglycemia, 338–339
metabolism of, 219
oxidative (NADPH/02-dependent) metabolite
of, 187
in placenta and breast milk, 250–251
during pregnancy, 231–232
serum lipid concentrations, 337–338
teratogenicity
and glucocorticoid receptor, 189
MCM risk, 205, 208–209
reactive free radical intermediates
modulating, 188
Phospholipase inhibitory proteins (PLIPs), 189
PHT. *See* Phenytoin
Physicians desk reference (PDR), 407
Pituitary MRI, role of, 144
Placental associated pregnancy protein A
(PAPP-A), 277
Plan B®, 125
Polycystic ovarian syndrome, 135, 144–148
definition of, 95
risk of, 95
Polytherapy, 205
vs. monotherapy MCM risk, 209
POPs. *See* Progestin-only oral contraceptive pills
Postmenopausal hormone therapy, effects
of, 46–47
Postnatal day 15 (PND15), 30
Postpartum depression, 418

Postpartum eclampsia, 266
Preeclampsia, 266–267
Pregabalin, 333, 404, 412
Pregnancy registry, 285, 419
to close registry, 302
design of, 286–290
committee for data monitoring, 290
comparison group, selection of, 287–288
critical elements to consider, 287
data collection and presentation, 289–290
eligibility requirements, 288
exposure and outcome data, 288
FDA guidance, 286
objectives and sample size, 286–287
patient privacy and human subject data
protection, 290
pregnancy outcomes, to include, 288–289
future roles and responsibility, 302–303
guidelines, to establish, 286
Pregnant women with epilepsy
AED treatment and
safety of new drugs, 177–178
time of exposure to, 175–176
maternal factors associated with birth defects
alcohol and tobacco, 174
endocrine conditions, 173
folic acid deficiency, 173–174
risk factors associated with, 169–170
congenital malformations, 171–172
epileptic seizures and AED, 172
genetic make-up and environmental
exposure, 173
syncope and nonepileptic seizures, 171
teratogenesis, experimental models
of, 176–177
Primidone (PRM), 117, 176, 231, 244, 352, 359,
404
in placenta and breast milk, 250
during pregnancy, 234
Progesterone (P). *See also* Combined oral
contraceptive
antiseizure properties of, 38–40
biosynthesis and metabolism, pathway of, 44
metabolite and seizure disorders, 40–42
therapy for catamenial epilepsy, 86–87
Progestin, 30, 40, 46–47, 50–51, 55, 114,
116–117, 121. *See also* Oral contraceptives
Progestin-only oral contraceptive pills, 122
Protriptyline, 403
Psychiatric comorbidity and epilepsy, 334–335

Psychiatric disorders, 348, 350, 373, 398–399
Psychotropic and antiepileptic drugs, on sexual
        dysfunction, 157–163
PTH. *See* Parathyroid hormone
Puberty and menopause, in women with
        epilepsy, 138–139

R

5α-Reductase inhibitor finasteride therapy, 47
Registry design impact, on data interpretation,
        293–299. *See also* AED pregnancy registries;
        Pregnancy registry
    choice of comparator, 297–299
    exclusion of chromosomal abnormalities
        from, 296
    exposed pregnancies lost or withdrawn, 295
    length of follow-up, in registry, 297
    loss to follow-up rate, in NAAED, 296
    outcome ascertainment/
        classification, 296–297
    patient recruitment and data
        collection, 294–296
    potential bias on risk estimation, 294
Relative infant dose (RID), 246
Renal stones and antiepileptic drugs,
        association, 342
Renal tubular acidosis, 340–341
Reproductive health and endocrinal
        disturbances
    difficulties of pregnancies in, 97
    disorders, in women with epilepsy, 141–144
    dysfunctions and epilepsy, 35–36
    menstrual irregularities, 94
    oral contraception failure risk, 96–97
    PCOS, 95
    sexual dysfunction, 96
Reproductive hormones, impact on bone, 308
Retinoid Pregnancy Prevention
        Program, 174–175
Rickets, 313–314, 341
Risperidone, 162–163, 358, 411–413
Rochester epidemiologic project, 15–18

S

SB. *See* Spina bifida
Schizophrenia, 360, 410
SE. *See* Status epilepticus
Seizure disorders, 27–30

acute stress-induced steroid biosynthesis
        and, 50–52
    androgens in, 30–33
    changes in women with epilepsy, 387–389
    factors affecting, 54–55
    frequency and AED concentrations, 228–229
    GABA transmitter system, 47–50
    HPG role in, 33–36
    menopause and HRT in animal
        models, 391–392
    in pregnancy, 260–261
        assessment of control of, 275
        eclampsia, 265–268
        fetal anatomical defect screening, 277–278
        in nonepileptic patients, 262–265
        obstetrical risks and management in
            labor, 278–281
        prenatal care, 277
        vitamin supplementation, 276–277
    progestins role in, 55–56
    reproductive events and, 36–37
        biosynthesis/metabolism of 3α,
            5α-THP, 42–45
        estrogens effects on, 37–38
        postmenopausal hormone therapy
            effects, 46–47
        progesterone metabolites and, 38–42
        3α, 5α-THP variations in, 45–46
        stress-induced changes in, 52–54
Selective serotonin reuptake inhibitors, 101,
        159–160, 354, 400–403, 409, 413
Serotonin-norepinephrine reuptake
        inhibitors, 353, 357, 401–402, 405
Sertraline, 161, 402–403
Serum lipid concentrations and AEDs, 335–338
Sex hormone binding globulin, 84, 117, 123,
        146, 149–150, 158
Sexual dysfunction in women, with epilepsy
    antiepileptic and psychotropic drugs effect
        on, 157–158
        antidepressant drugs, 158–162
        antiepileptic drugs, 158
        antipsychotic drugs, 162–163
    treatment for, 163–164
SHBG. *See* Sex hormone binding globulin
Signals interpretation, 299–302. *See also*
        Pregnancy registry
    FDA guidance, 299
    logistical issues associated with, 301
    pregnancy registry data, use of, 299–301

multiple registries, for woman to AED, 300
rolling case control studies, 301
signal, define, 299
Slone rolling case control study and
    EUROCAT network, 301
validation of birth defect data, 301–302
Sildenafil, 161–162, 164
SNRIs. *See* Serotonin-norepinephrine reuptake
    inhibitors
Sodium/multivitamin transporter (SMVT), 244
Sodium valproate, 335, 403, 405. *See also*
    Valproate
Spike-wave discharges, progesterone in, 55
Spina bifida, 175, 177, 181, 209, 277
    association of carbamazepine and, 195
    following valproate exposure, 194
SSRIs. *See* Selective serotonin reuptake inhibitors
Standardized mortality ratio (SMR), 21, 351
Status epilepticus, 12–13, 259, 341, 358, 391
    incidence of, 22–23
    in pregnancy, 261
    prevention of, 275
Steroid Hormones and AEDs, interactions
    of, 56–57
Stevens-Johnson syndrome (SJS), 219, 222
Subarachnoid hemorrhage, in
    pregnanacy, 263–264
Substantia nigra pars reticulata (SNR), 30
Sudden unexpected death in epilepsy
    (SUDEP), 12, 21–22
Suicide risk, 101–102
Swedish Medical Birth Register, 293
Systemic lupus erythematosus (SLE), 7

T

TCAs. *See* Tricyclic antidepressants
Temporal lobe epilepsy (TLE), 29, 139
Teratogenesis, models of congenital
    malformation risk, 176–177
Teratogenicity, AED-related
    criteria for assessing, 206–207
    cyclic adenosine monophosphate and, 189
    epoxide metabolites
        detoxification, 186
        phenytoin, 187
    folate deficiency, 190–192
    free radical intermediates, 188
    hypoxia and reoxygenation, 188–189
    modifiers lowering risk of, 215

phenytoin and homeobox (HOX) genes, 189
    VPA, CBZ, and PHT exposure, 210–211
Testosterone (T), 147
    and AEDs, 413
    replacement in women, 163
    in seizure disorders, 31–32
    VPA elevating serum concentrations of, 138
Thalidomide disaster, 284
Thioridazine, 412
Tonic–clonic seizures (TCS), 136
Topiramate, 121, 413
    and hyperglycemia, 339
    metabolic acidosis and, 341–342
    in placenta and breast milk, 253–254
    and renal stones, association of, 342
    weight loss associated with, 334
Tourette's syndrome, 410
Toxic epidermal necrolysis (TEN), 222
Tricyclic antidepressants, 159, 399–401
Trifluoperazine, 362, 411
T4 serum concentrations, 407
Type-II diabetes mellitus, 413

U

UDP-glucuronyl transferase (UGT), 1, 5,
    244–245, 403, 405
Uridine diphosphate-glucuronosyltransferase
    (UGT), 1, 4, 230, 244, 390

V

Valproate, 158. *See also* Valproic acid
    association of NTDs with, 193–194
    and CBZ, MCM risk with, 208
    epileptic young women treatment with
        anovulatory cycles, 94
    metabolism of, 220–221
    PPAR-δ activation, 222
    teratogenicity mechanism of, 195
Valproic acid, 119, 121, 176, 189, 220, 229, 231,
    315–316, 320, 359, 362, 364, 406
    associated weight gain, 332
    and hyperglycemia, 339–340
    in placenta and breast milk, 251
    during pregnancy, 234
    and serum lipid concentrations, 335–338
    therapy in women, 138–139
VPA exposure
    in neonates, 251

Valproic acid, *(cont.)*
  NTDs and, 192–195
  in utero, 205
Venlafaxine, 159, 402, 404
Vitamin D, 305, 307, 317–319, 322
Vitamin D3 metabolism, 307–308
Vocational disabilities, role of gender in, 418
VPA. *See* Valproic acid

W

Women's Health Initiative (WHI), 389
Women with epilepsy (WWE), 260. *See also*
    Epilepsy syndrome
  AED treatment for elderly, 392–393
  early perimenopause and menopause
      symptoms in, 386–387
  evaluation for reproductive endocrine
      disorders, 141–144
  fertility of, 139–141
  HPRL and, 144
  HRT in menopausal, 389–391
  psychosocial consequences for (*see also* Patients
      with epilepsy)
    depression, impact of, 365

  stigma of epilepsy, 365–366
  puberty and menopause in, 138–139
  risk of MCMs with AEDs among, 205
    valproate exposure, 207–208
  seizures changes in, 387–389
  sexual dysfunction
    antiepileptic and psychotropic drugs effect
        on, 157–163
    treatment for, 163–164
  weight gain and endocrine disorders in,
      137, 148

Y

Yohimbine, 161

Z

Zonisamide, 119, 242, 412
  linked to depression, 352
  in placenta and breast milk, 254
  and renal stones, association of, 342
  renal tubular acidosis and, 341

CONTENTS OF RECENT VOLUMES

Volume 37

Section I: Selectionist Ideas and Neurobiology

Selectionist and Instructionist Ideas in Neuroscience
  Olaf Sporns

Population Thinking and Neuronal Selection: Metaphors or Concepts?
  Ernst Mayr

Selection and the Origin of Information
  Manfred Eigen

Section II: Development and Neuronal Populations

Morphoregulatory Molecules and Selectional Dynamics during Development
  Kathryn L. Crossin

Exploration and Selection in the Early Acquisition of Skill
  Esther Thelen and Daniela Corbetta

Population Activity in the Control of Movement
  Apostolos P. Georgopoulos

Section III: Functional Segregation and Integration in the Brain

Reentry and the Problem of Cortical Integration
  Giulio Tononi

Coherence as an Organizing Principle of Cortical Functions
  Wolf Singerl

Temporal Mechanisms in Perception
  Ernst Pöppel

Section IV: Memory and Models

Selection versus Instruction: Use of Computer Models to Compare Brain Theories
  George N. Reeke, Jr.

Memory and Forgetting: Long-Term and Gradual Changes in Memory Storage
  Larry R. Squire

Implicit Knowledge: New Perspectives on Unconscious Processes
  Daniel L. Schacter

Section V: Psychophysics, Psychoanalysis, and Neuropsychology

Phantom Limbs, Neglect Syndromes, Repressed Memories, and Freudian Psychology
  V. S. Ramachandran

Neural Darwinism and a Conceptual Crisis in Psychoanalysis
  Arnold H. Modell

A New Vision of the Mind
  Oliver Sacks

INDEX

Volume 38

Regulation of GABA$_A$ Receptor Function and Gene Expression in the Central Nervous System
  A. Leslie Morrow

Genetics and the Organization of the Basal Ganglia
  *Robert Hitzemann, Yeang Olan,
  Stephen Kanes, Katherine Dains,
  and Barbara Hitzemann*

Structure and Pharmacology of Vertebrate GABA$_A$ Receptor Subtypes
  *Paul J. Whiting, Ruth M. McKernan,
  and Keith A. Wafford*

Neurotransmitter Transporters: Molecular Biology, Function, and Regulation
  Beth Borowsky and Beth J. Hoffman

Presynaptic Excitability
  Meyer B. Jackson

Monoamine Neurotransmitters in Invertebrates
and Vertebrates: An Examination of the Diverse
Enzymatic Pathways Utilized to Synthesize and
Inactivate Biogenic Amines
  B. D. Sloley and A. V. Juorio

Neurotransmitter Systems in Schizophrenia
  Gavin P. Reynolds

Physiology of Bergmann Glial Cells
  Thomas Müller and Helmut Kettenmann

INDEX

Volume 39

Modulation of Amino Acid-Gated Ion Channels
by Protein Phosphorylation
  Stephen J. Moss and Trevor G. Smart

Use-Dependent   Regulation   of   GABA$_A$
Receptors
  Eugene M. Barnes, Jr.

Synaptic Transmission and Modulation in the
Neostriatum
  David M. Lovinger and Elizabeth Tyler

The   Cytoskeleton   and   Neurotransmitter
Receptors
  Valerie J. Whatley and R. Adron Harris

Endogenous Opioid Regulation of Hippocampal
Function
  Michele L. Simmons and Charles Chavkin

Molecular Neurobiology of the Cannabinoid
Receptor
  Mary E. Abood and Billy R. Martin

Genetic Models in the Study of Anesthetic Drug
Action
  Victoria J. Simpson and Thomas E. Johnson

Neurochemical Bases of Locomotion and
Ethanol Stimulant Effects
  Tamara J. Phillips and Elaine H. Shen

Effects of Ethanol on Ion Channels
  Fulton T. Crews, A. Leslie Morrow,
  Hugh Criswell, and George Breese

INDEX

Volume 40

Mechanisms of Nerve Cell Death: Apoptosis or
Necrosis after Cerebral Ischemia
  R. M. E. Chalmers-Redman, A. D. Fraser,
  W. Y. H. Ju, J. Wadia, N. A. Tatton, and
  W. G. Tatton

Changes in Ionic Fluxes during Cerebral Ischemia
  Tibor Kristian and Bo K. Siesjo

Techniques   for   Examining   Neuroprotective
Drugs in Vitro
  A. Richard Green and Alan J. Cross

Techniques   for   Examining   Neuroprotective
Drugs in Vivo
  Mark P. Goldberg, Uta Strasser, and Laura L. Dugan

Calcium Antagonists: Their Role in Neuroprotection
  A. Jacqueline Hunter

Sodium and Potassium Channel Modulators:
Their Role in Neuroprotection
  Tihomir P. Obrenovich

NMDA Antagonists: Their Role in Neuroprotection
  Danial L. Small

Development   of   the   NMDA   Ion-Channel
Blocker, Aptiganel Hydrochloride, as a Neuro-
protective Agent for Acute CNS Injury
  Robert N. McBurney

The Pharmacology of AMPA Antagonists and
Their Role in Neuroprotection
  Rammy Gill and David Lodge

GABA and Neuroprotection
  Patrick D. Lyden

Adenosine and Neuroprotection
  Bertil B. Fredholm

Interleukins and Cerebral Ischemia
  Nancy J. Rothwell, Sarah A. Loddick,
  and Paul Stroemer

Nitrone-Based Free Radical Traps as Neuropro-
tective Agents in Cerebral Ischemia and Other
Pathologies
  Kenneth Hensley, John M. Carney,
  Charles A. Stewart, Tahera Tabatabaie,
  Quentin Pye, and Robert A. Floyd

Neurotoxic and Neuroprotective Roles of Nitric Oxide in Cerebral Ischemia
Turgay Dalkara and Michael A. Moskowitz

A Review of Earlier Clinical Studies on Neuro-protective Agents and Current Approaches
Nils-Gunnar Wahlgren

INDEX

Volume 41

Section I: Historical Overview

Rediscovery of an Early Concept
Jeremy D. Schmahmann

Section II: Anatomic Substrates

The Cerebrocerebellar System
Jeremy D. Schmahmann and Deepak N. Pandya

Cerebellar Output Channels
Frank A. Middleton and Peter L. Strick

Cerebellar-Hypothalamic Axis: Basic Circuits and Clinical Observations
Duane E. Haines, Espen Dietrichs,
Gregory A. Mihailoff, and
E. Frank McDonald

Section III. Physiological Observations

Amelioration of Aggression: Response to Select-ive Cerebellar Lesions in the Rhesus Monkey
Aaron J. Berman

Autonomic and Vasomotor Regulation
Donald J. Reis and Eugene V. Golanov

Associative Learning
Richard F. Thompson, Shaowen Bao, Lu Chen,
Benjamin D. Cipriano, Jeffrey S. Grethe,
Jeansok J. Kim, Judith K. Thompson, Jo Anne Tracy,
Martha S. Weninger, and David J. Krupa

Visuospatial Abilities
Robert Lalonde

Spatial Event Processing
Marco Molinari, Laura Petrosini,
and Liliana G. Grammaldo

Section IV: Functional Neuroimaging Studies

Linguistic Processing
Julie A. Fiez and Marcus E. Raichle

Sensory and Cognitive Functions
Lawrence M. Parsons and
Peter T. Fox

Skill Learning
Julien Doyon

Section V: Clinical and Neuropsychological Observations

Executive Function and Motor Skill Learning
Mark Hallett and Jordon Grafman

Verbal Fluency and Agrammatism
Marco Molinari, Maria G. Leggio, and
Maria C. Silveri

Classical Conditioning
Diana S. Woodruff-Pak

Early Infantile Autism
Margaret L. Bauman, Pauline A. Filipek, and
Thomas L. Kemper

Olivopontocerebellar Atrophy and Fried-reich's Ataxia: Neuropsychological Conse-quences of Bilateral versus Unilateral Cerebellar Lesions
Thérèse Botez-Marquard and
Mihai I. Botez

Posterior Fossa Syndrome
Ian F. Pollack

Cerebellar Cognitive Affective Syndrome
Jeremy D. Schmahmann and Janet C. Sherman

Inherited Cerebellar Diseases
Claus W. Wallesch and Claudius Bartels

Neuropsychological Abnormalities in Cerebellar Syndromes—Fact or Fiction?
Irene Daum and Hermann Ackermann

Section VI: Theoretical Considerations

Cerebellar Microcomplexes
Masao Ito

Control of Sensory Data Acquisition
James M. Bower

Neural Representations of Moving Systems
Michael Paulin

How Fibers Subserve Computing Capabilities: Similarities between Brains and Machines
Henrietta C. Leiner and
Alan L. Leiner

Cerebellar Timing Systems
  Richard Ivry

Attention Coordination and Anticipatory
Control
  *Natacha A. Akshoomoff, Eric Courchesne, and
  Jeanne Townsend*

Context-Response Linkage
  W. Thomas Thach

Duality of Cerebellar Motor and Cognitive
Functions
  James R. Bloedel and Vlastislav Bracha

Section VII: Future Directions

Therapeutic and Research Implications
  Jeremy D. Schmahmann

Volume 42

Alzheimer Disease
  Mark A. Smith

Neurobiology of Stroke
  W. Dalton Dietrich

Free Radicals, Calcium, and the Synaptic
Plasticity-Cell Death Continuum: Emerging
Roles of the Trascription Factor NFκB
  Mark P. Mattson

AP-I Transcription Factors: Short- and Long-
Term Modulators of Gene Expression in the
Brain
  Keith Pennypacker

Ion Channels in Epilepsy
  Istvan Mody

Posttranslational Regulation of Ionotropic Glu-
tamate Receptors and Synaptic Plasticity
  *Xiaoning Bi, Steve Standley, and
  Michel Baudry*

Heritable Mutations in the Glycine, GABA_A,
and Nicotinic Acetylcholine Receptors Provide
New Insights into the Ligand-Gated Ion Channel Receptor Superfamily
  Behnaz Vafa and Peter R. Schofield

INDEX

Volume 43

Early Development of the *Drosophila* Neuromus-
cular Junction: A Model for Studying Neuronal
Networks in Development
  Akira Chiba

Development of Larval Body Wall Muscles
  *Michael Bate, Matthias Landgraf,
  and Mar Ruiz Gmez Bate*

Development of Electrical Properties and Synaptic Transmission at the Embryonic Neuromuscular Junction
  Kendal S. Broadie

Ultrastructural Correlates of Neuromuscular
Junction Development
  *Mary B. Rheuben, Motojiro Yoshihara,
  and Yoshiaki Kidokoro*

Assembly and Maturation of the *Drosophila*
Larval Neuromuscular Junction
  L. Sian Gramates and Vivian Budnik

Second Messenger Systems Underlying Plasticity
at the Neuromuscular Junction
  Frances Hannan and Yi Zhong

Mechanisms of Neurotransmitter Release
  *J. Troy Littleton, Leo Pallanck, and
  Barry Ganetzky*

Vesicle Recycling at the *Drosophila* Neuromuscular Junction
  Daniel T. Stimson and Mani Ramaswami

Ionic Currents in Larval Muscles of *Drosophila*
  Satpal Singh and Chun-Fang Wu

Development of the Adult Neuromuscular
System
  Joyce J. Fernandes and Haig Keshishian

Controlling the Motor Neuron
  *James R. Trimarchi, Ping Jin, and
  Rodney K. Murphey*

Volume 44

Human Ego-Motion Perception
  A. V. van den Berg

Optic Flow and Eye Movements
  M. Lappe and K.-P. Hoffman

The Role of MST Neurons during Ocular Tracking in 3D Space
  K. Kawano, U. Inoue, A. Takemura, Y. Kodaka, and F. A. Miles

Visual Navigation in Flying Insects
  M. V. Srinivasan and S.-W. Zhang

Neuronal Matched Filters for Optic Flow Processing in Flying Insects
  H. G. Krapp

A Common Frame of Reference for the Analysis of Optic Flow and Vestibular Information
  B. J. Frost and D. R. W. Wylie

Optic Flow and the Visual Guidance of Locomotion in the Cat
  H. Sherk and G. A. Fowler

Stages of Self-Motion Processing in Primate Posterior Parietal Cortex
  F. Bremmer, J.-R. Duhamel, S. B. Hamed, and W. Graf

Optic Flow Analysis for Self-Movement Perception
  C. J. Duffy

Neural Mechanisms for Self-Motion Perception in Area MST
  R. A. Andersen, K. V. Shenoy, J. A. Crowell, and D. C. Bradley

Computational Mechanisms for Optic Flow Analysis in Primate Cortex
  M. Lappe

Human Cortical Areas Underlying the Perception of Optic Flow: Brain Imaging Studies
  M. W. Greenlee

What Neurological Patients Tell Us about the Use of Optic Flow
  L. M. Vaina and S. K. Rushton

INDEX

Volume 45

Mechanisms of Brain Plasticity: From Normal Brain Function to Pathology
  Philip. A. Schwartzkroin

Brain Development and Generation of Brain Pathologies
  Gregory L. Holmes and Bridget McCabe

Maturation of Channels and Receptors: Consequences for Excitability
  David F. Owens and Arnold R. Kriegstein

Neuronal Activity and the Establishment of Normal and Epileptic Circuits during Brain Development
  John W. Swann, Karen L. Smith, and Chong L. Lee

The Effects of Seizures of the Hippocampus of the Immature Brain
  Ellen F. Sperber and Solomon L. Moshe

Abnormal Development and Catastrophic Epilepsies: The Clinical Picture and Relation to Neuroimaging
  Harry T. Chugani and Diane C. Chugani

Cortical Reorganization and Seizure Generation in Dysplastic Cortex
  G. Avanzini, R. Preafico, S. Franceschetti, G. Sancini, G. Battaglia, and V. Scaioli

Rasmussen's Syndrome with Particular Reference to Cerebral Plasticity: A Tribute to Frank Morrell
  Fredrick Andermann and Yuonne Hart

Structural Reorganization of Hippocampal Networks Caused by Seizure Activity
  Daniel H. Lowenstein

Epilepsy-Associated Plasticity in gamma-Amniobutyric Acid Receptor Expression, Function and Inhibitory Synaptic Properties
  Douglas A. Coulter

Synaptic Plasticity and Secondary Epileptogenesis
  Timothy J. Teyler, Steven L. Morgan, Rebecca N. Russell, and Brian L. Woodside

Synaptic Plasticity in Epileptogenesis: Cellular Mechanisms Underlying Long-Lasting Synaptic Modifications that Require New Gene Expression
  Oswald Steward, Christopher S. Wallace, and Paul F. Worley

Cellular Correlates of Behavior
  Emma R. Wood, Paul A. Dudchenko, and Howard Eichenbaum

Mechanisms of Neuronal Conditioning
David A. T. King, David J. Krupa, Michael R. Foy, and Richard F. Thompson

Plasticity in the Aging Central Nervous System
C. A. Barnes

Secondary Epileptogenesis, Kindling, and Intractable Epilepsy: A Reappraisal from the Perspective of Neuronal Plasticity
Thomas P. Sutula

Kindling and the Mirror Focus
Dan C. McIntyre and Michael O. Poulter

Partial Kindling and Behavioral Pathologies
Robert E. Adamec

The Mirror Focus and Secondary Epileptogenesis
B. J. Wilder

Hippocampal Lesions in Epilepsy: A Historical Review
Robert Naquet

Clinical Evidence for Secondary Epileptogensis
Hans O. Luders

Epilepsy as a Progressive (or Nonprogressive "Benign") Disorder
John A. Wada

Pathophysiological Aspects of Landau-Kleffner Syndrome: From the Active Epileptic Phase to Recovery
Marie-Noelle Metz-Lutz, Pierre Maquet, Annd De Saint Martin, Gabrielle Rudolf, Norma Wioland, Edouard Hirsch, and Christian Marescaux

Local Pathways of Seizure Propagation in Neocortex
Barry W. Connors, David J. Pinto, and Albert E. Telefeian

Multiple Subpial Transection: A Clinical Assessment
C. E. Polkey

The Legacy of Frank Morrell
Jerome Engel, Jr.

Volume 46

Neurosteroids: Beginning of the Story
Etienne E. Baulieu, P. Robel, and M. Schumacher

Biosynthesis of Neurosteroids and Regulation of Their Synthesis
Synthia H. Mellon and Hubert Vaudry

Neurosteroid 7-Hydroxylation Products in the Brain
Robert Morfin and Luboslav Stárka

Neurosteroid Analysis
Ahmed A. Alomary, Robert L. Fitzgerald, and Robert H. Purdy

Role of the Peripheral-Type Benzodiazepine Receptor in Adrenal and Brain Steroidogenesis
Rachel C. Brown and Vassilios Papadopoulos

Formation and Effects of Neuroactive Steroids in the Central and Peripheral Nervous System
Roberto Cosimo Melcangi, Valerio Magnaghi, Mariarita Galbiati, and Luciano Martini

Neurosteroid Modulation of Recombinant and Synaptic GABA$_A$ Receptors
Jeremy J. Lambert, Sarah C. Harney, Delia Belelli, and John A. Peters

GABA$_A$-Receptor Plasticity during Long-Term Exposure to and Withdrawal from Progesterone
Giovanni Biggio, Paolo Follesa, Enrico Sanna, Robert H. Purdy, and Alessandra Concas

Stress and Neuroactive Steroids
Maria Luisa Barbaccia, Mariangela Serra, Robert H. Purdy, and Giovanni Biggio

Neurosteroids in Learning and Memory Processes
Monique Vallée, Willy Mayo, George F. Koob, and Michel Le Moal

Neurosteroids and Behavior
Sharon R. Engel and Kathleen A. Grant

Ethanol and Neurosteroid Interactions in the Brain
A. Leslie Morrow, Margaret J. VanDoren, Rebekah Fleming, and Shannon Penland

Preclinical Development of Neurosteroids as Neuroprotective Agents for the Treatment of Neurodegenerative Diseases
Paul A. Lapchak and Dalia M. Araujo

Clinical Implications of Circulating Neurosteroids
Andrea R. Genazzani, Patrizia Monteleone,
Massimo Stomati, Francesca Bernardi,
Luigi Cobellis, Elena Casarosa, Michele Luisi,
Stefano Luisi, and Felice Petraglia

Neuroactive Steroids and Central Nervous System Disorders
Mingde Wang, Torbjörn Bäckström,
Inger Sundström, Göran Wahlström,
Tommy Olsson, Di Zhu, Inga-Maj Johansson,
Inger Björn, and Marie Bixo

Neuroactive Steroids in Neuropsychopharmacology
Rainer Rupprecht and Florian Holsboer

Current Perspectives on the Role of Neurosteroids in PMS and Depression
Lisa D. Griffin, Susan C. Conrad, and
Synthia H. Mellon

INDEX

Volume 47

Introduction: Studying Gene Expression in Neural Tissues by in Situ Hybridization
W. Wisden and B. J. Morris

Part I: In Situ Hybridization with Radiolabelled Oligonucleotides
In Situ Hybridization with Oligonucleotide Probes
Wl. Wisden and B. J. Morris

Cryostat Sectioning of Brains
Victoria Revilla and Alison Jones

Processing Rodent Embryonic and Early Postnatal Tissue for in Situ Hybridization with Radiolabelled Oligonucleotides
David J. Laurie, Petra C. U. Schrotz,
Hannah Monyer, and Ulla Amtmann

Processing of Retinal Tissue for in Situ Hybridization
Frank Müller

Processing the Spinal Cord for in Situ Hybridization with Radiolabelled Oligonucleotides
A. Berthele and T. R. Tölle

Processing Human Brain Tissue for in Situ Hybridization with Radiolabelled Oligonucleotides
Louise F. B. Nicholson

In Situ Hybridization of Astrocytes and Neurons Cultured in Vitro
L. A. Arizza-McNaughton, C. De Felipe,
and S. P. Hunt

In Situ Hybridization on Organotypic Slice Cultures
A. Gerfin-Moser and H. Monyer

Quantitative Analysis of in Situ Hybridization Histochemistry
Andrew L. Gundlach and Ross D. O'Shea

Part II: Nonradioactive in Situ hybridization

Nonradioactive in Situ Hybridization Using Alkaline Phosphatase-Labelled Oligonucleotides
S. J. Augood, E. M. McGowan, B. R. Finsen,
B. Heppelmann, and P. C. Emson

Combining Nonradioactive in Situ Hybridization with Immunohistological and Anatomical Techniques
Petra Wahle

Nonradioactive in Situ Hybridization: Simplified Procedures for Use in Whole Mounts of Mouse and Chick Embryos
Linda Ariza-McNaughton and Robb Krumlauf

INDEX

Volume 48

Assembly and Intracellular Trafficking of GABA$_A$ Receptors Eugene
Barnes

Subcellular Localization and Regulation of GABA$_A$ Receptors and Associated Proteins
Bernhard Lüscher and Jean-Marc Fritschy D$_1$ Dopamine Receptors
Richard Mailman

Molecular Modeling of Ligand-Gated Ion Channels: Progress and Challenges
Ed Bertaccini and James R. Trudel

Alzheimer's Disease: Its Diagnosis and Pathogenesis
    Jillian J. Kril and Glenda M. Halliday

DNA Arrays and Functional Genomics in
Neurobiology
    Christelle Thibault, Long Wang, Li Zhang, and
    Michael F. Miles

INDEX

Volume 49

What Is West Syndrome?
    Olivier Dulac, Christine Soufflet,
    Catherine Chiron, and Anna Kaminski

The Relationship between encephalopathy and
Abnormal Neuronal Activity in the Developing
Brain
    Frances E. Jensen

Hypotheses from Functional Neuroimaging
Studies
    Csaba Juhász, Harry T. Chugani,
    Ouo Muzik, and Diane C. Chugani

Infantile Spasms: Unique Sydrome or General
Age-Dependent Manifestation of a Diffuse
Encephalopathy?
    M. A. Koehn and M. Duchowny

Histopathology of Brain Tissue from Patients
with Infantile Spasms
    Harry V. Vinters

Generators of Ictal and Interictal Electroenceph-
alograms Associated with Infantile Spasms:
Intracellular Studies of Cortical and Thalamic
Neurons
    M. Steriade and I. Timofeev

Cortical and Subcortical Generators of Normal
and Abnormal Rhythmicity
    David A. McCormick

Role of Subcortical Structures in the Pathogenesis of Infantile Spasms: What Are Possible
Subcortical Mediators?
    F. A. Lado and S. L. Moshé

What Must We Know to Develop Better
Therapies?
    Jean Aicardi

The Treatment of Infantile Spasms: An
Evidence-Based Approach
    Mark Mackay, Shelly Weiss, and
    O. Carter Snead III

ACTH Treatment of Infantile Spasms: Mechanisms of Its Effects in Modulation of Neuronal
Excitability
    K. L. Brunson, S. Avishai-Eliner, and
    T. Z. Baram

Neurosteroids and Infantile Spasms: The Deoxy-
ycorticosterone Hypothesis
    Michael A. Rogawski and Doodipala S. Reddy

Are there Specific Anatomical and/or Transmitter Systems (Cortical or Subcortical) That
Should Be Targeted?
    Phillip C. Jobe

Medical versus Surgical Treatment: Which
Treatment When
    W. Donald Shields

Developmental Outcome with and without
Successful Intervention
    Rochelle Caplan, Prabha Siddarth,
    Gary Mathern, Harry Vinters, Susan Curtiss,
    Jennifer Levitt, Robert Asarnow, and
    W. Donald Shields

Infantile Spasms versus Myoclonus: Is There a
Connection?
    Michael R. Pranzatelli

Tuberous Sclerosis as an Underlying Basis for
Infantile Spasm
    Raymond S. Yeung

Brain Malformation, Epilepsy, and Infantile
Spasms
    M. Elizabeth Ross

Brain Maturational Aspects Relevant to Pathophysiology of Infantile Spasms
    G. Auanzini, F. Panzica, and
    S. Franceschetti

Gene Expression Analysis as a Strategy to
Understand the Molecular Pathogenesis of
Infantile Spasms
    Peter B. Crino

Infantile Spasms: Criteria for an Animal Model
    Carl E. Stafstrom and Gregory L. Holmes

INDEX

Volume 50

Part I: Primary Mechanisms

How Does Glucose Generate Oxidative Stress In Peripheral Nerve?
   Irina G. Obrosova

Glycation in Diabetic Neuropathy: Characteristics, Consequences, Causes, and Therapeutic Options
   Paul J. Thornalley

Part II: Secondary Changes

Protein Kinase C Changes in Diabetes: Is the Concept Relevant to Neuropathy?
   Joseph Eichberg

Are Mitogen-Activated Protein Kinases Glucose Transducers for Diabetic Neuropathies?
   Tertia D. Purves and David R. Tomlinson

Neurofilaments in Diabetic Neuropathy
   Paul Fernyhough and Robert E. Schmidt

Apoptosis in Diabetic Neuropathy
   Aviva Tolkovsky

Nerve and Ganglion Blood Flow in Diabetes: An Appraisal
   Douglas W. Zochodne

Part III: Manifestations

Potential Mechanisms of Neuropathic Pain in Diabetes
   Nigel A. Calcutt

Electrophysiologic Measures of Diabetic Neuropathy: Mechanism and Meaning
   Joseph C. Arezzo and Elena Zotova

Neuropathology and Pathogenesis of Diabetic Autonomic Neuropathy
   Robert E. Schmidt

Role of the Schwann Cell in Diabetic Neuropathy
   Luke Eckersley

Part IV: Potential Treatment

Polyol Pathway and Diabetic Peripheral Neuropathy
   Peter J. Oates

Nerve Growth Factor for the Treatment of Diabetic Neuropathy: What Went Wrong, What Went Right, and What Does the Future Hold?
   Stuart C. Apfel

Angiotensin-Converting Enzyme Inhibitors: Are there Credible Mechanisms for Beneficial Effects in Diabetic Neuropathy?
   Rayaz A. Malik and
   David R. Tomlinson

Clinical Trials for Drugs Against Diabetic Neuropathy: Can We Combine Scientific Needs With Clinical Practicalities?
   Dan Ziegler and Dieter Luft

INDEX

Volume 51

Energy Metabolism in the Brain
   Leif Hertz and Gerald A. Dienel

The Cerebral Glucose-Fatty Acid Cycle: Evolutionary Roots, Regulation, and (Patho) physiological Importance
   Kurt Heininger

Expression, Regulation, and Functional Role of Glucose Transporters (GLUTs) in Brain
   Donard S. Dwyer, Susan J. Vannucci, and
   Ian A. Simpson

Insulin-Like Growth Factor-1 Promotes Neuronal Glucose Utilization During Brain Development and Repair Processes
   Carolyn A. Bondy and Clara M. Cheng

CNS Sensing and Regulation of Peripheral Glucose Levels
   Barry E. Levin, Ambrose A. Dunn-Meynell, and
   Vanessa H. Routh

Glucose Transporter Protein Syndromes
   Darryl C. De Vivo, Dong Wang,
   Juan M. Pascual, and
   Yuan Yuan Ho

Glucose, Stress, and Hippocampal Neuronal Vulnerability
   Lawrence P. Reagan

Glucose/Mitochondria in Neurological Conditions
  John P. Blass

Energy Utilization in the Ischemic/Reperfused Brain
  John W. Phillis and Michael H. O'Regan

Diabetes Mellitus and the Central Nervous System
  Anthony L. McCall

Diabetes, the Brain, and Behavior: Is There a Biological Mechanism Underlying the Association between Diabetes and Depression?
  A. M. Jacobson, J. A. Samson,
  K. Weinger, and C. M. Ryan

Schizophrenia and Diabetes
  David C. Henderson and Elissa R. Ettinger

Psychoactive Drugs Affect Glucose Transport and the Regulation of Glucose Metabolism
  Donard S. Dwyer, Timothy D. Ardizzone, and Ronald J. Bradley

INDEX

Stress and Secretory Immunity
  Jos A. Bosch, Christopher Ring,
  Eco J. C. de Geus, Enno C. I. Veerman, and
  Arie V. Nieuw Amerongen

Cytokines and Depression
  Angela Clow

Immunity and Schizophrenia: Autoimmunity, Cytokines, and Immune Responses
  Fiona Gaughran

Cerebral Lateralization and the Immune System
  Pierre J. Neveu

Behavioral Conditioning of the Immune System
  Frank Hucklebridge

Psychological and Neuroendocrine Correlates of Disease Progression
  Julie M. Turner-Cobb

The Role of Psychological Intervention in Modulating Aspects of Immune Function in Relation to Health and Well-Being
  J. H. Gruzelier

INDEX

Volume 52

Neuroimmune Relationships in Perspective
  Frank Hucklebridge and Angela Clow

Sympathetic Nervous System Interaction with the Immune System
  Virginia M. Sanders and Adam P. Kohm

Mechanisms by Which Cytokines Signal the Brain
  Adrian J. Dunn

Neuropeptides: Modulators of Immune Responses in Health and Disease
  David S. Jessop

Brain–Immune Interactions in Sleep
  Lisa Marshall and Jan Born

Neuroendocrinology of Autoimmunity
  Michael Harbuz

Systemic Stress-Induced Th2 Shift and Its Clinical Implications
  Ibia J. Elenkov

Neural Control of Salivary S-IgA Secretion
  Gordon B. Proctor and Guy H. Carpenter

Volume 53

Section I: Mitochondrial Structure and Function

Mitochondrial DNA Structure and Function
  Carlos T. Moraes, Sarika Srivastava,
  Ilias Kirkinezos, Jose Oca-Cossio,
  Corina van Waveren, Markus Woischnick,
  and Francisca Diaz

Oxidative Phosphorylation: Structure, Function, and Intermediary Metabolism
  Simon J. R. Heales, Matthew E. Gegg, and
  John B. Clark

Import of Mitochondrial Proteins
  Matthias F. Bauer, Sabine Hofmann, and
  Walter Neupert

Section II: Primary Respiratory Chain Disorders

Mitochondrial Disorders of the Nervous System: Clinical, Biochemical, and Molecular Genetic Features
  Dominic Thyagarajan and Edward Byrne

Section III: Secondary Respiratory Chain Disorders

Friedreich's Ataxia
J. M. Cooper and J. L. Bradley

Wilson Disease
C. A. Davie and A. H. V. Schapira

Hereditary Spastic Paraplegia
Christopher J. McDermott and Pamela J. Shaw

Cytochrome c Oxidase Deficiency
Giacomo P. Comi, Sandra Strazzer, Sara Galbiati, and Nereo Bresolin

Section IV: Toxin Induced Mitochondrial Dysfunction

Toxin-Induced Mitochondrial Dysfunction
Susan E. Browne and M. Flint Beal

Section V: Neurodegenerative Disorders

Parkinson's Disease
L. V. P. Korlipara and A. H. V. Schapira

Huntington's Disease: The Mystery Unfolds?
Åsa Petersén and Patrik Brundin

Mitochondria in Alzheimer's Disease
Russell H. Swerdlow and Stephen J. Kish

Contributions of Mitochondrial Alterations, Resulting from Bad Genes and a Hostile Environment, to the Pathogenesis of Alzheimer's Disease
Mark P. Mattson

Mitochondria and Amyotrophic Lateral Sclerosis
Richard W. Orrell and Anthony H. V. Schapira

Section VI: Models of Mitochondrial Disease

Models of Mitochondrial Disease
Danae Liolitsa and Michael G. Hanna

Section VII: Defects of β Oxidation Including Carnitine Deficiency

Defects of β Oxidation Including Carnitine Deficiency
K. Bartlett and M. Pourfarzam

Section VIII: Mitochondrial Involvement in Aging

The Mitochondrial Theory of Aging: Involvement of Mitochondrial DNA Damage and Repair
Nadja C. de Souza-Pinto and Vilhelm A. Bohr

INDEX

Volume 54

Unique General Anesthetic Binding Sites Within Distinct Conformational States of the Nicotinic Acetylcholine Receptor
Hugo R. Ariaas, William, R. Kem, James R. Truddell, and Michael P. Blanton

Signaling Molecules and Receptor Transduction Cascades That Regulate NMDA Receptor-Mediated Synaptic Transmission
Suhas. A. Kotecha and John F. MacDonald

Behavioral Measures of Alcohol Self-Administration and Intake Control: Rodent Models
Herman H. Samson and Cristine L. Czachowski

Dopaminergic Mouse Mutants: Investigating the Roles of the Different Dopamine Receptor Subtypes and the Dopamine Transporter
Shirlee Tan, Bettina Hermann, and Emiliana Borrelli

Drosophila melanogaster, A Genetic Model System for Alcohol Research
Douglas J. Guarnieri and Ulrike Heberlein

INDEX

Volume 55

Section I: Virsu Vectors For Use in the Nervous System

Non-Neurotropic Adenovirus: a Vector for Gene Transfer to the Brain and Gene Therapy of Neurological Disorders
P. R. Lowenstein, D. Suwelack, J. Hu, X. Yuan, M. Jimenez-Dalmaroni, S. Goverdhama, and M.G. Castro

Adeno-Associated Virus Vectors
   E. Lehtonen and
   L. Tenenbaum

Problems in the Use of Herpes Simplex Virus as
a Vector
   L. T. Feldman

Lentiviral Vectors
   J. Jakobsson, C. Ericson,
   N. Rosenquist, and C. Lundberg

Retroviral Vectors for Gene Delivery to Neural
Precursor Cells
   K. Kageyama, H. Hirata, and J. Hatakeyama

Section II: Gene Therapy with Virus Vectors for
Specific Disease of the Nervous System

The Principles of Molecular Therapies for
Glioblastoma
   G. Karpati and J. Nalbatonglu

Oncolytic Herpes Simplex Virus
   J. C. C. Hu and R. S. Coffin

Recombinant Retrovirus Vectors for Treatment
of Brain Tumors
   N. G. Rainov and C. M. Kramm

Adeno-Associated Viral Vectors for Parkinson's
Disease
   I. Muramatsu, L. Wang, K. Ikeguchi, K-i Fujimoto,
   T. Okada, H. Mizukami, Y. Hanazono, A. Kume,
   I. Nakano, and K. Ozawa

HSV Vectors for Parkinson's Disease
   D. S. Latchman

Gene Therapy for Stroke
   K. Abe and W. R. Zhang

Gene Therapy for Mucopolysaccharidosis
   A. Bosch and J. M. Heard

INDEX

Volume 56

Behavioral Mechanisms and the Neurobiology of
Conditioned Sexual Responding
   Mark Krause

NMDA Receptors in Alcoholism
   Paula L. Hoffman

Processing and Representation of Species-
Specific Communication Calls in the Audi-
tory System of Bats
   George D. Pollak, Achim Klug, and
   Eric E. Bauer

Central Nervous System Control of Micturition
   Gert Holstege and Leonora J. Mouton

The Structure and Physiology of the Rat
Auditory System: An Overview
   Manuel Malmierca

Neurobiology of Cat and Human Sexual
Behavior
   Gert Holstege and J. R. Georgiadis

INDEX

Volume 57

Cumulative Subject Index of Volumes 1–25

Volume 58

Cumulative Subject Index of Volumes 26–50

Volume 59

Loss of Spines and Neuropil
   Liesl B. Jones

Schizophrenia as a Disorder of Neuroplasticity
   Robert E. McCullumsmith, Sarah M. Clinton, and
   James H. Meador-Woodruff

The Synaptic Pathology of Schizophrenia: Is
Aberrant Neurodevelopment and Plasticity to
Blame?
   Sharon L. Eastwood

Neurochemical Basis for an Epigenetic Vision of
Synaptic Organization
   E. Costa, D. R. Grayson, M. Veldic,
   and A. Guidotti

Muscarinic Receptors in Schizophrenia: Is
There a Role for Synaptic Plasticity?
   Thomas J. Raedler

Serotonin and Brain Development
  Monsheel S. K. Sodhi and Elaine Sanders-Bush

Presynaptic Proteins and Schizophrenia
  William G. Honer and Clint E. Young

Mitogen-Activated Protein Kinase Signaling
  Svetlana V. Kyosseva

Postsynaptic Density Scaffolding Proteins at Excitatory Synapse and Disorders of Synaptic Plasticity: Implications for Human Behavior Pathologies
  Andrea de Bartolomeis and Germano Fiore

Prostaglandin-Mediated Signaling in Schizophrenia
  S. Smesny

Mitochondria, Synaptic Plasticity, and Schizophrenia
  Dorit Ben-Shachar and Daphna Laifenfeld

Membrane Phospholipids and Cytokine Interaction in Schizophrenia
  Jeffrey K. Yao and Daniel P. van Kammen

Neurotensin, Schizophrenia, and Antipsychotic Drug Action
  Becky Kinkead and Charles B. Nemeroff

Schizophrenia, Vitamin D, and Brain Development
  Alan Mackay-Sim, François Féron, Darryl Eyles, Thomas Burne, and John McGrath

Possible Contributions of Myelin and Oligodendrocyte Dysfunction to Schizophrenia
  Daniel G. Stewart and Kenneth L. Davis

Brain-Derived Neurotrophic Factor and the Plasticity of the Mesolimbic Dopamine Pathway
  Oliver Guillin, Nathalie Griffon, Jorge Diaz, Bernard Le Foll, Erwan Bezard, Christian Gross, Chris Lammers, Holger Stark, Patrick Carroll, Jean-Charles Schwartz, and Pierre Sokoloff

S100B in Schizophrenic Psychosis
  Matthias Rothermundt, Gerald Ponath, and Volker Arolt

Oct-6 Transcription Factor
  Maria Ilia

NMDA Receptor Function, Neuroplasticity, and the Pathophysiology of Schizophrenia
  Joseph T. Coyle and Guochuan Tsai

INDEX

Volume 60

Microarray Platforms: Introduction and Application to Neurobiology
  Stanislav L. Karsten, Lili C. Kudo, and Daniel H. Geschwind

Experimental Design and Low-Level Analysis of Microarray Data
  B. M. Bolstad, F. Collin, K. M. Simpson, R. A. Irizarry, and T. P. Speed

Brain Gene Expression: Genomics and Genetics
  Elissa J. Chesler and Robert W. Williams

DNA Microarrays and Animal Models of Learning and Memory
  Sebastiano Cavallaro

Microarray Analysis of Human Nervous System Gene Expression in Neurological Disease
  Steven A. Greenberg

DNA Microarray Analysis of Postmortem Brain Tissue
  Károly Mirnics, Pat Levitt, and David A. Lewis

INDEX

Volume 61

Section I: High-Throughput Technologies

Biomarker Discovery Using Molecular Profiling Approaches
  Stephen J. Walker and Arron Xu

Proteomic Analysis of Mitochondrial Proteins
  Mary F. Lopez, Simon Melov, Felicity Johnson, Nicole Nagulko, Eva Golenko, Scott Kuzdzal, Suzanne Ackloo, and Alvydas Mikulskis

Section II: Proteomic Applications

NMDA Receptors, Neural Pathways, and Protein Interaction Databases
  Holger Husi

Dopamine Transporter Network and Pathways
  Rajani Maiya and R. Dayne Mayfield

Proteomic Approaches in Drug Discovery and Development
  Holly D. Soares, Stephen A. Williams,

Peter J. Snyder, Feng Gao, Tom Stiger,
Christian Rohlff, Athula Herath, Trey Sunderland,
Karen Putnam, and W. Frost White

Section III: Informatics

Proteomic Informatics
Steven Russell, William Old, Katheryn Resing, and
Lawrence Hunter

Section IV: Changes in the Proteome by
Disease

Proteomics Analysis in Alzheimer's Disease: New
Insights into Mechanisms of Neurodegeneration
D. Allan Butterfield and Debra Boyd-Kimball

Proteomics and Alcoholism
Frank A. Witzmann and Wendy N. Strother

Proteomics Studies of Traumatic Brain Injury
Kevin K. W. Wang, Andrew Ottens,
William Haskins, Ming Cheng Liu,
Firas Kobeissy, Nancy Denslow,
SuShing Chen, and Ronald L. Hayes

Influence of Huntington's Disease on the Human
and Mouse Proteome
Claus Zabel and Joachim Klose

Section V: Overview of the Neuroproteome

Proteomics—Application to the Brain
Katrin Marcus, Oliver Schmidt, Heike Schaefer,
Michael Hamacher, André van Hall, and Helmut
E. Meyer

INDEX

Volume 62

GABA_A Receptor Structure–Function Studies: A
Reexamination in Light of New Acetylcholine
Receptor Structures
Myles H. Akabas

Dopamine Mechanisms and Cocaine Reward
Aiko Ikegami and Christine L. Duvauchelle

Proteolytic Dysfunction in Neurodegenerative
Disorders
Kevin St. P. McNaught

Neuroimaging Studies in Bipolar Children and
Adolescents

Rene L. Olvera, David C. Glahn, Sheila C. Caetano,
Steven R. Pliszka, and Jair C. Soares

Chemosensory G-Protein-Coupled Receptor
Signaling in the Brain
Geoffrey E. Woodard

Disturbances of Emotion Regulation after Focal
Brain Lesions
Antoine Bechara

The Use of *Caenorhabditis elegans* in Molecular
Neuropharmacology
Jill C. Bettinger, Lucinda Carnell, Andrew G. Davies,
and Steven L. McIntire

INDEX

Volume 63

Mapping Neuroreceptors at work: On the Definition and Interpretation of Binding Potentials
after 20 years of Progress
Albert Gjedde, Dean F. Wong, Pedro Rosa-Neto, and
Paul Cumming

Mitochondrial Dysfunction in Bipolar Disorder:
From ^{31}P-Magnetic Resonance Spectroscopic
Findings to Their Molecular Mechanisms
Tadafumi Kato

Large-Scale Microarray Studies of Gene Expression in Multiple Regions of the Brain in Schizophrenia and Alzheimer's Disease
Pavel L. Katsel, Kenneth L. Davis, and Vahram
Haroutunian

Regulation of Serotonin 2C Receptor PRE-
mRNA Editing By Serotonin
Claudia Schmauss

The Dopamine Hypothesis of Drug Addiction:
Hypodopaminergic State
Miriam Melis, Saturnino Spiga, and Marco Diana

Human and Animal Spongiform Encephalopathies are Autoimmune Diseases: A Novel Theory
and Its supporting Evidence
Bao Ting Zhu

Adenosine and Brain Function
Bertil B. Fredholm, Jiang-Fan Chen, Rodrigo A.
Cunha, Per Svenningsson, and Jean-Marie Vaugeois

INDEX

Volume 64

Section I. The Cholinergic System
John Smythies

Section II. The Dopamine System
John Symythies

Section III. The Norepinephrine System
John Smythies

Section IV. The Adrenaline System
John Smythies

Section V. Serotonin System
John Smythies

INDEX

Volume 65

Insulin Resistance: Causes and Consequences
Zachary T. Bloomgarden

Antidepressant-Induced Manic Conversion: A Developmentally Informed Synthesis of the Literature
Christine J. Lim, James F. Leckman, Christopher Young, and Andrés Martin

Sites of Alcohol and Volatile Anesthetic Action on Glycine Receptors
Ingrid A. Lobo and R. Adron Harris

Role of the Orbitofrontal Cortex in Reinforcement Processing and Inhibitory Control: Evidence from Functional Magnetic Resonance Imaging Studies in Healthy Human Subjects
Rebecca Elliott and Bill Deakin

Common Substrates of Dysphoria in Stimulant Drug Abuse and Primary Depression: Therapeutic Targets
Kate Baicy, Carrie E. Bearden, John Monterosso, Arthur L. Brody, Andrew J. Isaacson, and Edythe D. London

The Role of cAMP Response Element–Binding Proteins in Mediating Stress-Induced Vulnerability to Drug Abuse
Arati Sadalge Kreibich and Julie A. Blendy

G-Protein–Coupled Receptor Deorphanizations
Yumiko Saito and Olivier Civelli

Mechanistic Connections Between Glucose/Lipid Disturbances and Weight Gain Induced by Antipsychotic Drugs
Donard S. Dwyer, Dallas Donohoe, Xiao-Hong Lu, and Eric J. Aamodt

Serotonin Firing Activity as a Marker for Mood Disorders: Lessons from Knockout Mice
Gabriella Gobbi

INDEX

Volume 66

Brain Atlases of Normal and Diseased Populations
Arthur W. Toga and Paul M. Thompson

Neuroimaging Databases as a Resource for Scientific Discovery
John Darrell Van Horn, John Wolfe, Autumn Agnoli, Jeffrey Woodward, Michael Schmitt, James Dobson, Sarene Schumacher, and Bennet Vance

Modeling Brain Responses
Karl J. Friston, William Penny, and Olivier David

Voxel-Based Morphometric Analysis Using Shape Transformations
Christos Davatzikos

The Cutting Edge of fMRI and High-Field fMRI
Dae-Shik Kim

Quantification of White Matter Using Diffusion-Tensor Imaging
Hae-Jeong Park

Perfusion fMRI for Functional Neuroimaging
Geoffrey K. Aguirre, John A. Detre, and Jiongjiong Wang

Functional Near-Infrared Spectroscopy: Potential and Limitations in Neuroimaging Studies
Yoko Hoshi

Neural Modeling and Functional Brain Imaging: The Interplay Between the Data-Fitting and Simulation Approaches
Barry Horwitz and Michael F. Glabus

Combined EEG and fMRI Studies of Human Brain Function
  V. Menon and S. Crottaz-Herbette

INDEX

Volume 67

Distinguishing Neural Substrates of Heterogeneity Among Anxiety Disorders
  Jack B. Nitschke and Wendy Heller

Neuroimaging in Dementia
  K. P. Ebmeier, C. Donaghey, and N. J. Dougall

Prefrontal and Anterior Cingulate Contributions to Volition in Depression
  Jack B. Nitschke and Kristen L. Mackiewicz

Functional Imaging Research in Schizophrenia
  H. Tost, G. Ende, M. Ruf, F. A. Henn, and A. Meyer-Lindenberg

Neuroimaging in Functional Somatic Syndromes
  Patrick B. Wood

Neuroimaging in Multiple Sclerosis
  Alireza Minagar, Eduardo Gonzalez-Toledo, James Pinkston, and Stephen L. Jaffe

Stroke
  Roger E. Kelley and Eduardo Gonzalez-Toledo

Functional MRI in Pediatric Neurobehavioral Disorders
  Michael Seyffert and F. Xavier Castellanos

Structural MRI and Brain Development
  Paul M. Thompson, Elizabeth R. Sowell, Nitin Gogtay, Jay N. Giedd, Christine N. Vidal, Kiralee M. Hayashi, Alex Leow, Rob Nicolson, Judith L. Rapoport, and Arthur W. Toga

Neuroimaging and Human Genetics
  Georg Winterer, Ahmad R. Hariri, David Goldman, and Daniel R. Weinberger

Neuroreceptor Imaging in Psychiatry: Theory and Applications

W. Gordon Frankle, Mark Slifstein, Peter S. Talbot, and Marc Laruelle

INDEX

Volume 68

Fetal Magnetoencephalography: Viewing the Developing Brain In Utero
  Hubert Preissl, Curtis L. Lowery, and Hari Eswaran

Magnetoencephalography in Studies of Infants and Children
  Minna Huotilainen

Let's Talk Together: Memory Traces Revealed by Cooperative Activation in the Cerebral Cortex
  Jochen Kaiser, Susanne Leiberg, and Werner Lutzenberger

Human Communication Investigated With Magnetoencephalography: Speech, Music, and Gestures
  Thomas R. Knösche, Burkhard Maess, Akinori Nakamura, and Angela D. Friederici

Combining Magnetoencephalography and Functional Magnetic Resonance Imaging
  Klaus Mathiak and Andreas J. Fallgatter

Beamformer Analysis of MEG Data
  Arjan Hillebrand and Gareth R. Barnes

Functional Connectivity Analysis in Magnetoencephalography
  Alfons Schnitzler and Joachim Gross

Human Visual Processing as Revealed by Magnetoencephalographys
  Yoshiki Kaneoke, Shoko Watanabe, and Ryusuke Kakigi

A Review of Clinical Applications of Magnetoencephalography
  Andrew C. Papanicolaou, Eduardo M. Castillo, Rebecca Billingsley-Marshall, Ekaterina Pataraia, and Panagiotis G. Simos

INDEX

Volume 69

Nematode Neurons: Anatomy and Anatomical Methods in Caenorhabditis elegans
David H. Hall, Robyn Lints, and Zeynep Altun

Investigations of Learning and Memory in Caenorhabditis elegans
Andrew C. Giles, Jacqueline K. Rose, and Catharine H. Rankin

Neural Specification and Differentiation
Eric Aamodt and Stephanie Aamodt

Sexual Behavior of the Caenorhabditis elegans Male
Scott W. Emmons

The Motor Circuit
Stephen E. Von Stetina, Millet Treinin, and David M. Miller III

Mechanosensation in Caenorhabditis elegans
Robert O'Hagan and Martin Chalfie

Spectral Processing in the Auditory Cortex
Mitchell L. Sutter

Processing of Dynamic Spectral Properties of Sounds
Adrian Rees and Manuel S. Malmierca

Representations of Spectral Coding in the Human Brain
Deborah A. Hall, PhD

Spectral Processing and Sound Source Determination
Donal G. Sinex

Spectral Information in Sound Localization
Simon Carlile, Russell Martin, and Ken McAnally

Plasticity of Spectral Processing
Dexter R. F. Irvine and Beverly A. Wright

Spectral Processing In Cochlear Implants
Colette M. McKay

INDEX

Volume 70

Spectral Processing by the Peripheral Auditory System Facts and Models
Enrique A. Lopez-Poveda

Basic Psychophysics of Human Spectral Processing
Brian C. J. Moore

Across-Channel Spectral Processing
John H. Grose, Joseph W. Hall III, and Emily Buss

Speech and Music Have Different Requirements for Spectral Resolution
Robert V. Shannon

Non-Linearities and the Representation of Auditory Spectra
Eric D. Young, Jane J. Yu, and Lina A. J. Reiss

Spectral Processing in the Inferior Colliculus
Kevin A. Davis

Neural Mechanisms for Spectral Analysis in the Auditory Midbrain, Thalamus, and Cortex
Monty A. Escab and Heather L. Read

Volume 71

Autism: Neuropathology, Alterations of the GABAergic System, and Animal Models
Christoph Schmitz, Imke A. J. van Kooten, Patrick R. Hof, Herman van Engeland, Paul H. Patterson, and Harry W. M. Steinbusch

The Role of GABA in the Early Neuronal Development
Marta Jelitai and Emília Madarasz

GABAergic Signaling in the Developing Cerebellum
Chitoshi Takayama

Insights into GABA Functions in the Developing Cerebellum
Mónica L. Fiszman

Role of GABA in the Mechanism of the Onset of Puberty in Non-Human Primates
Ei Terasawa

Rett Syndrome: A Rosetta Stone for Understanding the Molecular Pathogenesis of Autism
Janine M. LaSalle, Amber Hogart, and Karen N. Thatcher

GABAergic Cerebellar System in Autism: A Neuropathological and Developmental Perspective
  Gene J. Blatt

Reelin Glycoprotein in Autism and Schizophrenia
  S. Hossein Fatemi

Is There A Connection Between Autism,
Prader-Willi Syndrome, Catatonia, and GABA?
  Dirk M. Dhossche, Yaru Song, and Yiming Liu

Alcohol, GABA Receptors, and Neurodevelopmental Disorders
  Ujjwal K. Rout

Effects of Secretin on Extracellular GABA and
Other Amino Acid Concentrations in the Rat
Hippocampus
  *Hans-Willi Clement, Alexander Pschibul, and
  Eberhard Schulz*

Predicted Role of Secretin and Oxytocin in the
Treatment of Behavioral and Developmental
Disorders: Implications for Autism
  Martha G. Welch and David A. Ruggiero

Immunological Findings in Autism
  Hari Har Parshad Cohly and Asit Panja

Correlates of Psychomotor Symptoms in Autism
  *Laura Stoppelbein, Sara Sytsma-Jordan, and
  Leilani Greening*

GABRB3 Gene Deficient Mice: A Potential
Model of Autism Spectrum Disorder
  Timothy M. DeLorey

The Reeler Mouse: Anatomy of a Mutant
  Gabriella D'Arcangelo

Shared Chromosomal Susceptibility Regions
Between Autism and Other Mental Disorders
  Yvon C. Chagnon index

INDEX

Volume 72

Classification Matters for Catatonia and Autism
in Children
  Klaus-Jürgen Neumärker

A Systematic Examination of Catatonia-Like
Clinical Pictures in Autism Spectrum Disorders
  Lorna Wing and Amitta Shah

Catatonia in Individuals with Autism Spectrum
Disorders in Adolescence and Early Adulthood:
A Long-Term Prospective Study
  Masataka Ohta, Yukiko Kano, and Yoko Nagai

Are Autistic and Catatonic Regression Related?
A Few Working Hypotheses Involving GABA,
Purkinje Cell Survival, Neurogenesis, and ECT
  Dirk Marcel Dhossche and Ujjwal Rout

Psychomotor Development and Psychopathology in Childhood
  Dirk M. J. De Raeymaecker

The Importance of Catatonia and Stereotypies
in Autistic Spectrum Disorders
  *Laura Stoppelbein, Leilani Greening, and
  Angelina Kakooza*

Prader–Willi Syndrome: Atypical Psychoses and
Motor Dysfunctions
  Willem M. A. Verhoeven and Siegfried Tuinier

Towards a Valid Nosography and Psychopathology of Catatonia in Children and Adolescents
  David Cohen

Is There a Common Neuronal Basis for Autism
and Catatonia?
  *Dirk Marcel Dhossche, Brendan T. Carroll, and
  Tressa D. Carroll*

Shared Susceptibility Region on Chromosome
15 Between Autism and Catatonia
  Yvon C. Chagnon

Current Trends in Behavioral Interventions for
Children with Autism
  Dorothy Scattone and Kimberly R. Knight

Case Reports with a Child Psychiatric Exploration of Catatonia, Autism, and Delirium
  Jan N. M. Schieveld

ECT and the Youth: Catatonia in Context
  Frank K. M. Zaw

Catatonia in Autistic Spectrum Disorders: A
Medical Treatment Algorithm
  Max Fink, Michael A. Taylor, and Neera Ghaziuddin

Psychological Approaches to Chronic Catatonia-Like Deterioration in Autism Spectrum Disorders
  Amitta Shah and Lorna Wing

Section V: Blueprints
Blueprints for the Assessment, Treatment, and Future Study of Catatonia in Autism Spectrum Disorders
  Dirk Marcel, Dhossche, Amitta Shah, and Lorna Wing

INDEX

Volume 73

Chromosome 22 Deletion Syndrome and Schizophrenia
  Nigel M. Williams, Michael C. O'Donovan, and Michael J. Owen

Characterization of Proteome of Human Cerebrospinal Fluid
  Jing Xu, Jinzhi Chen, Elaine R. Peskind, Jinghua Jin, Jimmy Eng, Catherine Pan, Thomas J. Montine, David R. Goodlett, and Jing Zhang

Hormonal Pathways Regulating Intermale and Interfemale Aggression
  Neal G. Simon, Qianxing Mo, Shan Hu, Carrie Garippa, and Shi-Fang Lu

Neuronal GAP Junctions: Expression, Function, and Implications for Behavior
  Clinton B. McCracken and David C. S. Roberts

Effects of Genes and Stress on the Neurobiology of Depression
  J. John Mann and Dianne Currier

Quantitative Imaging with the Micropet Small-Animal Pet Tomograph
  Paul Vaska, Daniel J. Rubins, David L. Alexoff, and Wynne K. Schiffer

Understanding Myelination through Studying its Evolution
  Rüdiger Schweigreiter, Betty I. Roots, Christine Bandtlow, and Robert M. Gould

INDEX

Volume 74

Evolutionary Neurobiology and Art
  C. U. M. Smith

Section I: Visual Aspects

Perceptual Portraits
  Nicholas Wade

The Neuropsychology of Visual Art: Conferring Capacity
  Anjan Chatterjee

Vision, Illusions, and Reality
  Christopher Kennard

Localization in the Visual Brain
  George K. York

Section II: Episodic Disorders

Neurology, Synaesthesia, and Painting
  Amy Ione

Fainting in Classical Art
  Philip Smith

Migraine Art in the Internet: A Study of 450 Contemporary Artists
  Klaus Podoll

Sarah Raphael's Migraine with Aura as Inspiration for the Foray of Her Work into Abstraction
  Klaus Podoll and Debbie Ayles

The Visual Art of Contemporary Artists with Epilepsy
  Steven C. Schachter

Section III: Brain Damage

Creativity in Painting and Style in Brain-Damaged Artists
  Julien Bogousslavsky

Artistic Changes in Alzheimer's Disease
  Sebastian J. Crutch and Martin N. Rossor

Section IV: Cerebrovascular Disease

Stroke in Painters
  H. Bäzner and M. Hennerici

Visuospatial Neglect in Lovis Corinth's Self-Portraits
  Olaf Blanke

Art, Constructional Apraxia, and the Brain
  Louis Caplan

Section V: Genetic Diseases

Neurogenetics in Art
  Alan E. H. Emery

A Naïve Artist of St Ives
  F. Clifford Rose

Van Gogh's Madness
  F. Clifford Rose

Absinthe, The Nervous System and Painting
  Tiina Rekand

Section VI: Neurologists as Artists

Sir Charles Bell, KGH, FRS, FRSE (1774–1842)
  Christopher Gardner-Thorpe

Section VII: Miscellaneous

Peg Leg Frieda
  Espen Dietrichs

The Deafness of Goya (1746–1828)
  F. Clifford Rose

INDEX

Volume 75

Introduction on the Use of the *Drosophila* Embryonic/Larval Neuromuscular Junction as a Model System to Study Synapse Development and Function, and a Brief Summary of Pathfinding and Target Recognition
  Catalina Ruiz-Cañada and Vivian Budnik

Development and Structure of Motoneurons
  Matthias Landgraf and Stefan Thor

The Development of the *Drosophila* Larval Body Wall Muscles
  Karen Beckett and Mary K. Baylies

Organization of the Efferent System and Structure of Neuromuscular Junctions in *Drosophila*
  Andreas Prokop

Development of Motoneuron Electrical Properties and Motor Output
  Richard A. Baines

Transmitter Release at the Neuromuscular Junction
  Thomas L. Schwarz

Vesicle Trafficking and Recycling at the Neuromuscular Junction: Two Pathways for Endocytosis
  Yoshiaki Kidokoro

Glutamate Receptors at the *Drosophila* Neuromuscular Junction
  Aaron DiAntonio

Scaffolding Proteins at the *Drosophila* Neuromuscular Junction
  Bulent Ataman, Vivian Budnik, and Ulrich Thomas

Synaptic Cytoskeleton at the Neuromuscular Junction
  Catalina Ruiz-Cañada and Vivian Budnik

Plasticity and Second Messengers During Synapse Development
  Leslie C. Griffith and Vivian Budnik

Retrograde Signaling that Regulates Synaptic Development and Function at the *Drosophila* Neuromuscular Junction
  Guillermo Marqués and Bing Zhang

Activity-Dependent Regulation of Transcription During Development of Synapses
  Subhabrata Sanyal and Mani Ramaswami

Experience-Dependent Potentiation of Larval Neuromuscular Synapses
  Christoph M. Schuster

Selected Methods for the Anatomical Study of *Drosophila* Embryonic and Larval Neuromuscular Junctions
  Vivian Budnik, Michael Gorczyca, and Andreas Prokop

INDEX

Volume 76

Section I: Physiological Correlates of Freud's Theories

The ID, the Ego, and the Temporal Lobe
  Shirley M. Ferguson and Mark Rayport

ID, Ego, and Temporal Lobe Revisited
  Shirley M. Ferguson and
  Mark Rayport

Section II: Stereotaxic Studies

Olfactory Gustatory Responses Evoked by Electrical Stimulation of Amygdalar Region in Man Are Qualitatively Modifiable by Interview Content: Case Report and Review
  Mark Rayport, Sepehr Sani, and Shirley M. Ferguson

Section III: Controversy in Definition of Behavioral Disturbance

Pathogenesis of Psychosis in Epilepsy. The "Seesaw" Theory: Myth or Reality?
  Shirley M. Ferguson and Mark Rayport

Section IV: Outcome of Temporal Lobectomy

Memory Function After Temporal Lobectomy for Seizure Control: A Comparative Neuropsychiatric and Neuropsychological Study
  Shirley M. Ferguson, A. John McSweeny, and
  Mark Rayport

Life After Surgery for Temporolimbic Seizures
  Shirley M. Ferguson, Mark Rayport, and
  Carolyn A. Schell

Appendix I
  Mark Rayport

Appendix II: Conceptual Foundations of Studies of Patients Undergoing Temporal Lobe Surgery for Seizure Control
  Mark Rayport

INDEX

Volume 77

Regenerating the Brain
  David A. Greenberg and Kunlin Jin

Serotonin and Brain: Evolution, Neuroplasticity, and Homeostasis
  Efrain C. Azmitia

Therapeutic Approaches to Promoting Axonal Regeneration in the Adult Mammalian Spinal Cord
  Sari S. Hannila, Mustafa M. Siddiq, and
  Marie T. Filbin

Evidence for Neuroprotective Effects of Antipsychotic Drugs: Implications for the Pathophysiology and Treatment of Schizophrenia
  Xin-Min Li and Haiyun Xu

Neurogenesis and Neuroenhancement in the Pathophysiology and Treatment of Bipolar Disorder
  Robert J. Schloesser, Guang Chen, and
  Husseini K. Manji

Neuroreplacement, Growth Factor, and Small Molecule Neurotrophic Approaches for Treating Parkinson's Disease
  Michael J. O'Neill, Marcus J. Messenger,
  Viktor Lakics, Tracey K. Murray, Eric H. Karran,
  Philip G. Szekeres, Eric S. Nisenbaum, and
  Kalpana M. Merchant

Using *Caenorhabditis elegans* Models of Neurodegenerative Disease to Identify Neuroprotective Strategies
  Brian Kraemer and Gerard D. Schellenberg

Neuroprotection and Enhancement of Neurite Outgrowth With Small Molecular Weight Compounds From Screens of Chemical Libraries
  Donard S. Dwyer and Addie Dickson

INDEX

Volume 78

Neurobiology of Dopamine in Schizophrenia
  Olivier Guillin, Anissa Abi-Dargham, and
  Marc Laruelle

The Dopamine System and the Pathophysiology of Schizophrenia: A Basic Science Perspective
  Yukiori Goto and Anthony A. Grace

Glutamate and Schizophrenia: Phencyclidine, *N*-methyl-D-aspartate Receptors, and Dopamine–Glutamate Interactions
  Daniel C. Javitt

Deciphering the Disease Process of Schizophrenia: The Contribution of Cortical GABA Neurons
  David A. Lewis and Takanori Hashimoto

Alterations of Serotonin Transmission in Schizophrenia
  Anissa Abi-Dargham

Serotonin and Dopamine Interactions in Rodents and Primates: Implications for Psychosis and Antipsychotic Drug Development
  Gerard J. Marek

Cholinergic Circuits and Signaling in the Pathophysiology of Schizophrenia
  Joshua A. Berman, David A. Talmage, and Lorna W. Role

Schizophrenia and the α7 Nicotinic Acetylcholine Receptor
  Laura F. Martin and Robert Freedman

Histamine and Schizophrenia
  Jean-Michel Arrang

Cannabinoids and Psychosis
  Deepak Cyril D'Souza

Involvement of Neuropeptide Systems in Schizophrenia: Human Studies
  Ricardo Cáceda, Becky Kinkead, and Charles B. Nemeroff

Brain-Derived Neurotrophic Factor in Schizophrenia and Its Relation with Dopamine
  Olivier Guillin, Caroline Demily, and Florence Thibaut

Schizophrenia Susceptibility Genes: In Search of a Molecular Logic and Novel Drug Targets for a Devastating Disorder
  Joseph A. Gogos

INDEX

Volume 79

The Destructive Alliance: Interactions of Leukocytes, Cerebral Endothelial Cells, and the Immune Cascade in Pathogenesis of Multiple Sclerosis
  Alireza Minagar, April Carpenter, and J. Steven Alexander

Role of B Cells in Pathogenesis of Multiple Sclerosis
  Behrouz Nikbin, Mandana Mohyeddin Bonab, Farideh Khosravi, and Fatemeh Talebian

The Role of CD4 T Cells in the Pathogenesis of Multiple Sclerosis
  Tanuja Chitnis

The CD8 T Cell in Multiple Sclerosis: Suppressor Cell or Mediator of Neuropathology?
  Aaron J. Johnson, Georgette L. Suidan, Jeremiah McDole, and Istvan Pirko

Immunopathogenesis of Multiple Sclerosis
  Smriti M. Agrawal and V. Wee Yong

Molecular Mimicry in Multiple Sclerosis
  Jane E. Libbey, Lori L. McCoy, and Robert S. Fujinami

Molecular "Negativity" May Underlie Multiple Sclerosis: Role of the Myelin Basic Protein Family in the Pathogenesis of MS
  Abdiwahab A. Musse and George Harauz

Microchimerism and Stem Cell Transplantation in Multiple Sclerosis
  Behrouz Nikbin, Mandana Mohyeddin Bonab, and Fatemeh Talebian

The Insulin-Like Growth Factor System in Multiple Sclerosis
  Daniel Chesik, Nadine Wilczak, and Jacques De Keyser

Cell-Derived Microparticles and Exosomes in Neuroinflammatory Disorders
  Lawrence L. Horstman, Wenche Jy, Alireza Minagar, Carlos J. Bidot, Joaquin J. Jimenez, J. Steven Alexander, and Yeon S. Ahn

Multiple Sclerosis in Children: Clinical, Diagnostic, and Therapeutic Aspects
  Kevin Rostásy

Migraine in Multiple Sclerosis
  Debra G. Elliott

Multiple Sclerosis as a Painful Disease
  Meghan Kenner, Uma Menon, and Debra Elliott

Multiple Sclerosis and Behavior
  James B. Pinkston, Anita Kablinger, and Nadejda Alekseeva

Cerebrospinal Fluid Analysis in Multiple Sclerosis
  Francisco A. Luque and Stephen L. Jaffe

Multiple Sclerosis in Isfahan, Iran
  Mohammad Saadatnia, Masoud Etemadifar, and Amir Hadi Maghzi

Gender Issues in Multiple Sclerosis
  Robert N. Schwendimann and Nadejda Alekseeva

Differential Diagnosis of Multiple Sclerosis
  Halim Fadil, Roger E. Kelley, and
  Eduardo Gonzalez-Toledo

Prognostic Factors in Multiple Sclerosis
  Roberto Bergamaschi

Neuroimaging in Multiple Sclerosis
  Robert Zivadinov and Jennifer L. Cox

Detection of Cortical Lesions Is Dependent on Choice of Slice Thickness in Patients with Multiple Sclerosis
  Ondrej Dolezal, Michael G. Dwyer, Dana Horakova,
  Eva Havrdova, Alireza Minagar,
  Srivats Balachandran, Niels Bergsland, Zdenek Seidl,
  Manuela Vaneckova, David Fritz, Jan Krasensky,
  and Robert Zivadinov

The Role of Quantitative Neuroimaging Indices in the Differentiation of Ischemia from Demyelination: An Analytical Study with Case Presentation
  Romy Hoque, Christina Ledbetter, Eduardo Gonzalez-
  Toledo, Vivek Misra, Uma Menon, Meghan Kenner,
  Alejandro A. Rabinstein, Roger E. Kelley,
  Robert Zivadinov, and Alireza Minagar

HLA-DRB1*1501, -DQB1*0301, -DQB1*0302, -DQB1*0602, and -DQB1*0603 Alleles Are Associated with More Severe Disease Outcome on MRI in Patients with Multiple Sclerosis
  Robert Zivadinov, Laura Uxa, Alessio Bratina,
  Antonio Bosco, Bhooma Srinivasaraghavan,
  Alireza Minagar, Maja Ukmar, Su yen Benedetto,
  and Marino Zorzon

Glatiramer Acetate: Mechanisms of Action in Multiple Sclerosis
  Tjalf Ziemssen and Wiebke Schrempf

Evolving Therapies for Multiple Sclerosis
  Elena Korniychuk, John M. Dempster,
  Eileen O'Connor, J. Steven Alexander,
  Roger E. Kelley, Meghan Kenner, Uma Menon,
  Vivek Misra, Romy Hoque, Eduardo C. Gonzalez-
  Toledo, Robert N. Schwendimann, Stacy Smith, and
  Alireza Minagar

Remyelination in Multiple Sclerosis
  Divya M. Chari

Trigeminal Neuralgia: A Modern-Day Review
  Kelly Hunt and Ravish Patwardhan

Optic Neuritis and the Neuro-Ophthalmology of Multiple Sclerosis
  Paramjit Kaur and Jeffrey L. Bennett

Neuromyelitis Optica: New Findings on Pathogenesis
  Dean M. Wingerchuk

INDEX

Volume 79

Epilepsy in the Elderly: Scope of the Problem
  Ilo E. Leppik

Animal Models in Gerontology Research
  Nancy L. Nadon

Animal Models of Geriatric Epilepsy
  Lauren J. Murphree, Lynn M. Rundhaugen, and
  Kevin M. Kelly

Life and Death of Neurons in the Aging Cerebral Cortex
  John H. Morrison and Patrick R. Hof

An In Vitro Model of Stroke-Induced Epilepsy: Elucidation of the Roles of Glutamate and Calcium in the Induction and Maintenance of Stroke-Induced Epileptogenesis
  Robert J. DeLorenzo, David A. Sun, Robert E. Blair,
  and Sompong Sambati

Mechanisms of Action of Antiepileptic Drugs
  H. Steve White, Misty D. Smith, and Karen S. Wilcox

Epidemiology and Outcomes of Status Epilepticus in the Elderly
  Alan R. Towne

Diagnosing Epilepsy in the Elderly
  R. Eugene Ramsay, Flavia M. Macias, and A. James
  Rowan

Pharmacoepidemiology in Community-Dwelling Elderly Taking Antiepileptic Drugs
  Dan R. Berlowitz and Mary Jo V. Pugh

Use of Antiepileptic Medications in Nursing Homes
  Judith Garrard, Susan L. Harms, Lynn E. Eberly,
  and Ilo E. Leppik

Differential Diagnosis of Multiple Sclerosis
Halim Fadil, Roger E. Kelley, and Eduardo Gonzalez-Toledo

Prognostic Factors in Multiple Sclerosis
Roberto Bergamaschi

Neuroimaging in Multiple Sclerosis
Robert Zivadinov and Jennifer L. Cox

Detection of Cortical Lesions Is Dependent on Choice of Slice Thickness in Patients with Multiple Sclerosis
Ondrej Dolezal, Michael G. Dwyer, Dana Horakova, Eva Havrdova, Alireza Minagar, Srivats Balachandran, Niels Bergsland, Zdenek Seidl, Manuela Vaneckova, David Fritz, Jan Krasensky, and Robert Zivadinov

TheRole ofQuantitativeNeuroimaging Indices in the Differentiation of Ischemia from Demyelination: An Analytical Study with Case Presentation
Romy Hoque, Christina Ledbetter, Eduardo Gonzalez-Toledo, Vivek Misra, Uma Menon, Meghan Kenner, Alejandro A. Rabinstein, Roger E. Kelley, Robert Zivadinov, and Alireza Minagar

HLA-DRB1*1501, -DQB1*0301,-DQB1*0302,-DQB1*0602, and -DQB1*0603 Alleles Are Associated with More Severe Disease Outcome on MRI in Patients with Multiple Sclerosis
Robert Zivadinov, Laura Uxa, Alessio Bratina, Antonio Bosco, Bhooma Srinivasaraghavan, Alireza Minagar, Maja Ukmar, Su yen Benedetto, and Marino Zorzon

Glatiramer Acetate: Mechanisms of Action in Multiple Sclerosis
Tjalf Ziemssen and Wiebke Schrempf

Evolving Therapies for Multiple Sclerosis
Elena Korniychuk, John M. Dempster, Eileen O'Connor, J. Steven Alexander, Roger E. Kelley, Meghan Kenner, Uma Menon, Vivek Misra, Romy Hoque, Eduardo C. Gonzalez-Toledo, Robert N. Schwendimann, Stacy Smith, and Alireza Minagar

Remyelination in Multiple Sclerosis
Divya M. Chari

Trigeminal Neuralgia: A Modern-Day Review
Kelly Hunt and Ravish Patwardhan

Optic Neuritis and the Neuro-Ophthalmology of Multiple Sclerosis
Paramjit Kaur and Jeffrey L. Bennett

Neuromyelitis Optica: New Findings on Pathogenesis
Dean M. Wingerchuk

INDEX

Volume 81

Epilepsy in the Elderly: Scope of the Problem
Ilo E. Leppik

Animal Models in Gerontology Research
Nancy L. Nadon

Animal Models of Geriatric Epilepsy
Lauren J. Murphree, Lynn M. Rundhaugen, and Kevin M. Kelly

Life and Death of Neurons in the Aging Cerebral Cortex
John H. Morrison and Patrick R. Hof

An In Vitro Model of Stroke-Induced Epilepsy: Elucidation of the Roles of Glutamate and Calcium in the Induction and Maintenance of Stroke-Induced Epileptogenesis
Robert J. DeLorenzo, David A. Sun, Robert E. Blair, and Sompong Sambati

Mechanisms of Action of Antiepileptic Drugs
H. Steve White, Misty D. Smith, and Karen S. Wilcox

Epidemiology and Outcomes of Status Epilepticus in the Elderly
Alan R. Towne

Diagnosing Epilepsy in the Elderly
R. Eugene Ramsay, Flavia M. Macias, and A. James Rowan

Pharmacoepidemiology in Community-Dwelling Elderly Taking Antiepileptic Drugs
Dan R. Berlowitz and Mary Jo V. Pugh

Use of Antiepileptic Medications in Nursing Homes
Judith Garrard, Susan L. Harms, Lynn E. Eberly, and Ilo E. Leppik

Age-Related Changes in Pharmacokinetics: Predictability and Assessment Methods
Emilio Perucca

Factors Affecting Antiepileptic Drug Pharmacokinetics in Community-Dwelling Elderly
James C. Cloyd, Susan Marino, and Angela K. Birnbaum

Pharmacokinetics of Antiepileptic Drugs in Elderly Nursing Home Residents
Angela K. Birnbaum

The Impact of Epilepsy on Older Veterans
Mary Jo V. Pugh, Dan R. Berlowitz, and Lewis Kazis

Risk and Predictability of Drug Interactions in the Elderly
René H. Levy and Carol Collins

Outcomes in Elderly Patients With Newly Diagnosed and Treated Epilepsy
Martin J. Brodie and Linda J. Stephen

Recruitment and Retention in Clinical Trials of the Elderly
Flavia M. Macias, R. Eugene Ramsay, and A. James Rowan

Treatment of Convulsive Status Epilepticus
David M. Treiman

Treatment of Nonconvulsive Status Epilepticus
Matthew C. Walker

Antiepileptic Drug Formulation and Treatment in the Elderly: Biopharmaceutical Considerations
Barry E. Gidal

INDEX

Volume 82

Inflammatory Mediators Leading to Protein Misfolding and Uncompetitive/Fast Off-Rate Drug Therapy for Neurodegenerative Disorders
Stuart A. Lipton, Zezong Gu, and Tomohiro Nakamura

Innate Immunity and Protective Neuroinflammation: New Emphasis on the Role of Neuroimmune Regulatory Proteins
M. Griffiths, J. W. Neal, and P. Gasque

Glutamate Release from Astrocytes in Physiological Conditions and in Neurodegenerative Disorders Characterized by Neuroinflammation
Sabino Vesce, Daniela Rossi, Liliana Brambilla, and Andrea Volterra

The High-Mobility Group Box 1 Cytokine Induces Transporter-Mediated Release of Glutamate from Glial Subcellular Particles (Gliosomes) Prepared from In Situ-Matured Astrocytes
Giambattista Bonanno, Luca Raiteri, Marco Milanese, Simona Zappettini, Edon Melloni, Marco Pedrazzi, Mario Passalacqua, Carlo Tacchetti, Cesare Usai, and Bianca Sparatore

The Role of Astrocytes and Complement System in Neural Plasticity
Milos Pekny, Ulrika Wilhelmsson, Yalda Rahpeymai Bogestål, and Marcela Pekna

New Insights into the Roles of Metalloproteinases in Neurodegeneration and Neuroprotection
A. J. Turner and N. N. Nalivaeva

Relevance of High-Mobility Group Protein Box 1 to Neurodegeneration
Silvia Fossati and Alberto Chiarugi

Early Upregulation of Matrix Metalloproteinases Following Reperfusion Triggers Neuroinflammatory Mediators in Brain Ischemia in Rat
Diana Amantea, Rossella Russo, Micaela Gliozzi, Vincenza Fratto, Laura Berliocchi, G. Bagetta, G. Bernardi, and M. Tiziana Corasaniti

The (Endo)Cannabinoid System in Multiple Sclerosis and Amyotrophic Lateral Sclerosis
Diego Centonze, Silvia Rossi, Alessandro Finazzi-Agrò, Giorgio Bernardi, and Mauro Maccarrone

Chemokines and Chemokine Receptors: Multipurpose Players in Neuroinflammation
Richard M. Ransohoff, LiPing Liu, and Astrid E. Cardona

Systemic and Acquired Immune Responses in Alzheimer's Disease
Markus Britschgi and Tony Wyss-Coray

Neuroinflammation in Alzheimer's Disease and Parkinson's Disease: Are Microglia Pathogenic in Either Disorder?
Joseph Rogers, Diego Mastroeni, Brian Leonard, Jeffrey Joyce, and Andrew Grover

Cytokines and Neuronal Ion Channels in Health and Disease
Barbara Viviani, Fabrizio Gardoni, and Marina Marinovich

Cyclooxygenase-2, Prostaglandin E$_2$, and Microglial Activation in Prion Diseases
Luisa Minghetti and Maurizio Pocchiari

Glia Proinflammatory Cytokine Upregulation as a Therapeutic Target for Neurodegenerative Diseases: Function-Based and Target-Based Discovery Approaches
Linda J. Van Eldik, Wendy L. Thompson, Hantamalala Ralay Ranaivo, Heather A. Behanna, and D. Martin Watterson

Oxidative Stress and the Pathogenesis of Neurodegenerative Disorders
Ashley Reynolds, Chad Laurie, R. Lee Mosley, and Howard E. Gendelman

Differential Modulation of Type 1 and Type 2 Cannabinoid Receptors Along the Neuroimmune Axis
Sergio Oddi, Paola Spagnuolo, Monica Bari, Antonella D'Agostino, and Mauro Maccarrone

Effects of the HIV-1 Viral Protein Tat on Central Neurotransmission: Role of Group I Metabotropic Glutamate Receptors
Elisa Neri, Veronica Musante, and Anna Pittaluga

Evidence to Implicate Early Modulation of Interleukin-1β Expression in the Neuroprotection Afforded by 17β-Estradiol in Male Rats Undergone Transient Middle Cerebral Artery Occlusion
Olga Chiappetta, Micaela Gliozzi, Elisa Siviglia, Diana Amantea, Luigi A. Morrone, Laura Berliocchi, G. Bagetta, and M. Tiziana Corasaniti

A Role for Brain Cyclooxygenase-2 and Prostaglandin-E$_2$ in Migraine: Effects of Nitroglycerin
Cristina Tassorelli, Rosaria Greco, Marie Therèse Armentero, Fabio Blandini, Giorgio Sandrini, and Giuseppe Nappi

The Blockade of K+-ATP Channels has Neuroprotective Effects in an *In Vitro* Model of Brain Ischemia
Robert Nisticò, Silvia Piccirilli, L. Sebastianelli, Giuseppe Nisticò, G. Bernardi, and N. B. Mercuri

Retinal Damage Caused by High Intraocular Pressure-Induced Transient Ischemia is Prevented by Coenzyme Q10 in Rat
Carlo Nucci, Rosanna Tartaglione, Angelica Cerulli, R. Mancino, A. Spanò, Federica Cavaliere, Laura Rombolà, G. Bagetta, M. Tiziana Corasaniti, and Luigi A. Morrone

Evidence Implicating Matrix Metalloproteinases in the Mechanism Underlying Accumulation of IL-1β and Neuronal Apoptosis in the Neocortex of HIV/gp120-Exposed Rats
Rossella Russo, Elisa Siviglia, Micaela Gliozzi, Diana Amantea, Annamaria Paoletti, Laura Berliocchi, G. Bagetta, and M. Tiziana Corasaniti

Neuroprotective Effect of Nitroglycerin in a Rodent Model of Ischemic Stroke: Evaluation of Bcl-2 Expression
Rosaria Greco, Diana Amantea, Fabio Blandini, Giuseppe Nappi, Giacinto Bagetta, M. Tiziana Corasaniti, and Cristina Tassorelli

INDEX